M000250016

Neural Organization

Michael A. Arbib, Péter Érdi,
and János Szentágothai

Neural Organization

Structure, Function, and Dynamics

A Bradford Book
The MIT Press
Cambridge, Massachusetts
London, England

© 1998 Massachusetts Institute of Technology

All rights reserved. No part of this book may be reproduced in any form by any electronic or mechanical means (including photocopying, recording, or information storage and retrieval) without permission in writing from the publisher.

This book was set in Palatino on the Monotype "Prism Plus" PostScript Imagesetter by Asco Trade Typesetting Ltd., Hong Kong and was printed and bound in the United States of America.

Library of Congress Cataloging-in-Publication Data

Arbib, Michael A.
  Neural organization : structure, function, and dynamics / Michael
  A. Arbib, Péter Érdi, and János Szentágothai.
      p.   cm.
  "A Bradford Book."
  Includes bibliographical references and index.
  ISBN 0-262-01159-X (hardcover : alk. paper)
  1. Neurosciences—Methodology. 2. Brain—Research—Methodology.
I. Érdi, Péter. II. Szentágothai, János. III. Title.
QP356.A765   1997
612.8—dc21   96-44543
                                                            CIP

To Alice Szentágothai
in affectionate memory of her strong support for János,
his colleagues, and this volume

Contents

Preface

Both experiment and theory in neuroscience are in a constant state of flux. A "good" model is responsive to available data; an "interesting" set of data will test hypotheses that are theory-laden, whether the theory be formal or not. New data lead to new models; new models suggest the design of new experiments. This book provides a comprehensive view of neural organization in the spirit of that cooperative development of theory and experiment. Our task is not to provide final models or a complete unified theory of the brain. Rather, we seek to show how theory and experiment can supplement each other in an integrated, evolving account of structure, function, and dynamics. Much of modern neuroscience seems to us excessively reductionist, focusing on the study of ever smaller microsystems to the exclusion of an appreciation of their contribution to the behaving organism. We do not reject the data gained in this way but are concerned with restoring some equilibrium between systems neuroscience, cellular neuroscience, and molecular neuroscience. For example, one of the book's recurrent themes will be to bridge different levels of organization by linking the learning rules that structure a variety of brain regions both to the functional roles of these regions and to the emerging understanding of the neurochemistry of synaptic plasticity and its variation from region to region. This is but one of many ways in which we seek to exemplify how theory and experiment may be intricately intertwined in a continuing cycle of analysis and synthesis. With this general viewpoint, we now briefly characterize the three approaches—structural, functional, and dynamical—that inform our account of neural organization.

Structural Approach

Studies of brain function and dynamics build on and contribute to an understanding of many brain regions and of the neural circuits that constitute them. Thus, we review anatomical data that integrate the overall spatial relations between a variety of brain regions with a selection of critical details of neural morphology and synaptic connectivity. This analysis of neural structure is guided by a developmental view that approaches the complexity of the adult nervous system through an understanding of the way in which that complexity emerges during embryogenesis, thus linking the structural approach to dynamical models of self-organization. The developing nervous system can generate movement before it becomes responsive to sensory stimuli, consonant with the emphasis on action-oriented perception in our functional studies that analyze the ways in which sensory systems are specialized to serve a variety of behaviors. As a basis for our functional and dynamical analysis of a variety of systems, later chapters progress through regions of the brain that, singly or in combination, underlie these systems: the segmented part of the neuraxis (discussed as a case study in chapter 2), the olfactory system, the hippocampus, the thalamus, the cerebral cortex, the cerebellum and, finally, the basal ganglia.

Functional Approach

First, we approach such complex functions as the control of eye movements, reaching and grasping, the use of a cognitive map for navigation, and the roles of vision in these behaviors, by the use of *schemas* in the sense of units that provide a *functional* decomposition of the overall skill or behavior. A schema account becomes a brain model when we offer hypotheses as to how each schema is implemented through the interaction of specific brain regions. A brain-based schema model may be tested by analysis of the behavior of animals with localized lesions or with reversible inactivation of specific brain regions or by human brain imaging; such a model provides the basis for modeling the overall function by neural networks that plausibly implement (usually in a distributed fashion) the schemas in the brain. Further analysis then may proceed bottom up (as the neural data drive further research) as well as top down (as we refine our schema-theoretical formulations).

We stress that the models in this book use *neural networks in the sense of computational neuroscience*, in which the structure of the network and the function of the neurons are constrained, at some appropriate level of detail, by the data of neuroanatomy and neurophysiology. This stands contrast to *neural networks in the sense of connectionism*, in which the structure of the network is generic (e.g., a multilayered feedforward network or a fully connected network) and the connections are determined by some "learning rule" that may be nonbiological (e.g., backpropagation) rather than constrained by anatomical data.

Dynamical Approach

Dynamic systems theory offers a conceptual and mathematical framework to analyze spatiotemporal neural phenomena occurring at different levels of organization, such as oscillatory and chaotic activity both in single neurons and in (often synchronized) neural networks, the self-organizing development and plasticity of ordered neural structures, and learning and memory phenomena associated with synaptic modification. We discuss a variety of rhythms (and arrhythmia) found in the olfactory bulb and olfactory cortex, in the hippocampus, and in the thalamocortical system. In most cases, we relate these rhythms to memory functions. Also, we study learning rules in both developmental processes (self-organization) and the acquisition of a variety of behaviors. In this way, we ground our functional analysis of neural organization in a dynamic systems analysis of the neural networks that implement the basic schemas.

Organization of the Book

Part I of the book, Overviews, opens with a chapter on the many themes of neural organization, which expands on the foregoing discussion of structure, dynamics, and function to introduce a variety of themes that weave in and out of subsequent chapters, binding the book into a moderately coherent whole. We then devote three chapters to detailed overviews of our three methods for understanding neural organization: a structural overview, a functional overview, and a dynamical overview.

Part II, Interacting Systems of the Brain, uses a structural organization to order our integrated approach to structure, function, and dynamics. Almost all of chapters 5–10 begin with a structural analysis of a specific brain region as the prelude to our account of the dynamics of the neural circuits and of the function of the region. Learning, memory, and plasticity are discussed in this functional and dynamical context. In this way, we look at the role of rhythm generation and chaotic patterns in both olfactory bulb and olfactory cortex, and we analyze rhythm generation in, and memory functions of, hippocampus and provide an extensive account of cognitive maps in the rat and declarative memory in humans. We offer a primarily structural account of the thalamus, emphasizing that, far from being simply a set of relay structures, it binds the cerebral cortex in a variety of subtle loops to sensory systems, cerebellum, and the basal ganglia. We study the modular structure and self-organization of visual cortex; we study the role of different thalamocortical oscillatory rhythms in the transition between sleeping and waking; and we model the interaction of multiple cortical regions in vision, saccade control, and cortically guided reaching and grasping. Finally, we extend our understanding of cerebral cortex by showing how its function can be understood fully only through analysis of its *cooperative computation* with the cerebellum and basal ganglia. We analyze the role of the cerebellum in both motor control and classical conditioning and provide an account of the role of the basal ganglia in motor coordination and learning, contrasting its role with that of cerebellum and emphasizing the important role of the dopamine system in its functioning.

In this way, we provide for many important brain regions a structural analysis that is integrated with models of a number of the functions that these regions serve, both singly and in concert, and of the dynamics of their neural networks. We study a variety of systems involved in sensory analysis (especially for olfaction and vision), rhythm generation, sensorimotor integration (with special attention to visual guidance of eye, arm, and hand movements), and for learning and memory and an account of the self-organization of several components of the nervous system. Part II concludes with chapter 11, Prospects for a Neuroscience of Cognition, which both summarizes the progress exhibited in the preceding chapters and points the way for the broader use of our methodology in the future development of a cognitive neuroscience. The appendixes then introduce the Neural Simulation Language (NSL), in which a number of the functional models described in this volume are programmed, and show the reader how to access these models on the World Wide Web via a database called Brain Models on the Web (being developed as part of the University of Southern California Brain Project).

Acknowledgement

In preparing the book for publication, we have benefited greatly from the helpful comments of a number of colleagues who read parts of an earlier draft. These colleagues include Michel Baudry, Ted Berger, Jim Bloedel, Neil Burgess, Joaquin Fuster, Mel Goodale, John Hertz, Bruce McNaughton, Tom McNeill, Almut Schüz, Larry Swanson, Richard Thompson, and Steven Wise. Also helpful were Ildikó Aradi, György Barna, and Tamás Gröbler, and University of Southern California students Amanda Bischoff, Jason Chu, Fernando Corbacho, Michael Crowley, Alex Guazzelli, Mathew Lamb, Ilya Ovsiannikov, Yuri Pryadkin, Osman Qamar, Paul Rothemund, and Jacob Spoelstra. We also thank all those colleagues whose contributions are cited in references made to the work either of us has done with them.

János Szentágothai: In Memoriam

The idea of writing this book was formed when its three authors took part in the first week of a school organized by Francesco Ventriglia on "Neural Modeling and Neural Networks" held on the Isle of Capri in October 1992, a week that included the celebration of John Szentágothai's eightieth birthday. Szentágothai and Arbib had coauthored *Conceptual Models of Neural Organization* (MIT Press 1975), which inspired (but very much differs from) the present volume, and Szentágothai and Érdi had written articles together on the self-organization of the nervous system. These collaborations provided the basis for the present volume. A lengthy draft of the book had been completed by the time of John Szentágothai's death in September 1994. In fact, John was working on the book that very morning. In view of this history, we thought it appropriate to complete this preface with a short account of John's seminal career in neuroscience.

John Szentágothai (1912–1994) is known for his many pioneering contributions to neuroanatomy. His scientific career began in the midthirties, during which time he helped verify the neuron doctrine against the reticular theory. (His early papers appeared under his original family name of Schimert.) In the late thirties and early forties, he elaborated his secondary degeneration method as a technique to detect pathways between brain regions. Szentágothai served in the Chair of Anatomy at Pécs University Medical School from 1946 to 1963. Combining anatomical and physiological methods, he made pioneering studies on the vestibulo-ocular reflex arc, then worked on the functional anatomy of spinal cord, brainstem, and cerebellum. Furthermore, he was involved in neuroembryological and neuroendocrinological research. In 1963, John Szentágothai moved to the First Department of Anatomy of the Semmelweis University Medical School, Budapest, where he worked until the last day of his life. Szentágothai's anatomical discoveries in the cerebellum, together with the physiological findings of J. C. Eccles and M. Ito, led to a fruitful cooperation and an epoch-making monograph, *The Cerebellum as a Neuronal Machine* (Springer-Verlag 1967). From the late sixties, Szentágothai's activity concentrated on the functional organization of the cerebral cortex. He formulated (and refined in the light of new data) the modular architectonic principle of the cerebral cortex as the anatomical basis for physiologically defined cortical modules. John Szentágothai searched for "the essence of the neural" and hoped to find it in the self-organization of spontaneous (random) activity into biologically significant spatiotemporal activity. A very characteristic autobiography entitled "Too 'Much' and Too 'Soon'" was written for a Festschrift dedicated to his seventieth birthday (Szentágothai 1982). For a brief summary of his activity, including most of his publications and written for his eightieth birthday, see Záborszky et al. (1992). His final reflections on neuroscience are preserved in the present volume, especially in chapter 2 (except for the last section), chapter 7 (except for the last section), section 8.1, section 9.1, and much of section 9.2. We thank Tamas Freund, Attila Gulyás, Miklós Réthelyi, György Székely, and especially Jozsef Takacs for their help in editing portions of this material. As we have completed the other sections, our continuing "conversations" with John, based on many earlier interactions, have influenced our work strongly.

Michael Arbib
Los Angeles

Peter Érdi
Budapest

Part I

Overviews

Part I provides overviews of the three perspectives that structure our approach to neuroscience: structural (chapter 2), functional (chapter 3), and dynamical (chapter 4). As the introductory chapter 1 and many cross-references in chapters 2, 3, and 4 make clear, the different perspectives are presented within an integrative framework that supports efforts at a synthesis yielding an understanding greater than would be possible with overreliance on a single methodology.

The Many Themes of Neural Organization

Recent years have seen a tremendous explosion of knowledge pertaining to the brain. This has led to an ever-increasing sense of the complexity not only of the brain's circuits but of the individual neurons that compose them. Much of this new understanding has involved a reductionist program focusing on the biophysics of the cell membrane and the neurochemistry of the synaptic mechanisms that underlie the plasticity of the brain. However, the true fascination of the brain is with the many functions it serves, such as perception and the control of action, memory, and thought. It is a commonplace that the gaps between the levels of perception and action and the levels of biophysics and neurochemistry are too immense to be bridged with a single span. Rather, the analysis of many levels from the molar to the molecular are required.

But how are these levels to be defined? One approach is *structural*, seeking to find units of analysis—we use the general term *module*—as a bridge between brain regions and the neurons that comprise them, these neurons in turn being subdividable into structural components to be treated at the level of biophysics or neurochemistry. Another approach is *functional*, looking for functional entities—we call them *schemas*—into the "cooperative computation" of which we may refine the overall function of a set of interacting brain regions; the functions of individual schemas, in turn, then may be played out over one or more neural circuits. *Dynamics* provides yet another bridge, this time between the perspectives of structure and function. Whether at the highest or the lowest level, we may use the general language of dynamic systems theory to tease apart the convergence of a neural system's state to some fixed point, or the oscillations of the system, or even chaotic behavior.

This, then, provides the rationale for our volume: to help the reader to understand how the multilevel analysis of both structure and function and the unifying conceptual analysis of dynamics allow us to begin the integration of an immense diversity of facts into a more systematic understanding of the functioning of the brain. Of course, there are many facts that do not find their unification yet in the present state of neuroscience, let alone within the confines of this single volume. Even within this book, there will be places at which we will explore beautiful anatomical structures whose function, if any, is not well-understood. For some of the human capabilities and animal behaviors that attract our attention, excellent models of neural functioning are available, but in other cases only the most preliminary of connectionist models can be offered now. In the same fashion, we will find a number of cases in which the rhythmogenesis in, or the self-organization of, different anatomical structures, or a number of paradigms for learning, can be illuminated by a careful dynamical analysis rooted in a powerful mathematical framework; yet in other cases, our appreciation of dynamical properties, such as the deterministic chaos that we can describe in a number of our models, is not paired yet with an understanding of whether they have functional significance for the normal activity of the brain. Nonetheless, we share the belief that the bridging of different perspectives that we offer here—the attempt to solve complex puzzles by attacking them from several angles—is a necessary complement to the reductionist program in empirical neuroscience. Only by integrating diverse facts into systems models can we infuse those facts with meaning and gain some approximation of true understanding.

In light of this background, a brief account of the contents of this book provides a rationale going beyond the mere enumeration of the contents chapter by chapter or section by section. In chapters 2–4, we provide three overviews of our methodology: a structural overview, a functional overview, and a dynamical overview, respectively. Having agreed to start with three perspectives on the brain, we had to face the complex issue of how best to order and select later chapters so that each would exemplify, to a greater or lesser extent, the integration of these perspectives. The metalevel decision was to adopt structure as the means of defining individual chapters. And thus, for reasons to be explored later, we move through the olfactory system, the hippocampus, the thalamus, the cerebral cortex, and the cerebellum to end with the basal ganglia. In each chapter, we present our perspective of the insights to be gained from a structural, a functional, and a dynamical perspective. Where possible, we go beyond this perspective to show how the structures lead to dynamical modes of operation and contribute to the function of the given brain region, a function often best understood in terms of the interaction of that region with others. Clearly, the book could have been organized around different principles of dynamics, or we could have devoted each chapter to some functional system for which we could have explored both the structures involved and the dynamical pro-

cesses needed to realize the given function. In a sense, then, the reader must treat this book as an exercise in "virtual hypertext" in which many different paths can be chosen to further one's understanding of the material. To help the reader to find such paths, in addition to keeping track of the many aspects of the different chapters as they occur in the present linear order, we devote the remainder of this introduction to stating explicitly a number of themes that are introduced first in the next three chapters but occur again and again as the rest of the book unfolds. The concluding perspective, chapter 11, will then look back in a way that builds on the insights the reader will have gained through reading this book, so as to assess the point at which we have arrived for each of these themes; then it will suggest that we can build on them in a rich fashion to construct a cognitive neuroscience that embraces many systems beyond those we analyze in this book.

1.1 Structure

Our approach to structure is very much wrapped up with our concern with dynamics: We not only ask what the structure of an adult brain is but also ask how it came to be. Thus, on many occasions, our analysis of anatomical structure is complemented by an analysis of phylogeny and ontogeny: how the structure evolved and the embryological basis for its emergence in the adult. In this volume, we will gain insights into function from an evolutionary perspective, but we will not offer models of the evolutionary process per se. On the other hand, the process of embryological development will not only yield insights into adult structure and function but will also be the subject of formal dynamic systems modeling, both in section 4.4, which introduces the study of self-organization, and in section 8.2, which studies the process of self-organization of both ocular dominance and orientation columns in visual cortex. Our embryological study also will make the point that motility occurs in the developing nervous system before it becomes sensitive to environmental influences. This will fit in very much with a general methodological perspective in our functional analysis: Rejecting a simple chain of causality in which stimulus leads directly to response, we will emphasize the action-perception cycle in which the internal state of the organism usually is more potent than are current stimuli in determining action and in which stimuli often will result from the exploratory actions of the animal. The action-perception cycle provides one of the ways in which we may analyze the organism in terms of a circular causality, the other being based on the multiple loops that integrate circuitry in different regions in the brain so as to deny any view of a one-way flow from sensory periphery up to some top level of cortex and from there down in linear fashion to the motor periphery.

Our second structural theme is that of hierarchical levels of analysis, most specifically embodied in the *modular architectonics principle*: Each distinctive region of the brain can be analyzed in terms of a variety of "modules," such as columns, stripes, and layers. Each of these modules can in turn be analyzed in terms of some basic pattern of a small number of neurons of well-defined types, and a neuron of each type then may be analyzed further in terms of its distinctive pattern of dendrites, cell body, and axons and the distinctive pattern of synapses that they form. Reversing the order, we may move up the scale from neural compartments and synapses to neurons and then to networks and, finally, to integrated systems. What brings these structures to life is, in particular, the specialization of different connections for excitation and inhibition, thus allowing different patterns of dynamical behavior to emerge. To this basic mode of neural interaction we can add today a list of further properties, such as the pacemaker activity of some cells, and the ability of certain neurotransmitters to act as neuromodulators rather than as the providers of simple, transient excitatory or inhibitory messages.

We reiterate the point that again and again we see patterns of reciprocal interaction that bind structural units together into functional wholes. For example, in cerebral cortex, the columnar organization is a striking property of at least the sensory cortices. However, equally striking is the pattern of horizontal connections that allow the columns within a single cortical region to influence one another strongly, and the longer-range intracortical connections that form different parts of cortex into functional systems. Even more dramatically, we will reject the simplistic view of thalamus acting as a relay station that simply transfers sensory information upward to primary sensory areas of cerebral cortex, and instead we will touch (all too briefly) on the wealth of information that shows the role of the thalamus in diverse systems of loops: loops from sensory thalamus to sensory cortex and back again; loops from cortex to basal ganglia to thalamus and back to cortex; and loops from cerebral cortex to cerebellum to thalamus and back to cortex once more. Thus, rather than seeing the cerebral cortex as being at the top of a pyramid, we see it as involved in the "cooperative computation" that integrates the competition and cooperation of many different regions as the action-perception cycle progresses. These considerations motivated the ordering of the chapters that follow chapter 4. First we study the olfactory system and hippocampus to provide a parallel study of both rhythmogenesis and learning in two systems whose properties can be studied without explicit reference to the thalamus. Then we study the thalamus itself and follow with a study of the cerebral cortex. Finally we study cerebellum and basal ganglia by emphasizing the loops that link them to the cerebral cortex via thalamus, so as to stress that the functions of cerebral cortex can be understood fully only within the rich context of cooperative computation.

1.2 Function

We have already noted a hierarchy of structural levels from neurons to networks to integrated systems, and one may certainly seek to analyze the function of each such system. However, given our emphasis on cooperative computation, on the way in which many different structural systems may be tightly coupled into a functional whole, it becomes clear that we need the ability to analyze functions more general than those that can be associated with a single structural unit. For this reason, the functional overview of chapter 3 will introduce the terminology of a *schema* as a unit of function, leaving open to further analysis whether in fact that function is played out in one structural unit at a given level of analysis or over a network of such units. Also to be resolved is the question of whether a given brain region is dedicated to implementing a single schema or may play a role within a set of diverse schemas.

Our concern with phylogeny will be repeated in our functional analysis as we attack a too cerebrocentric view of human brain function by stressing the important role of subcortical structures. We will use the comparison of frog and monkey in chapter 3, and of rat and human in chapter 6, to probe the extent to which cerebral cortex can best be understood, not in terms of the adding of completely new functions to "primitive" ones but rather in terms of the evolutionary modulation of functions whose basic form may persist through evolution but which also become capable of an increasingly rich repertoire of means of expression.

The grand themes of function that will occur again and again throughout the following chapters will involve the way in which the animal can use sensory information, particularly (but not only) visual information, to guide its actions, including the ways in which learning and memory can build a "model of the world" within the brain, allowing the animal to act on the basis of experience rather than in terms of simple emission of responses to stimuli. To apply an important corrective to the emphasis on vision that dominates most of our consideration of function, we devote chapter 5 to the olfactory system. In chapter 6, we will try to learn from a comparison of the role of the hippocampus in the formation of cognitive maps in rats and its role in declarative memory in humans. This study of declarative memory will be contrasted with the "procedural memory" that we will see exemplified in our studies of visuomotor conditional learning and of cerebellum and basal ganglia in chapters 8, 9, and 10, respectively.

Two subthemes will carry forward the general theme of the relationship of vision to action and the involvement of memory—both working memory and long-term memory. The first of these will be the control of saccadic eye movements; the second will be the coordination of arm and hand in reaching and grasping. These are both systems in which a wealth of data in monkey neurophysiology can be used to constrain models that then can provide insight into the new results on human brain imaging so crucial to the current emergence of cognitive neuroscience. For each of these two themes, we will start with a basic functional perspective in terms of interacting schemas in chapter 3 and will proceed to elaborate on the story as we look at the roles of cortex, cerebellum, and basal ganglia in chapters 8, 9, and 10, respectively. We shall address briefly the more cognitive functions of visual perception, episodic memory, planning, and language in chapters 3, 6, 8, and 11, respectively.

We should also note that, although it plays only a minor role in the present volume, the phenomenon of disease provides both a major motivation for the study of the brain and a major source of data to inspire and test models of brain function. We shall relate briefly our models of the role of cerebellum to studies of the effects of cerebellar damage on motor control and its adaptation; also, we will strengthen our insight into the functions of the basal ganglia by noting the effect on a variety of behaviors of the diseases of the basal ganglia, especially Parkinson's disease.

1.3 Dynamics

The past 25 years have seen the increasing importance of analyzing the brain as a dynamical system at both a variety of time scales and a variety of structural levels. The dynamical overview of chapter 4 will present the basic vocabulary of systems analysis within which this

variety of time scales and structures can be analyzed. Basically, a dynamical system's state develops through time, either autonomously (i.e., without the influence of external inputs) or in a fashion affected by the availability of environmental inputs. Much attention has been given to three basic modes of autonomous behavior. A dynamical system, when left to itself, may exhibit unstable behavior, but if its trajectory is stable, it will either converge to a single fixed point at which the state will remain unless influenced by changing inputs; it will traverse repeatedly a "limit cycle" (in other words, exhibit oscillations); or it will traverse what is called a *strange attractor* whereby a deterministic system may exhibit that appearance of randomness referred to as *deterministic chaos*.

The models that we will offer for dynamic analysis will tend to be at either of two *structural scales*: Either they will be neural networks in which the state of each neuron is represented by a single real number, such as its membrane potential or its firing rate, or a single neuron may be analyzed by subdividing the dendrites and the cell body into compartments, each of which can be considered to be at a relatively uniform membrane potential or in a relatively uniform neurochemical state. These compartmental models rest on an even more basic form of dynamical analysis, corresponding to the Hodgkin-Huxley model and its various descendants. Each of these levels will be introduced in chapter 4, which will also introduce the different *temporal scales* of analysis.

At the fastest time scale, we may take a neural network whose connections have already been determined and ask how this network will behave, either autonomously or in response to some input. We will devote particular attention to oscillatory behavior—both rhythmogenesis and synchronization—studying electrical activity patterns in the olfactory system, theta rhythm, sharp waves, and epileptic seizure activity in the hippocampus, and thalamocortical oscillations in chapters 5, 6, and 8, respectively. Also, we shall see that the retrieval of stored patterns in a network often may be analyzed in terms of the movement of a trajectory toward a stable fixed point, or attractor. Finally, we shall see some cases in which neural networks exhibit chaotic behavior and shall offer a rather preliminary account of the extent to which such chaotic behavior may or may not play an important functional role.

At the next time scale, that of learning, we ask how a network with an overall architecture already fixed may, through experience, vary the strength of its connections to exhibit some form of memory. The basic paradigm we will present here is known as *Hebbian learning* in honor of Donald Hebb, who offered his hypothesis on general theoretical grounds in his pioneering analysis of neuropsychology in *The Organization of Behavior*. We shall see a number of explicit learning rules for the adjustment of synaptic strengths that can be considered variations on a Hebbian theme. Also, we shall explore three major variations in learning style: *unsupervised learning*, in which a network extracts correlations from its input structure; *supervised learning*, in which this process may be shaped by rather explicit error messages from a "teacher" (which may be an external organism or simply some other, supervisory, network); and *reinforcement learning*, in which an entire network gets a generalized signal (from a "critic") on whether its response was "good" or "bad" without any neuron receiving an explicit quantitative error message. Our later functional models will employ different learning rules of these kinds as we seek to explain how the function of a particular structure, or its role within some overall system organization, may be shaped by experience. For example, we will see examples of supervised Hebbian learning in our study of hippocampus in chapter 6, of reinforcement learning in our studies of cerebral cortex and basal ganglia in chapters 8 and 10, respectively, and of supervised, error-based learning in our study of the cerebellum in chapter 9.

When learning phenomena occur on the time scale of minutes or hours, we do indeed refer to them as *learning* mechanisms. However, when they occur over a period of hours or days or weeks during the early stages of the life of the organism, we refer to them as *developmental* mechanisms; and to the extent that they involve mechanisms whereby the organism extracts structure from its environment rather than shaping itself in response to the explicit instructions of the teacher, we refer to the process involved as *self-organization*. In fact, it is in models of the self-organization that occurs during development that variations on the Hebbian learning rule for unsupervised learning have had some of their most important applications. We shall sample this in chapter 4, in which we study retinotectal connections, and in chapter 8, wherein we look at the basic development of the modular structure in visual cortex, both for ocular dominance and for orientation sensitivity.

The compartmental modeling that we have mentioned briefly will be exemplified in the study of individual neurons and some small circuits in the olfactory system, the hippocampus, the thalamocortical system, and the cerebellum (chapters 5, 6, 8, and 9, respectively). The study of learning rules offers another bridge to the microworld from neurons described in a rather compact way appropriate to the study of dynamics of very large circuits. In this case, the microworld is even smaller than that of a compartment within a compartmental model of a neuron; it is the microworld of neurochemistry. Today, much detailed investigation of the brain focuses on the question of how receptors in the postsynaptic membrane may undergo kinetic changes that serve to increase or decrease the efficacy of a synapse. Thus, when we are hypothesizing that a particular learning rule expressed in the form of a relatively simple dynamical equation underlies the learning of the neural networks in some region of the brain, we are at the same time suggesting high level hypotheses on the kinetics of molecules in the synapse and its membranes. Although most details of neurochemistry are outside the scope of the present volume, nonetheless it will be illuminating to assess briefly the extent to which current studies of long-term depression and long-term potentiation (currently focusing on hippocampus, cerebral cortex, cerebellum, and basal ganglia) are consistent with the learning rules hypothesized in our models of these regions, and to what extent our learning rules go beyond consistency to suggest important properties of synaptic plasticity that must challenge future studies in neurochemistry. In this fashion, we will make clear how the systems level of analysis—uniting structure, function, and dynamics—can provide a framework in which the meaning of even the finest details of neural function can be illuminated.

A Structural Overview

Modern neuroanatomical methods have made it possible to define practically any neuron along three dimensions:

1. *Anatomically*, by the shape and location of the cell body, by dendritic arborizations, by a considerable part of the axonal arborizations, and by the synapses received from and given to other neurons (or other tissue elements).

2. *Physiologically*, especially by spiking activity under suitable experimental conditions, by biophysical conditions prevailing on the outside or the inside of the neuronal membrane, and by the number and location as well as distribution of ionic channels, and so forth. The situation is somewhat more difficult in neurons that lack spiking activity and have to be assumed to convey changes of state electrotonically, but the sign of synaptic action, whether excitatory or inhibitory, usually can still be defined.

3. *Biochemically*, by identification of the mediator(s) through which one neuron can influence other neurons with which they are connected synaptically. In addition to mediators that act on a millisecond time scale, there are neuromodulators that can modify the function of a neuron on time scales lasting from seconds to minutes or more.

Beyond these classic properties, current investigations are uncovering the molecular and genetic mechanisms that underlie the anatomical, physiological, and biochemical properties of neurons.

Considering the extreme complexity of structure and function of any piece of neural tissue, we have to start with a clear objective so as not to lose our way from the very beginning. The classic approach of the neuroanatomist was, and probably will always remain, to give reasonable descriptions of the structure of neuron networks. In this volume, we will build on the *structural* framework of anatomy to address functional data on the role of different brain regions, singly or in concert, in a variety of animal and human behaviors. Also, we will address physiological descriptions of network dynamics to provide realistic, albeit simplified, models of neuron networks, giving life to such models either by mathematical analysis or by simulation experiments. This chapter provides a structural overview from the neuro-anatomist's viewpoint. Chapter 3 will give a functional overview of modeling strategies for relating the activity of neural networks to ongoing animal behavior, and chapter 4 will provide a dynamical overview of the use of dynamic system analysis to study both the physiological dynamics of the brain and the dynamics of self-organization in development and learning. The remaining chapters then will integrate structural, functional, and dynamical perspectives on different key regions of the mammalian brain.

Neuronal connectivity in most neural centers is sufficiently specific to permit disassembly of the entire network into distinct pieces (or units) of characteristic internal connectivity that are arranged into larger structures by repetition of similar architectural units. These units have been termed *neuronal modules*, and this architectural principle is referred to by speaking of the *modular architectonic principle* of neural centers. This chapter will illustrate this principle in various parts of the central nervous system (CNS) of vertebrates, starting with the spinal cord, and the changes that occur in the lower brainstem. Subsequently, we shall address briefly the examples of the cerebellum, the neocortex and, as a special case of the cortex, to its archaic part, the limbic lobe, and its highly specialized structure, the hippocampus. We will elaborate on much of this material in later chapters, which also will discuss the olfactory system and the basal ganglia.

A theme to be established in this chapter, and to which we shall return in a number of the anatomical excursions of later chapters, is that the complexity of adult structure often can be approached best through the embryology of the structure to make clear crucial relationships that may be obscured in the adult form. One insight of this approach will be the clear understanding that the embryonic nervous system is able to generate movement before it is able to respond to sensory stimuli. This view supports an action-oriented view of brain function that is far from a view grounded in reflexes or stimulus-response behaviorism. Also, we shall pay some attention to the evolution of the mammalian brain, seeing how (as the brain evolves) basic structures become overlaid with more and more complex structures that can both inhibit and coordinate what has evolved before. Though current forms are, by definition, all contemporary, there is a very important logic of comparative neuroscience that relates actual current forms to a putative evolutionary sequence, allowing us a much more informed analysis of the mammal, primate, or human.

Section 2.1 introduces the theme that structure often can be illuminated by the study of phylogeny and ontogeny: seeing how the structure evolved or developed. We provide an evolutionary grounding for brain structure in segmentation, the repetition of similar structural units along the main body axis, one of the most basic building principles of multicellular animal bodies. Because we deal with neural centers of vertebrates, we use the segmented part of the neuraxis (i.e., the spinal cord and lower brainstem) to ground discussion of the progressive loss of segmentation in the upper brainstem, including the diencephalon (sec. 2.1.1). The neuraxis itself is not really segmented but is more of a structural continuum on which segmentation is to some extent superimposed by the somites.

Motor pattern generators (MPGs) augment the central circuitry of central pattern generators (CPGs), which can produce only a crude sketch of the motor pattern, with the sensory feedback crucial to shaping this "sketch" into coordinated activity. Embryological studies show that motility of embryos begins well ahead of the development of afferent systems (sec. 2.1.2). This provides the basis for later exploration of complex behaviors in terms of the coordinated activity of more and more neural subsystems. We view the elementary source of neural activity to be oscillatory, whether resulting from tight coupling of auto-oscillators or the self-organization of quasi-random networks of excitatory and inhibitory interneurons. This does not, however, imply that motility is an end in itself. Rather, this "motor foundation" serves to ground the later development of sensory maps and sensorimotor representations in a self-directed manner more expressive of the evolved structure of the organism than it is responsive to the buffeting of sensory stimuli. Moreover (sec. 2.1.3), the development of vertebrate motoneurons can be traced by the techniques of modern molecular genetics and biology and by experimental labeling techniques for retrograde identification of motoneurons from their axons in studying the ontogeny and structural basis of tetrapod locomotion.

Section 2.2 introduces the structural theme of providing an architectonic basis for the analysis of function and dynamics of circuitry. We approach a hierarchy of levels of analysis—neurons, networks, integrated system—by presentintg data that support the modular architectonic principle: Neuronal connectivity in a typical neural center is sufficiently specific to permit disassembly of the whole network into neuronal modules of characteristic internal connectivity, and the larger structure can be reconstituted by repetition of these modules. In section

2.2.1, we visualize the spinal gray matter as a double-barrel structure, then consider the remaining parts of the cord as dorsal, ventral, and (in some places) lateral appendages attached to the perimeters of the barrels. Viewing the double-barrel core and adjacent white matter as two columns of coins (the boundaries between coins are chosen for convenience of analysis) reveals a segmental structure with respect to which the spatial orientation of dendrites and terminal axonal arborizations can be made clear. Section 2.2.2 then shows that the lower brainstem (medulla oblongata, pons, and midbrain) is arranged in essentially the same quasi-segmental (stacked-discs) pattern. However, only the serotoninergic neurons really fit into the segmental architecture, whereas catecholaminergic and dopaminergic neurons more often are concentrated in separate cell groups (e.g., the locus ceruleus). A fundamental change of the design involves nuclear masses connecting the longitudinal arrangement of the neuraxis with higher centers, notably the cerebellum and the tectum. However (sec. 2.2.3), the upper diencephalic and telencephalic parts of the brainstem do not retain the quasi-segmental arrangement of the lower neuraxis, save that elements of the basic architectural principle of the neuraxis are preserved in the hypothalamus in longitudinally oriented fiber tracts and transversely oriented quasi-discs of neuropil. In section 2.2.4 we treat the importance in many structures of local circuit neurons and of the complex synaptic arrangements (called *glomeruli*) with their synaptic triads in, for example, the cerebellar cortex, the olfactory bulb, and some of the anterior thalamic nuclei.

In section 2.3, we continue the search for a hierarchy of levels of analysis of neurons, networks, and integrated systems and show how various regions (to be studied more fully in later chapters) each have their own distinctive internal modules while also being embedded within loops traversing many brain regions (a theme to be developed in our study of thalamocortical loops and cooperative computation, sec. 7.3).

In section 2.3.1, we introduce the beautiful quasi-crystalline structure of the cerebellar cortex and the embedding of this cortex in the cerebellar system, the links of which ("upstream" with the cerebral cortex and "downstream" with the spinal cord) are closed not in the cortex but in the cerebellar nuclei to which the output cells of cerebellar cortex project. The fact that this output is purely inhibitory ties into the theme that the passage from structure to function often is based on understanding the patterns of interplay of excitation and inhibition. In this case, the inhibition from cerebellar cortex serves to modulate the activity in the cerebellar

nuclei, which (as we shall see in chap. 9) serve in turn to tune and coordinate MPGs located upstream and downstream in the nervous system.

In section 2.3.2, we present the modular architectonics principle as applied to the cerebral cortex. It links observations of anatomical regularities to the observations of Mountcastle (1957) on physiological "columns" in somatosensory cortex and the later observations of Hubel and Wiesel (1959) on visual cortex. Several earlier forms of relatively simple modules were built around the arborizations of the specific sensory afferents or corticocortical connections; an entire hierarchy of highly regular modularities now can be defined within the primary visual cortex of the monkey. Finally, in section 2.3.3, we review the basic neuron chains of the hippocampus, noting both the classically known pathways and the more recently discovered inhibitory interneurons. In this way, we sample a number of the basic neural circuitries that will occupy our attention in part II as we link structure, function, and dynamics for these brain regions and for others besides.

2.1 An Embryological Perspective on Neural Structure and Motility

In this section, we introduce an embryological perspective on neural structure. This theme will be developed further in discussions of intermediate embryonic stage of developing brain (see figure 7.1), the development of sensory systems (part of sec. 7.2.2), the development of cerebral cortex (sec. 8.1.1), ontogeny of the cerebellum (sec. 9.1), and striatal compartmentalization (sec. 10.3). It also will find resonances in our discussion of the dynamical theme of self-organization in chapters 4 and 8.

2.1.1 Segmentation and the Neuraxis

To provide an evolutionary grounding for our structural overview, we note that *segmentation* (i.e., a stringlike repetition of similar structural units along the main body axis) is one of the most basic and consequently retained (or reappearing) building principles of multicellular animal bodies. Its recent analysis by Gehring (1987) and others by molecular genetic techniques has led to the general homeobox principle for explaining the design of multicellular animal phyla (worms, arthropods, and vertebrates) in terms of a key set of genes, the homeotic genes (see Lawrence 1992, Chapter 5, for an exposition). The monoaxial and bilateral symmetry of body design is by no means all-encompassing. There are pentaxial symmetrics (e.g., in the echinodermata: starfish and sea urchins) and bilateral or helicoid symmetries (e.g., in the molluscs: bivalves, gastropods, and cephalopods). This type of body design depends on the homeotic genes that bind to portions of other genes and eventually regulate the production of specific proteins giving rise to the development of such body parts as eyes, antennae, limbs, or any other organ or body tissue.

Because this book deals almost exclusively with neural centers of vertebrates, we shall use a discussion of the segmented part of the neuraxis (i.e., the spinal cord and lower brainstem) to ground discussion of the progressive loss of segmentation in the upper brainstem, including the diencephalon, where some of the architectonic elements can still be recognized in their remnants, and will close the chapter with a preview of other structures to be treated at length in later chapters. It has to be borne in mind that the segmental arrangement in the vertebrates differs fundamentally from the segmentation in invertebrate phyla. In invertebrates, segmentation belongs to the essence of the building plan, whereas in the vertebrates, the neuraxis itself is not really segmented but is more of a structural continuum on which segmentation is quasi-superimposed by the somites (i.e., by the segmentation of the medial strip of the mesoderm) or partially by the branchial arches. Despite this, the secondarily imposed segmentation serves as an important system of landmarks for the description of spinal cord architecture.

Within this general framework, we now address the most basic facts concerning the embryology of the CNS. The original primordium of the CNS of the vertebrates—the medullary tube—is simply a tube built of pseudostratified cylindrical epithelium, in which all cells have their two points of attachment at the inner and outer surfaces of the primary ectoderm, points that originally were the outer and inner surfaces (looking toward the interior of the early gastrula), respectively, before the neural tube forms from the neural crest (figure 2.1A). The early movements of the cell nuclei are now known to be crucial steps of cellular differentiation (Jacobson 1970), serving to prepare for cell divisions that take place exclusively while the nuclei are positioned close to the inner lining of the epithelium. Hence, this inner zone is called the *germinative* (or ventricular) *zone*, whereas the middle zone of the medullary tube, containing the nuclei of the primordial cells as they move up and down to position themselves for the stage of their final division, is called the *mantle zone.* The outermost layer of the tube, practically devoid of cell nuclei, is termed the *marginal zone.*

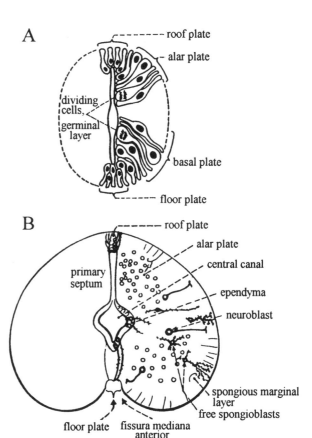

Figure 2.1
(A) The original primordium of the central nervous system of the vertebrates, the medullary tube, which is simply a tube built of pseudostratified cylindrical epithelium. All cells have their two points of attachment at the inner—originally the outer surfaces (looking toward the interior of the early gastrula)—before the neural tube forms from the neural crest. (B) The original sagittal slotlike lumen of the central canal becomes obliterated in its dorsal third by the progressive shortening of the ependymal cells in the so-called roof plate.

In the development and formation of cell lines in the more expanded rostral parts of the medullary tube, giving rise to the cerebellum and the cerebral cortex, the birth and exodus of specific cell types can be observed readily. In the early morphogenetic steps of the rhombencephalon (giving rise to the medulla oblongata, the pons, and the cerebellum), the early processes of development have been studied under relatively favorable conditions (Altman 1982; Sidman 1970). By analogy with these processes, we may reconstruct the essential steps of the origin and timing of genetic specification of the nerve cells in the spinal cord and the lower brainstem, going back to the early observations of spinal cord tissue development by the classical authors of the nineteenth century (His, Koelliker, Retzius, v. Lenhossek, and many others). At that time it was, of course, out of the question to identify different cell lines or clones with any degree of confidence; thus, we may consider the classic observations only relevant for what could be seen directly in histological preparations. We still may assume by analogy that neurons as well as glial cells of the dorsal horn were derived from the dorsal part (dorsal to the sulcus limitans) of the medullary tube epithelium. The majority of nerve and glial cells of the intermediate zone and the ventral horn were derived from neuroepithelial cells positioned ventrally from the sulcus limitans. The original sagittal slotlike lumen of the central canal becomes obliterated in its dorsal third by the progressive shortening of the ependymal cells in the so-called roof plate (i.e., the place where the closure of the two margins of the medullary plate has originally occurred; (see figure 2.1B). By the later development of the two halves of the dorsal (white) funiculi, the dorsal surface of the spinal cord becomes totally closed; the site of this second closure is marked only by a dorsal median septum. Conversely, on the ventral side, the so-called floor plate persists and is occupied later by the ventral white commissure. The two ventral white funiculi never come together completely, so that a deep ventral fissure persists throughout the entire length of the spinal cord.

Figure 2.2 (right side) pictures the radiate glial system as described by the classical neurohistologists (Retzius 1891; v. Lenhossek 1891). By indicating the later border between gray and white matter in Figure 2.2. and relying on the analogy of the process of birth and emigration of neuroblasts and free gliablasts (better known from the development of the cerebral and cerebellar cortex; see chapters 8 and 9), we may assume that their sites of origin in the germinative zone and their paths of emigration toward their later locations can be deduced safely from the "scaffolding" (Rakic 1981) of the medullary tube tissue afforded by the radiate glia. Several successive generations of neuroblasts (and free glioblasts) are born and start to emigrate from the same sites of the germinative zones, so that the life histories of virtually all nerve cells can be indicated (as putatively shown for the ventral horn on the left side of figure 2.2). Having no direct information for the dorsal horn, the cell architecture of which is more complicated than in the intermediate and ventral region, we refrain from further theorizing regarding the cells of the dorsal horn. We have one relevant datum based on tracing certain proteins characteristic for motoneurons by molecular genetic methods (Chen and Chiu 1992) suggesting that the motoneurons are the cells first born in the ventral part of the germinative zone and the first to emigrate toward their final positions. When similar data are gathered for

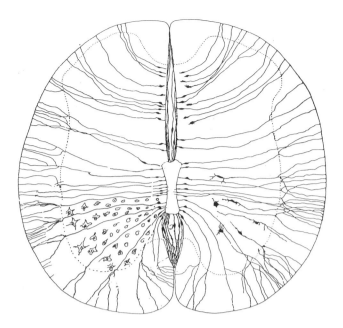

Figure 2.2
A Retzius drawing illustrating early development of the radiate glia (ependymal) cells in a 3-cm human embryo. The right side shows the emigration from the internal germinative layer of a few glioblasts that still have not lost their attachment to the outer surface. The position of radiate glial cells on both sides of the dorsal septum indicates that the dorsal part of the original medullary tube lumen becomes gradually obliterated. The left ventral quadrant has been redrawn by the author to illustrate the process of emigration of neuroblasts from their sites of origin in the inner cell lining of the medullary tube and to suggest the role that the radial glia plays as a "scaffolding" for later cell movements.

other specific cell types of the spinal cord, we will be in a position to define the life histories of these cells also.

2.1.2   The Onset of Motility Prior to Sensation

Now we supplement this embryological view of developing structure in the spinal cord by reviewing the elementary structures involved in motion and later shall address the sensory aspects of reflexes as a basis for the overlay of more complex structures.) Embryological studies show that motility and coordinated motor activity provides a basic structure on top of which sensory refinements later develop. This ties in with a key notion in the motor control literature. It is common to talk of CPGs for intrinsic circuitry that has been shown capable of producing structured motor patterns in adult creatures. However, the consensus now is to view MPGs as augmenting this central circuitry, which can produce only a crude sketch of the motion, with the sensory feedback crucial to shaping this basic rhythm or other movement into coordinated activity (Dean and Cruse 1995). Thus, the basic studies of "autonomous motility" that we develop here provide the basis for later work in the book exploring complex behaviors in terms of the coordinated activity of more and more neural subsystems. This section focuses on the importance of neuroembryology in revealing basic connections between structure and function.

The very first elements of neural activity during ontogenesis are on the motor side. Already in the nineteenth century (Pryer 1885), it was known that motility of embryos begins well ahead of the development of afferent systems. The careful studies of Hamburger, Wenger, and Oppenheene (1966; Hamburger 1977) gave experimental evidence for the fact that primary sensory elements do not play any role in the early movements of the chick embryo before day 18. Thus the inescapable conclusion is that the most basic conditions of motility are not sensory input but autogenic activities of elementary neural networks around motoneurons and, of course, the early muscle elements innervated by them. This was shown in tissue recombination experiments that used a technique originally devised by Weiss (1950) but fully exploited only later by Székely and Szentágothai (1962), whose first experiments were designed to ensure that the tissue recombination material contained very small fragments only of ventral quadrant neural tube tissue and of limb buds acting as indicators of movement but of no sensory elements whatsoever. The early experiments of Weiss (1950) had shown that muscles of the supernumerary limbs developing from the limb buds could be innervated exclusively by prospective motoneurons, because the cholinergic transmission mechanism was available in the segmented neuraxis exclusively in prospective motoneurons. Now we know that the motoneurons of the ventral quadrant of the medullary tube always were surrounded by a mixed population of excitatory and inhibitory interneurons. It appears that as few as 10 interneurons of excitatory and inhibitory nature are sufficient to generate the "epileptiform" movements, a term used to characterize the strange apparently random nature (in time and character) of the movements of the indicator limb (figure 2.3A).

Somewhat later, Székely and Czéh (1971) found that the minimal conditions under which quasi-natural (i.e., stepping) movements of the implanted limb could occur (see figure 2.3B) were that (1) the deplanted neural tube fragment had an intact part of the central canal, which was essential for orderly (natural) neuron network arrangement and (2) that the deplanted tube part was taken from the "limb innervating segments" of the tube. However, no part of the dorsal (i.e., sensory) horn was required for quasi-orderly movement (i.e., showing rudi-

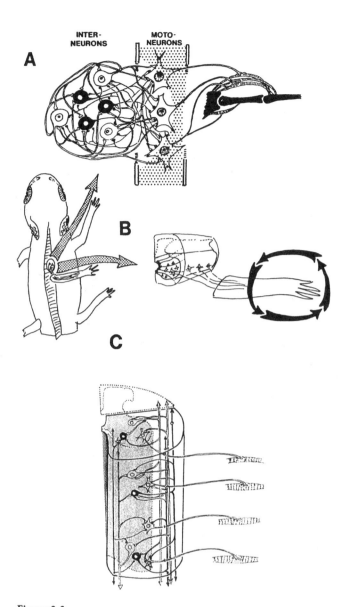

Figure 2.3
Diagram of the tissue recombination experiments described in the text. The general experimental situation (implantation of a limb and a portion of the neural tube) is given at left of (B). (A) Illustration of the original experiment of Székely and Szentágothai (1962). Motoneurons innervating the muscles of the grafted limb were separated from the interneurons (excitatory in outlines; inhibitory in full black), whereas both cell types were present in the tranplantations. (B) The ventral quadrant of a limb-bearing spinal segment that could move a transplanted limb in "stepping sequences" (Székely and Czéh 1971). The sequence of movements is shown by the circle of large arrows. C. The local spinal network in situ that is needed for the results observed by Székely and Czéh 1971 (Modified after Szentágothai 1987, 1993.)

ments of stepping sequences) of the deplanted limb. Figure 2.3C gives an impression of the interneuronal apparatus of the ventral horn as deduced from our histological studies (Szentágothai and Réthelyi 1973; Szentágothai 1981, 1983).

The conclusions that can be drawn from the observations summarized in figure 2.3 are (1) that haphazardly interconnected interneurons of excitatory and inhibitory nature can produce only haphazard (quasi-random) activity patterns, whereas (2) orderly connected interneurons as exist in the limb-bearing segments of the ventral medullary tube can guarantee limb-type (stepping-sequence) movements in complete lack of any sensory input. Using more sophisticated tissue (brain slice) culturing experiments, Gähwiler (1980, 1981, 1988) showed by direct recording from large hippocampal pyramid cells that this principle can be generalized to other parts of the CNS: Mutually interconnected neurons of excitatory and inhibitory nature can produce (quasi)-natural rhythms of activity. This probably extends to any part of the CNS. We shall return briefly to this subject in discussing the dentate-hippocampal formation in chapter 6. We also see strong linkages here to work on oscillators and self-organization (to be discussed in chapter 4).

So far, however, we have described only the phenomenology. What can be said about the causes of this kind of original activity of motility prior to sensation? One fact is clear: There is nothing involved here that would even remotely resemble the traditional cartesian view of the reflex. If there is no neural input to an active system—and that is what the foregoing studies tried to exclude from the very beginning—we may deny safely the primacy of the classic paradigm, the reflex principle. As far as we know, there are two causal explanations for the observed phenomena: One is that of Rodolfo R. Llinás (1987), and another is by Szentágothai (1984, 1987b).

According to Llinás, "auto-oscillators" are the ultimate (earliest and most elementary) source of neural activity. There are both structural and biophysical considerations that suggest the primary role of auto-oscillators.

First, it is observed generally that at the earliest stages of synaptogenesis, the connections between different neurons have the structural characteristics of electrical synapses. Synapses with the usual structural criteria of those acting by chemical mediation begin to appear later and only gradually replace the earlier "electric"-type contacts.

In addition, low-threshold calcium spikes and electrical synapses have been observed by Llinás and Yarom (1981) in the inferior olive of the cat, and the causal relations of the two in the physiological function of the

olive have been demonstrated. Subsequently, many similar organizations and coincidences have been shown to exist in other parts of the CNS.

Further, from a review of the electroresponsive properties of single neurons in the mammalian CNS, it could be deduced (Llinás 1988) that in many of these cells the ionic conductances responsible for their excitability endow them with autorhythmical electrical oscillatory properties. Chemical or electrical synaptic contacts between these neurons often result in network oscillations.

In such networks, autorhythmical neurons may act as true oscillators (pacemakers) or resonators (responding preferentially to certain firing frequencies). Oscillations and resonance in the CNS were proposed to have diverse functional roles, such as determining global functional states (sleep-wakefulness or attention), timing in motor coordination, and specifying connectivity during development.

Szentágothai's hypothesis was based simply on the assumption that the raw material for intrinsic rhythms of neural tissue was the spontaneous discharges of individual nerve cells in isolated pieces of neuron networks containing mutually coupled inhibitory and excitatory neurons. As suggested by the early tissue recombination models, this in itself would suffice for the emergence by self-organization of activity bursts or cycles. As shown about a decade later by simulation experiments and mathematical analysis (Anninos et al. 1970; Harth et al. 1970; Wilson and Cowan 1972, 1973), the ubiquitous conditions in all parts of the CNS of mutually and reversibly interconnected excitatory and inhibitory neurons can lead to various types of cyclic activities. The basic conditions for the existence of such neuron connections were predicted long ago by Lorente de Nó (1933, 1938) by his two laws: (1) "multiplicity" and (2) "reversibility of neural connections," although the existence of specific inhibitory interneurons was not known at that time. In the theoretical models of Wilson and Cowan (1972, 1973), spontaneous activity of the individual cell constituents was not envisaged, and stimuli were assumed to have to come from some outside source. Because outside sources were excluded in the aforementioned embryological tissue recombination experiments, and could be excluded *ab initio* in activities observed in nervous tissue cultures (Crain 1973; Legendre et al. 1988) as well as the more sophisticated experiments of Gähwiler (1980, 1981), the origin of the activity from spontaneous discharges was the more likely assumption. Admittedly, neither of these experiments would disprove the existence of auto-oscillators in the sense assumed by Llinás, but self-organization from random discharges of single cells would be the assumption that is in better conformation with the law of parsimony. It does have, additionally, the advantage of bringing the theory of self-organizing systems almost automatically into theorizing about neural phenomena (Szentágothai 1984, 1987b; Szentágothai and Erdi 1989; Szentágothai 1993). Though these comments have stressed the differences between Szentágothai's ideas and those of Llinás, an integration of the two viewpoints is indeed conceivable because, in invertebrate preparations, network oscillators may depend on intrinsic bursters or interactions between nonburster cells (see sec. 4.2.1). Endogenous oscillation, plateau properties, and postinhibitory rebound are crucial for the dynamic properties of invertebrate oscillators (Marder and Selverston 1992); these properties also are present in vertebrate neurons (Hounsgaard and Kjaerulff 1992). In any case, the issue of rhythmogenesis will be a recurrent theme in the dynamic analysis in later chapters, though the functional implications of such rhythms is not always clear. For now, let us sum up the major points of understanding reached so far by examining the very beginning of motor neural functions.

1. We think the basic raw material from which neurally driven motility arises is spontaneous discharges in individual nerve cells (i.e., neural "noise"). (The causes of such spontaneous discharges may be manifold; let it suffice that spontaneous discharges do occur in many isolated cells or in small assemblies of cells.)

2. Given the ubiquitous condition that neurons of excitatory and inhibitory nature are coupled mutually with one another (and possibly with themselves, although the question of autosynapses is still far from being proved or disproved), this may lead through self-organization to the emergence of cyclical activities as they are commonly observed in neurally isolated groups of nerve cells.

3. Such cyclic activities appears to be random or at least biologically senseless if the arrangement and connectivity of the neurons is haphazard.

4. Ordered activity appears when the types of neurons and their connectivity are ordered.

5. Ordered (or in fact any) sensory neural input does not belong to the elementary conditions of neurally driven motility. Of course, there are many different nonneural (or preneural) motilities that may have very different mechanisms and that are biologically highly useful (e.g., in bacteria, protozoa, smooth- and heart-muscle tissues), but they do not belong to the phenomena being discussed in this book.

Essentially similar principles were recognized by Maturana and Varela (1980), although on the basis of an entirely different approach. It is remarkable that such a fundamental concept as autopoiesis of neural functions should emerge from two entirely different approaches that were virtually unconnected. The tissue recombination experiments were made well before Maturana and Varela developed their concept; the convergence of the two concepts became apparent only much later. The important finding that sensory neural input does not belong to the elementary conditions of neurally-driven motility does not, however, imply that motility is an end in itself. Rather, this "motor foundation" serves to ground the later development of sensory maps and sensorimotor representations in a self-directed manner more expressive of the evolved structure of the organism than it is responsive to the buffeting of sensory stimuli. Having said this, we will make clear the subtle interactions of "nature" and "nurture" in our treatment of self-organization in section 4.4.

2.1.3 The Phylogenesis of Motoneurons and Motility in the Vertebrate Phylum

Having concluded that the primary sources of neural motility are to be traced back to motoneurons and their surround of interneurons, we look at the phylogenesis of various types of motoneurons in the vertebrates. There are two (as yet) separate lines of research leading to the understanding of the development (both ontogenetic and phylogenetic) of vertebrate motoneurons. Unfortunately (again for the time being), we have markers, or footholds for marking, only for the motoneurons themselves, so that the other necessary constituents logically assumed for the development of motor activity (the interneuron "surround" of motoneurons) cannot be traced by any direct method. We have to assume simply that wherever there are motoneurons, they are automatically joined by a surround of such interneurons. One way of tracing motoneurons backward is given by the techniques of modern molecular genetics and biology. The other approach is indirect and makes use of experimental labeling techniques for retrograde identification of motoneurons from their axons.

It was mentioned earlier that motoneurons are the first neurons to appear in the medullary tube and that they do so at a relatively early stage (Chen and Chiu 1992), during embryonic days 10 and 11 (E10 and E11) of the chick (H-H stages 36–37; Hamburger and Hamilton 1951). Neurofilament protein was the earliest marker (day E10), followed by neural cell adhesion molecule

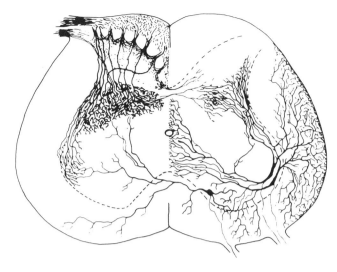

Figure 2.4
Székely drawing (1989) of the frog lumbosacral region. The left side illustrates the typical arborizations of dorsal root collaterals; the right side illustrates the characteristic dendritic arborizations of a "primary" motoneuron (lower right-hand side) innervating the axial (swimming) musculature and of two representative secondary motoneurons (somewhat to the right and above the primary motoneuron) innervating the limb muscles. Comparison of the two drawings reveals the preferential synaptic relations of the two different motoneuron types. (Reprinted with permission from Székely 1989.)

(NCAM) (day E11) and choline acetyltransferase (day E11.5). Motoneurons in the chick embryo express a homeobox gene, islet-1, soon after their final division (Ericson et al. 1992); the signals arise from inductive influences localized in the floor plate and the motochord (beginning with H-H stages 15–16).

There is a huge body of evidence available from classic experimental embryology on the ontogeny and structural basis of tetrapod (quadrupedal) locomotion. A most illuminating and comprehensive summary of the field was given by George Székely (1989), who has contributed to the whole story with several coworkers. In essence, there are two different movement generators in the urodele (salamander and newt) larvae that can be considered as some kind of prototype for quadruped movement. The first is for swimming movements, using an early set of primary motoneurons. A second set of motoneurons (the so-called secondary motoneurons) having radically different modes of dendritic arborization and later connections with the primary sensory afferents become established (determined) in the early tailbud stadium in the urodele and on the second day of incubation in the chicken embryo. The two types of motoneurons, their characteristically different dendritic arborization patterns, and some of their later relations with primary efferents are summarized in figure 2.4. This secondary set of motoneurons is available only in the limb-bearing

segments of the neuraxis. In the earliest stages of their determination, the segments for the forelimbs and the hindlimbs already have their own specific differences, but both use the descending waves generated for swimming movements by the spinal network of interneurons associated with the primary motoneurons (Székely 1965; Kling and Székely 1968; Ádám 1968; Kling 1971). The characteristic diagonal alternation of limb movements in the basic quadruped gait depends on the function of the rhythmic swimming movement generator. (A brief mathematical analysis of chains of oscillators responsible for rhythmic swimming is presented in section 4.2.2.)

At least one-third of the spinal cord is needed for normal alternating movements in both the forelimb and hindlimb segments. (In normal development, the alternating movement of the brachial segments requires the presence of the medulla. However, this can be replaced in recombination experiments by a group of transplanted thoracic segments sufficiently long to correspond to one-third of the entire cord length; Brändle and Székely 1973). In the frog and in the chicken, the specific movement patterns for both the brachial and the lumbosacral segments need specific further differentiations for which afferent input may become progressively necessary, relating to our earlier observation that CPGs need afferent input to form fully effective MPGs. In this way, we see how the basic emergence of motility in the embryo provides the basis for the later development of sensory refinements that allow the CNS to express its full range of function and dynamics.

2.1.4 Somatotopic Projections and the Problem of the Crossing of Neural Connections

The problem of the crossing of neural pathways has always fascinated neuroscientists. Virtually all authors, both in classic treatises of such general questions and even in more recent ones, approach the question from the teleological viewpoint: "What is the crossing good for?" Many recent authors appear to be conscious of the pitfalls of teleological reasoning and try to dissimulate even if their argument is influenced by the teleological views. In fact, teleological arguments always and everywhere are at the background of our thinking, irrespective of whether this is on the surface or in a highly abstract sphere as expressed, for example, in the anthropic principle of creation. However, here we offer a contrary view that, in the spirit of this chapter, sees the crossing as a result of embryological processes. We argue that this is a case where form does not follow function, though function well may follow form.

Weiss (1934) had clearly shown that the major factors in giving direction to the growth of nerve processes are the macromolecular orientation of the media in which the growth occurs. Between two foci of expansive growth (e.g., between two neighboring tissue colonies), the macromolecular structure of the medium is oriented automatically in parallel to the line connecting the centers of the two foci. Because the embryonic primordium of the CNS has a bilateral symmetry and because both halves undergo expansive growth (by cell division and outgrowth of processes), the connecting commissures (i.e., the roof plate and the bottom plate of the medullary tube) are subjected to transversal stresses; hence, the microcellular matrix comes under transversal stresses irrespective of the original radiate direction of the neural tube epithelium and the later emerging radiate glia (see figure 2.2). Further, it is here that developing fibers (and dendrites) preferentially cross.

The same applies to all upper parts of the medullary tube, where, especially on the ventral side, the commissure between the two halves of the CNS primordium remains uninterrupted throughout the later development. This is not so simple on the dorsal side of the cranial part of the medullary tube, where a large part of the roof of the fourth and third ventricle becomes defective, and commissures occur only in and at both ends of the mesencephalon and in the cerebellar velum. A preferential site of commissures is the rostral end of the anterior cerebral vesicle (lamina terminalis), where the decussation of the optic nerves takes place near the bottom, and the anterior commissure develops somewhat above. However, the development of the other telencephalic commissures, the corpus callosum and the hippocampal commissure, vividly illustrate how crude an oversimplification it would be if all tract crossings were reduced to fiber tracts being caught in the transverse stresses developing between two rapidly expanding halves of the central organ.

The developmental causes we study here are the residue of evolutionary processes that can bias or choose between different patterns of tract formation. Thus, though we see here what types of structure in the embryo can guide the growth of fibers, we do not resolve the issue of why some tracts are crossed and others are uncrossed. Braitenberg (1984) offers a provocative essay (mixing speculations on teleology and evolution) on how a variety of crossed and uncrossed pathways first might serve approach and withdrawal behaviors and then provide the basis for the evolution of ever more complex pathways. Here, however, we focus on embryological issues that may guide naturally the formation of path-ways connecting different neural regions. Our study of self-organization in section 4.4 will address the question, "Once the fibers get to their target region, how do they sort themselves out to form an orderly projection?" This question leads back to the specific analysis of the courses of optic nerve fibers.

Szentágothai and Székely (1956b) realized that in complete cyclopic malformation (of the type studied by Mangold in 1931) caused by destruction of the prechordal plate, we find the extreme of a continuum. In the case of complete fusion of the eye cups and one central lens, the optic fibers do cross virtually completely behind the posterior surface of the lens, so that retinal fibers originating from the right half of the retina entered the cell layers of the developing retina on the left side and vice versa (figure 2.5A). Lacking a choroidal fissure, there was no recognizable guiding medium of the optic fibers, and on reaching the outer pigment epithelium, the fibers were stopped and did not grow outside the closed eye cup. In cases with incomplete fusion of the two eye cups (semifused eye cups and two lenses, see figure 2.5B) or closely adjacent but separate eye cups, when usually there were choroidal fissures, the retinal fibers were guided into them and into the rudimentary optic stalks surrounded by pigment cell precursors. Depending on the position of the separate but closely adjacent "semicyclopic" eye cups, the majority of the optic fibers did cross at the floor of the diencephalon. However, in some cases, when the abnormal eyes were more dorsally positioned, the optic fibers entered the side of the diencephalon and continued their route to the ipsilateral tectum. In a few cases, the uncrossed optic fibers ran caudalward and found a more posterior part of the diencephalic floor plate, where they could cross and eventually reach their proper controlateral side of the tectum. We can deduce from these experiments that primary axis orientation of the retinal axons was a major factor in determining the direction of the outgrowth of axons but that preformed guiding structures (choroidal fissure, optic stalk, and their surround of pigment cells) soon take over as decisive factors in finding their proper targets.

Turning from the optic crossing to the role of primary axon axis orientation in the development of somatotopic projections, Szentágothai and Székely (1956b) discussed in the same paper what they called the *elementary crossings* of both sensory and motor roots (summarized diagrammatically in figure 2.6). Part A was assembled from the data of Angulo (1951), and part B was taken from the observations of the authors on embryos of *Lacerta viridis*. Part C is reproduced from a drawing of v. Lenhossek (1895) illustrating the crossing of the Ia afferent

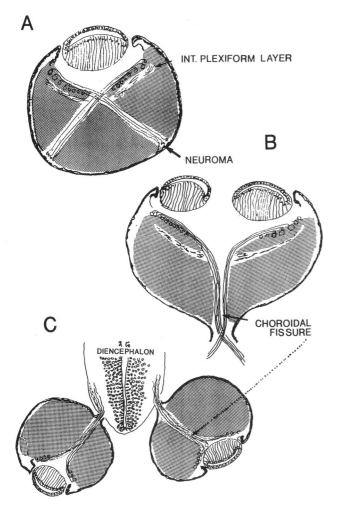

A

INT. PLEXIFORM LAYER

B

NEUROMA

C

CHOROIDAL FISSURE

DIENCEPHALON

Figure 2.5
Summary of various types of optic fiber crossings in experimental cyclopoid malformations (Szentágothai and Székely, 1956a,b). (A) In a complete fusion of the two eye cups in a Mangold-type cyclop with one lens, the optic fibers from both retinal halves cross behind the lens and, in the absence of a preformed choroidal fissure, penetrate as solid bundles though the retinal layers, stopping on reaching the close outer pigment layer of the cup. (B) Incompletely fused eye cups having a single central choroidal fissure and two lenses. The optic nerves cross in the optic stalk immediately behind the eye. (C) Malformation with two complete eye cups, shifted to a more dorsal position. In such cases, the optic fibers may lack the opportunity to cross at the bottom of the diencephalon and so continue their courses toward the tectum on the ipsilateral side (retinal tissue stippled).

(so-called reflex) collaterals. These collaterals directed to the interneurons for the axial muscles penetrate through the dorsal horn more laterally and those for the limb muscles more medially. As a result, the reversed projection of the sensory segment on the dorsal horn (Szentágothai and Kiss 1949; Szentágothai and Réthelyi 1973) becomes reversed again in the ventral horn, where the motoneurons for the axial muscles are positioned medially and those for the muscles are supplied by the

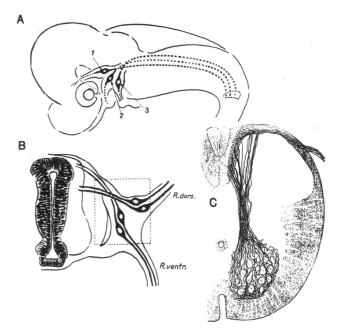

A

B

R.dors.

R.ventr.

C

Figure 2.6
Illustration of the crossings at the entrance into the neuraxis of sensory root axons. (A) Axis orientation of 1, the ophthalmic neurons; 2, the maxillary neurons; and 3, the mandibular neurons, giving rise to the known reverse Bregman localization in the spinal tract of the trigeminus of the fibers arising from the main sensory fields. (B) The same principle of "crossing" observed in embryos of *Lacerta viridis*. (C) An early observation of v. Lenhossek on the crossing of the Ia afferent (reflex collaterals) for adapting to one another the reverse somatotopic projections of the sensory segments in the dorsal and the motor segment in the ventral horn. There are more impressive drawings of the collateral crossings by Ramón y Cajal (1909), but these show the original observation.

ventral branches of the spinal nerves more laterally. Szentágothai and Székely (1956b) generalized this to a somewhat mechanistic camera obscura principle of the projection between periphery and center (figure 2.7). However crude this simplification may be, the agreement between the facts and what the hypothesis predicts is too good to be rejected out of hand. (It would be easy to cite hundreds of examples for the camera obscura principle from the huge body of observations in comparative neuroanatomy.) All this should not be taken too literally. The growth of axons is guided by many factors, and primary axis orientation is only one among many. Axons may grow and find their appropriate targets (as seen from numerous facts in experimental neuroembryology) despite gross changes of both their sources and their targets; however, such elementary geometry has prevailed throughout the entire course of phylogeny, and the nervous system had to (and in fact did) adapt to and incorporate these geometrical bases into the unfolding developmental program.

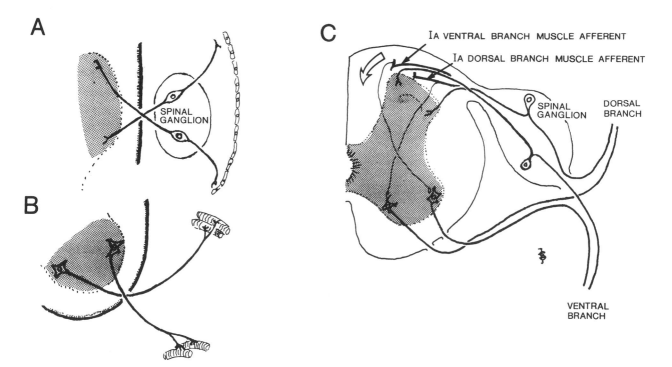

Figure 2.7
The camera obscura principle of somatotopic projections. (A) Dorsal horn. (B) Ventral horn. (C) The later shifts in tissue mass caused by the development of the dorsal funiculi (large outline below). The two spinal neurons shown in the diagram are cutaneous afferents; the courses of two (dorsal and ventral branch) large-muscle [Ia] afferents are added to show the crossing of the stretch reflex collaterals.

2.2 The Modular Architectonics Principle

An examination of the modular architectonics principle —that neuronal connectivity in most neural centers is sufficiently specific to permit disassembly of the entire network into neuronal modules of characteristic internal connectivity, and the larger structure can be reconstituted by repetition of these modules—must start with an analysis of the spinal cord and brainstem.

2.2.1 Spinal Cord and Brainstem

The spinal cord of vertebrates has three major functions: (1) to generate basic patterns of movement (as was seen in sec. 2.1); (2) to apply sensory stimuli in modulating these motor patterns to integrate neural (reflex and other) functions in one or a few neighboring segments of the body; and (3) to serve as a conducting medium along the entire body axis. These basic functions cannot be separated completely, because intersegmental mechanisms bridging only minor or even major parts of the body axis often share pathways with connections between the higher parts of the CNS and the spinal segmental level. The brainstem regions (from rostral to caudal, the medulla oblongata, pons, and mesencephalon) preserve the essential architectural principle of the cord but are widened gradually by being "blown up" by new neuron systems that, besides acting as centers for higher coordination of body posture and movement, also serve the increased demand for central structures by the concentration of specific sense organs (equilibrium, audition, vision) on the head. They also act as structures connecting the CNS axis with highly specialized centers (e.g., the cerebellum) in all vertebrates and the lateral lobes subserving specific electrical senses and lateral line organs that were developed in the fish but gradually disappeared in the upper vertebral classes.

We may reduce the strange form of the spinal gray matter—two dorsal and two ventral gray columns, connected before and behind the central canal by two gray commissures—to a more schematic representation of the spaces occupied by the cell and neuropil material in which the central core of the gray matter is visualized as a double-barrel structure resembling the shape of a hunting rifle (figure 2.8). Then we may consider the remaining parts of the cord as dorsal and ventral (in some parts of the cord also as lateral) appendages attached to the dorsal, lateral, and ventrolateral perimeters of the barrels (Szentágothai 1967). This architecture was not apparent for the early students of the CNS, because the classic Golgi procedures could best be applied to very young animals in which the double-barrel structure has not be-

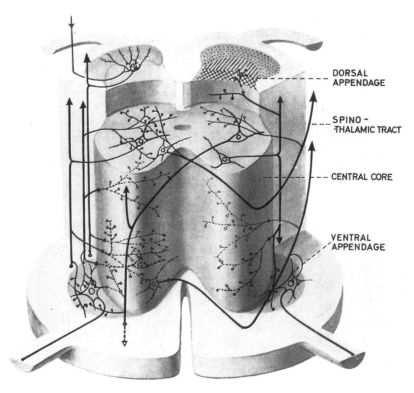

Figure 2.8
The original drawing of the concept of double-barrel architecture of the spinal cord intermediate zone (Szentágothai 1967) based on circumstantial evidence from synaptology but later corroborated by the Golgi studies of Réthelyi (1976). The simple terminal branches of axon arborizations in the intermediate zone (central core) stand in clear contrast to the elaborate axon trees in the "appendages."

come apparent. It is only during postnatal development that the neuropil is expanded by ingrowing arborizations of preterminal and terminal arborizations. This became clear only when the application of Golgi-type methods by perfusion made the study of adult material possible (Réthelyi, 1976).

Fig. 2.9 (from Szentágothai and Réthelyi 1973; see also Szentágothai 1983) shows the fine architecture of the spinal gray matter in full detail, indicating also where the double-barrel concept fits with the cytoarchitectonic divisions of Rexed (1954) discussed further. Both dendrites of the interneurons and axonal arborizations appear to be compressed into flat cylinders from which it is easy to deduce that synapses are established with the largest probability between terminal axons that enter any given flat cylinder and the interneurons, the bodies of which lie in (and the dendritic arborizations of which are confined to) the same cylinder. The neuropil of the ventral horn also is restricted, although with much less rigor, to half-moon-shaped extensions in the ventrolateral direction of these discs. The motoneurons not only are much larger than the interneurons but are oriented with the longer axes of their bodies and their dendrites parallel to the spinal cord axis, so that they may

receive synapses from the preterminal axon arborizations within four or five neighboring discs. The neuropil architecture of the dorsal gray column differs considerably from that of the ventral gray column in that it is very clearly layered into cell sheets lying parallel to the dorsal surface of the dorsal horn.

On this basis, the entire spinal gray matter was subdivided by Rexed (1954) into 10 layers, generally labeled in the dorsoventral direction by Roman numerals I–IX. (We show regions I–IV and IX in figure 2.9.) For practical purposes, especially in physiological experiments, Rexed's subdivision is quite useful. However, a view into cross-sections of the cord makes apparent that only laminae I–IV really can be considered as a laminated structure in the strict sense; the intermediate region and the ventral horn cannot be pressed into this scheme, apart from the motoneurons that are recognizable simply from the sizes of their bodies. Lamina I has its neuropil (both dendritic arborizations and terminal axon ramifications) arranged parallel to the dorsal surface of the dorsal column gray matter. Consequently, this layer is crucial for receiving and transmitting the impulses entering the cord via the medium-size A_δ fibers. These fibers serve a variety of sensory functions, including that of fast conducted

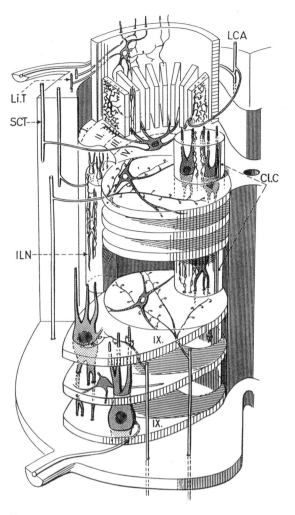

Figure 2.9
The modular building block (tissue spaces of simple geometrical character) architecture of the spinal cord gray matter after, Szentágothai and Rethélyi (1973). The building blocks are defined chiefly by the overall orientation of the dendritic trees and axon arborizations: surface parallel in lamina I (of Rexed 1954), slender blocks in lamina II and (partially) III, and transversely oriented stacked "coins" in the central core (intermediate region) and in the half-moon-shaped transverse disc of lamina IX. The orientation of both neuropil and dendrites is longitudinal in Clarke's column (Cl.C) and the intermediolateral column (ILN). Fiber tracts include large caliber afferents (LCA), Lissauer's tract (Li.T), and spinocervical tract (SCT).

pain. Conversely, the neuropil of laminae II and III is arranged in lobuli in radiate direction (i.e., vertical to the dorsal surface of the gray matter). The lobuli are narrower and more numerous in lamina II and somewhat wider (in the mediolateral direction) in lamina III, but the relation between the neuropil of the two layers is not clear, as the lobuli become intermixed at the border of the two laminae. There are two specific territories of the spinal gray matter in which the neuropil is oriented longitudinally: in Clarke's column and in the so-called

intermediolateral nucleus, containing the majority of the sympathetic preganglionic neurons.

Many important functional conclusions can be drawn from this curious combination in spatial orientation of the neuropil. Here, however, we enlarge on a single point that we believe to be the most important for understanding the essence of the segmental apparatus. Imagine the double-barrel central core of the spinal cord and the tracts of the white matter—especially the short intersegmental connection located close to the border of the gray matter in the so-called lateral and ventral fundamental fasciculi—as two columns of coins, one stacked on the other. We stress that the boundaries between coins are chosen for convenience of analysis; though the spinal cord may be divided on the basis of the nerve roots for each vertebra, the internal circuitry shows no corresponding discontinuities in its structure. Though there are places in the brain in which modules are defined naturally (e.g., the ocular dominance columns of sec. 8.3.2), there are many other cases where it is the anatomist's task to define modules that reveal the overall repetitive structure of a brain region as the basis for functional and dynamic study and yet overlap in such a way that the choice of "cuts" between the modules may be somewhat arbitrary. In the present case, a modular analysis allows us clearly to specify patterns of neural connectivity. The spatial orientation of dendrites and terminal axonal arborizations already was understood by the authors of the early classical period of neuroanatomy in the years from 1888 until shortly after 1900, notably by Ramón y Cajal (1894), as the most important cue for understanding the synaptic relations in any part of the neuropil. Figure 2.10 shows the principle for the case of the dorsal root fibers that, after entering the cord, bifurcate into an ascending and a descending branch. Of these, only the main ascending branch serves direct forward conduction toward the dorsal column nuclei of the medulla oblongata (as well as indirectly to the cerebellum and to the ventrobasal nuclear complex of the thalamus). The descending branch and the initial part of the ascending branch give rise to collaterals oriented transversely to the spinal cord axis. These collaterals arborize in the flat transversely oriented discs of the central core and directly contact either interneurons or motoneurons. They also mainly serve local segmental reflexes. This principle is illustrated for the central core and the ventral horn in figure 2.11 (from Szentágothai 1981) which, for the sake of simplicity, entirely neglects the dorsal root collaterals. As seen from the lower, longitudinally cut part of the diagram, the principle shown

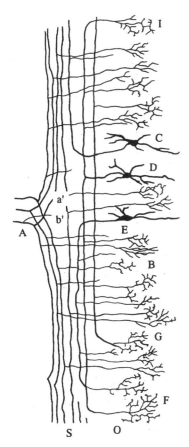

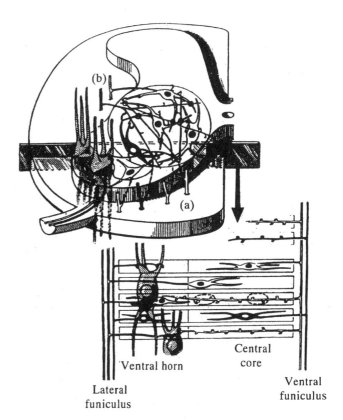

Figure 2.10
Ramón y Cajal drawing (1894) illustrating the entrance of dorsal root (A) and its branching into an ascending and descending main brain in the dorsal funiculus. Collaterals (a', b') are transversally oriented interneurons C, D, and E, giving similarly oriented transversal collaterals (sagittal longitudinal section). (Other labels denote fiber terminations.)

by Ramón y Cajal (1911) for the dorsal root fiber holds also for the axons of local interneurons that enter into and bifurcate in the lateral and ventral (white) funiculi and give transversely oriented preterminal branches confined to the aforementioned flat discs. Although this diagram is simplified radically and selectively, it may convey the basic principle of segmental design. Our earlier discussion of embryonic transplantation and tissue recombination experiments (Székely and Szentágothai 1962; Székely and Czéh 1971) showed the importance of this architecture of the spinal segmental apparatus. We saw that fragments of the early medullary tube, lacking the dorsal horn and any sensory input, spontaneously (i.e., without any external input) may generate walking-like movements in supernumerary limbs implanted nearby, as

Figure 2.11
Stacked-chips architecture principle of the intermediate zone (center core) of the spinal cord, in the form of flat discs (represented as a circle in the upper transverse section diagram and as brick-shape compartments in the lower longitudinal section diagram). Interneurons assumed excitatory are indicated in outlines, inhibitory in full black; motoneurons are stippled. Note the straight courses of interneuron axon collaterals penetrating through the flat neuropil discs, by which they may establish synaptic contacts with any element encountered on their way. Certain potential contacts are considered forbidden by some mismatch between the respective elements (indicated by small circles), for example, between excitatory interneuron axon a and inhibitory interneuron axon b.

long as the structure illustrated in figure 2.11 (and only that) remained intact, and we saw that the medullary tube fragment was taken from spinal cord segments designed for innervating limbs.[1]

2.2.2   The Lower Brainstem

The lower brainstem (medulla oblongata, pons, and midbrain) is arranged essentially in the same quasi-segmental (transversely oriented disc) pattern. This was first recognized and most elegantly illustrated by Scheibel and Scheibel (1958), whose work was basic to one of the

---

1. Figures 2.9–2.11 provide a wealth of material on which future modeling should be based, exploiting this modular architecture. However, current models of spinal cord are concerned primarily with simple reflex circuits or with a minimal set of neurons and interneurons to represent physiological data on simple patterns of locomotion (see Bullock [1995] and Williams and Sigvardt [1995] for reviews).

earliest models of modular architecture in the nervous system (Kilmer, McCulloch, and Blum 1969). In fact, it was the Golgi studies of the Scheibels in which the fundamental (stacked-discs) principle of the entire neuraxis first was recognized, although the consequences could not be stated explicitly then. An entirely new principle, this time of chemoarchitectonic nature, extends the segmental principle here. Groups of specific monoaminergic neurons are built into the brainstem. However, only the serotoninergic neurons really fit into the segmental stacked-chips architecture, whereas catecholaminergic and dopaminergic neurons more often than not are concentrated in separate cell groups (e.g., in the locus ceruleus) that belong to the new structures appearing in the brainstem. The specific sensory and motor (and also vegetative) nuclei of the cranial nerves are subdivided into separate entities in the brainstem, but the continuity of sensory and motor columns can still be recognized and traced upward until the mesencephalon (see Székely 1989).

A fundamental change of the design occurred with the appearance in the lower brainstem of larger nuclear masses connecting the longitudinal arrangement of the neuraxis with higher centers, notably the cerebellum and the tectum, which have developed, even in very early stages of the vertebrate phylogeny, for auxiliary (although very highly specialized and essential) functions.[2] The two main nuclear formations for connection with these higher (auxiliary) centers are the inferior olive of the medulla oblongata and the nuclei of the pons. This is a crude oversimplification, because the pathways feeding into the cerebellum arise also from the spinal cord itself (spinocerebellar tracts, spinocervicocerebellar tracts) and from the medulla oblongata (dorsal column nuclei).

According to the traditional view, two main groups of somatomotor nuclei can be separated, both arranged more or less in a column of individual nuclei that are interrupted in stringlike fashion. The so called dorsomedial column consists in the caudocranial direction of the hypoglossus, the abducens, the trochlear, and the oculomotor nuclei. The position of the nuclei and the courses of their axons remain fairly stable in the phylogeny of the vertebrates.

The ventrolateral column is built of the branchial motor nuclei, in caudocranial direction of the accessorius, vagus, glossopharyngeus, facial, and trigeminal nucleus. The position of these nuclei, the shape and dendritic ar-

borization patterns of their motoneurons, and the initial courses of their axons, are subject to major changes during the phylogenesis from amphibia to the mammalians.

Figure 2.12 gives a schematic figure of the arrangement of the various nuclei, whereas figure 2.13, based on studies by Székely and Matesz (1989) using retrograde labeling of the motoneurons from the motor nerves by cobalt, illustrates the gradual separation of two distinct nuclei, the accessory trigeminal and the facial nuclei in the mammalians—as cell groups separate from the main nuclei and having the function of jaw-openers—from the still unseparated nuclei in the amphibia and reptilea having two different cell types for jaw closure and opening. The existence of an accessory abducens nucleus mainly for the innervation of the retractor bulbi and the position of its cells more resembling that of the branchial nuclei (Matesz and Székely 1977) may indicate that the separation of the two dorsomedial and branchial motor columns is not as radical as assumed earlier. It is most unfortunate that transplantation experiments comparable to those performed on the spinal part of the medullary tube have not been made, because they might contribute to our insight into the very earliest beginnings of motility in the head region.

The inferior olive deserves our special attention, because it supplies the most specific afferent system of the cerebellum, the so-called climbing fibers. All other afferent systems of the cerebellar cortex (and nuclei) terminate in the mossy fibers, whose collaterals reach the cerebellar nuclei and which terminate in the cerebellar cortex in a more diffuse manner via the parallel fibers of the granule cells driven by the mossy fibers. The climbing fibers are highly selective in that a Purkinje cell is contacted by only one climbing fiber but with synaptic connections that (if activated) ensure effective transmission. In addition, the olivary nuclei receive massive afferent input both from ascending spinal pathways and from descending pathways. This usually does not occur with the pontine nuclei, although it occurs with the dorsal column nuclei.

2.2.3 Hypothalamus

The upper diencephalic and telencephalic (the striatum and putamen of the basal ganglia) parts of the brainstem do not retain anything resembling the quasi-segmental arrangement of the lower neuraxis. However, there is a

---

2. The mesencephalic tectum has become reduced in mammalian phylogeny so that the mammalian brain has only remnants from earlier phylogenic history of the optic lobes (seen in amphibia, reptiles, and birds) and the acoustic lobes (seen in some genera of all classes of vertebrates with a highly organized sense of hearing).

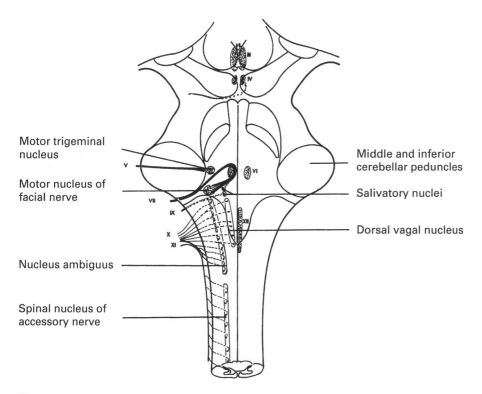

Motor trigeminal
nucleus

Motor nucleus of
facial nerve

Nucleus ambiguus

Spinal nucleus of
accessory nerve

Middle and inferior
cerebellar peduncles

Salivatory nuclei

Dorsal vagal nucleus

Figure 2.12
Diagrammatic posterior view of the brainstem and upper spinal medulla to show the position of the cranial nerve motor nuclei and the
course of their fibers to the surface. (*Left*) Motor nuclei of the branchial

nerves (ventrolateral column); (*right*) motor nuclei of the dorsomedial
column. (From Romanes 1991.)

small part of the diencephalon—the so-called hypothalamus (i.e., the ventralmost part of the diencephalon)—in
which elements of the basic architectural principle of the
neuraxis are preserved in longitudinally oriented fiber
tracts and transversely oriented (coronal) quasi-discs of
neuropil (Makara et al. 1980; Szentágothai 1983). The
longitudinal fiber systems are concentrated in a medial
periventricular bundle and in a more lateral (but still
medial in name) so-called medial forebrain bundle. The
transverse (coronal) orientation of the neuropil still can
be detected here, but this facility applies less to the cells,
(generally organized in nuclei) than to the terminal axon
arborizations. However, these barely recognizable architectural properties are of little use for the model builder
unless the details of neurochemistry are included in the
models, because connectivity (although still important)
yields pride of place to a very sophisticated system of
chemical information processing. Transmission is effected
in this part of the brain by a system of more than 20
(known today) neuropeptide transmitters and modulators that, moreover, do not act exclusively or even
predominantly synaptically; thus, the classic neuroanatomical approach becomes secondary to considerations
based on peptide biochemistry and its background of
molecular biology and genetics.

2.2.4 Complex Synaptic Systems

Kievit and Kuypers (1977) discovered an entirely new
principle of somatotopic architecture: the overall somatotopic relation of gross frontal (coronal) discs of the
cerebral cortex and of the striatum to discs of the thalamus diverging in the (sagittal) anterior direction. However, this will not be discussed further here because its
consequences have not yet been expanded nor has any
general functional consideration been attached to this
curious, probably very meaningful relation.

However, there is one aspect of the thalamic system
that has not received any legitimate physiological explanation thus far, in spite of gallant efforts, first by Rakic
(1975), then in more elaborate form by Schmitt, Dev
and Smith (1976) who called them local circuit neurons.
Having only relatively short axonal arborizations, local
neurons, already were known to the early classical neurohistologists and have been labeled as Golgi type II
neurons (or simply Golgi-type neurons). The classic
neuron type has one relatively long axon, was first described by Deiters in 1865 (Deiters first distinguished
between the two kinds of fibers that later were called
axons and *dendrites*), and hence is called a *Deiters-type
neuron* in the German literature. However, in distinction

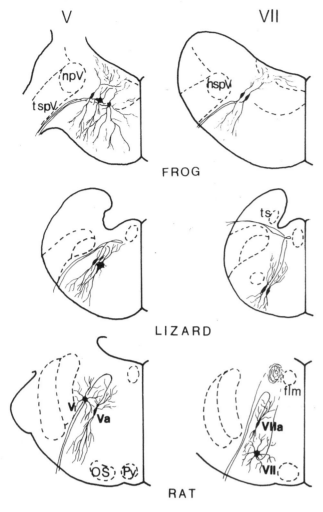

V   VII

FROG

LIZARD

RAT

Figure 2.13
Schematic representation of the different types of motoneurons of the branchial nerves V and VII, as seen in frog, lizard, and mammal. npV, principal nucleus of the trigeminal nerve; tspV, spinal tract of the trigeminal nerve; nspV, spinal nucleus of the trigeminal nerve; ts, solitary tract; OS, superior olive; Py, pyramidal tract; flm, longitudinal medial fasciculus. (Reprinted from Székely and Matthesz 1989.)

to Golgi type II neurons, neurons of this type are called Golgi type I neurons because the long axon of most neurons became clearly recognizable only in the classic studies of Camillo Golgi (1873).

By the term *synaptic glomeruli*, the classic neuro-histologists understood the combination of several synaptic structures in what appeared to be islands of the neuropil (in the cerebellar cortex, the olfactory bulb, and some of the anterior thalamic nuclei). Much later, beginning in the mid-1960s, electron-microscopic studies showed that such neuropil islands may be surrounded and almost completely enclosed by glial envelopes (in which case they were labeled *encapsulated zones*) or may lie virtually free in the general neuropil. Such complex

synaptic arrangements may not even be recognizable as specific islands. What is standard in the complex synaptic arrangements are so-called synaptic triads (i.e., at least three synaptically connected, terminal elements are combined in characteristic arrangements). Although found in a vast number of combinations, the most general (or basic) type of these triads contains (1) a main input element, excitatory by structural and transmitter biochemistry standards (i.e., presynaptic) to (2) a dendrite (appendage) of a forward-conducting (projective) cell and also presynaptic to (3) a presynaptic dendrite element (usually appendage) of a local, generally Golgi type II cell that is inhibitory both by transmitter biochemical (GABAergic) and by structural standards (flattened or at least not clearly spherical synaptic vesicles, and giving symmetrical synapses [i.e., synapses lacking postsynaptic densities]). The third element is always presynaptic (again based on structural criteria) to the second. These three synaptic contacts rarely are more distant from one another than a couple of microns. It should be emphasized, though, that this is only the most common combination of synapses; there are many exceptions and additional complications that we will not discuss further. These synaptic arrangements have been the subject of theoretical studies based on logic networks by Lábos (1977a; Lábos, Hámori, and Isomura 1980; see also an attempt to express them in realistic anatomical terms by Szentágothai 1983), and they will be discussed in chapter 7.

2.3 Multiple Models of Modularity

To conclude this chapter, we briefly examine diverse attempts to understand neural structure at a level above that of the individual neuron but below that of an overall brain region or a complex of such regions. First we look at the quasi-crystalline, rectangular lattice structure of the molecular layer of cerebellar cortex, foreshadowing the discussion in chapter 9 of the "microcomplex" as a unit of cerebellar analysis uniting a microzone of cerebellar cortex with the patch of nucleus to which it projects. Then we continue the discussion of columnar architectonics in cerebral cortex. Finally, we look at the basic organization of hippocampal circuitry revealed in the cross-section of a "lamella."

2.3.1 The Cerebellar System

The cerebellar cortex has been the most favored anatomical structure since the classic study of Ramón y

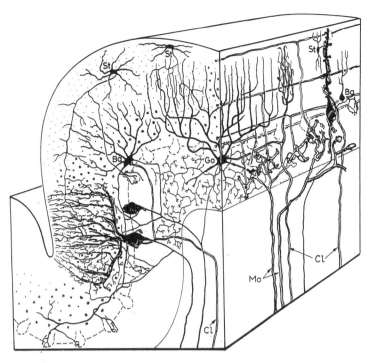

Figure 2.14
Stereodiagrammatic illustration of a tissue block taken from a cerebellar folium. The section surface at left is a transversal, at right a longitudinal section through the folium axis. Ba, basket cells; St, stellate cells; Go, Golgi cells; Cl, climbing fibers; Mo, mossy fibers contacting granule cells in the granular layer below the row of Purkinje cells, which in turn give rise to the parallel axons running parallel to the folium axis. (From Eccles, Ito, and Szentágothai 1967.)

Cajal (1888) of the bird cerebellar cortex. This was due primarily to the quasi-crystalline, rectangular lattice structure of the most important synaptic stratum, the molecular layer, and to the clear stratification of the cerebellar cortex into very distinct layers: the (outermost) molecular layer; a single layer of the main output cells, the Purkinje cells; and an inner layer of the granule cells. This enabled investigators to see immediately and exactly the point at which they were in any microscopical field.

As is well-known, the only output of the cerebellar cortex is provided by the Purkinje cells, which provide inhibitory input to the cerebellar nuclei. The neurotransmitter for this inhibition is γ-aminobutyric acid (GABA), but in some Purkinje cells, motilin also may be a neurotransmitter. The function of this inhibition is best understood by seeing how activity of a Purkinje cell modulates the activity of the cerebellar nucleus to which it projects (see the discussion of microcomplexes in sec. 9.4.3). Cerebellar cortex contains four major neuron types in addition to the Purkinje cells: basket, stellate, Golgi, and granule cells. The cortex has four types of afferents: the mossy and climbing fibers (discussed in chapter 9) and fibers containing noradrenaline and serotonin.

The basic neuronal connections of the cerebellar cortex are summarized in figure 2.14 (a simplified version of the color diagram given in Eccles, Ito, and Szentágothai 1967, figure 2.1), which exhibits the characteristic rectangular lattice structure of the cerebellar cortex. It diagrams a small piece of a cerebellar cortex folium, showing one surface cut to run at right angles to, and the other cut to be parallel with, the folium axis. For the sake of convenience, a Golgi cell is positioned at the edge of the two cuts to demonstrate that the dendritic tree of the Golgi cells has no preference for either of the two planes. Many of the characteristic dendrite and axon arborizations of this diagram have been copied directly from the original drawings of Ramón y Cajal. Among the many puzzling features of cerebellar cortex structure, probably the most remarkable is the confinement of the dendritic arborizations of the Purkinje cells to flat, non-overlapping boxes roughly $300 \times 250 \times 6$ µm in size (in cat). Section 9.1.2 will offer some speculations about the mechanism by which this might be achieved.

Once the existence of specific inhibitory interneurons became known, it was inevitable that students of the cerebellar cortex would begin to speculate about possible operational mechanisms of such neuron networks. Szentágothai (1963, 1965) had speculated on the anat-

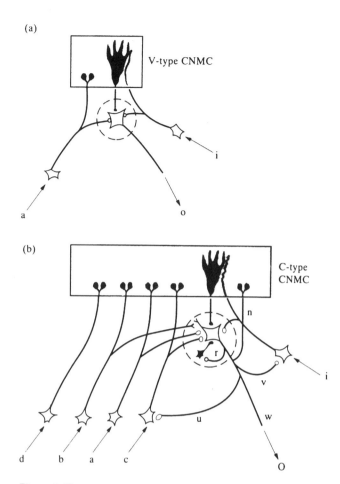

(a)

V-type CNMC

i

a   o

(b)

C-type
CNMC

n

r

i

v

u   w

d   b   a   c   O

Figure 2.15
(A) Elementary circuits. (B) More realistic complex relations between cerebellar nuclear cells (in dashed circles) and the cerebellar cortex (stippled).

omy of cerebellar cortex, noting the relation of climbing fibers to Purkinje cells and suggesting that interneurons were inhibitory to Purkinje cells and that Purkinje cells were inhibitory to cells of the cerebellar nuclei. This caught the interest of Eccles who, because the origin of the climbing fibers in the inferior olive was already known at that time, tested the basic assumption of these speculations and (with Ito) found it to work in physiological experiments, yielding a coherent hypothesis of the operational features of the cerebellar cortex neuron network (Eccles, Ito, and Szentágothai 1967). However, this was insufficient to provide real insight into the functions of the cerebellum simply because it does not address one of our main structural themes: the embedding of the region (in this case, the cerebellar cortex) in loops

and pathways integrating it with other regions. The cerebellar system, into which paths descending from the cerebral cortex and ascending from the spinal cord and the more complex sense organs are detoured (into a "side loop"), is closed not in the cerebellar cortex but in the cerebellar nuclei. The cerebellar cortex serves only as a very sophisticated modulator of the activity in the cerebellar nuclei, extended over an extremely large two-dimensional but intricately folded sheet of neural tissue. It is as if it were superimposed on the basic nuclear reflex level so as to supply it with a fine-grained control system. This cerebellar cortical control system is peculiar in the following three ways:

1. In having little detailed association in space (i.e., along the two dimensions of the enormous surface), though we shall see in chapter 9 that a crude somatotopy may be important for its role in motor coordination.

2. In containing an enormous number of nerve cells (the granule cells of the cerebellum probably contribute the majority of nerve cells in the body of the higher mammals, including cetaceans, and hence give the system an extremely high degree of redundancy.

3. In exercising its influence on the nuclear level exclusively by inhibition, the Purkinje cells being inhibitory.

However this may be, the cerebellar system can be understood more completely by two diagrams of Ito (1984) shown with some modifications in figure 2.15. The simpler diagram (A) shows the elementary circuit, whereas B tries to convey an impression of the more complex real neuron circuit. As we shall see in chapter 9, the neuron network of the cerebellum is a garden of delights for the model builder working on many levels: from molecular neuroanatomy through single-cell and neuron circuit models and into the realm of more ambitious holistic models of the acquisition of basic motor skills,[3] and finally the almost mysterious ability of the human to develop social motor skills from the survival technologies of so-called primitive societies, various forms of artistic expression, and professionally overbred sports and acrobatics, to (most importantly) articulated speech.

2.3.2 Cerebral Cortex

A quick look through the light microscope at a histological specimen stained for cells reveals the only appar-

---

3. Motor skill acquisition occurs in the postnatal development of many animals, but the few exceptions (e.g., the guinea pig, which is born as a miniature adult) serve to caution us against rash generalizations.

ent but undoubtedly striking feature of the cerebral cortex: its clear separation in most brain regions into six distinct layers parallel to the surface, some of which in certain regions of the brain can be subdivided again into sublayers. This is the *cytoarchitectonic* picture. Corresponding but different layers can be seen in stains for myelin sheaths of the intracortical fibers, yielding what is called *myeloarchitectonics*. Another architectonic picture can be observed in cortex specimens stained for lipids, yielding *lipid architectonics*. For the time being, only the cytoarchitectonic picture really is useful for practical work. The Golgi picture, showing various cell types with their very characteristic dendritic arborizations, seems to make things more obscure rather than contributing to our understanding, because it shows only fragments of the arborization of incoming or local axons. We have been able to gain important insights during the past 20 years with the help of modern neural tracing methods, particularly with the reconstruction of the local arborizations (both dendritic and axonal) of single cells impaled with microelectrodes, studied in physiological experiments, and eventually labeled by the injection of either horseradish-peroxidase or phaseolus lectin. We have learned much that is new about many of the hitherto known neuron types and their anatomical and synaptic connections (both locally and at longer distances) and have come closer to a real understanding of the multiple mediators and modulators involved in synaptic transmission.

Figure 2.16 conveys the state of knowledge at the end of the 1970s, when the concept of the cortical module (an architectural unit, a cylinder of some 200–300 µm in diameter and approximately 3 mm in height extending vertically through the entire depth of the cortex) first became solidified, even though the present level of characterization of various cell types was still in its beginnings. This figure deals with the module based primarily on corticocortical connectivity, probably the soundest basis yet available. The major cylinder, therefore, is built around an arborization of a corticocortical afferent.

The concept of modular architectonics of the cerebral cortex arose originally from the early physiological observation of Mountcastle (1957) of a vertical columnar organization of the somatosensory cortex, soon followed by an analogous architectural principle in the visual cortex found by Hubel and Wiesel (1959). Anatomical studies in continuation of the classic observations of Ramón y Cajal (1899) and the then-revolutionary insight of Lorente de Nó (1938b) into the predominantly vertical orientation of neuron chains were taken up by Szentágothai (1962), who used an entirely new approach of

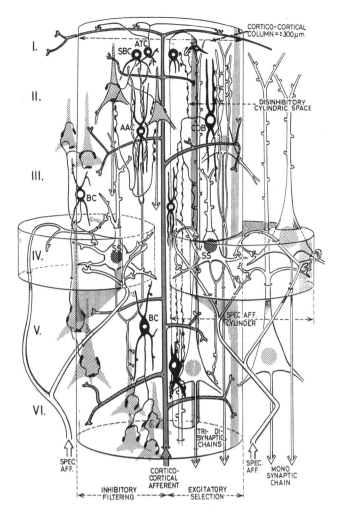

Figure 2.16
Relatively early stereodiagrammatic view from Szentágothai (1978c), with layering in Roman numerals at left margin. BC, basket cells; SS, spiny stellate cells; ATC, axonal tuft cell; SBC, small basket cell; AAC, axoaxonic cell; CDB, cellule double bouquet. Excitatory cells and fibers in outlines, inhibitory cells in full black.

chronically isolated cortical tissue slabs (a technique made available to the Western readership only in 1966 by Colonnier). Szentágothai's first anatomically based neuron circuit model (1969) was still very much under the influence of the earlier circuit model of the cerebellar cortex. It is not as if the early specific sensory cortex model had to be abandoned. This is incorporated by the two flat cylinders located at both sides of figure 2.16 in lamina IV so that the corticocortical module model simply is a more realistic application of the model based on specific sensory afferents to a more general architectonic principle holding true in the several regions of the neocortex.

The whole concept of the module principle has been questioned by Swindale (1990), who argued that continuity in the surface parallel direction would be more in

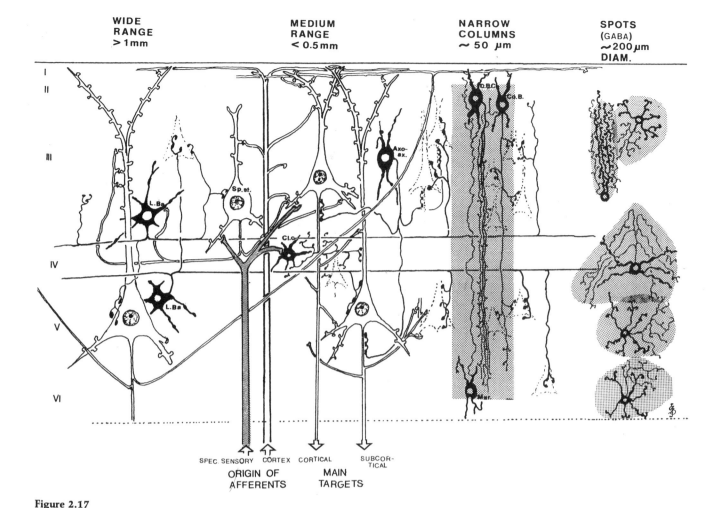

SPEC. SENSORY CORTEX   CORTICAL   SUBCOR-
                                        TICAL
        ORIGIN OF   MAIN
        AFFERENTS   TARGETS

Figure 2.17
Highly simplified diagram illustrating the main known types of internal connections of the cerebral cortex. Excitatory neurons and their connections are drawn in outlines, inhibitory neurons in full black. Relatively large distance (1–5 mm) excitatory connections are given by a special type of large pyramidal cells of layer V. The large basket cells (L.Ba) are causing tangential inhibition at distances of 1 mm and slightly above. The excitatory spiny stellate cells (Sp.st) act mainly at medium range distances, but may run up to several (up to 5) mm. The two main input lines (specific sensory afferents, indicated by hatching and corticocortical afferents) act directly at medium range. Medium range inhibitory interneurons, like the so-called clutch cells (Cl.c), are specific for layer IV; axo-axonic interneurons (Axo.ax) are most frequent in layer III, but occur in all layers. The collaterals of the pyramid cells act also mainly at medium range distances. Vertically oriented inhibitory interneurons appear to establish narrow strips of vertical inhibition between layers II and VI. The known cell types are columnar basket cells (Co.B), the double bouquet cells of Ramón y Cajal (D.B.C.) although their main characteristics are the narrow vertical (horsetail shape) axonal strands. The vertically ascending inhibitory interneurons occur in all layers of the cortex and in a large variety of forms and patterns of arborization. Their action is restricted to spotlike regions usually less than 200 μm in diameter (stippling). The outlines of many pyramidal cells are shown in dotted outlines to give indication for synaptic targets. Remember that all of these cells and connections coexist in the same space of cortical tissue; many more cells with little-known connections had to be omitted to keep the diagram intelligible. (From Szentágothai 1993.)

accordance with reality than with modularity. Earlier forms of relatively simple modules were built around the arborizations of the specific sensory afferents or corticocortical connections; more subtle analysis discerns an entire hierarchy of highly regular modularities within the primary visual cortex of the monkey. The architecture of the visual cortex of the primate is more sophisticated in reality than could have been imagined earlier. The hierarchy consists of at least three different types of regularities (modules) built into each other in a rather regular crystalline-like structure. Figure 2.17 makes the duality of continuity and discontinuity (i.e., modularity) intelligible. This diagram tries to show the various ranges within which neurons are connected with each other over distances of a couple of millimeters, that is, still locally. The local arborizations of various types of individual neurons have been drawn to scale to indicate how the several types of architecture units (modules) fit together so that there is no conflict whatever between continuity and discontinuity.

2.3.3 The Dentate Gyrus–Hippocampus System

The hippocampal system, including its gateway of the dentate gyrus (or fascia dentata), is the most important formation of the archicortex from both the functional and the anatomical points of view. It has been argued that its main physiological function is in being instrumental in memory functions, not in the sense that it would directly contain the traces, if memory were based on gathering and encoding traces (engrams) of past experience (probably not the case), but in issuing the order for any functional event to be imprinted on (or fixed in) some other part or parts of the brain. It also has been implicated in the formation of "cognitive maps." (We return to these functional issues in chapter 6.)

Although clearly a cortical structure, the hippocampal formation shares with the cerebellar cortex the crucial advantage that its layering separates cells and neuropil, with an additional advantage that even the neuropil and fiber strata radiating into or out from the hippocampal formation are separated into various distinct layers or sheets of fibers. This renders the entire hippocampal formation an exceptionally favored ground for combined anatomical, physiological, and immunohistological analysis.

The essential features of the hippocampal formation already were understood from the Golgi studies of the classical period as magnificently summarized by the beautiful drawing of Ramón y Cajal (1911; reproduced here in figure 2.18). The figure and its legend are largely self-explanatory. The input channels were not understood sufficiently at the time, although the two main fiber systems are indicated correctly. One is the so-called perforant path, arising in the entorhinal cortex and entering the dentate gyrus through its convexity. What was thought to be (and indeed is) the main output line of the hippocampal formation, the fornix, supplies the other main input path, both of the dentate gyrus and the hippocampus proper, with strong afferent systems from both sides of the septum. Hence, coming from the hippocampal commissure, this second path also is labeled the *commissural path*. What was not known in Ramón y Cajal's time was the sophisticated system of short GABAergic (hence inhibitory) interneurons. Only the basket cells, with their axonal terminations directed preferentially to the cell bodies of the pyramidal cells of the hippocampus proper and of the dentate gyrus granule cells, were known to early authors. Even so, the neuron chains

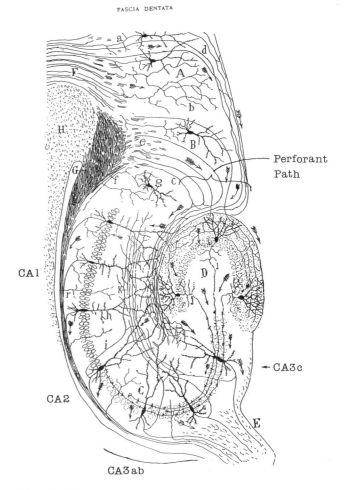

FASCIA DENTATA

Figure 2.18

Hippocampal-dentate formation from a Ramón y Cajal drawing (1911). A, entorhinal cortex; B, cells of the subiculum giving rise to perforant path fibers; D, hylus of the dentate gyrus with the origin of the mossy fibers; j, axons arising from a single but multicellular layer of the dentate granule cells; i, Schaffer collateral; K, stratum of the Schaffer collaterals; C, row of hippocampal pyramidal cells (the several parts of which—CA1, CA2, CA3ab, and CA3C—are indicated around the perimeter of the hippocampus.

entorhinal cortex → perforant path → dentate gyrus granule cells → mossy fibers → pyramidal cells of the proximal CA3 (adjacent to the dentate gyrus) → Schaffer collaterals → pyramidal cells of the distal CA2 and CA1 regions of the hippocampus proper → eventually, the pyramidal cell main axons entering the fornix

already were well known and illustrated correctly in the classic figure (see figure 2.18) of Ramón y Cajal. It was much later that the axoaxonic interneuron was discovered first in the hippocampus proper and later in the dentate gyrus. However, it took still more time and considerable technical refinements before additional interneuron types were recognized, and it took new immunocytochemical methods before the crucial importance of the inhibitory interneurons in the regulation of hippocampal neuronal operations began to dawn on us (and about which we shall have much more to say in chapter 6).

Apart from providing deeper insight into the possible neural mechanisms involved in memory and cognition (and it is hoped, also into the pathological mechanisms of epileptic seizures), the great advantage in studying the hippocampal formation is the basis it provides for understanding neuron coupling mechanisms in the neocortex. The analyses possible in the hippocampal formations need further development to lead to an improved insight into the intricacies of the complex network of the many types of inhibitory interneurons in the neocortex. The diverse forms of modularity exhibited in cerebellum, cerebral cortex, and hippocampus exemplify the richness of structure exhibited in different regions of the mammalian brain (and will be addressed in more detail in part II of the book).

A Functional Overview

As we have seen in chapter 2, neuroscience has a well-established terminology for levels of *structural* analysis (e.g., brain region; layer, module, column, circuit; neuron; compartment; channel). However, less attention has been paid to the need for a *functional* vocabulary. It is usual to pick some overall function (e.g., vision) and then immediately seek a structural grounding for its analysis, trying to establish the role of specific regions or circuits in achieving that function. This chapter presents *schema theory* as a framework for the rigorous analysis of behavior that requires no prior commitment to hypotheses on the localization of each *schema* (unit of functional analysis) but can be linked to a structural analysis as and when it becomes appropriate.

To make sense of the brain, we may divide it into functional systems—the motor system, the visual system, and so on—or into structural subsystems, from the spinal cord and the hippocampus to the various subdivisions of the prefrontal cortex. The problem for functional neuroscience is to achieve congruence between these two types of analysis. Schema-based modeling may be based purely on behavioral data but becomes part of functional neuroscience when it is constrained by data provided by, say, human brain mapping, clinical neurology, or studies of the effects of brain lesions on animal behavior. The resulting model may constitute an adequate explanation in itself or may provide the framework for modeling at the level of neural networks or below. Such a *neural* schema theory provides a functional-structural decomposition, in strong contrast with models employing learning rules for training a single, otherwise undifferentiated neural network to respond as specified by some training set.

In figure 3.1, the top level considers the brain or behavior of the organism as a whole. The second level diverges: Our structural overview provides the vocabulary of brain regions, layers, modules, columns, and the like for an intermediate level of structural analysis; the task of the present functional overview is to show how schemas provide the corresponding level of *functional* analysis. Structure and function then meet at the level of neural networks, where we show how the competition and cooperation of schemas may be implemented in

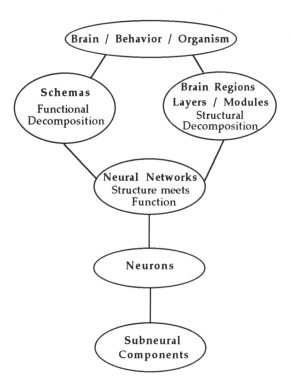

Figure 3.1
Structural and functional levels of analysis of brain and behavior, highlighting the role of schemas as an intermediate level of functional analysis.

neural circuitry. Moreover, in the dynamical overview of chapter 4, we introduce the use of dynamic system analysis to link structure and function. We consider the neuron as the basic unit of function and of structure, but append a lower level to figure 3.1 to emphasize that much work in computational neuroscience (and our work in several sections of later chapters) seeks to explain the complex functionality of real neurons in terms of yet finer units, such as membrane compartments, channels, spines, and synapses.

What makes our work in linking structure and function so challenging is that, in general, a functional analysis proceeding top down from some overall behavior need not map directly onto a bottom up analysis proceeding upward from the neural circuitry (the correct assignment of function to structure may not be at first apparent) so that several iterations from the middle out may be required to bring the structural and functional accounts into consonance. The schemas that serve as the functional units in our initial hypotheses about the decomposition of some overall function well may differ from the more refined hypotheses which provide an account of structural correlates as well.

Section 3.1 introduces schema theory, starting in section 3.1.1 with a historical analysis of the schema as con-

ceptualized by such writers as Kant, Piaget, Head and Holmes, and Bartlett and including a brief review of current usage of the term in such fields as cognitive psychology. This sets the stage for our own approach to schema theory, which emphasizes the modeling of action-oriented perception, and the constraints imposed by linking schema theory to functional neuroscience. Section 3.1.2 provides a quasi-formal introduction to the basic concepts of this version of schema theory, namely perceptual and motor schemas, coordinated control programs, cooperative computation, and schema assemblages. Section 3.1.3. uses a simple account of approach and avoidance behavior in frogs to illustrate the use of perceptual and motor schemas, shows how they may be linked, and addresses what is involved in making a schema-based account of a function into a neural model. Section 3.1.4 illustrates the notion of a coordinated control program with an introduction to the visual control of reaching and grasping. Section 3.1.5 uses a schema-based model of visual perception to provide a perspective on short-term and long-term memory by using the notion of schema assemblage.

Section 3.2 builds on section 3.1.3 to present a few examples from *Rana computatrix*, a set of models of visuomotor coordination in frog and toad. Sections 3.2.1. and 3.2.2 present a study of approach, avoidance, and detour behavior to show how perception may demand the mutual refinement of one perceptual schema by another, how multiple motor schemas may act together to yield complex motor behaviors, and how brain function can be analyzed in a process of evolutionary refinement in which basic systems serve as the substrate for the designed evolution of more refined systems (New schemas often arise as "modulators" of existing schemas, rather than as new systems with independent functional roles.) Section 3.2.3 focuses on neural mechanisms of avoidance behavior to provide our first example of how neural modeling can be used to replace schemas with neural networks of equivalent functionality.

The next two sections take us from frog and toad to monkey, as we introduce schemas involved in the basic functions for looking, reaching, and grasping. These sections will define challenges for neural modeling that will be taken up in chapters 8, 9, and 10 as we consider the roles of cerebral cortex, thalamus, cerebellum, and basal ganglia in the realization and refinement of these functions. Section 3.3 is devoted to the rapid eye movements called saccades and focuses on the homology between the tectum in frog and toad and the superior colliculus in primates—the whole body movement of the frog toward its prey corresponding to the monkey's orienting of gaze toward a visual target. Just as section 3.2 showed how basic schemas for approach and avoidance could be extended by other schemas to yield detour behavior in frog and toad, we now study how schemas for working memory and for dynamic remapping may extend the monkey's saccadic repertoire to include saccades to remembered targets or to two targets in succession.

In studying the role of perception in mediating behavior, we stress that there is in general no complete and objective percept of an object but rather a set of partial characterizations (including parameters that we may not be able to represent symbolically in any explicit fashion) related to the current set of goals and motivations of the observer and which may keep unfolding as interaction with, or contemplation of, the object continues. Section 3.4 illustrates this concept by using the schemas involved in reaching and grasping. In section 3.4.1 we present the concepts of virtual fingers and opposition space that allow us to offer a precise but compact description of the degrees of freedom involved in a number of grasping movements. In section 3.4.2, a series of experiments reveals flaws in our preliminary model of reaching and grasping. This leads us (via a discussion of the roles of optimality, feedback, and feedforward in motor control) to a new, coordinated control program that explicitly involves a coordinating schema as well as perceptual and motor schemas. This again demonstrates that much is to be learned at the level of schema analysis prior to, or in concert with, the analysis of neural circuitry. However, we shall indeed present a neural analysis of these schemas in later chapters. In chapters 8 and 10, the schemas involved in looking, reaching, and grasping will be shown to be distributed across cerebral cortex and basal ganglia, whereas chapter 9 will show the role of cerebellum in their adaptation and coordination.

3.1 Schema Theory and Functional Neuroscience

Our structural overview was grounded in the reality of the brain, stained, sliced, dissected, viewed, and visualized in a variety of ways. However, the empirical work of the neuroanatomist is not mere description of every detail but rather the search for pattern, for a compact description of form that reveals order within complexity. The modular architectonics principle offers one such de-

scription, but we have noted other patterns, seen ways in which ontogeny and phylogeny may aid the description of the mammalian nervous system, and discussed the problems of relating structure to function.

Where should a functional overview begin? Most neurophysiological experiments to date have been limited to the analysis of one brain region at a time, with stimulation of and recordings from single cells being used to determine the response of cells to natural and artificial stimuli, their plasticity, and correlations of cell activity with overt behavior. A visual region, then, is one where the firing of certain cells covaries with certain parameters of visual stimulation, and the region may be given a functional label, such as *movement region* or *color region*. However, it is rare for a neurophysiologist to start with an analysis of, say, the role of color perception in the behavioral ecology of an animal and then systematically to survey multiple brain regions and their interactions so as to elucidate the overall realization of this function in the brain.[1] Thus, although one can imagine a functional overview focusing on current technology and listing the functional correlates of the activity of neurons that now can be measured in the laboratory, we instead take a far more ambitious approach aimed at elucidating the overall realization of mental function and behavior in the brain. More specifically, we present *schema theory* as a language in which one may analyze the full range of mental function, regardless of whether it can be related to neuronal function. The theory is rooted in the *Critique of Pure Reason* of Immanuel Kant (1781/1929) and is well developed in cognitive psychology and kinesiology (the study of motor skills) where thought and behavior are viewed "from the outside." Our contribution has been to provide a schema theory that can bridge from the external characterization of function to the interactions of brain regions and the inner workings of neural circuitry.

In most of this book, we will attend to a range of visuomotor functions for which sufficient neurophysiological data are available so as to constrain our functional analysis of brain mechanisms. Recent developments in human brain imaging (see Footnote 1) extend the range of neurological data concerning cognitive functions, though at present neurology focuses more on correlating regional activity with different functions than on causal accounts of the neural interactions subserving

---

1. However, human brain imaging, though still limited in spatial and temporal resolution, now offers ways of assessing brain regions the activation of which differs significantly in execution of one task as compared to the other. How, then, might the overall assessment of brain activity in such imaging be reconciled with the detailed analysis of circuitry offered by neurophysiological study of single-cell activity in animal brains? One methodology that directly addresses this issue is "Synthetic PET" (Arbib et al. 1995 cf. section 8.4.3).

these functions. We shall see some hints on how to address such data in the chapters on hippocampus (chapter 6) and cerebral cortex (chapter 8) and will evaluate the prospects for a broader cognitive neuroscience in our concluding chapter (chapter 11). First we examine various notions of schema in a quasi-historical perspective, then we make explict the schema theory that we use in this book and outline why we believe it is a proper part of the vocabulary of neuroscience. The rest of this chapter will develop neural schema theory further, and we will return to it where appropriate later in the book.

3.1.1 Schemas: History and Comparisons

The concept of the schema in Western thought goes back at least to its use by Immanuel Kant in the 1780s. The twentieth century has seen a diversity of notions of schema, which more or less overlap with the concept as developed in this volume. Schemas have played an important role (as has control theory) in attempting to define units of behavior as a basis for analyzing their development, interaction, and mechanism. Thus, the term *schema* arises in such fields as neurology (Head and Holmes 1911; Fredericks 1969), cognitive psychology (Bartlett 1932; Mandler 1985; Neisser 1976; Oldfield and Zangwill 1942, 1943; see Rumelhart et al. 1986 for a rapprochement with connectionism), developmental psychology (Piaget 1971), motor control and kinesiology (Schmidt 1975, 1976), neuroethology (Ewert 1989), and neuropsychology (Shallice 1988) and appears in artificial intelligence under such names as *frames* and *scripts* (Minsky 1975; Schank and Abelson 1977). In this subsection, we review a number of these concepts and those leading up to a variant of the notion (Arbib, 1975, 1981, 1992) more tightly constrained by the need to explain the neural basis of behavior.

How is it that we may intuit the pure concept of the circle from experience with a particular wheel? Kant posited that the transcendental schema makes possible the application of the category to the appearance. In modern terms, one might be tempted to think of such a schema as a pattern recognition device: Input a visual pattern to the circle schema to receive a binary output; "Yes, the object is circular" or "No, it is not." However, in several ways this falls vastly short of what Kant intends.

First, simply labeling something as circular does not entail understanding circularity in, say, the sense in which the properties of circles may be characterized richly by Euclidean geometry.

Also, Kant (1781/1929, p. 183) distinguishes the image as "a product of the empirical faculty of reproductive imagination" from the schema as "a product ... of pure a priori imagination, through which, and in accordance with which, images themselves become possible." In a famous passage (p. 182), he observes that "No image could ever be adequate to the concept of a triangle in general. It would never attain that universality of concept which renders it valid of all triangles, whether right-angled, obtuse-angled, or acute-angled ... The schema of the triangle can exist nowhere but in thought. It is a rule of synthesis of the imagination, in respect to pure figures in space."

Further, Kant's schemas include far more than schemas for such "universals" as circles and triangles or even dogs, as we can see from such passages as "[T]he pure *schema* of magnitude (*quantitas*), as a concept of the understanding, is *number*" (p. 183); "The schema of substance is permanence of the real in time" (p. 184); and "The schema of cause, and the causality of a thing in general, is the real upon which, whenever posited, something else always follows" (p. 185).

For Kant, knowledge is grounded in a priori principles (pp. 195–196). "Even natural laws, viewed as principles of the empirical employment of understanding, carry with them an expression of necessity, and so contain at least the suggestion of a determination from grounds which are valid a priori and antecedently to all experience. The laws of nature, one and all, without exception, stand under higher principles of understanding."

In the account of schema theory to be given in these pages, we shall build on Kant's notion of schema and image for objects of perception so as to develop the notion of a *perceptual schema* and an instance thereof, and shall introduce the complementary notion of the *motor schema* in an account of action. In terms of current neurophysiology, we can explore the form of understanding involved in the linkage of perception and action, but for now we must relinquish the studies of such schemas as those of magnitude, substance, and cause to a psychology little constrained as yet by the data of neuroscience. However, the real disagreement with Kant is not over the shifting divide between what we can and cannot neuralize but rather over the notion of the a priori. Whereas an eighteenth century philosopher could see the postulates of euclidean geometry as a priori truths, we in the twentieth century see them as providing a compact basis for the inference of many facts about the geometry of limited regions of space, although from the work of Einstein and others we know them to be inadequate to describe many spatial phenomena of the physical universe. Thus, we can entertain the idea of euclidean geometry as a convenient approximation. Moreover, we now understand that much (if not all) of spatial behavior of animals is controlled by their brain-body-environment interactions and that if these interactions rest on both nature and nurture, then the nature is not one of a priori structure but rather a contingent structure shaped by evolution through natural selection. Such an "innate nature," moreover, is not expressed directly in adult behavior but, rather, sets a developmental pathway whose unfolding may be more or less influenced by the experience of the organism (see Waddington's 1957 notion of the epigenetic landscape for the embryological perspective). This leads us to look at schemas not as immutable objects expressive of a priori principles but rather as biologically rooted entities that evolve and develop to adapt more effectively the behavior of the animal, and the thought of the human, to its world.

Central to our approach is the notion of the *active organism*, which does not so much react to the world as search out from the world the information it needs to pursue its chosen course of action. To highlight this concept, we describe the organism not in stimulus-response terms, wherein stimulus leads to response, but rather in terms of the *action-perception cycle* (Arbib 1981) inspired by the perceptual cycle of Neisser (1976; see his figures 2.2, 6.4). In the continuing *action-oriented perception* that it serves, current sensory input is itself a function of the subject's active exploration of the world, which is directed by *anticipatory schemas*, which Neisser defines to be plans for perceptual action and readiness for particular kinds of sensory structure. The information thus picked up modifies the perceiver's anticipations of certain kinds of information that, thus modified, direct further exploration. For example, to tell whether any coffee is left in a cup, you may reach out and tilt the cup to make the interior visible and keep tilting the cup further and further as you fail to see any coffee until you either see the coffee at last or conclude that the cup is empty. Perception is linked inextricably with the organism's interaction with its environment. The organism is perceiving as it is acting and acting as it is making, executing, and updating plans. We may say that *perception* activates (defining a search space; drawing a map), whereas *planning* concentrates (laying out the route to be followed). The organism must remain tuned to its spatial relationship with its immediate environment, anticipating facets of the environment before they come into view. The information gathered during ego-motion must be systematically integrated into its internal model of the world (see our discussion of "cognitive maps" in chapter 6), which is not so much a mental picture of the environment as an active, information-seeking process.

Of course, the notion of action-oriented perception is inextricable from perception-oriented action, as exemplified in eye movements. In many mammals (and especially in humans), the retina is nonuniform, with a fovea that provides particularly detailed information about the visual scene. Thus, the successive fixations must be integrated, with the information acquired with the eyes in one position remapped as the eyes move. Other sensory modalities, such as audition and touch, also must be integrated into this evolving representation of the visually perceived world. In like manner, the actions that scan the environment are themselves constrained by the subject's plan of action. We perceive the environment to the extent that we are prepared to interact with it in some reasonably structured fashion. For example, our perception of a cat need involve no conscious awareness of its being a cat per se (e.g., when it jumps on our lap while we are reading, and we simply classify it by the action we take: "something to be stroked" or "something to be pushed off").

Our action-oriented view resonates with one of the best-known uses of the term *schema*, that of the Swiss developmental psychologist Jean Piaget, who wrote: "Any piece of knowledge is connected with an action... [T]o know an object or a happening is to make use of it by assimilation into an action schema...[namely] whatever there is in common between various repetitions or superpositions of the same action" (Piaget 1971, pp. 6–7). As you act on the basis of an action schema, you do so with the expectation of certain consequences. When you recognize something, you "see" in it things that will guide your interaction with it, but there is no claim of infallibility, no claim that the interactions will always proceed as expected. Piaget talks both of *assimilation*, the ability to make sense of a situation in terms of the current stock of schemas, and of *accommodation*, the way in which the stock of schemas may change over time as the expectations based on assimilation to current schemas are not met. To the extent that our expectations are false, our schemas can change, we learn. Piaget traced the cognitive development of the child, starting from reflexive or instinctive schemas that guide its motoric interactions with the world. Piaget sees the child starting with such schemas for basic survival as breathing, eating, digesting, and excreting and such basic sensorimotor schemas as suckling, grasping, and rudimentary eye-hand coordination. Objects are secondary to these primary schemas, and such schemas pave the way for more global concepts, such as the schema for object permanence, the recognition that when an object disappears from view, the object still exists and is there to be searched for. This schema develops to allow the use of extrapolation: inferring where a moving object that has passed from sight is likely to reappear. Piaget argued that such schemas lead to further development until the child has schemas for language and logic—for abstract thought—no longer rooted in the sensorimotor particularities. The later stages bring to the child such schemas as those of magnitude, substance, and cause posited by Kant, but now they are the outcome of a developmental process rather than the direct embodiment of the a priori. For this reason, Piaget has referred to his work as *genetic epistemology*.

Earlier, the term *schema* had entered the neurological literature through the work of Head and Holmes (1911) who spoke of the *postural schema* (or *body schema*) that underlies the perception of one's own body: "By means of perpetual alterations in position we are always building up a postural model of ourselves which constantly changes. Every new posture or movement is recorded on this plastic schema, and the activity of the cortex brings every fresh group of sensations evoked by altered posture into relation with it." They also add that "Anything which participates in the conscious movement of our bodies is added to the model of ourselves and becomes part of those schemata: a woman's power of localization may extend to the feather of her hat." A person with damage to the parietal lobe on one side might lose awareness that the body on the opposite side actually belonged to him or her, not only ignoring painful stimuli but even neglecting to dress that half of the body. Damage to the thalamus and the somatosensory system also may produce disorders of the body schema. Frederiks (1969) provides a thorough review of the neurological literature, including an analysis of the insights into the body schema afforded by phantom limb phenomena.

Frederick Bartlett, a student of Head, took up the notion of schemas in his study of *Remembering* (1932), carrying this idea into the realm of cognitive psychology. Though not happy with the word *schema*—its association with the adjective *schematic* carried the suggestion that a schema was a vaguely outlined theory rather than an active, developing pattern or organized setting— Bartlett adopted the term in the sense of "an active organization of past reactions, or of past experiences, which must always be supposed to be operating in any well-adapted organic response." With this as background, Bartlett stressed the constructive character of remembering. He found that when people try to recall a story they have heard, they reconstitute the story in their own terms, relating what they experience to a familiar set of schemas rather than by rote memorization of arbi-

trary details. Condensation, elaboration, and invention are common features of remembering and often involve the mingling of materials from different schemas. Instead of thinking of ideas as impressions of sense-data, schema theory posits an active and selective process of schema formation (cf. Piaget's notion of assimilation), which in some sense constructs reality as much as it embodies it. Bartlett viewed the repetition of basic sequences of activity in lower animals as the maintenance of a few schemas, whereas in social creatures who have a means of communication, the schema-based reactions of one creature are constantly both checked and facilitated by those of others. Because Bartlett has characterized the schema as "an active organization of past reactions...operating in any well-adapted organic response," an important part of our following work' is to make clear the sense in which there can be different schemas acting in concert to determine the behavior of an animal or the mental activity in the human. A neurally compatible schema-based theory of visuomotor coordination in lower animals and primates will be a recurring theme of this book. The social dimension of schema theory is beyond the scope of this volume, but Arbib and Hesse (1986) develop philosophical analyses linking the schemas of the individual to the social construction of reality (including an account of consciousness and free will).

Kenneth Craik's 1943 essay, *The Nature of Explanation*, criticized kantian "a priorism" and offered the hypothesis that the brain creates a "model" of the world that allows a person to try out alternatives prior to action. He emphasizes the three processes of translation, inference, and retranslation: "the translation of external events into some kind of neural patterns by stimulation of the sense organs, the interaction and stimulation of other neural patterns as in 'association,' and the excitation by these of effectors or motor patterns." Here Craik's paradigm of stimulus-association-response allows the response to be affected by association with the person's current model but does not invoke sufficently the active control of its stimuli by the organism. Though Craik seemed not to have used the word *schema*, his notion of the brain as providing "internal models of the world" (see also Minsky 1961; MacKay 1966; Gregory 1969) certainly finds resonance with Piaget's discussion of the adaptive nature of action schemas. In a related usage, Schmidt (1975, 1976) offered a schema theory of discrete motor skill learning. Through experience, the subject builds up a recall schema that pairs the response specifications of a movement with the actual outcome. Later, this recall schema can be consulted to infer, from a desired outcome, the response specification that will produce it. Similarly, the recognition schema pairs the desired outcome with the expected sensory consequences of each movement. The recall schema is what now is known in the literature of motor control as an *inverse model*—it goes from a desired response to a command that achieves it rather than taking the "direct" causal path from command to action—whereas the recognition schema corresponds to Neisser's anticipatory schema.

The notion of motor schema is related to other attempts to extract the patterns underlying motor behavior. In describing the movement of a horse, we do not normally speak of the independent contraction of thousands of muscle fibers but instead specify the gait—a walk, trot, or canter, say—and the speed at which the horse is moving. This suggests a more general strategy: to describe the control of movement in terms of selecting one of a relatively short list of modes of activity and then, within each mode, to specify the few parameters required to tune the movement. This strategy was borne out by experiments of the Russian school of Bernstein (1967), Gel'fand et al. (1971), Shik, Severin, and Orlovskii (1966a, b), and Orlovskii (1970, 1972a, b), who suggested that movement be analyzed in terms of synergies in the sense of relatively standard patterns of coordinated activity in some ensemble of muscles; a synergy in this sense is the dynamic of muscles acting in concert. In similar fashion, we see the problem of motor control as one of sequencing and coordinating *motor schemas* rather than of directly controlling the vast number of degrees of freedom offered by the independent activity of all the motor units. To use the language of Greene (1972), we have to get the system "into the right ballpark" and then to tune activity within the ballpark: the dual problems of activation and tuning.

The schema theory used in this volume to provide a functional analysis of brain mechanisms of visuomotor coordination owes much to the work of Warren McCulloch and Walter Pitts (see Lettvin 1989 for an appreciation). McCulloch and Pitts's 1943 formal theory of neural networks laid the basis for automata theory and (via such papers as those in Shannon and McCarthy 1956) artificial intelligence, whereas Pitts and McCulloch (1947) wrote a study, "How We Know Universals," a theoretical construction of neural networks for pattern recognition showing how visual input could control motor output via the distributed activity of a layered neural network without the intervention of executive control, perhaps the earliest example of what we shall refer to as *cooperative computation*. One of the classics of single-cell neurophysiology, "What the Frog's Eye Tells the Frog's Brain" (Lettvin et al. 1959), is acknowledged to be an outgrowth of "How We Know Universals," even though the processes found in frog tectum are not those predicted for mammalian cortex. What the later paper did confirm, however, were the notions that (1) an important method of coding information in the brain is by topographically organized activity distributed over layers of neurons, (2) that computation may be carried out in a distributed way by a collection of neurons without the intervention of a central executive, and (3) the retina begins the process of transformation that extracts from the visual input information that is relevant to the action of the organism (in this case, the frog's need to get food and evade predators no matter how bright or dim it is about him).

Lettvin et al. (1959) concluded:

By transforming the image from a space of simple discrete points to a congruent space where each equivalent point is described by the intersection of particular qualities in its neighborhood, we can then give the image in terms of distributions of combinations of those qualities. In short, every point is seen in definite contexts. The character of these contexts, genetically built in, is the physiological synthetic a priori.

The schema theory developed later will build on these lessons but will restrict its investigations of "the physiological synthetic a priori" neither to the retina nor to neural functions that are determined completely by genetic processes. An important notion will be that a schema expresses a function that need not be coextensive with the activity of a single neuronal circuit. This view was foreshadowed in the work of Kilmer, McCulloch, and Blum (1969). They built on the observation by Scheibel and Scheibel (1958, already noted in sec. 2.2.2) that the reticular formation is essentially arranged as a stack of "poker-chip" modules and on the functional observation that the reticular formation is involved in switching the organism from sleep to wakefulness (Moruzzi and Magoun, 1949). This notion posed the more general question of how the nervous system could set the organism's "overall mode of behavior" through the cooperative computation (again, without executive control) of modules that each aggregate the activity of many neurons. We may say that the schema of mode selection is distributed across an entire series of modules.

Around 1970, Arbib and Didday addressed the key issue of the "generativity of the world." Neither a frog confronted with a novel arrangement of prey, predators, and obstacles nor a human deciding how to act in relation to current goals in a novel and complex situation can base its actions on the activation of a single familiar schema; rather, action must depend on a set of schemas configured to express the novelty of the situation. Arbib and Didday (1971) developed the slide-box metaphor as a setting for a general view of the role of visual perception in the guidance of action, whereas Didday's thesis (1970, 1976) started the work on *Rana computatrix* (e.g., see Arbib 1987, 1991b), which models data on visuomotor coordination in frog and toad so as to study the integration of action and perception. As noted above, Bernstein (1967) studied synergies as units of motor control, and his work on the development of the coordination and control of movements inspired further work on early acquisition of skill (see Thelen and Smith 1994). All this led to the analysis of visual perception and motor control in terms of "slides" and "output feature clusters" (Arbib 1972), which Arbib later (1975, 1981) refined and renamed as *perceptual schemas* and *motor schemas* in response to the observation of Richard Reiss (personal communication) regarding the continuity of concerns of this approach with the discussion of schemas by Bartlett, among others.

Mandler (1985, pp. 35–45) provided a convenient summary of schema theory from the viewpoint of cognitive psychology, evoking similarities with the usages of Bartlett (1932) and Piaget (1971). He viewed schemas as those cognitive structures used primarily to organize experience and distinguished them from "logical devices, syntactic structures and purely procedural mechanisms," a distinction that we find less useful than Mandler takes it to be. Schemas are built up in the course of interaction with the environment so as to represent organized experience ranging from discrete features to general categories. Moreover, Mandler addressed the issue of generativity, stating:

[I]nput from the environment is coded selectively in keeping with the schemas currently operating, while that input also selects relevant schemas....A chair activates not only the "chair schema" but also the more general schemas, such as "furniture" and possibly "things to sit on." At the same time, the activation of a schema also involves the inhibition of other competing schemas (Mandler 1985, p. 37).

Shallice (1988) offered a similar view, while stressing (p. 308n) that the schema "not only has the function of being an efficient description of a state of affairs—as in, say, Bartlett's usage—but also is held to produce an output that provides the immediate control of the mechanisms required in one cognitive or action operation. The usage is thus more analogous to Piaget's view than to Bartlett's original concept."

Finally, we note that there is much work that contributes to schema theory in the sense developed here, even

though the scientists involved do not use this term. For example, Minsky (1985) espoused a *Society of Mind* analogy in which "members of society," the agents, are analogous to schemas. Brooks (1986) controlled robots with layers made up of asynchronous modules that can be considered as a version of schemas. This work shares with our schema theory, with its mediation of action through a network of schemas, the point that no single, central, logical representation of the world need link perception and action (Arbib 1972, p. 168), while sharing with Walter (1953) and Braitenberg (1965, 1984) the study of the "evolution" of simple "creatures" with increasingly sophisticated sensorimotor capacities.

3.1.2 A Quasi-Formal Overview of Schema Theory

This section provides a quasi-formal introduction to the basic concepts of the schema theory developed in this volume, namely perceptual and motor schemas, coordinated control programs, cooperative computation, and schema assemblages. The next three sections then flesh out the story as follows:

1. A simple account of approach and avoidance behavior in frogs illustrates the use of perceptual and motor schemas, shows how they may be linked, and addresses what is involved in making a schema-based account of a function into a neural model. *Rana computatrix*, an evolving family of models of frog visuomotor coordination, will be discussed further later in this chapter to provide something of an evolutionary counterpoint for our usual emphasis on mammals in general and primates in particular.

2. A simple model of the visual control of reaching and grasping illustrates the notion of a coordinated control program. We present a more subtle schema-based model later in the chapter and then address neural-based models of this functionality in later chapters (cerebral cortex, chapter 8; cerebellum, chapter 9; and basal ganglia, chapter 10).

3. A simple model of visual perception provides a perspective on short-term and long-term memory that uses the notion of schema assemblage. The theme of memory will recur in many subsequent chapters, but the further investigation of visual perception in its more cognitive aspects (as distinct from the control of a focused behavioral repertoire) will not recur until its brief revival at the end of chapter 8.

Because this section is somewhat abstract, the reader may find it useful to skim it on a first reading, then return for a second reading after viewing the next three sections.

In seeking to bridge from mind to neuron, we can either move, as it were, from the *bottom up*, viewing the neurons as our building blocks and asking how to put them together to do interesting things, or we can work from the *top down*, starting with the person, the mind, or linguistic and visual behavior and asking how to decompose it into the functional interaction of various subsystems. The *schema* is going to be that unit that, together with other such units, forms a network at the mental level. Such things as the knowledge of how to use a word, recognize a dog, drive a car, or read a book are embedded in a network of schemas.

Schemas are composable programs in the mind. A schema is like a computer program but with the special property that its instances can be combined with other simultaneously active programs to provide the ability of an organism or robot to perceive, and act within, its world. A schema represents a generalized skill (rather than a rigid stereotyped behavior) that can adapt itself to many situations. However, a schema differs from a serial computer program in that *schema instances* (simultaneously active copies of schemas) continually pass messages to each other to solve some problem cooperatively rather than being successively activated one at a time. A schema is not a module if this is identified with a discrete region or circuit of the brain. On the contrary, it is a *functional entity*. The activity of a given schema may involve the deployment of a number of modules; conversely, a given module may contribute to the implementation of many schemas. Schema activations are largely task-driven, reflecting the goals of the animal and the physical and functional requirements of the task, and may require the ability to maintain several different instances, each suitably tuned, of a schema simultaneously. As a result, we cannot think of the linkage of schema instances in an assemblage as always corresponding to fixed anatomical connections between the circuitry implementing the given schemas. This latter point is related to Lashley's discussion (1951) of the problem of repetition of action in a sequence of behaviors (taken up in the context of "motor set" in sec. 8.5.1).

There is no formalism that captures all aspects of current and future work in schema theory (any more than there is a uniform account of all current styles of computer program). Nonetheless, it may be useful to outline one formal approach (Lyons and Arbib 1989). A schema constitutes the "long-term memory" of a perceptual or motor skill or the structure coordinating such skills, whereas the process of perception or action is controlled

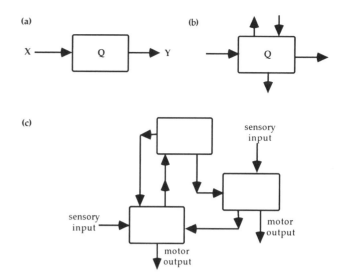

Figure 3.2
(a) A discrete-time automaton. (b) A port automaton is like an ordinary automaton, except that it may have multiple input and output ports. (c) Port automata embedded in a network. Either ports are unconnected (providing the inputs and outputs for the overall network), or output ports are connected to input ports. X, set of inputs; Y, set of outputs, Q, set of states.

by active copies of schemas called *schema instances*. A schema may be instantiated to form multiple schema instances as active copies of the process to apply that knowledge. For example, given a schema that represents generic knowledge about some object, we may need several active instances of the schema, each suitably tuned to subserve our perception of a different instance of that object. For certain behaviors, there may be no distinction between schema and instance; a single neural network may embody the skill memory and provide the processor that implements it. However, in more complex behaviors, the different mobilizations of a given "skill-unit" must be distinguished carefully. A *schema assemblage* is a network of schema instances, and its characteristics are similar to that of a single schema.

A *port automaton* generalizes the concept of a discrete-time dynamic system (figure 3.2a). The latter is characterized by sets X of inputs, Q of states, and Y of outputs, together with a state-transition function $\delta: Q \times X \to Q$ and an output function $\beta: Q \to Y$. The idea is that each time the system is in state q and receives input x, it changes state to $\delta(q, x)$ and emits output $\beta(y)$. A port automaton is generalized from this as follows (figure 3.2b): Instead of one input line, it may have several input ports; instead of one output line, it may have several output ports. In forming an assemblage, these ports are to be thought of as tied to communication channels linking one schema instance to another. At any moment, a given channel may or may not contain a message en route from an output port to some input port (figure 3.2c). We will adopt here the convention that each channel can hold at most one message. A schema assemblage forms a network of schema instances and may itself be considered a schema for further processes of assemblage formation, and the schema instance network in general will be dynamic, growing and shrinking as various instantiations and deinstantiations occur (see below). A schema assemblage tells us how to put schemas together in a way independent of how the behavior of a constituent is given, whether directly (as in a basic schema) or indirectly (as when the schemas constituting an assemblage are themselves schema assemblages). Thus, it is simple to extend the present automaton-based scheme to a neural net specification by making it possible in the basic schemas to define the behavior directly in terms of a neural network. Like a basic schema, an assemblage also has communication ports, but its behavior is defined through the interactions of a network of schema instances.

The behavior of each automaton is defined by a set of transitions

(a configuration of messages on some of its input ports, an old state) $\Rightarrow$ (a new state, a configuration of messages on some of its output ports).

The port automaton changes state when it can apply one of these quadruples. As there are many ports, more than one may be applicable at a given time, so the automaton is nondeterministic. In addition to the foregoing transitions, a schema instance may execute transitions of the form

(a configuration of messages on some of its input ports, an old state) $\Rightarrow$ (a new state, W)

where W is an instantiation or deinstantiation operation. An *instantiation* operation creates a new instance of some specified schema, makes designated connections to link it into the current schema assemblage, and uses the initiation of variables and the prior values on the port to which the new automaton is connected to establish its initial full state (i.e., its internal state together with any messages currently held on its input and output lines). The full state of all other automata in the network remains unchanged. Conversely, the *deinstantiation* operation specifies that a given schema instance is to be deinstantiated so that it no longer plays any role in the transactions of the current network of schema instances. Deinstantiation and instantiation operations, respectively, capture the notion that as action and perception pro-

gress, certain schema instances need no longer be active, whereas new ones are added as new objects are perceived and new plans of action are brought into play. With this, we return to our general, informal discussion of schema theory.

Perceptual schemas are those used for perceptual analysis. They embody the processes whereby the system determines whether a given domain of interaction is present in the environment. They not only serve as pattern-recognition routines but also can provide the appropriate parameters concerning the current relationship of the organism with its environment. Schema instances have an activity level that indicates its current salience for the ongoing computation. If a schema is implemented as a neural network, all the schema parameters would be implemented via patterns of neural activity. Thus, it is important to distinguish "activity level" as a particular parameter of a schema from the "neural activity" that will vary with different neural implementations of the schema. The activity level of a perceptual schema signals the credibility of the hypothesis that what the schema represents is indeed present, whereas other schema parameters represent such other salient properties as size, location, and motion of the perceived object. Given a perceptual schema, we may need several schema instances, each suitably tuned, to subserve our perception of several instances of its domain.

Motor schemas provide the control systems that can be coordinated to effect the wide variety of movement. A set of basic motor schemas is hypothesized to provide simple, prototypical patterns of movement. The activity level of a motor schema may signal its degree of readiness to control some course of action, thus enriching somewhat the related notion of motor pattern generators (MPGs) from the motor control literature.

The key for analyzing the brain, with its many different regions active at the same time, is also crucial to the design of large, complex systems: to understand how local interactions can integrate themselves to yield some overall result without explicit executive control. As we saw in figure 3.2c, schema instances may be combined (possibly with those of more abstract schemas, including coordinating schemas) to form schema assemblages. For example, an assemblage of perceptual schema instances provides an estimate of environmental state with a representation of goals and needs. New sensory input and internal processes update the schema assemblage as the action-perception cycle progresses. The internal state also is updated by knowledge of the state of execution of current plans made up of motor schemas. We use the term *coordinated control program* (Arbib 1981) for a schema assemblage that processes input via perceptual schemas and delivers its output via motor schemas, interweaving the activations of these schemas in accordance with the current task and sensory environment to mediate more complex behaviors. The notion of a coordinated control program is a combination of control theory and the computer scientist's notion of a program suited to the analysis of the control of movement: It combines mechanisms for the passing of control parameters between schemas with the phasing in and out of patterns of coactivation.

Schema theory uses the paradigm of *cooperative computation*, a shorthand for "computation based on the competition and cooperation of concurrently active agents," as its style of interaction. Cooperation yields a pattern of strengthened alliances between mutually consistent schema instances and allows them to achieve high activity levels to constitute the overall solution of a problem (as perceptual schemas become part of the current short-term model of the environment or motor schemas contribute to the current course of action). It is as a result of competition that instances that do not meet the evolving (data-guided) consensus lose activity and thus are not part of this solution (though their continuing subthreshold activity well may affect later behavior). In general, a schema network does not need a top-level executor, because schema instances can combine their effects by distributed processes of competition and cooperation (i.e., interactions that, respectively, decrease and increase the activity levels of these instances) rather than by the operation of an inference engine on a passive store of knowledge. This may lead to apparently emergent behavior, owing to the absence of global control.

Schema theory thus provides a distributed model of computation, supporting many concurrent activities for recognition of objects and the planning and control of different activities. The use, representation, and recall of knowledge is mediated through the activity of a network of interacting computing agents—the schema instances—that between them provide processes for going from a particular situation and a particular structure of goals and tasks to a suitable course of action. Such "action" may be overt or covert (as when learning occurs without action or the animal changes its state of readiness). The dynamics of schema instances may involve passing of messages, changes of state (including activity level), instantiation to add new schema instances to the network, and deinstantiation to remove instances.

Schemas, then, provide abilities for recognition and guides to action, but schema theory is a learning theory also. As already noted in our discussion of Piaget, sche-

mas must provide expectations about what will happen so that we may choose our actions appropriately. These expectations may be wrong, and so it is that sometimes we learn from our mistakes. In a general setting, there is no fixed repertoire of basic schemas. Rather, new schemas may be formed as assemblages of old schemas, but once formed, a schema may be tuned by some adaptive mechanism. This tunability of schema assemblages allows them to start as composite but emerge as primitive, much as a skill is honed into a unified whole from constituent pieces. For this reason, a model expressed in a schema-level formalism may only approximate the behavior of a model expressed in a neural net formalism. When used in conjunction with neural networks, schema theory provides a means of providing a functional-structural decomposition and is to be contrasted with models that employ some learning rule to train an otherwise undifferentiated network to respond as specified by some training set.

Schemas, and their connections with each other, change through the processes of accommodation. These processes adjust the network of schemas so that over time one well may be able to handle more capably a wide range of situations. In many ways, these processes are reminiscent of how a scientific community modifies and develops its theories on the basis of the pragmatic criterion of successful prediction and control (Hesse 1980; Arbib and Hesse 1986). An early example of a computational learning theory formalizing the ideas of Piaget is the work of Cunningham (1972), whereas subsequent work includes that of Drescher (1989). Arbib, Conklin, and Hill (1987) studied language perception and generation and offer a "computational, neo-piagetian" approach to language acquisition (Hill 1983). In a related vein, Rumelhart et al. (1986) suggest how schemas may be seen as emergent properties of adaptive, connectionist networks.

In the rest of this section, we chart informally how schema theory views human memory, perception, and action; thereby, we set the stage for the more formal accounts in chapters 6, 8, and 11. Note that the scientist's explicit analysis of schemas does not imply that we normally have explicit, conscious access to all, or even most, of the schemas that direct our behavior. Moreover, the schema theorist seeks to understand the overall network of schemas by looking at some subnetwork in isolation, always aware that this is an approximation to an incredibly complex whole.

We view the *short-term memory* (STM) of an organism as a schema assemblage combining an estimate of environmental state based on a variety of instances of perceptual schemas with a representation of goals and needs. *Long-term memory* (LTM) is provided by the stock of schemas from which STM may be assembled. New sensory input and internal processes can update STM. The internal state also is updated by knowledge of the state of execution of current plans that specify a variety of coordinated control programs for possible execution. To comprehend a situation, we may call on tens or hundreds of schemas in our current schema assemblage, but this STM puts together instances of schemas drawn from an LTM that encodes a lifetime of experience in a vast network of interconnected schemas.

This personal "encyclopedia" of hundreds of thousands of schemas ranges from perceptual schemas for words and objects through memories of many specific episodes to skills and belief systems that themselves weave together a multitude of other schemas. However, we do not have a different schema for every different object of every different size or position in space, because each schema may be tuned by parameters (size, speed, color, and on and on) that adapt its generalities to the specifics of the current situation. Our knowledge is neither certain nor neatly compartmentalized. Schemas do not correspond to isolated facts but may be linked to subsidiary schemas, as when the skill of riding a bike incorporates our ability to judge distances to potential obstacles. Also, one schema may generalize another, as in the relationship between the ability to recognize houses in general and the ability to recognize our own house in particular. Thus our knowledge forms a tangled skeinwork.

Perception involves a continual updating of our initial comprehension of the more salient aspects of the current environment/situation by noting discrepancies between what we expect and what our senses now tell us. We view STM as a working memory of data organized for their possible relevance to the organism's current behavior—a schema assemblage combining an estimate of environmental state with a representation of goals and needs. ("Pure" perception and action are but two points on a continuum, and most schemas are not purely perceptual or motor but intermesh perceptual and motor skills with more abstract forms of knowledge.) This is different from some psychologists' view of STM as simply a repository for traces of recent stimuli. Research on the brain has revealed such working memory, exemplified in delayed reaction tasks in monkeys in which activity in specific brain regions correlated with the desired response persists precisely for the period from the presentation of the cue that specifies the response to the emission of the response on presentation of a neutral trigger stimulus (Fuster, Bauer, and Jervey 1982;

Goldman-Rakic 1991; Fuster 1995). We will offer a neural model for a possible corticothalamic mechanism for working memory in section 8.3.2.

To relate the dynamics of STM to LTM (or, in piagetian terms, to relate assimilation to accommodation), consider that each time a schema is instantiated in STM, it can be annotated (either through changes in the schema itself or through changes in contextual connections to other schemas) with information about actions taken at that time and about the consequences of such action. Such data can be consolidated over time to provide useful guides to action, helping update LTM by editing existing schemas and adding new ones. Though new schemas initially may enter LTM as assemblages of old schemas, they may (once formed) be tuned to form a new integral schema (e.g., for a well-practiced skill). In the initial stage of driving a car, the foot pedals, steering wheel, and passing scene all seem to require minute and conflicting attention to fit into an ill-learned assemblage specified by verbal rules that only outline what is necessary to survive in traffic. Practice yields an integrated schema that can operate in tandem with conversation in all but the most trying of traffic situations. Not only have separate driving-related motor schemas for eyes, hands, and feet been acquired and combined, but the new composite schema, the coordinated control program, has been tuned to form a whole in which each part is so adapted to the others that their integration no longer engages our conscious effort. Learning processes can meld the pieces smoothly, like a carpenter planing, sanding, and varnishing an assemblage of blocks of wood to achieve a single smooth unity in a piece of furniture.

Through learning, a complex schema network arises that can mediate first the child's and then the adult's reality. Through being rooted in such a network, schemas are interdependent, so that each finds meaning only in relation to others. For example, a house is defined in terms of parts such as a roof, yet a roof may be recognized because it is part of a house recognized on the basis of other criteria, such as "people live there." Each schema enriches and is defined by the others (and may change when a formal linguistic system allows explicit, though partial, definition). Though processes of schema change may affect only a few schemas at any time, such changes may "cohere" to yield dramatic changes in the overall pattern of mental organization. There is change yet continuity, with many schemas held in common yet changed, because now they must be used in the context of the new network. Arbib and Hesse (1986) offered an epistemology rooted in this view of schema theory and showed how it may be expanded to link schemas in the head with the social schemas that form the collective representations (to use Durkheim's phrase) shared by a community.

3.1.3 Perceptual Schemas, Motor Schemas, and Neural Schema Theory

Having soared to the higher, more cognitive aspects of schema theory, we now return to action and perception and discuss the linking of perceptual and motor schemas to specific brain structures. Though the brain may be considered as a network of interacting boxes (i.e., anatomically distinguishable structures), there is no reason to expect each such box to mediate a single function that is well-defined from a behavioral standpoint. For example, an experimentalist might approach the cerebellum by postulating that it serves for learning elemental movements, mediating feedforward, timing action and perception, or rendering movement more graceful. It may do one or more of these things, but it is more likely that it does none of them by itself, rather, participating in each and more besides. The language of schemas lets us express hypotheses about the various functions that the brain performs without a necessary commitment to localization of any one function in any one region. These hypotheses nonetheless can allow us to express the way in which many regions participate in a given function, whereas a given region may participate in many functions.

Defined functionally, a given schema may be distributed across more than one brain region; conversely, a given brain region may be involved in many schemas. Hypotheses about the localization of schemas in the brain may be tested by lesion experiments or functional imaging, with possible modification of the model (e.g., replacing one schema by several interacting schemas with different localizations) and further testing. Given robust hypotheses about the neural localization of schemas, we may model a brain region by seeing whether its known neural circuitry can indeed be shown to implement the posited schema. When the model involves properties of the circuitry that have not been tested yet, it lays the ground for new experiments.

A schema model becomes a biological model (as distinct from a purely functional model) when explicit hypotheses are offered as to how the constituent schemas are played over particular regions of the brain. To exemplify this, consider approach and avoidance in the toad. To simplify rather drastically, we may say that the frog's or toad's ability to find food and escape enemies can be reduced to the ability to tell small moving objects from large moving objects. A frog surrounded by dead flies

will starve to death, but the frog will snap with equal enthusiasm at a moving fly or a pencil tip wiggled in a flylike way. On the other hand, a larger moving object can trigger an escape reaction. Thus, a highly simplified model of the functioning of the brain of the toad has signals from the eye routed to two basic pattern-recognition routines (perceptual schemas), one for recognizing small moving objects (foodlike stimuli) and one for recognizing large moving objects (enemylike stimuli). If the small-moving-object schema is activated, it in turn will trigger the motor schema (our term for an automaton or control system for controlling action) to get the animal to approach what apparently is its prey. If the perceptual schema for large-moving-object is activated, it will trigger the motor schema for avoidance, causing the animal to escape an apparent enemy (figure 3.3A).

The schemas have *activation levels* that measure some degree of confidence, and it is the more active of the two perceptual schemas that will trigger the appropriate motor schema to yield the appropriate response. We may say that the perceptual schemas *compete* to control the behavior of the animal, a very simple example of the type of competition and cooperation that can be exhibited by a network of schemas. In general, multiple motor schemas may be coactivated to control subtle behaviors. Moreover, perceptual schemas provide a parametric description that can be used in tuning motor behavior. When it recognizes prey, the animal does not simply respond with a launch in a standard or random direction; rather, it snaps at just the position in three-dimensional space where the prey is located. Similarly, when the animal sees a predatorlike stimulus, it must find an escape direction that will have a good likelihood of taking it out of the path of the predator.

However, to make a biological model, we must relate these schemas to the anatomy. Each eye of the frog projects to the opposite half of the brain, especially to the important visual midbrain region called the *tectum*. This projection from the retina to a layered structure of the brain preserves the neighborhood relationships of the visual field; it is called a *retinotopic map*. (The self-organizing formation and plastic behavior of retinotopic mapping has been the subject of many modeling studies; see sec. 4.4.2.) Another retinotopic map goes to the *pretectum* (so called because it is in front of the tectum). If we make the hypothesis that the small-moving-object schema is in the tectum whereas the large-moving-object schema is in the pretectum, the preceding model predicts that animals with a pretectal lesion would continue to approach small moving objects just as the normal animal would but would not respond at all to large moving

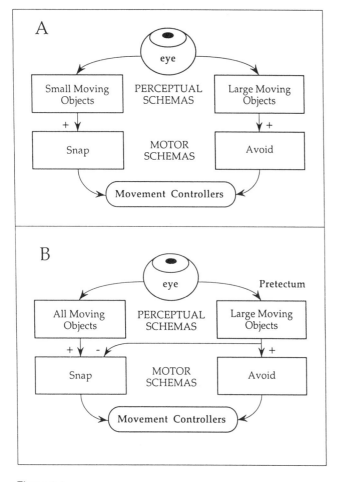

Figure 3.3
(A) A "naive" schema program that represents the perceptual and motor schemas for frog approach behavior (snap at small moving objects) as completely separated from those for avoidance. (B) A schema program for approach and avoidance that takes into account data on the effect of lesioning the pretectum. In particular, the approach schema is not localized in the tectum alone, because it depends on pretectal inhibition for its integrity.

objects. However, this is false. Peter Ewert studied toads in which the pretectum had been lesioned (see Ewert 1987 for a review). He found not only that the toads responded to small moving objects with approach behavior; they also responded to large moving objects with approach behavior. This observation leads to the new schema-level model shown in figure 3.3B. The new data tell us that in the absence of the pretectum, the animal must be able to respond to all moving objects with approach. Thus, we replace the perceptual schema for *small* moving objects by a perceptual schema for *all* moving objects. On the other hand, in the normal toad, recognition of large moving objects triggers avoidance, so we leave the right hand column the way it was. However, although now we have explained the response of the lesioned animal to all moving objects and the re-

sponse of the normal animal to large moving objects, it remains to tune the model so that the normal animal will respond to small moving objects with approach but not avoidance. We can achieve this by having an inhibitory pathway running from the perceptual schema for large moving objects (in the pretectum) to the approach schema—or, equivalently, to the schema for all moving objects. This model explains our small database by the behavior of both normal animals and those with a lesion of the pretectum.

Thus, we have shown how hypotheses about neural localization of subschemas may be tested and refined by lesion experiments. The important point is that biological models can be expressed at the level of a network of interacting schemas and that these really can be biological models in the sense that they can be subjected to test at the level of such a coarse-grained network, irrespective of whether data or hypotheses are available about the fine-grain implementation of those schemas in neural networks.

3.1.4 Coordinated Control Programs and Motor Schemas

As the hand moves to grasp a ball, it is preshaped so that when it has almost reached the ball, it is of the right shape and orientation to enclose the ball prior to gripping it firmly. Moreover (to a first approximation), the movement can be broken into a fast initial movement and a slow approach movement, with the transition from the fast to the slow phase of transport coming just before closing of the fingers from the preshape so that touch may take over in controlling the final grasp (Jeannerod 1984). Figure 3.4 shows the original coordinated control program (Arbib 1981) for this behavior; solid lines indicate the transfer of data from one schema to another, and dashed lines indicate the transfer of activation. Note that the schemas are akin to the blocks in a conventional block diagram for a control system but have the special property that they can be activated and deactivated. Thus, whereas control theory usually examines the properties of a fixed control system, schema theory allows the control system to expand and contract, adding and deleting subschemas in a task- and data-dependent manner.

The top half of the figure shows three perceptual schemas; successful location of the object activates schemas for recognizing the size and orientation of the object. The outputs of these perceptual schemas are available for the control of the hand movement by concurrent activation of two motor schemas, one controlling the arm to transport the hand towards the object and the other preshaping the hand, with finger separation and orientation

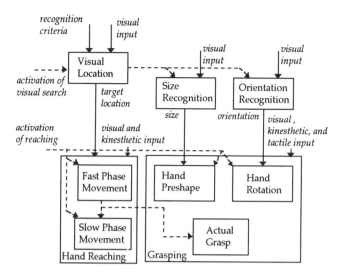

Figure 3.4
Hypothetical coordinated control program for reaching and grasping. Note that different perceptual schemas are required for the control of reaching (arm transport ≈ hand reaching) and grasping (controlling the hand to conform to the object). Also, note the timing relations posited here within the hand reaching motor schema and between the motor schemas for hand reaching and grasping. Dashed lines, activation signals; solid lines, transfer of data. (Adapted from Arbib 1981.)

guided by the output of the appropriate perceptual schemas. Once the hand is preshaped, it is only the completion of the fast phase of hand transport that "wakes up" the final stage of the grasping schema to shape the fingers under control of tactile feedback.

Crucially, then, schemas can be combined to form coordinated control programs that control the phasing in and out of patterns of schema coactivation and the passing of control parameters from perceptual to motor schemas. The notion of schema is thus *recursive*: A schema defined functionally may be analyzed later as a coordinated control program of finer schemas and so on until such time as a secure foundation of neural localization is attained. Moreover, perceptual and motor schemas may be embedded in coordinated control programs embracing more abstract schemas to yield accounts of cognition and language that link psychology to neuroscience (see sec. 3.1.5, and the forward pointers given there). A corollary to this is that knowledge receives a distributed representation in the brain. A multiplicity of different representations must be linked into an integrated whole, but such linkage may be mediated by distributed processes of competition and cooperation.

3.1.5 Visual Scene Interpretation

We use a model of the computations underlying visual perception to show how schema theory extends to more "cognitive" realms than the basic patterns of sensori-

motor coordination presented earlier. The approach to schema-based interpretation in the VISIONS computer vision system (Draper et al. 1989) is an important exemplification of schema theory within artificial intelligence (i.e., there is no claim to model the brain in their work). The main idea is that an object's characteristics determine the best way to recognize it (though in general, schema theory would go further to stress the extraction of parameters relevant to a current task, rather than mere recognition); thus, a schema for an object class has an object-specific control strategy for efficient context-dependent object and scene recognition.

As in most computer vision systems, *low-level vision* takes an image (e.g., a color photograph) and, working independently of object-specific knowledge, extracts multiple representations, including regions, lines, surfaces, and vertices tagged with features such as color, texture, shape, size, and location. Given a pair (or sequence) of images, other processes could yield further information, such as depth and motion. The result is an *intermediate representation* (a set of partial representations) of the image, which may be updated as interpretation proceeds. The interacting schemas that encode recognition routines for houses and walls and trees provide the processes by which different features of the intermediate representation are accessed and the overall interpretation of the image is devised.

In the VISIONS system, *high-level vision* depends on the knowledge required for interpretation which is stored in LTM as a network of schemas, whereas the state of interpretation of the particular scene unfolds in STM (working memory) in the form of a network of schema instances. VISIONS embodies the perception cycle in that the treatment of current input depends on the current state of STM. Section 8.6, From Action-Oriented Perception to Cognition, will suggest how VISIONS might be extended to model the action-perception cycle in a manner consistent with our current understanding of the primate brain.

The user starts the interpretation process by invoking an arbitrary number of initial schemas. These may reflect general visual goals, such as "interpret this image as a road scene," or more specific needs, such as "find the sidewalk in this image." Each schema instance has an associated activity level (or confidence level) that changes on the basis of interactions with other units in the (dynamically reconfigurable) STM network. The STM network makes context explicit: Each object represents a context for further processing, using to advantage the relations among objects. When a schema instance is activated, it is linked with an associated area of the image and an associated set of local variables. Different instances of a given schema may be associated with separate portions of the image. The structure of STM is constrained further in part by relationships encoded within LTM—both those between schemas for interobject relations and those within a schema for geometric relations of parts.

In addition to its schema instances, the STM contains hypotheses and goals. A *hypothesis* asserts that a particular object provides the interpretation of a portion of the image. The hypothesis is registered when the relevant schema instance achieves a threshold in its confidence level and then will include parameters descriptive of the object so recognized—contrast schema activation (when an instance starts to process) with schema "firing" or propagation (when an instance posts a hypothesis that can affect the activity of other schemas). A schema instance may set as a *goal* the confirmation that a certain context applies, and posting the goal in turn may lead to the forming of a schema instance to check whether a posited object occurs in a certain portion of the image (in the following example, recognizing a roof sets the goal of finding a wall-region beneath it in the image).

Active schema instances set out to accomplish their goals as independently acting agents. As part of recognizing their particular scene or object, schemas may invoke other schemas to recognize subparts of their object or to recognize spatially, functionally, or contextually related objects. The set of schemas that another schema invokes is flexible. A schema for recognizing houses, for example, may only invoke a schema for recognizing a wall if one of its hypotheses needs additional support. Otherwise, it may never invoke the wall schema. Thus, instantiation of a schema may be either data-driven or goal-driven (i.e., on the basis of data extracted from the image or on the basis of goals set by the context of other hypotheses and instances). In a data-driven interpretation routine for the sky (other routines can use contextual cues to determine that a region is skylike), measures of goodness of fit (m_i) are calculated for a region for such features as location, color, shape, and texture. Then a region r is adjudged more skylike, if a specified linear combination $m_{sky}(r)$ of the $m_i(r)$s takes on a larger value. Such measures have proved effective in assigning a confidence level to an initial data-driven classification of a region on the basis of local cues (Riseman and Hanson 1987). In general, this will be only the first step and in no way forces the final interpretation.

Processing can create errors and ambiguities. The problem is to ensure that the schema interactions usually will sort themselves out into a useful interpretation so that what may be wrong to start with will be removed and replaced by better hypotheses en route to the final analysis.

To see how the system works, imagine how schemas might process an image of an outdoor scene in which a house is set against a wintry sky such that a lack of contrast leads low-level vision to overlook a crucial edge separating wall and sky. The sky schema runs on the segmented image and finds a region reasonably high in the image and with a high value for m_{sky}. However, because the segmentation left out the crucial edge, the "sky" in fact includes one of the walls of the house. The slate-colored roof region also has skylike properties, but because it is lower in the image, the color is not quite sky, and it has more texture, its $m_{sky}(r)$ is much lower. Meanwhile, an instance of the roof schema finds that the roof region has just the right geometrical characteristics and is in the right position of the image to yield a high value of m_{roof} and thus posts the hypothesis that it is indeed the roof. As a result, the low-confidence hypothesis that it might be sky does not play any further part in the computation.

The roof hypothesis leads to formation of a house hypothesis, and this in turn leads to the goal of finding confirming context, invoking an instance of the wall schema to search underneath the posited roof to see if the criteria for a wall are met, as indeed they are. However, because of the missing edge in the roofline, there is now a big region that is interpreted both as wall and as sky. We saw in the case of the roof that if one confidence level were much stronger than another, further interactions would tend to ignore the low-confidence schema instance; but here, both hypotheses are too strong to be ignored. One solution is to reprocess the sensory data to extract missing details (e.g., to resegment the offending region with a lower threshold for edges). Instances of the sky and wall schemas now can compete over just these regions to yield quickly their contribution to the final interpretation. Other schemas then can continue their competition and cooperation to yield the overall interpretation (see Arbib 1989; sec. 5.2 for further exposition).

3.2 Schemas for *Rana computatrix*

To further our perspective of how schemas may be used to model the brain, we build on the simple model presented in section 3.1.3 to consider a few further examples from *Rana computatrix*, "the frog that computes." Section 3.2.1. advances our understanding of schema assemblages and coordinated control programs by showing how perception may demand the mutual refinement of one perceptual schema by another and how multiple motor schemas may act together to yield complex motor behaviors. Section 3.2.2 uses the study of detours and path planning to show how brain function can be analyzed in a process of evolutionary refinement in which basic systems serve as the substrate for the evolution of more refined systems. (This is not the actual path of evolution by natural selection but rather an attempt to understand a complex behavior by the designed "evolution" of successively more complex models to approximate more and more fully the neural realization of that function. We may contrast the phylogenic approach to neural structure introduced in section 2.1.3.) The key point here is that new schemas often arise as modulators of existing schemas rather than as new systems with independent functional roles. Section 3.2.3. closes our discussion of *Rana computatrix* with a study of neural mechanisms of avoidance behavior to provide our first example of how neural modeling can be used to replace schemas with neural networks of equivalent functionality.

3.2.1 Approach and Avoidance in Frog and Toad

In section 3.1.3, we presented the simplest schema-based model of approach and avoidance behavior in the toad consistent with data on lesion of the pretectum. We may think of each basic schema in figure 3.3 as having its own dedicated neural circuitry. More complex schemas, such as that for recognizing small moving objects, are schema assemblages realized by patterns of activity across the circuits that realize the schemas of the coordinated control program that defines it. If the same basic schema occurs more than once in some coordinated control program, it must be made clear whether the program will require the activity of only one of these instances at any one time. For example, although a more elaborate version (Cobas and Arbib 1992) of the schema for prey capture and predator avoidance contains the "orient" motor schema in the subschemas for both prey capture and predator avoidance, the overall schema is so structured that at most one of those subschemas is active at any one time; thus, the circuitry for the orient schema will be activated either with parameters for orienting toward the prey or with parameters for orienting away from the predator. Moreover, should the competition between the prey-capture and predator-avoidance sub-

schemas be unsuccessful in such a way that both activate the orient schema, it will mean simply that the same circuitry receives simultaneous, conflicting, commands—in which case it might, for example, orient the animal to the "average" direction.

Cobas and Arbib (1992) modelled prey catching and predator avoidance at the level of maps and schemas,[2] which is the correct level at which to capture and extend data from lesion and behavioral experiments (they did not offer neural network models). The motor schemas are driven by specific internal "maps" that between them constitute a distributed internal representation of the world. These maps collectively provide the transition from topographically coded sensory information to population-coded inputs to the diverse motor schemas that drive muscle activity. However, whereas stimulus and response direction are the same for prey, different maps are involved for predator location and escape direction. Thus, they distinguish between the Positional Heading hypothesis (heading codes the position of the object) and the Motor Heading hypothesis (each system has a separate projection pathway converging in a different way onto a heading map coding the required motor response). They follow the latter hypothesis, with motor actions constructed through the interaction of different motor schemas via competition and cooperation. It is not necessary for control of action to devolve to a single motor schema. Two or more schemas (e.g., approach and orient) may cooperate to yield the final motor pattern. The model generates for prey-catching behavior different motor zones that match those observed in normal conditions and in studies of lesioned animals and offers predictions for experiments on both approach and avoidance behaviors.

Next we present two models for the insight they offer into the processes of competition and cooperation. The Didday model of prey selection (Didday 1976) embodies pure competition (i.e., the neuron that "wins" the competition determines which prey the frog will snap at); the Dev (1975) model of stereopsis embodies both competition (between neurons encoding different depths in a given direction) and cooperation (so that neurons encoding similar depths in nearby directions will excite each other, thus favoring stable states that encode surfaces rather than rapid fluctuations in depth with changing visual direction). Each of these models presents a single neural network.

---

2. In these studies of frogs and in the related work on saccades discussed later, a map is simply a neural network the activity of which encodes one or more targets in some "action space." More general notions of "map" and the question, "Is a map a schema?" will be taken up in section 6.4.

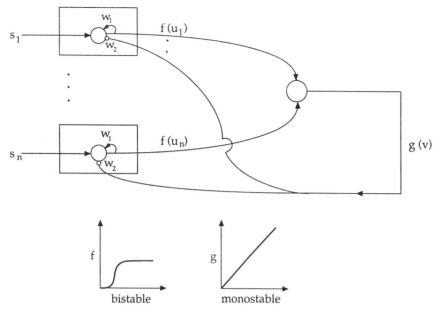

Figure 3.5
Maximum selector (winner-take-all) network. All excitatory cells receive sensory input, self-excitation, and global inhibition and each contributes equally to this global inhibition. If all excitatory cells start with equal activity, and if certain conditions are met by the network parameters, only the excitatory cell with largest input will remain active when the network reaches equilibrium. $s_1, \ldots, s_n$ inputs; $f(u_i)$ output of ith excitatory neuron; $g(v)$ output of inhibitory neuron; w_1, w_2 synaptic weights for self-excitation and inhibition, respectively. (From Amari and Arbib 1977.)

A Model of Prey Selection

In much visually guided behavior, an animal does not simply respond to a single stimulus but rather to some property of the overall configuration. For example, consider the snapping behavior of frogs confronted with one or more flylike stimuli. Ingle (1968) found that it is only in a restricted region around the head of a frog that the presence of a flylike stimulus elicits a snap (i.e., the frog turns so that its midline is pointed at the stimulus and then captures the prey with its tongue). There is a larger zone in which the frog only orients, and beyond that zone the stimulus elicits no response at all. When confronted with two flies within the snapping zone, either of which is vigorous enough that alone it could elicit a snapping response, the frog exhibits one of three reactions: It snaps at one of the flies, it does not snap at all, or it snaps in between at the "average fly." Didday (1976) offered a simple model of this choice behavior; figure 3.5 shows a variant due to Amari and Arbib (1977). Either may be considered as protypical for what has become known as a *winner-take-all* (WTA) *network* (Yuille and Geiger 1995), which receives a variety of inputs and (under ideal circumstances) suppresses the representation of all but one of them. The one that remains is the "winner" that will play the decisive role in further processing. In figure 3.5, each cell receives an excitatory input (the value that determines the winner) and contributes to the excitation level of an inhibitory cell. It is through this inhibition that cells compete with each other: As cellular interactions proceed, cells with less input activity are suppressed. With appropriate parameter settings, at most one cell remains active when the network reaches equilibrium for a given setting of the input activities.

A Model for Stereopsis

Between them, a point on each of the two retinas determines a single point in space, the intersection of the corresponding rays. Given that these retinal points are x and $x + d$, we call d the *disparity* between the retinal projections. Given x and d, we can find the corresponding point in space. However, given several similar stimuli, the brain must solve the *stimulus-matching* (also known as the *correspondence*) problem of determining for each left-eye stimulus which is the corresponding right-eye stimulus. False matches can lead to the detection of "ghost-images." Arbib, Boylls, and Dev (1974) designed a neural net cooperative computation model for solving the correspondence problem so as to build a depth map "guided by the plausible hypothesis that our visual world is made up of relatively few connected regions." Each cell of the neural manifold of this model had a firing

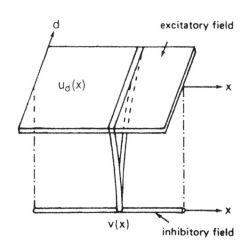

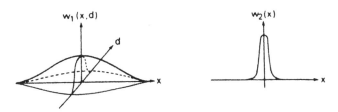

Figure 3.6
A model of stereopsis (from Dev 1975). For each visual direction as seen from the left eye, the network functions like a maximum selector network (see figure 3.5). However, excitation between nearby "direction stripes" is designed to embody the constraint that the world is made up of surfaces and that points with similar retinal coordinates should have the same or similar disparity if they lie on the same surface. See text for details.

level representing a degree of confidence that a point was located at a corresponding position in three-dimensional space, and each cell received retinal input from cells with this point in their visual field. The neurons were so connected via inhibitory interneurons as to embody the principle that cells that coded for nearby direction in space and similar depth should excite each other, whereas cells that corresponded to nearby direction in space and dissimilar depth should inhibit each other. More precisely, this so-called Dev model receives input from two one-dimensional retinas, each with coordinate axis x. It comprises (figure 3.6) a two-dimensional excitatory field wherein the membrane potential $u_d(x, t)$ of the cell at position (x, d) represents the confidence level at time t that there is a feature in direction x on the left retina the disparity of which on the right retina is d; and a one-dimensional inhibitory field with $v(x, t)$ the activity of the cell at position x at time t. We use a finite set of disparities d. The cross-section along the d-axis for a fixed x is like the Amari-Arbib version of Didday's maximum selector circuit. The idea is this: "The world is made up of surfaces; points with similar x should have

the same or similar d if they lie on the same surface." Because we have quantized d, we remove "similar" here: A surface gets approximated by a set of steps. Excitatory cross-coupling between points of nearby x with the same d ensures that nearby maximum selectors are biased to be more likely to choose similar d; thus, the effect of the overall network is to segment the image into patches of constant d for nearby values of x. Dev (1975) showed by computer simulation, and Amari and Arbib (1977) later established by mathematical analysis, that this system did indeed yield a segmentation of the visual input into connected regions. Later, a variant of this model was published by Marr and Poggio (1977), and in subsequent writings, Marr took our "plausible hypothesis that our visual world is made up of relatively few connected regions" and showed how it could be developed into an elegant mathematical theorem relating the structure of a depth-perception algorithm to the nature of surfaces in the physical world. A similar model was developed by Nelson (1975), who provided the first attempt to link such a cooperative model to a plausible neurophysiological substrate, adding cooperation in the orientation domain, so that processes tend not only to build up surfaces but to couple edge hypotheses that can cooperate to form continuous curves. Moreover, he structured the network explicitly in terms of orientation-specific columns (see sec. 8.2) grouped together and sharing spatial location and disparity.

We now build on the foregoing work to see the utility of multiple neural networks working together. The previous work established that depth maps could be constructed by a method of cooperative computation based on the hypothesis that the world was made up of surfaces. (A current review of work in this area is given by Frisby 1995.) However, the cooperative computation algorithms discussed earlier exhibited the problem of false minima. Consider, for example, a picket fence. Suppose by pure chance that the system starts by matching a number of fence posts presented to one eye with the images of their neighbors one to the left presented to the other eye. In the cooperative computation model, this initial mismatch could coopt the possible choices of neighbors and end up with a high confidence estimate that the fence was at a depth different from that at which it actually occurred. This provides a local "energy minimum" for the algorithm. The question then arises: How could one come up with an algorithm that would avoid at least some of these false minima? The cue interaction model (House 1989) solves this problem by coupling two copies of the Dev schema, one driven by disparity and the other by accommodation, giving an example of cooperation between schemas to yield an intramodal form of "sensor fusion." An accommodation-driven field, M, receives information about accommodation (the sharper the image at a particular depth in a given direction the greater the activity of the neuron corresponding to that spatial position), whereas a stereo-driven field, S, uses disparity information as input. The initial state of the accommodation field is blurred, representing the lack of fine tuning offered by accommodation. Targets are more precisely tuned in the stereopsis field, but they offer ghost images (due to matches between discordant images on the two retinas) in addition to the correct images. However, the systems are so intercoupled that a point in the M field will excite the corresponding point in S, and vice versa. As a result, ghost targets are suppressed whereas accommodation information is sharpened. Localization now is precise and unambiguous and can be used to guide the behavior of the animal. This shows how the binocular cue of disparity and the monocular cue of accommodation may be used to complement each other to yield a system that achieves more accurate depth estimates than could a system relying on a single cue.

3.2.2 Detours and Path Planning

Our task now is to see how brain function can be analyzed in a process of evolutionary refinement in which basic systems serve as the substrate for the evolution of more refined systems. We offer a disclaimer: This "evolutionary path" is *not* substantiated as the actual path of evolution by natural selection that shaped the brains of the frogs and toads that we can study today. Rather, it is an attempt to show how the methodology of schema theory may help us to understand a complex behavior by the evolutionary design of successively more complex models to approximate more accurately the neural realization of that function. The same methodology will be used in relating cortical functions in mammals to the subcortical functions that are more closely homologous to certain nonmammalian forms; it also will be used in refining mammalian models by the successive addition of more brain regions to those that can offer a first approximation to the given function. However, in the latter case, the order of addition will reflect a strategy of modeling or exposition with no claim that the regions evolved one after another in the given order.

The motivation for this work is the behavior of frogs (Ingle 1976) and toads (Collett 1982) observing a worm through a semitransparent grating or barrier. Instead of launching directly at its prey (as would occur if no bar-

rier were present), the frog often reacts "appropriately," detouring around the barrier to get its prey. This behavior already extends the schema picture of figure 3.3. Now, the perceptual schema for recognizing prey must be augmented by the perceptual schema for recognizing a barrier, and there no longer can be a simple direct path from prey recognition to the triggering of approach behavior. Rather, there must be some way for this path to be modulated by the recognition of the barrier so as to yield an indirect detour rather than the direct response.

In the situation under consideration, the animal not only must recognize prey and barrier but must locate them in space. If it can recognize that the prey is in front of the barrier or at most a tongue's length behind, the animal will indeed snap directly. However, if the prey is further behind the barrier, the animal must use its recognition of where the prey is and where the barrier is to come up with a path that will carry it around the barrier toward the prey.

Even if, soon after its initial movement, the toad no longer can see the worm, it nonetheless proceeds along a trajectory the final stage of which clearly indicates that the animal has retained an accurate representation of its position. However, the final approach is aborted by the lack of adequate stimuli. Epstein (1979) adapted Didday's simple model of the tectum as a row of neurons selecting its maximal stimulus by positing that each visible preylike stimulus provides a tectal input with a sharp peak at the tectal location corresponding retinotopically to the position of the stimulus in the visual field, with an exponential decay away from the peak. A barrier, on the other hand, provides a trough of inhibition whose tectal extent is slightly greater, retinotopically, than the extent of the barrier in the visual field. Epstein's model can exhibit choice of a target in the direction of the prey or the barrier edge but not the spatial structure of the behavior.

Given that the behavior of the toad—whether approaching the prey directly or detouring around the barrier—depends on how far behind the barrier the worms are, a full model of this behavior must incorporate an analysis of the animal's perception of depth. To address this, Arbib and House (1987) gave two models for detour behavior that make use of separate depth maps for prey and barriers. Lara et al. (1984) offered an alternative model of detour behavior in the presence of barriers with gaps, in which the recognition of gaps is an explicit step in detour computation. The same paper also offers models (at the level of interacting schemas rather than of layers of neuronlike elements) for prey acquisition in environments containing chasms and barriers and for predator avoidance.

In the first Arbib and House (1987) model, the Orientation model, the retinal output of both eyes is processed for barrier and worm recognition so as to provide separate depth mappings for barrier and worm. We suggest that the animal's behavior reflects the combined effects of prey attraction and barrier repulsion. Formally generalizing Epstein's model, the barrier map B is convolved with a mask I that provides a (position-dependent) inhibitory effect for each fencepost, whereas the worm-depth map W is convolved with a mask E that provides an excitatory effect for each worm. The resultant map

$$T = B^*I + W^*E$$

then is subject to further processing that will determine the chosen target. E is an excitatory mask that projects broadly laterally and somewhat less broadly toward the animal; I is an inhibitory mask with a short distance behind the edge where there is little inhibition but beyond this inhibition is equally strong at all distances. The total excitation, T, is summed in each direction, then a winner-take-all (maximum selector) network chooses the direction with maximal activity. If this corresponds to the prey, the animal will approach and snap; otherwise, further processing is required. We postulate that each component of the detour behavior (sidestep, orient, snap) is governed by a specific motor schema. Ingle (1983) offers some clues as to their localization; he finds that a lesion of the crossed tectofugal pathway will remove orienting, lesioning the crossed pretectofugal pathway will block sidestepping, and lesions of the uncrossed tectofugal pathway will block snapping.

In their second model, the Path-Planning model, Arbib and House (1987) associate with each point of the depth map a two-dimensional vector. In place of a single scalar indicating a measure of confidence that there is a target for the first move at the corresponding position in the visual field, the vector is to indicate the preferred direction in which the animal should move were it to find itself at the corresponding position. The model specifies how this vector field is generated and begins to specify how the vector field is processed so as to determine the appropriate parameters for the coordinated activation of motor schemas. Each prey sets up an attractant field, whereas each fencepost sets up a field for a predominantly lateral movement relative to the position of the post from the viewpoint of the animal. Arbib and House suggest that in the case of a "tracking creature," such as the gerbil, the vector field is integrated to yield a variety of trajectories, with a weight factor for each trajectory; whereas in a "ballistic creature," such as the frog or toad, processing yields a map of motor targets, appropriately

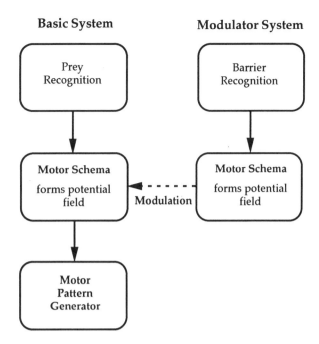

Figure 3.7
Detour behavior modeled as an evolutionary refinement of prey approach obtained by using a potential field representing barrier location to modulate the basic system for approaching prey. (From Arbib and Liaw 1995.)

labeled as to type. The current model uses vectors encoding components of forward and lateral motion; future work will explore the hypothesis that a particular vector would have components governing side-stepping, turning, and snapping. It is an open question whether the components of the vector would be expressed in adjacent nerve cells or distributed across different regions of the brain.

It is not our claim here that the brainstem of the frog implements the foregoing potential field algorithm in its neural circuitry. Rather, the crucial point is that we have an evolutionary account of how such a system might arise (figure 3.7): First, the elements of the prey-recognition system (perceptual schema, motor schema, and MPG) coevolve so that activity in the prey schema can represent a goal in such a way that the approach schema provides the right control signals for the MPG to determine a path to the prey. Then the detour system evolves by combining a perceptual schema for stationary objects with a motor schema that modulates the effect that the approach schema has on the MPG.

Section 3.1.3 presented our first example of the evolving subtlety of the schema interactions. We started with two basic systems for response to small and large moving objects, respectively; then, to match the biological lesion data, moved on to the more subtle interactions shown in figure 3.3B. Here, recognition of small moving objects is a system property involving the modulation of the tectum by the pretectum. Now we have extended the complexity of the environment to which the animal responds; it no longer contains a single prey or a single predator to which the animal may respond with the most basic forms of the survival behaviors of feeding or fleeing. Now it contains the more subtle structure of obstacles that can block the animal's path and around which the animal must be equipped to detour. In evolutionary terms, this corresponds to expansion of the ecological niche in which the animal is well-suited to survive.

The Path-Planning model shows how a toad confronted by a worm behind a semitransparent barrier can "choose" whether to approach the worm directly or to make a detour. The important methodological point here is that the Path-Planning model demands separate schemas for mapping the location of barriers and for locating a prey but does not depend on the use of a specific neural network to implement them.

New schemas often arise as modulators of existing schemas, rather than as new systems with independent functional roles. Further examples of this may be seen in the lesion-based analysis of schemas for approach and avoidance behavior (Cobas and Arbib 1992). The implications of such work for computational neuroethology and robot design were reviewed by Cliff (1995) and Arkin (1995), respectively. Recently, Corbacho and Arbib (1995) have offered a study of how frogs learn to detour as the first step toward a general theory of schema-based learning. This theory attempts to show how the search space for learning can be drastically reduced when learning builds on partially successful schemas rather than starting ab initio with an unstructured neural network.

Our focus on visually guided behavior in frog and toad has provided core examples of schema models, whereas Arbib (1987, 1991b) reviewed models based on interacting layers of neuronlike units and of neural network models closely coupled to detailed data from neuroanatomy and neurophysiology (see also the next section). Besides illustrating these types of models and the give-and-take between them, the examples also suggest the excitement of incrementally evolving an integrated account of a single animal, seeing the challenges posed by combining different aspects of vision with mechanisms for the control of an expanding repertoire of behavior.

Increasing attention to mechanisms of neural function has made *Aplysia* and other invertebrates invaluable in the study of basic cellular mechanisms of facilitation and habituation and in the study of the coupling of neurons

for rhythm generation, for example. However, if creatures that have evolved by chance can provide insight into cellular mechanisms, "creatures" that "evolve" in the computer can provide opportunities for understanding organizational principles. These are not to be sought solely in terms of cellular mechanisms but in terms of structural constructs (layers and modules), functional constructs (schemas), and computational strategies (cooperative computation, competition and cooperation in neural nets, and the like). *Rana computatrix* is thus a test-bed not only for the incorporation of specific data on neural circuitry but also for the development of organizational principles. Thus, data on frog and toad do not exhaust the implications of *Rana computatrix*. Rather, the better we understand the relation of detailed neural circuitry to models that are more schematic (in both senses of the word) the better we can adapt these models to provide insight into analogous systems in other organisms and into the design of "neurally inspired" computers and robots.

3.2.3 Neural Mechanisms of Avoidance Behavior

A study of the escape behaviors of frogs (Ingle 1976) provides a fairly detailed example of how neural modeling can fill in the schemas.

If a stimulus is looming directly at the frog, its escape direction will be a compromise between the direction away from the stimulus and the forward direction of the frog. However, Ingle and Hoff (1990) showed that the behavior is more subtle than a fixed relation between the position of the predator and the direction of escape. If, instead of moving directly toward the animal, the stimulus is on a trajectory that will carry it in front of the animal, the animal will not respond on the basis solely of the position of the looming stimulus, for in this case the animal would jump on a collision path with the predator, making it highly likely to be captured. Instead, the animal exhibits a highly adaptive "cutback" behavior that carries it on a path well away from that being pursued by the looming object. Here again, we note an evolutionary refinement going from simple recognition of a predator to recognition of the trajectory that the predator is following to finding an escape direction based on this extra information. Clearly, an interesting question is to ask how evolutionary pressure could produce an animal able to exhibit this more subtle repertoire. However, in this section, our concern is with the neural mechanisms that provide the frog with this functional repertoire. Unlike previous sections in which we have sought simply a specification of schemas (regardless of whether they have been analyzed in terms of specific brain regions) to provide a functional analysis of the behavior, now we look at the availability of neurophysiological data.

Lettvin et al. (1959) classified the ganglion cells of the frog retina, those that send their axons back to the brain, into four different classes; these four classes of cells were found to project to different depths in the tectum, forming four specific retinotopic maps. Even more excitingly, these maps appeared to be tied to the behavioral repertoire of the animal. If we call the four classes R1, R2, R3, and R4 (remember that each one is a spatially arrayed population of cells in the "output layer" of the retina), we find that the R3 cells seem to respond best to small moving objects—as if they were bug detectors—whereas the R4 cells seemed to respond best to the large moving objects—as if they were enemy detectors (recall our discussion of the synthetic a priori in sec. 3.1.1). Fortunately or unfortunately, research over subsequent years has shown that the story is not so simple and that the frog really does need a brain and not just a retina to determine whether to feed or flee. For example, it has been shown that the activity of the R3 cells is quite complicated. To a first approximation, it can be viewed as responding to the leading edge of a moving object entering its receptive field (the region of the visual field in which activity can affect the activity of the cell) rather than as the presence of a preylike object within the receptive field. Again (as was already recognized by Lettvin et al. 1959), the activity of the R4 cell can be interpreted more suitably as just a measure of dimming, but clearly (by casting a larger shadow) a predator will dim the receptive field more than will prey and thus excite the R4 cell more strongly.

Many studies of visual processing or visually guided behavior ignore the particular transformations conducted by the retina or simply reduce them to a contrast enhancement difference-of-gaussians lateral inhibition mask. However, Liaw and Arbib (1993) have taken as a starting point the properties of the R3 and R4 neurons. Recall that the R3 and R4 neurons form an array that stretches across the output layer of the retina. If we consider the effect of a dark looming stimulus, we will see greatest activity among those R3 cells the receptive fields of which include the leading edge or expanding boundary of that looming stimulus, whereas the R4 cells that will respond most strongly are those contained within the interior of that expanding pattern. Then we can combine these cells to provide a model of the T3 cells (so called because they are type 3 among cells of the tectum as characterized by their physiological response). The T3 cell will

respond more and more strongly as a stimulus looms to a position at the center of its receptor field if the connections from R3 cells to the T3 cell are radially symmetric but with a sort of inverted gaussian form in which activity toward the periphery is more effective than is activity at the center. The larger the looming stimulus the further out the pattern of R3 activity (and thus the stronger the input to the T3 cell). Because the T3 cells also form a retinotopic array, many cells will be activated by this looming stimulus, but the T3 cell with its receptive field centered on the center of the looming stimulus will have the strongest response. To complete the design of the T3 cell and to make it responsive to a large looming stimulus (but not to several small objects flying apart from each other or to an expanding ring), we give the R4 cells a standard gaussian projection to the T3 cells so that darkness at the center of the receptive field of the T3 cell will increase its response.

This analysis (although not showing all the details) explains how the presence of a looming stimulus can be represented by a peak of activity in an array of neurons and uses circuitry with cells whose firing rates provide a good model of firing rates actually observed neurophysiologically. In this neural network, the current position of the looming stimulus on the retina implies the preferred direction of escape. However, to provide the necessary perceptual schema for the cutback response, we must find cells that recognize the direction of motion across the retina. It turns out that the T2 neurons (also in tectum) do have this sensitivity. However, we have no information as to how these cells actually might be wired up, so we resort to a standard model of directional selectivity to ensure that the passage of the stimulus from left to right will increase the likelihood of a T2 neuron firing, whereas a pattern moving in the opposite direction on the T3s will yield little or no T2 response.

This process provides all the perceptual information we need to complete our model. In figure 3.8a, we see the retinotopic map of T3 neurons (simplified from a two-dimensional to a one-dimensional retina for ease of comprehension) with an appropriate projection pathway from neurons in the T3 array to neurons in what we call the *motor heading map*, which will cause the animal to turn toward the retinotopically corresponding location. Unlike the projection from prey-recognition neurons to the motor heading map (in which retinotopically corresponding points are linked by the projection), here we make the connections so that each peak of activity on the T3 layer will have a peak of activity centered at that point which is a compromise between the forward direction and the direction away from the looming stimulus.

(a)

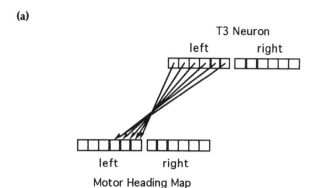

(b)

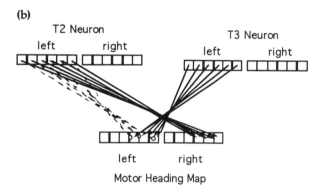

priate motor behavior in this case while avoiding the normal escape behavior. Worth stressing here is that the T3 neurons serve as the basis for the evolution of a more sophisticated set of neurons: the T2 neurons that signal both the presence of a looming stimulus and the presence of a looming stimulus moving on a particular type of trajectory. This new system then *modulates* T3 activity by projecting to the same motor heading map and competing there with the T3 input rather than acting on the T3 array itself. This is another instance of schema evolution and modulation.

We refer the reader to Liaw and Arbib (1993) for further details of the neurophysiological data that ground the model, further details of the circuitry involved in the model, and a number of analyses of the simulations that we have conducted. Here, we close by noting a general property of veretebrate neural control, namely that there may be no place prior to the MPG at which the different representations of the animal's situation are brought together. In general, a multiplicity of different representations must be linked into an integrated whole; however, this may be mediated by distributed processes of competition and cooperation. There need be no single place in the brain where an integrated representation of space plays the sole executive role in linking perception of the current environment to action. We stress that the representation of the world is the pattern of relationships between all its partial representations.

Figure 3.8
Gating of the tectal projection onto the motor heading map. For simplicity, only half of the projections are shown here. (a) The T3 neurons project to the heading map to indicate the escape trajectory for a looming object on a colliding trajectory. (b) When the stimulus is crossing the visual field, the T2 signal blocks the T3 signal while exciting the contralateral heading map, thus resulting in a cut-back jump. (From Liaw and Arbib 1993.)

This will control the MPGs so that the animal escape a directly looming threat.

We show how to model the cutback data in figure 3.8b. First we add the T2 array, which again is retinotopic but now is signaling not simply that there is a looming stimulus at that point of the retina but also there is a stimulus moving from left to right. (We will not look at the corresponding connections for a stimulus on the right half of the visual field moving to the left; this will be simply the mirror image). This activity must block the normal escape response; thus we see a projection from cells of the T2 array to the motor heading map, which is a replica of the projection from the T3 array to the motor heading map, but this new projection is inhibitory. Thus, if there is no T2 activity, the system will respond as in figure 3.8a but not if there is T2 activity. To complete this extended model, we must add a new excitatory pathway from the T2 neurons that project to the cutback direction, thus triggering the appro-

3.3   Schemas for Saccades

Having stressed how schemas may be modulated by new schemas to extend their functionality, we now study saccadic eye movements in the monkey to show how a schema can be extended by integration into an assemblage of other schemas. When a limb moves, it needs a burst of agonist contraction to accelerate the limb in the desired direction and must be followed by an appropriately timed antagonist burst to decelerate it to rest at the desired position (with a possible small agonist correction thereafter); a new resting level of muscle contraction holds the limb in its new position. By contrast, the eye has little inertia; thus, no antagonist burst is required, and the eye has no changing load to require feedback. Robinson (1964) showed that a saccade involved an initial pulse of force to move the eye (of fixed amplitude but increasing in duration with the size of the saccade) followed by a maintained force to hold the eye in its new position. These findings lead naturally into a brief review of the neurophysiology of the circuits controlling the ocular motoneurons for eye movements in the horizontal plane (Fuchs, Kaneko, and Scudder 1985). The excitatory burst neurons (EBNs), located in the paramedian pontine reticular formation, are thought to drive the burst of activity in ipsilateral motoneurons. The inhibitory burst neurons (IBNs) located in the dorsomedial medullary reticular formation inhibit the contralateral motor neurons, thus seeming to control the pause in motoneuron firing during movements in the off direction. Whereas the burst neurons seem involved in the control of the saccade, the tonic neurons (TNs) exhibit regular firing at a rate related (in a nonlinear way) to eye position during and after saccades. TN firing does vary with eye velocity in smooth pursuit of a target, as distinct from a rapid saccade to a target.

The gain of burst cells is very large so as to keep the duration of saccades as small as possible by generating a high-velocity movement when any appreciable motor error exists. In fact, the gain is so high that the model would be unstable were it not that the pulse generators are suppressed during fixation. This is done by the omnipause neurons (OPNs) which fire continuously except that they pause during saccades. There is strong evidence that pause cells inhibit burst cells and prevent them from generating a saccade until released. Another group of burst cells exhibits roughly the same discharge for all but the smallest ipsilateral saccades. These are thought to play a role in triggering a saccade and thus are called *trigger cells*.

These data led to several hypotheses about saccade control. When the OPNs fire (i.e., between saccades), they inhibit the burster neurons (both EBNs and IBNs), thus blocking the burst drive to the motoneurons. For a saccade, the trigger cells silence the OPNs, whereas the EBNs receive a signal to fire, thus raising the firing rate of ipsilateral motoneurons and, via the IBNs, silencing the contralateral motor neurons for the duration appropriate to the length of the saccade. Robinson (1975) suggested that the TNs integrate the firing of the EBNs

$$\text{TN}(t) = k \int^t \text{EBN}(\tau) \, d\tau$$

to obtain the desired eye position for maintaining the gaze after the saccade has occurred.

3.3.1 From Superior Colliculus to the Brainstem Saccade Generator

It is possible to trigger saccades by stimulation of the superior colliculus (SC), the mammalian homolog of the tectum the role of which we have just studied in the frog,

with the length and direction of the saccade encoded retinotopically on the collicular surface (with further subtleties to be explored later). The SC, the primary recipient of the projection from the retina to the midbrain, is a layered structure; activity of cells in the superficial layers of the SC indicates visual activity but with cells in the deep layers activated only for the target of the upcoming saccade. Both maps are retinotopic and in register (i.e., a hypothetical coordinate grid drawn on the retina may be related to a grid on the SC such that, given a point on the retina, a vertical penetration at the corresponding point of the SC will yield cells in the upper layers that are activated by stimulation of the retinal locus and yield cells in the deep SC the firing of which correlates with shift of gaze to a target in that retinal direction). Note that the SC commands an eye movement relative to the current direction of foveal gaze rather than giving commands in a head-centered or body-centered frame.

Deeper layers of monkey SC contain cells that fire before saccades. Each such neuron fires before a range of saccades, thus a large population fires before a particular saccade. Identical discharges by a given cell can precede a variety of saccades, but Sparks and Jay (1985) stated that "it is the location of the active neurons within the topographical map of movement fields, not their frequency of firing, that specifies the trajectory of the saccade," though current evidence suggests that the burst frequency of the ensemble of active collicular neurons affects saccade velocity. The colliculus is related intimately with the pulse generators; The projection from the SC to long-lead burster neurons (LLBNs) is monosynaptic, whereas the latency from deep SC activity to motoneurons is polysynaptic.

van Gisbergen, Robinson, and Gielen (1981) modeled the brainstem saccade burst generator (SG) as a control system that takes as input the desired position of the fovea and provides as output the control signal to the ocular motoneurons, whereas Scudder (1988) extended this model to address the issue of spatial coding in the SC. Saccades may be elicited by stimulation of deep layers of the SC, with target position coded by the position of a peak of activity in a neural map rather than by a single neural variable. The output of the SC is integrated by a neural integrator composed of LLBNs. The retinotopic code of saccade size in the SC is converted to an intensity code by weighting differentially the output of collicular neurons according to the eccentricity of each SC neuron's movement field. The first event is the onset of the SC discharge, which simultaneously begins to charge the LLBN-integrator and to inhibit the OPN by a long-latency indirect pathway. The firing rate envelope of the SC neurons is a simple Gaussian, having a standard deviation of 15 milliseconds. As excitation from the LLBN-integrator discharge increases and the inhibition from the OPN decreases, the net EBN input goes from inhibitory to excitatory. As the EBN fires, the IBN fires and further inhibits the OPN, causing a regenerative increase in EBN and IBN discharge rate. The firing of the IBN also inhibits the LLBN-integrator, causing it to begin to be discharged. Progressively, the LLBN-integrator firing rate decreases until the inhibition of the OPN by the IBN no longer exceeds the excitatory bias of the OPN. The OPN begins firing, and the burst ends. The model matches the physiological data for saccades up to 15 degrees. Scudder (1988) suggests a number of ways in which the model might be extended to fit the data more completely.

SC neurons burst prior to saccades in response to visual targets and also burst before saccades in response to auditory targets. Moreover, with each movement of the eyes in the orbit, the population of neurons responsive to a stationary auditory stimulus changes to a new location within the SC; the auditory input is remapped into retinotopic coordinates for the current eye position (i.e., coordinates that represent the eye movement required for fixation). Somatosensory input also is mapped into the SC. Note that these are very different inputs because the somatosensory input depends on the position of body and limbs, whereas position in auditory input is time-coded via the difference of arrival of signals at the two ears. Thus, mapping the input into visual coordinates seems complex in the former case, comparatively simple in the latter. Stein and Meredith (1993) offer a comprehensive account of such multimodal integration.

An especially interesting property of the maps in superior colliculus is that existing visual targets in superficial layers get remapped to deep layers when the eye moves. Sparks and Mays (1980) used trials in which an intervening saccade changed the position of the eyes after a brief visual target had been extinguished. They discovered quasi-visual cells the location of whose activity, even if the eyes had moved after the target disappeared, represented the current retinotopic position of the remembered target.

3.3.2 Working Memory and Remapping

The logic of modeling integrates both structural and functional considerations. As we saw in our discussion of *Rana computatrix*, the functional definition of a schema becomes refined further as we expand it to include neurophysiological and anatomical data on the brain region(s) posited to implement it, and our definition of particular schemas will be reshaped as this process of model extension proceeds. The use of the coarse functional description at the schema level and the detailed functional-structural description at the neural level is to maintain intelligibility as more and more neural details are incorporated into the model to explain a wider and wider body of behavioral-cognitive data. In this spirit, we consider a multischema view of the saccadic eye-control system. In chapters 8 and 10 we suggest how to replace the constituent schemas by neurophysiologically plausible networks in the cerebral cortex and basal ganglia. The discussion here addresses three types of saccade of increasing subtlety.

The simple-saccade task: A monkey fixates a spot of light that later disappears as another spot of light (target point) appears in another location. The monkey is rewarded for making a saccade to the new target at its onset.

The delayed-saccade task (Hikosaka and Wurtz 1983a): A peripheral target point is illuminated briefly during the display of the fixation point. The monkey is trained to make a saccade to the location of the previously flashed target only after removal of the fixation point, thus showing that it has remembered the location of this target during the period between the removal of the target and the removal of the fixation point.

The double-saccade task (Mays and Sparks 1980): Following offset of the initial fixation point (*F*), targets *A* and *B* are presented successively. The total duration of presentation is less than the time required to initiate the first saccade. Reward is contingent on successive saccades from *F* to *A* and then from *A* to *B*.

Our task is to show how to build on the classic models of saccade control by adding schemas to obtain an overall system able to yield the simple-, delayed- and double-saccade performances, building on the base model found in figure 3.9a. Leaving aside the "eye plant," this model has two schemas, the retinotopic mapper and the saccade burst generator (SG), but it also embodies the structural hypotheses that the retinotopic mapper is implemented by the SC, whereas SG is implemented by the brainstem.

The delayed saccade task requires that the target specification be held in some form of *working memory* rather than being derived from current retinal input. The double-saccade task exhibits a dissociation between the site of retinal stimulation and the metrics of the saccade it elicits. Whereas the initial retinotopic representation of the second target, *B*, in the colliculus would by itself drive a saccade from *F* to *B*, the saccade it elicits starts from *A*, suggesting that a *dynamic remapping* takes place during

(a)

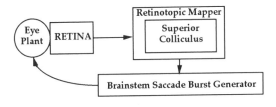

(b)

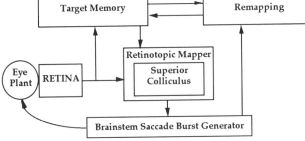

Figure 3.9

(a) The basic model for control of simple saccades. The model has two schemas, the retinotopic mapper and the saccade burst generator (SG), but it also embodies the structural hypotheses that the retinotopic mapper is implemented by the superior colliculus, whereas the SG is implemented by the brainstem. The input to SG codes the target position by the position of a peak of activity in a neural map rather than by a single neural variable. (b) An expanded schema model adds two new schemas, the target memory schema and the remapping schema, to accommodate data on delay saccades and double saccades.

the initial saccade to *B*, effectively subtracting vector **FA** from vector **FB** to yield the actual movement specified by the vector **AB**. This leads us to add the schema for remapping and that for target memory to form fig. 3.9b, but this is incomplete as a schema model. We must spell out in more detail the functionality of each schema. Before doing so, however, we note that even the diagram as it stands makes a number of strong assumptions, not all of which will stand in the light of analysis of further data. First, we assume that retinal input goes to target memory and not to remapping. Second, we assume that the output of target memory is routed to the retinotopic mapper. Finally, we assume that remapping depends on a corollary discharge from SG and has its effect by updating the representation in target memory. Going further, we may say that the target memory will hold a retinotopic target map until a saccade occurs and will make this map available to both remapping and the retinotopic mapper. When a saccade occurs, remapping will use its input from SG to delete the current target and shift the other targets to form a new map to be stored in target memory. In the present example, the schema assemblage may appear no different from a control sys-

tem, but even here we have phasing in and out of the schemas in a task-dependent aggregate of different active schemas, depending on whether a simple, delayed, or double saccade is to be executed.

Note that the foregoing model lacks the circuitry to implement the monkey's knowledge of the current task. In the simple-saccade task, the onset of the target provides both the data that the retinotopic mapper is to encode for SG and the trigger for initiation of a saccade. In the delayed-saccade task, the onset of the target provides the data that target memory is to maintain as input to the retinotopic mapper, but it is the extinction of the fixation point that triggers SG. Finally, for the double-saccade task, the initiation of the first saccade triggers remapping, and it is the completion of remapping that triggers the second saccade.

Chapters 8 and 10 will show how these schemas may be mapped onto the brain. The working memory is posited to be effected by a loop linking the frontal eye fields of cerebral cortex and the mediodorsal nucleus of thalamus, whereas remapping is posited to occur in posterior parietal cortex but with these neural systems augmented by subtle control mechanisms in the basal ganglia.

3.4 Schemas for Reaching and Grasping

We have noted that the role of tectum in directing whole-body movements in frog is analogous to the role of the SC in directing orienting movements in the monkey. The study by N. K. Humphrey (1970) entitled "What the frog's eye tells the monkey's brain" provided a famous example of the attempt to place human cognition in an evolutionary context rooted in mechanisms for instinctive behavior. It had been believed by neurologists that a monkey (or human) without a visual cortex was blind. However, Humphrey argued that a monkey without visual cortex should have at least as much visual ability as a frog but that such monkeys had not been taught to pay attention to available visual cues. He gave 2 years of attention training to a monkey without visual cortex, after which she was able to use visual cues to grab at moving objects and to use changes in luminance—such as an open door—for navigation, even though delicate processes of pattern recognition were never regained. Moreover, it was discovered that humans without visual cortex also could "see" in this sense, but, remarkably, they were not conscious that they could see. This phenomenon is referred to as *blindsight* (Weiskrantz 1974a, b). In section 8.4, we show how Goodale and Milner (1992) distinguish cortical substrates of visual perception in primates (monkeys and humans) from those underlying the visual control of actions, while noting the crosstalk that may integrate these systems in the overall behavior of the organism. Even if the two computations can proceed independently, it does not follow that normally there is no interaction between them. In fact, the planning of more elaborate actions involves the use of both representations (e.g., recognizing the nature of an object normally will affect the way we pick it up). There remains the question as to how information for visual perception "appends itself" to the type of information required for manipulating objects. We continue to emphasize the role of perception in mediating behavior, stressing that in general there is no complete and objective "percept" of an object. Rather a set of partial characterizations (including parameters that we may not be able to represent symbolically or explicitly) is related to the current set of goals and motivations of the observer and may continue unfolding as interaction with (or contemplation of) the object continues. In this section, we focus on an account of the schemas involved in reaching and grasping; it will set the stage for our discussion of cerebral mechanisms in chapter 8 and of related issues in chapters 9 and 10. Section 3.4.1 presents the concepts of virtual fingers and opposition space, allowing us to offer a precise but compact description of the degrees of freedom involved in a number of grasping movements. (Section 8.4 discusses the extent to which these relate to patterns of neural activity in parietal cortex and premotor cortex). Section 3.4.2 offers a series of experiments that reveal flaws in our preliminary model of reaching and grasping, and they lead us to a new coordinated control program that explicitly involves a coordinating schema in addition to perceptual and motor schemas.

3.4.1 Virtual Fingers and Opposition Space

Earlier we studied a coordinated control program that separates the motor schema for arm transport from those for preshaping and then enclosing the hand (see fig. 3.4). However, how is the preshape determined? For the purpose of the control of action, the task of the perceptual schemas is not so much to recognize the object as a ball or pencil in any generic sense as it is to anatomize the object in terms of parameters, such as size and orientation, that are crucial to the task of grasping. Then they can pass these parameters to the various motor schemas for moving and preshaping the hand. In that regard, two concepts, virtual fingers and opposition spaces, have been used to describe human grasping.

Arbib, Iberall, and Lyons (1985) analyzed the task of picking up a mug not directly in terms of what the five fingers do but rather in terms of three *virtual fingers*. The first (always the thumb) places itself on top of the handle. Virtual finger 2 goes through the handle and can contain one, two, three, or even four fingers. Whatever fingers remain constitute virtual finger 3. The concept of the virtual finger tells us how to replace analysis of hand movements directly based on the mechanical degrees of freedom of individual fingers by analysis of the functional roles of the forces being applied in carrying out some task. However, having agreed to analyze the hand in terms of these virtual fingers, how do we specify the movement of these units? Iberall, Bingham, and Arbib (1986) argued that a variety of *opposition spaces* (such as shown in figure 3.10) provides the appropriate coordinate systems.

Of course, when an object is grasped, the virtual fingers moving along the opposition axis may come to

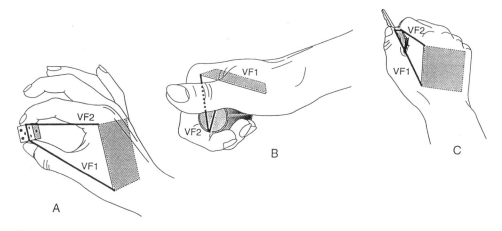

Figure 3.10
Opposition spaces, such as the (A) pad, (B) palm, and (C) side oppositions shown here, are posited to provide coordinates for the control of a variety of hand movements. VF, virtual finger. (Reprint from C. L. MacKenzie and T. Iberall, *The Grosping Hand*, 1994, with kind permission from Elsevier Science–NL, Sara Burgerhartstraat 25, 1055 KV Amsterdam, The Netherlands.)

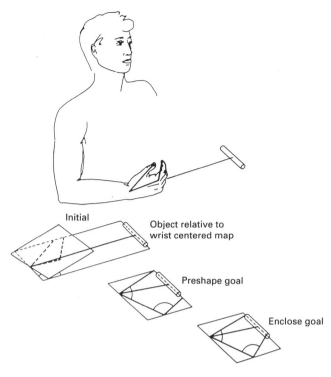

Figure 3.11
Planning the preshape changes the desired offset of the wrist from the center of the object to be grasped, and thus affects the plan for the arm trajectory.

Initial

Object relative to
wrist centered map

Preshape goal

Enclose goal

rest their opposing surfaces on the object between them rather than making direct contact with each other. This makes possible a theory of preshaping (figure 3.11). One task of vision is to determine from the retinal input an opposition space embedded in the object and serving as the target for the positioning of the appropriate opposition space of the hand. There is a safety margin extending the opposition space beyond the boundaries of the object. Preshaping forms the hand so that the opposing surfaces of the virtual fingers will be separated correspondingly. An approach vector between the origin of opposition space and the center of the opposition vector distinguishes the orientation and distance of the hand relative to the object. A virtual finger configuration must be moved from its current state to a desired state under the control of a motor schema. As the hand preshapes to meet this specification (the preshape schema), the arm transports it (the move-arm schema) and the wrist rotates it (the orient schema) to approximately the right position. Note that the target position of the wrist depends on the proposed preshape of the hand: The arm controller must know the offset of the wrist from the center of the opposition space as embedded in the object if it is to transport the hand successfully to its goal. Thereafter, the position of the hand is adjusted to align the two

opposition spaces (that in the hand with that in the object), then virtual fingers close along the aligned axes to grasp the object firmly under tactile control (the enclose schema).

3.4.2 Feedback Control of Reaching to Grasp

The coordinated control program for reaching and grasping can be refined in three stages:

1. We replace the original schema for transport (involving separate schemas for the fast and slow phases of movement) by a single schema that embodies an optimality principle within a feedback controller with delays, which acts like a feedforward controller unless perturbations occur and the delays give time enough to register them.

2. Then, we offer a similar schema for the enclose and preshape schemas that control the hand.

3. Finally, we provide a new schema for coordinating these motor schemas so as to explain empirical data more clearly than does the simple transfer of activation in the original model.

This section is devoted to step 1, whereas the next section continues with steps 2 and 3.

Our original model (see figure 3.4) distinguished two phases of arm movement: a fast phase controlled by a ballistic schema (i.e., one that moves rapidly to completion, unaffected by feedback) followed by a slow phase controlled by a schema that does admit error correction by use of sensory feedback. However, now there is evidence that reaching is subject to modification by sensory input even during the fast phase.

Goodale, Pelisson, and Prablanc (1986) perturbed the target of a pointing task at movement onset. The initial target was 30, 40, or 50 cm from the hand's starting position, and the perturbed target position was 10% farther away. Vision of each subject's hand was prevented, although the target was visible, and subjects consistently undershot the target. However, when the target was perturbed, the movement distance was increased by an amount corresponding to the perturbation. Also, the subject did not stop before moving on to the new target; rather, a smooth transition was made (without secondary accelerations) in midflight to a new trajectory terminating farther away. Thus, ballistic completion of the primary movement was not necessary before implementing a correction trajectory.

Paulignan et al. (1991b) perturbed the location of a vertically oriented dowel on initiation of a reaching movement toward the dowel. Recording the kinematics of reaching and grasping under normal and perturbed conditions, they noted trajectory adjustment within 100 msec (on the average) after target-location perturbation, without compromise of accuracy (i.e., there were no trials in which the subject failed to grasp the dowel). The movements that lasted approximately 500 unperturbed msec, lasted approximately 100 msec longer when the target was shifted at movement onset, indicating on-line incorporation of novel sensory information. Another interesting aspect of this study was that of variability during movement. The authors found that the standard deviation of position in the path reached a maximum of approximately 25 mm during the movement, whereas the standard deviation of the final position was approximately 5 mm. This finding implies that though motor variability causes significant deviation in the path during the movement, some feedback mechanism stabilizes the trajectory toward the end. This aspect of trajectory generation is not taken into account in such models as those fashioned by Schmidt, Zelaznik, and Frank (1977), in which movement variability is lumped into a few parameters of the overall movement (e.g., into the amplitude and duration of the impulse driving the movement, which uniformly scale the entire trajectory).

To address such data (and more), Hoff and Arbib (1992) incorporated an optimality principle into the design of a controller that can use feedback to resist noise and compensate for target perturbations, thus explaining speed-accuracy tradeoffs. The resultant controller (figure 3.12) also uses a predictor element to extrapolate feedback from the periphery (which is received with a delay) so as to get an estimate of the current state. Before proceeding, we should reflect briefly on the terms feedback and feedforward.

Traditionally, a feedback system is one in which, throughout the course of a behavior, measures of actual and desired performance are compared, with the error signal playing a large role in the choice of control signals designed to ensure that the controlled system behaves as desired. Conversely, a feedforward system is one in which the controller has a "model" of the controlled system that, given information about the initial state of the controlled system and a desired behavior, is good enough to generate a complete sequence of control signals that will cause the controlled system to perform as desired without depending on feedback signals. The model provided by Hoff and Arbib (1992) provides a hybrid: a feedback system that can act like a feedforward system in "well-modeled" situations, wherein the conditions of the desired behavior are not perturbed and where the accuracy requirements are such that "normal"

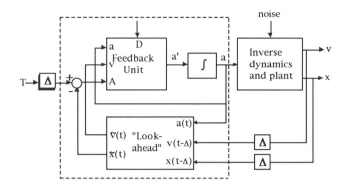

Figure 3.12
An arm transport controller using feedback to generate a time varying trajectory that is feedforward-like in a number of respects. It provides a mechanism for generating a state trajectory by mapping the current state and target into a control signal, $a'(t)$. Plant and inverse dynamics are "lumped together." Command to the plant is specified in terms of acceleration [$a(t)$]. The output of the trajectory generator (a') is in terms of the change in acceleration and is integrated to yield $a(t)$. Time delay for plant state feedback to the trajectory generator is indicated by Δ. Other variables are defined in the text. The controller accepts delayed feedback by calculating the estimates $\tilde{x}(t)$ and $\tilde{v}(t)$ of the present state from the efferent command to the plant, $a(t)$, and delayed feedback, $x(t - \Delta)$ and $v(t - \Delta)$. The "lookahead" for each of x and v is provided by a "sliding-window integrator" (details not shown) integrating its input over time for the past (Δ) time interval. Because noise is present in the plant, what is generated is only an estimate of the actual state. (From Hoff and Arbib 1992.)

errors in execution may be ignored - the error signal remains close enough to zero to have little or no effect on the unfolding behavior. However, when perturbations must be accommodated or when the precision required of the movement makes small errors intolerable, the feedback plays a crucial role in keeping the behavior close to that desired. A particular feature of the model is that it takes explicit account of delays in putting feedback into effect. One particular consequence of this is the explanation of Fitts' law effects in which increased movement accuracy can be obtained only at the price of a slower movement which allows sufficient time for feedback to be factored into the ongoing control.

Hoff and Arbib (1992) adopted the optimality principle used by Hogan (1984) to model the elbow rotations in pointing movements of monkeys toward a visually located target. Like other models in this section, his model takes target position as its input and yields acceleration of the hand endpoint as its output, thus ignoring the way in which motoneuron activity controls the dynamics of the muscle and skeleton of the limb. He proposed the minimum-jerk criterion: The arm's end point is moved in such a way that a trajectory of duration D will be such as to minimize the integral

3 A Functional Overview

$$\int_0^D \left[\frac{d^3x}{dt^3}\right]^2 dt$$

of the square of the *jerk*, the derivative of acceleration. This yields (by the calculus of variations) a position function of time given by a fifth-order polynomial, uniquely specified by the initial and final values of position, velocity, and acceleration. If the target is stationary at the start and end of the movement, then the hand's predicted path is a straight line, whereas the velocity profile is symmetrical and bell-shaped. This is a good match with the low-accuracy pointing movements of subjects performing unconstrained arm movements in the horizontal plane, holding a light-weight manipulandum (Flash and Hogan 1985). Because the trajectory depends only on the initial and final positions of the hand, these movement profiles are predetermined and then executed, as in the ballistic (fast-phase) schema that forms part of figure 3.4.

Hoff and Arbib built on this process. If the system state is $q = (x, v, a)^*$ (the ordered triple of position, velocity, and acceleration, where * denotes the transpose), the initial position is x_o, and the target position T, then the original minimum jerk formulation links the initial state $(x_o, 0, 0)^*$ and the final state $(T, 0, 0)^*$. For our model, we generalize the boundary conditions to allow a non-static initial state, $(x_o, v_o, a_o)^*$. Then, in considering the hand's acceleration (second derivative of position and hence a cubic polynomial), Hoff and Arbib showed (the nonmathematical reader may skip directly to the text following equation 4) that the boundary conditions yield the following expression:

$$a(t) = a_o[1 - 9\tau + 18\tau^2 - 10\tau^3] + v_o/D[-36\tau + 96\tau^2$$
$$- 60\tau^3] + (T - x_o)/D^2[60\tau - 180\tau^2 + 120\tau^3] \quad (1)$$

where the movement begins at $t = t_o$ and ends at $t = t_f$, so that $D = t_f - t_o$ is the duration and $\tau = (t - t_o)/D$ is the normalized time variable. Setting v_o and a_o to zero yields the acceleration component of the trajectory derived by Hogan (1984). As it stands, equation 1 offers no mechanism for responding to perturbations in the arm's state or the target location. Hoff and Arbib thus employ equation 1 to design a feedback controller which compensates inherently for perturbations during motion:

$$\frac{dq}{dt} = \mathbf{A}q + \mathbf{B}T, \quad (2)$$

where $q = (x, v, a)^*$ is the system state vector, the target position T is the input, and the matrix $\mathbf{A}$ and vector $\mathbf{B}$ embody the system dynamics. Because q', the rate of change of the state, depends on the current state, pertur-

bations in the state are reflected in the modified trajectory. Already we have the first two components for $q' = \frac{dq}{dt}$, namely $x' = v$ and $v' = a$, so it remains to compute a', the derivative of acceleration, which we do by differentiating equation 1,

$$\frac{da(t)}{dt} = a_o/D[-9 + 36\tau - 30\tau^2]$$
$$+ v_o/D^2[-36 + 192\tau - 180\tau^2]$$
$$+ (T - x_o)/D^3[60 - 360\tau + 360\tau^2]$$

which gives a' at any time from $t = t_o$ to t_f. Now let t_o, x_o, v_o, and a_o be the current values of time and state rather than the values at the beginning of movement. Then we can find the current value of a' by setting $t = t_o$, so $\tau = 0$:

$$\frac{da(t_o)}{dt} = -9a_o/D - 36v_o/D^2 + 60(T - x_o)/D^3 \quad (3)$$

where again D is the time remaining in the movement, $D = t_f - t$. Hence, the system can be described by equation 2, with

$$\mathbf{A} = \begin{bmatrix} 0 & 1 & 0 \\ 0 & 0 & 1 \\ -60/D^3 & -36/D^2 & -9/D \end{bmatrix},$$

$$\mathbf{B} = \begin{bmatrix} 0 \\ 0 \\ 60/D^3 \end{bmatrix} \quad (4)$$

The controller does not store an entire temporal trajectory, as in a feedforward system. Instead, it need generate only D, the time remaining, and monitor the current state q and target T. However, we need one more modification to obtain our new schema for reaching to grasp to replace the two subschemas of the reaching schema of figure 3.4. The foregoing formulas use instantaneous feedback, whereas in reality, the current target hand velocity and position v and x are sensed with some latency. Hoff and Arbib thus designed "look-ahead" units to estimate the plant's position and velocity from delayed feedback in the presence of noise by forming the integral of its input over the most recent time period, Δ. If the noise is unbiased, this is the most reasonable estimate of the current state. With no mechanical noise or unexpected perturbations of the hand, the look-ahead module gives a precise prediction. However, noise causes prediction (and hence control) error, so that slower movement is required to maintain accuracy. In

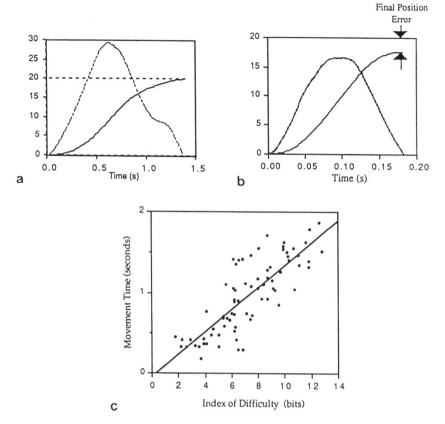

Figure 3.13

Sample simulations of slow (accurate) and fast (inaccurate) movements. (a) A slow (1,400-msec) one-dimensional reaching movement attained the target position within 0.7% when the hand first slowed to zero velocity. The monotonically increasing curve represents hand position in centimeters during the 20-cm reach. The other curve is velocity in centimeters per second. Horizontal broken line, the target position. (b) A fast (182-msec) movement undershot the target position by 12.3%. Hand position is, again, in centimeters, whereas velocity is calculated by multiplying by 10 cm/sec (e.g., peak velocity is 170 cm/sec). In each simulation, feedback delay is 250 milliseconds. Note that the low speed in *a* allows delayed feedback information to correct the movement, as is evident in the slowed deceleration visible in the velocity profile. (c) For 75 simulated movements, this is a plot of speed (represented as movement time) versus final position error [represented as index of difficulty: $\log_2(2T/|T - x_e|)$, where T is the target position and x_e is the actual final position of the system]. Also shown is the least-squares-fit line, which corresponds to Fitts' speed-accuracy tradeoff: MT = $-0.033 +$ 0.137 ID. (From Hoff and Arbib 1992.)

using look-ahead modules to compensate for latencies in receipt of sensory data, we have introduced a principle of *neural synchrony*. The brain may provide erroneous control signals unless there are explicit subnetworks to compensate for delays so as to give the brain the best estimate possible of the current state of the organism and its environment (see the general issue of extrapolation of time series in Wiener 1949).

To investigate the speed-accuracy tradeoff in such movements, Hoff and Arbib simulated a 20-cm reaching movement, using movement times ranging from 200 to 1400 msec, with noise added to the movement that increased as a function of velocity. Sensorimotor delay was assumed to be $\Delta = 250$ msec, the nominal reaction time to visual stimuli. Because the servo nature of the controller along with the nature of the mechanical model ensures zero error in every case if the movement is allowed

to proceed indefinitely, a movement-end criterion had to be imposed. Thus they simulated the movement until the hand velocity first decelerated to zero, at which moment they collected movement time and accuracy data for examination of speed-accuracy tradeoff. The anticipated effect of longer movement time is that the slower movements will have more time to take advantage of the feedback delayed by 250 msec, in addition to the fact that because of our formulation of mechanical noise, slower movements will have less variability. Figure 3.13 shows sample simulations of slow (accurate) and fast (inaccurate) movements. Figure 3.13a shows a slow (1400-msec) reaching movement that attained the target position within 0.7%. The monotonically increasing curve represents hand position in centimeters, during the 20-cm reach. The other curve is velocity in centimeters per second. Figure 3.13b shows a fast (182-msec) movement that undershot the target position by 12.3%. Note that the low speed in figure 3.13a allows delayed feedback information to correct the movement, compensating for earlier kinematic variability, as is evident in the slowing of deceleration visible in the velocity profile. This adjustment for accuracy during deceleration may be the source of asymmetry in the velocity profiles of the accurate movements discussed earlier, because slowing the rate of deceleration lengthens the tail of the velocity profile. Figure 3.13b duplicates the more symmetrical profile of a low-accuracy movement, as described by the minimum-jerk formulation of Hogan (1984).

Figure 3.13c shows the speed-accuracy relationship for 75 simulated movements of various speeds. Note the variation caused by our assumption of mechanical noise in the system. Speed is plotted in terms of movement time. Accuracy is plotted in terms of the index of difficulty (ID) in Fitts' law, which is defined as the logarithm of twice the ratio of movement amplitude (T) to target size (W) [i.e., ID = $\log_2(2T/W)$]. Hence, the ID is large when the target is small compared to the movement amplitude. For us, $W = |T - x_e|$ where x_e is the actual final position of the system. Clearly, there is an increasing relationship between the two variables in figure 3.13c. For comparison, the least-squares-fit line is shown, corresponding to the form of the relationship predicted by Fitts' law. Hoff and Arbib also showed that the model can address data from the target-perturbation experiments of Goodale, Pelisson, and Prablanc (1986) and Georgopoulos, Kalaska, and Massey (1981).

Given this analysis, how might the speed-accuracy tradeoff described by Fitts' law be learned? We suggest that through experience of carrying out movements at various speeds, we learn that different velocities yield different errors. Later, our mature behavior reflects the (perhaps implicit) use of this knowledge; given a desired accuracy, we slow down to a velocity known unconsciously to be highly likely to keep the error within the desired bounds. This will allow time to use the delayed-error signals at a rate that will keep them within acceptable bounds.

3.4.3 Coordination of Reach and Grasp

Figure 3.4 embodies another claim: that the transition from preshaping to enclosing is controlled by the slowing of the transport phase, but is not influenced by it. Recent data suggest the existence of subtle influences in both directions. For example, Paulignan et al. (1991a) found that when the hand has to open wider (if object size is increased during reach), transport slows by ap-

proximately 200 milliseconds. They also found (Paulignan et al. 1991b) that when target location is perturbed, the hand temporarily closes so that maximum aperture is delayed as transport takes longer to reach the new target. In this context, Hoff and Arbib (1993) modeled the schema for control of the grasp and its interaction with grasping to explain such data.

Basing their study of the preshape schema on that of the transport schema, these authors sought an appropriate optimality principle to use in place of the minimum-jerk criterion. Some smoothness criterion is needed to prevent discontinuous "jumps" in the preshape, whereas the partial reclosing of the hand during prolonged movement caused by location perturbation implies that there is some "cost" to having the hand open more than a certain amount. The relative importance of these two criteria is not known a priori. Thus, a weighting parameter is introduced, yielding the criterion

$$\int_0^D \left[x(t)^2 + w\left(\frac{d^2x}{dt^2}\right)^2 \right] dt$$

for preshape, where $x(t)$ is the hand's aperture and w controls the relative weighting of the two components; w is tuned empirically to best match the optimal trajectory of a typical data set. Our hypothesis is that for a trajectory of an expected length, the hand will open slowly during the preshape, thus reducing both terms in this optimality criterion. However, when the controller expects a short movement, by a given stage it will have opened the hand more than would be appropriate for a longer movement. Thus, if a perturbation then signals that a longer movement is required, the hand will close somewhat to reduce the cost of the first term and later will open again. Clearly, the value of w is crucial. If w were very large, the cost of changing the grip size would dominate the cost of maintaining the grip size, and there would be little decrease of the grip size, during a prolongation of movement. If, on the other hand, w were very small, the cost of holding the hand open would dominate, and we would see almost no preshape, with the hand staying in its relaxed state until the very last moment, when a sudden increase in size would adapt the hand to its target object.

The preceding paragraph already holds implicit the strategy for coordinating the motor schemas set forth in figure 3.14. Here, the enclose schema is a replica of the preshape schema, with the only exception that its starting point is the maximum aperture achieved by the preshape schema. The data suggest a linear relation between the actual object size and the maximum aperture achieved.

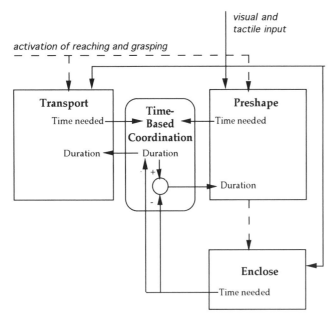

visual and
tactile input

activation of reaching and grasping

Transport

Time needed

Duration

Time-Based Coordination

Duration

+

-

Duration

Preshape

Time needed

Duration

Enclose

Time needed

Figure 3.14
Feedback controllers for transport and preshape. "Cooperative computation" between subprograms is mediated by a coordinating schema ensuring that both reaching and grasping have adequate movement time. (From Hoff and Arbib 1993.)

We require that the coordinating schema receive from each of the constituent schemas—transport, preshape, enclose—an estimate of the time that it needs to move from its current state to the desired final state (or, in the case of the enclose schema, from its *expected* initial state to its *expected* final state.) At the moment, we have only an ad hoc algorithm for estimating these durations, and we consider it a task for our future research to determine how the brain finds, represents, and transmits them. Nonetheless, here we can see that the basis for coordination is very simple: We compare the time needed for transport with the sum of the times needed for preshape and enclose. Also, we assume that the perturbations will not affect the enclose phase; thus, any adjustment will be provided either to the transport or to the preshape schemas. Simply put, whichever schema is going to take longer—Transport or Grasp (Preshape + Enclose), is given the full time it needs, whereas the other schema will be slowed down to apply its optimality criterion from its current state to completion over the longer time base. There is a satisfactory match between data and simulation.

With these and preceding results, we see again a truth better known in motor control than in other areas of neurophysiology: that much is to be learned at the level of schema analysis prior to, or in concert with, the "lower-level" analysis of neural circuitry. Though the

hypotheses developed in this section allow us to gain insight into the interaction of a number of different processes, they also pose major challenges for further neurophysiological investigation. Can we show that neural networks in the brain really do embody the look-ahead principles and the dynamic exemplification of the optimality principles that we have hypothesized? Is time represented in the brain, and if so, is it represented in a fashion that would allow the neural implementation of the time-based coordination of figure 3.14? We note that work on the many visual systems of the monkey (reviewed in sec. 8.4) shows us that separate visual pathways do exist for the information postulated in the perceptual schemas of figure 3.4. We also know from the classic studies of Brinkman and Kuypers (1972) that the transport and grasp motor schemas can be impaired differentially by lesions both in the sensory and in the motor pathways. For further investigation, we might suggest that the transport and grasp schemas are controlled through different cortical pathways, whereas the cerebellum plays a primary role in the coordination of these activities. However, even this parcellation of function is too simplistic, for we know that the basal ganglia also play an important role in the coordination of movement and thus must be included in the full story of the schemas for reaching and grasping (also true for the schemas involved in saccadic eye movements). We will return to many of these issues in chapters 8, 9, and 10.

3.5 Schemas Representing Space and Time

Modeling the brain in terms of interacting neurons is a well-established part of computational neuroscience. However, we have argued that cognitive neuroscience needs at least another level of analysis in which assemblages of schemas express the functional interactions underlying cognition and behavior at a more molar level. Our studies of frog and toad (and the study of neural mechanisms for looking, reaching and grasping to be elaborated in chapters 8, 9, and 10) show how behavioral and neurophysiological studies may be integrated to expand a schema analysis to an assemblage in which the function of specific schemas is delegated to particular regions of the brain. When a schema is provided with a precise functional characterization and a neurological localization, it sets the appropriate framework for neural network modeling.

These considerations have shown that the control of complex behavior cannot be embodied in a single neural network but must be analyzed in terms of a network of complex subsystems. A variety of control systems manage different subsystems but with subtle mechanisms of coordination to modulate the dynamics of these different components into a harmonious whole. Schema theory provides the language for representing the interaction between these systems, whereas neural networks (with or without adaptation) provide the implementation for these subsystems at some suitable level of refining schemas into subschemas. This background leads to a brief discussion of the neural representations of space and time that our studies have so far revealed.

Rana computatrix: We studied pattern recognition for Prey, Predators, and Barriers. The models revealed the following representations:

Regarding space, we saw retinotopic mapping to multiple brain regions and also saw that the animal's pattern of action may be based on the trajectory of objects (normal versus cutback avoidance behavior) and on the relative position of objects (i.e., that the maps for prey and barrier must be brought into register so that the animal will snap directly or detour, whichever is appropriate).

In the context of time, once behavior is triggered by perception, it proceeds to completion in the specified and appropriate order. This effect can be quite subtle. In their simulation of a neural network to detect looming objects, Liaw and Arbib (1993) found the behaviorally appropriate result that reaction time diminishes as the approach velocity of the looming predator increases.

The representation of the world is provided by the distributed interactions of a set of partial (incomplete, possibly inaccurate) representations.

In the **saccadic system**, the brainstem saccade generator converts space (retinotopic code) to time (firing of the excitatory burst neurons). The working memory holds a "plan" (the retinotopic position of targets) until it is executed, whereas dynamic remapping updates the plan as action proceeds.

The neural mechanisms in parietal cortex, frontal eye fields, thalamus, and basal ganglia underlying saccadic eye movements (to be discussed in chapters 8 and 10) provide simple examples of capabilities crucial to the development of intelligent behavior. Schemas allow an overall functional analysis of the system, but each brain region cooperates in the implementation of many schemas, and each schema may involve the competition and cooperation of many brain regions. Thus, each schema find its true meaning only through its embedding within the overall schema network. Our brains and our science proceed by successive approximations to reality.

Reaching and grasping encompass space and time. With regard to space, we may distinguish two spaces:

(1) the peripersonal, or body-centered, space in which an object must be located to guide the reaching movement and (2) the object-centered space in which the appropriate preshaping and orientation of the hand is determined. Section 8.4.3 contains a review of some recent data on the neural coding of these spaces, coding that occurs in parietal and premotor cortices.

As concerns time, we have seen that timing plays a crucial role here in at least two ways. First, in reaching, the speed of a movement must be reduced (i.e., the duration must be increased) as increasing demands are made on accuracy. Additionally, we offered a schema-theoretic model in which the coordination of reaching and grasping is mediated by an explicit representation of the duration of each movement. We saw also that the brain must take into account that neural signals may be based on sensory and motor events signaled with varying delays, so that some form of extrapolation or lookahead is needed to provide a coherent view of signals at each nexus wherein they are brought together.

The foregoing discussions highlight the multiplicity of "times" and "spaces" in the brain, so that euclidean space and newtonian time are an abstraction from our experience, which in turn is implemented through the interaction of a multiplicity of partial representations in the brain. In part II, we refine our schema analyses through the analysis of a wealth of neuroanatomical and neurophysiological data. Also, we look in detail at several examples of a most crucial example of timing: rhythmical behavior (or oscillations), an example of the dynamical systems behavior to whose overview we now turn.

A Dynamical Overview

In this chapter, we show why and how dynamical system theory provides mathematical tools for describing the spatiotemporal operation of the nervous system. A dynamical system operates in time. Typically, we take the time set T to be the real line $\mathscr{R}$ (a continuous-time system) or the set of integers $\mathbb{Z}$ (a discrete-time system). We then formalize an *autonomous system* as an ordered pair (Q, g), where Q is the state space, and $g : T \times Q \to Q$ is a function that assigns to each initial state $x_o \in Q$ the state $x = g(t, x_o)$, in which the system will be after a time interval t if it started in state x_o. A fundamental property of g, then, is the validity of the identity

$$g(t + s, x) \equiv g(s, g(t, x_o)) \text{ for all states } x, \text{ and times } t, s.$$

The behavior of a dynamic system may also depend on the time course of the input applied. Systems that take into account the effect of inputs are called non-autonomous systems. They have important neurobiological significance when the effect of the continuous sensory input is taken explicitly into consideration.

As we have seen, the brain is considered a prototype of hierarchical structures: Neural systems can be studied at one or more levels, such as the molecular, membrane, cellular, synaptic, network, and system levels. Similarly, mathematical models of dynamical systems can be classified into two groups: single-level and multilevel (hierarchical) models.

Two main neurodynamical problems are treated within these frameworks: Problems with fixed wiring, in which we study the dynamics of activity spreading through the entire network or the temporal change of activity at specific neurons; and problems in which modifiable synapses are taken into consideration in normal ontogenetic development as well as in learning, as a network is tuned by experience. The concept of state space, derived from the theory of mechanics and thermodynamics and generalized by mathematical system theory (e.g., Kalman, Falb, and Arbib 1969), is particularly useful in describing neural systems. A class of neurodynamical problems can be studied by single-level models that describe the temporal evolution of either the activation of the cells or the strengths of synaptic connections. However, many network models use two levels by coupling the levels of neuron activity and connectivity dynamics (synaptic modifiability). A two-level state space can be obtained by combining the activation space with the weight space of connectivities.

Section 4.1.1 introduces the key dynamical concept of an attractor, a pattern of activity that captures nearby states of an autonomous system. An attractor may be an equilibrium point, a limit cycle (oscillation), or a strange attractor (chaotic behavior). (A critique of an approach to neural computation based on attractors will follow in section 4.5.4.) Both ontogenetic development of neural structures and their plastic behavior often are considered as dynamic processes in the state space of synaptic connections. "Synaptic selection" is one form of such a dynamic process, but the "self-organization" of the nervous system is, in general, a broader process, including addition as well as removal of synapses, and the modification of synaptic strengths. As we shall see in detail in chapter 8, modular architectonics may be seen as a pattern of organization resulting from the dynamics of self-organization rather than being completely laid down in the genome.

Section 4.1.2 introduces some of the specific formalisms used to treat neurons and neural networks as dynamic systems. First, we recall the framework for the detailed treatment of the membrane potential dynamics of a patch of neuron—the neuronal cable equation and the Hodgkin-Huxley equation and its relatives. Synaptic currents provide external input to the system. An entire neuron may be represented by a multicompartment model, with compartments chosen to take into account the location of the entering synaptic currents or the geometry of dendritic branching, say, or as a single-compartment model characterized by a single membrane potential. The leaky integrator neuron is a popular model for the single-compartment case. The McCulloch-Pitts neuron is the simplest neural model, representing the neuron as a discrete-time binary-state element. Whatever the representation of the individual neuron, neural tissues may be modeled as networks of intricately connected neurons in which strengths w_{ij} of the synaptic connections may themselves be described by differential (or difference) equations, the learning rules that will be studied in section 4.5. The input to such a network is provided by the afferents that provide inputs to sensory neurons. Behavior of large networks of neurons may be studied by population theories.

In section 4.1.3, we look at the structure-function problem: For what overall patterns of connectivity will a network exhibit the simple behavior of passage to a stable equilibrium point. In general, the quantitative and qualitative effects of parameter changes are studied by sensitivity analysis and bifurcation theory, respectively. The Wigner-May theorem provides conditions on the eigenvalues of matrices associated with randomly connected networks, whereas other results focus on the signs of entries of the jacobian. Unfortunately, these results are suggestive rather than directly applicable to biologically realistic models of neural networks.

Section 4.2 introduces the topic of oscillatory behavior in neural systems. Section 4.2.1 notes three types of experimental data: evidence for single-cell oscillations resulting from the interplay of a few currents (e.g., low-threshold calcium conductance); central pattern generators (CPGs), in which network of neurons can produce rhythmical behavior in the absence of sensory input (either due to single-cell oscillations or neural interactions); and a preview of the oscillatory activity studied in more detail in later chapters—olfactory oscillations (chapter 5), hippocampal oscillations (chapter 6), and thalamocortical oscillations (chapter 8). Section 4.2.2 then introduces a number of mathematical techniques for studying oscillations. Variants of the Hodgkin-Huxley equation are used in the study of single-cell oscillators. Of particular interest are bifurcation analyses, which show a transition from equilibrium point to small-amplitude oscillation, or from oscillation to chaos, as some control parameter passes through a critical value. Picking up the theme of section 4.1.3, we turn to the network architecture of possible rhythm generators. First we consider qualitative criteria on the signs of synaptic couplings that guarantee that a network will oscillate. Then we study phase lags in chains of oscillators (mimicking data on the spinal cord of the lamprey), the importance of long-range coupling in the synchronization of more fully coupled networks (as in models of cortical structures), and bifurcation analysis of gait transitions in locomotion.

Section 4.3 addresses chaotic behavior in the nervous system. Though many models of neural systems have been proved to exhibit chaos, verification that an actual neural system exhibits chaos (rather than being random or deterministic in some complicated but nonchaotic way) often remains controversial. Section 4.3.1 notes that chaotic systems are characterized by sensitivity to initial conditions and relates this to positive Lyapunov exponents. Subsequent sections show that the structural conditions of chaos occur at different hierarchical levels of neural organization. Both periodic and chaotic temporal patterns can be generated at the single-neuron level (sec. 4.3.2). Basic phenomena can be modeled with membrane equations involving two functionally distinct currents, the slow and fast currents, in which a series of complex patterned activities (simple slow oscillation, bursting, bursting-chaos, beating-chaos, and beating) can be generated by changing the time constant of inactivation of the slow current.

Neurochemical synaptic transmission often is characterized as a random process, but section 4.3.3 notes that the dripping faucet model may be adapted to explain this apparent randomness as a case of deterministic chaos. Section 4.3.4 shows how chaos may emerge at the multicellular network level due to interactions among neurons, extending the qualitative conditions on connectivity of neural networks—the network architecture—defined earlier for convergence to a point equilibrium (sec. 4.1.3) and for rhythm generation (sec. 4.2.2). Section 4.3.5 notes that cortical dynamics, as seen at the global level in the electroencephalogram (EEG), also may exhibit chaotic behavior. Section 4.3.6 discusses "dynamical diseases," introducing the diagnosis and also the control of chaos associated with normal and pathological brain functions. Section 4.3.7 then closes this introduction to chaotic neural behavior by discussing the possible (controversial but intriguing) functional roles of chaos in normal brain activity, including perception and memory formation.

In section 4.4.1, we return to the analysis of self-organizing mechanisms related to normal ontogenetic development (sec. 4.4) and learning (sec. 4.5), emphasizing the trade-off between determinism and randomness. Section 4.4.2 then focuses on retinotectal connections, providing a clear discussion of specificity versus plasticity; genetically prespecified versus environmentally controlled wiring; marker theories versus activity-dependent mechanisms; decrease of synaptic strength by normalization rule only or by selective mechanism; deterministic versus stochastic models; sets of discrete nerve cells versus continuous neural fields; and positional information. The last part of this section reviews the choices made in a specific model that matches a range of data and shows the importance of noise-induced transitions.

Section 4.5 provides a general framework for considering learning as a dynamic process in the state space of synaptic connection weights. Section 4.5.1 introduces hebbian learning and its variations, which include means to avoid saturation of synaptic strengths, ways to accommodate various time delays, and differential learning mechanisms, as well as antihebbian rules to describe features of pattern dissociations. Section 4.5.2 focuses on synaptic matrix models of associative memory but concludes with a treatment of how invariant pattern recognition may be modeled using the dynamic-link architecture, in which hebbian plasticity is invoked on a fast

time scale for information processing as well as on a slow time scale for learning. Section 4.5.3 introduces Hopfield networks to show how much recent work on neural networks has been motivated by statistical mechanics, including ideas of "energy", "temperature", and the statistical distribution of patterns in relation to an attractor-based model of pattern recognition. In this model, passage of the system to a pattern recognition attractor depends only on the internal state of the system and not on the sensory input. This provides the essential background for the critique of computation with attractors in section 4.5.4. The many explicit and implicit modifications of Hopfield's classic scenario include consideration of limit cycles and strange attractors, analysis of dynamic equations for connectivity (including a time-dependent energy function), and a more general analysis of the change of the system as depending both on the internal state of the system and on the time-dependent sensory input. This leads to a discussion of continuous learning and dynamic categories. The chapter closes with section 4.5.5, which provides explicit pointers to the treatment, in later chapters, of the varieties of learning in the brain, including the relation of learning rules to long-term potentiation (LTP) and depression (LTD), examples of unsupervised learning in the development of the visual system (chapter 8), reinforcement learning due to neuromodulators (chapters 8 and 10), and supervised learning found in the cerebellum (chapter 9).

4.1 Neurodynamical System Theory

4.1.1 Neurodynamical Phenomena: Conceptual Frameworks

Dynamics and Attractors

Static and dynamic structures appear as distinct forms of the macroscopic world. *Static structures*, such as rocks, are maintained by the large interacting forces among their constituents. The perturbation of the environment causes only very slight effects, at least in the range of stability of the structure. More intensive perturbation yields the complete breakdown of the structure. The new "structureless" structure also is static.

Dynamic structures, in open systems such as living systems, are maintained by the interaction between the system and its environment. The system itself is in permanent material, energetic, and informational interaction with the external world.

For the time being, we will consider the case in which dynamic structures can be treated as autonomous systems

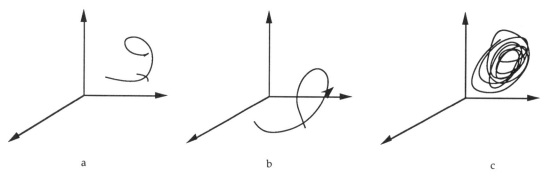

Figure 4.1
The visualization of three type of attractors, and the convergence of trajectories to them: (a) Point attractor. (b) Periodic attractor. (c) Strange attractor.

$g: T \times Q \to Q$ (i.e., we consider the case in which the external world may provide inputs that maintain the overall structure of the open system but we do not—for now—consider the case in which input patterns play a causal role in the system's dynamics). The borderline between static and dynamic structures is rather arbitrary: The static structures of the morphologist may be considered as dynamic ones from the thermodynamic point of view. More precisely, they might be interpreted as the final states (attractors) of real time-dependent structures.

An *attractor* is a subset A of the state space Q that "attracts" the trajectory of nearby states. More formally, A is an attractor if

1. $g(t, x) \in A$ for all x in A and all $t \geqslant 0$.

2. No proper subset of A has property (1).

3. Stability Property: For every $x \in A$ there exists $\varepsilon > 0$ such that each state y with distance from y to x satisfying $d(y, x) < \varepsilon$ has the property that $d(g(t, y), A) \to 0$ as $t \to \infty$ (i.e., every point "near enough" to A tends to move closer to A).

We then define the *basin of attraction* of A to be the set of all those states y such that $d(g(t, y), A) \to 0$ as $t \to \infty$. In the simplest case, trajectories of dynamic systems converge to a stable equilibrium point, as time tends to infinity. An equilibrium point is a state x in which the system stays at rest: $g(t, x) \equiv x$ for all $t \geqslant 0$, thus satisfying (1) and (2). To say an equilibrium point is stable is to say that it satisfies (3).

Closed curves also may serve as attractors, which then are called *limit cycles*. Nonlinear systems can possess these periodic attractors. Trajectories that do not tend to point or periodic attractors are called *strange attractors* and are associated with chaotic processes. *Chaotic processes* often are labeled as causal but unpredictable, and they are considered to be complexity producing. Chaotic phenomena have been found at almost all hierarchical

levels of the nervous system, from the membrane through the network to the system level. The three different types of attractors visualized in the state space are shown in figure 4.1. Convergence to equilibrium, oscillation, and chaos occurring in neural systems are the main subject of this chapter.

The formation and recognition of spatiotemporal and abstract patterns are essential aspects of information-processing devices. Biological pattern-generating mechanisms, occurring at different hierarchical levels (from molecular to ecological), may share common formal structures (Rosen 1981; Murray 1989). Ontogenetic development of neural structures and their plastic behavior often are considered as dynamic processes in the state space of synaptic connections, and both should be explained by common mechanisms. Both embryonic and postnatal development result from the interaction of a built-in connectivity pattern generator with environmental factors. Though the full genetic coding of brain structures cannot be excluded by algebraic arguments once basic regularities are taken into account, such complete coding is highly improbable since the complexity of anatomical structures increases much faster than that of the genome (Changeux, Heidmann, Patte 1984; see also Rager 1983).

The most popular pattern-forming theories offer a third option between two extreme hypotheses—the *preformationist*, which states that neural wiring is strictly prespecified genetically, and the *empiricist*, which overemphasizes the role of neural activities in specifying connectivities. Several such theories adopt the notion of selection. In the neurobiological context, this means that favorable (and dynamically modifiable) connections of neurons are selected by some mechanism. The selective stabilization hypothesis (Changeux, Courrege, and Danchin 1973; Changeux and Danchin 1976; Changeux 1985, pp. 227–229) argues that the genetic code sketches an initial connectivity pattern that is both exuberant (more connections are made initially than will eventually be retained) and subject to some random fluctuations. The subset of these synapses that are stabilized, (i.e., endure into the adult) then is determined by an activity-dependent selection process. What are the units of selection? Changeux, Heidmann, and Patte (1984) answer that spontaneous activity of neurons is selected, whereas Edelman (1987) speaks about the role of groups: Stages of selection of neural patterns are the group confinement (i.e., the limitations of group size), group selection, and group competition. The main conceptual advantage of the selective stabilization hypothesis is that it suggests a gene-saving mechanism for specifying ordered neural structures. Different mechanisms of synaptic elimination may occur in various structures: Cell death, axon retractions, and axon regrowth are characteristic examples (Clarke 1981). We agree with Stent (1981), who argued for the fundamental role of "developmental noise" (Waddington 1957) to produce phenotypical variation in the nervous system.

However, selection approaches may be misleading if they suggest that the genes have anticipated all possible demands of the organism by providing a prespecified set of neural structures from which a selection may be made. Rather, they may be seen as providing "sketches" for neural networks, first approximations on which synaptic plasticity may operate to yield a pattern of connectivity adapted to the particular pattern of organism-environment interaction. Synaptic selection is just one theoretical approach to self-organization, the ability of a system to change its structure on the basis of its own activity (which may or may not depend, in part, on a shaping role of the external world; see sec. 4.4.1 for further discussion). However, our approach to self-organization in this book will be broader than selective stabilization, in general corresponding to a combination of (1) structural changes due to the alteration of synaptic connectivity patterns, which may include addition as well as removal of synapses; and (2) the modification of synaptic strengths of the individual connections of the essentially unchanged network. Synaptic mobility occurs in the adult brain, too. Reactive synaptogenesis, like developmental synaptogenesis, is a highly complex process. Although the nervous system cannot generate new neurons to compensate for cell death (though there are exceptions, as in the song system of the male songbird), proliferation of new cell processes (e.g., axonal sprouting) can substitute functionally for those that have been lost. Dramatic structural changes occur in response to partial denervation (Cotman, Nieto-Sampedro, and Harris 1981)

and have been observed to yield functional reorganization in the somatosensory cortex (Merzenich and Kaas 1980; Merzenich et al. 1983; Merzenich 1987) and in the visual cortex (Kaas et al. 1990; Darian-Smith and Gilbert 1994).

Self-Organization in the Nervous System

Although vague in many respects, the idea of self-organization is nevertheless a powerful concept of modern theoretical sciences. The concept of self-organization is associated with more or less abstract notions, e.g. macroscopic order and disorder, pattern formation and recognition, emergence of complexity, noise-induced transition.

Both ontogenetic development and phylogenetic evolution are dynamic processes to be identified with self-organization phenomena. Motivated by the abstract concept of the replicator (Dawkins 1976), mathematical models for the prebiological evolution (Eigen and Schuster 1979) were extended to cover phenomena from other fields, such as population genetics, ecology, and sociobiology (Schuster and Sigmund 1983). Self-organization phenomena (and adaptation) in complex systems were found to be the key concept in explaining the origin of the biological order (Kaufmann 1993).

The convergence between empirical data of neurobiology with the results of dynamic system theory suggests that neural phenomena occurring at different hierarchical levels can be interpreted in terms of self-organization. Specifically, random spontaneous activity (on the macroscopic, i.e., supermolecular, level) might lead to temporal order (i.e., oscillatory type burst activity) by self-organization in the absence of any interference from the environment. These activity patterns may reach high levels of specificity, providing that the connectivity in these networks is not random but determined by some genetic mechanism. Its clockwork is being driven essentially by internal mechanisms (Szentágothai and Érdi 1989).

Self-organization phenomena have been demonstrated in cell culture experiments (Székely and Szentágothai 1962; see our chap. 2) that showed that randomly interconnected neurons, even without sensory input, might produce biologically significant behavior. The spontaneous activity of single neurons has a random character, so that coherent, organized activity is the result of some self-organizing mechanism. Given organoid (i.e., naturelike) connectivity of various type of neurons, highly specific output patterns—such as a stepping rhythm, or, with some additions, alternate stepping—can be produced in very elementary neural system models. Modern neurophysiological methods applying multiple electrode techniques can give information about the emergence of spatiotemporal coherence among the cells of neuron populations (Krueger 1983; Abeles 1991).

Self-organization is also a key concept in bridging the functional and dynamic approaches. Kelso (1995) summarizes the results of experiments on functional dynamics, including coordinated hand movement, coordination between organisms, intentional dynamics, behavioral development, learning dynamics, and perceptual dynamics. The models he presents are influenced strongly by Haken's synergetics (Haken 1977, 1996) and are, admittedly, phenomenological. Though Kelso beautifully demonstrates the emergence of self-organizing patterns at different levels of neural organization, the connection between the levels remains implicit. Synergetics describes single-level phenomena, assuming that lower levels can be eliminated; the intrinsic couplings between levels thus remain uncovered in this approach.

Molecular self-organizing mechanisms are responsible for such processes as the development of ion channels (Fromherz 1988), the rhythmical activity of single neurons (Llinás 1988), and the regulation of synaptic efficacy based on "receptor desensitization" (Heidmann and Changeux 1982).

Experimental facts from anatomy, physiology, embryology, and psychophysics give evidence of highly ordered repetitive structures composed of building blocks in the vertebrate nervous system, as noted in the modular architectonics principle (see chapters 2 and 8). Modular architecture is a basic feature of the spinal cord, the brainstem reticular formation, the hypothalamus, the subcortical relay nuclei, the cerebellar cortex and, especially, the cerebral cortex. After the so-called corticocortical columns were demonstrated anatomically (Goldman and Nauta 1977), it was suggested (Szentágothai 1978b) that the cerebral cortex might be considered on a large scale as a mosaic of vertical columns interconnected according to a pattern strictly specific to the species. Motivated by the pioneering work of Katchalsky, Rowland, and Blumenthal (1974) on the dynamic patterns of neural assemblies, Szentágothai (1987a) sought to interpret the cortical order in terms of dynamic structures instead of applying some crystallike approach. We respond in chapter 8 to qualms raised recently (Swindale 1990) regarding the modularity of cortex. The more precisely a system is prespecified, the greater is the danger of mistakes; such mistakes can be reduced when spatially ordered structures are the product of some self-organizing mechanism. Most of the evidence on activity-dependent reorganization of cortical connectivity during develop-

ment comes from experiments on the development and plasticity of visual cortex and is reviewed in chapter 8. "The essence of the neural" may be its self-organizing character (Szentágothai and Érdi 1989).

4.1.2 Neurodynamical Models: Technical Frameworks

Single-Cell Dynamics

The investigation of single-neuron dynamics received a new impetus from at least two different directions. First, with the development of anatomical and electrophysiological methods, both the axonal and dendritic branching patterns and the intrinsic physiological properties of different types of neurons became the subject of investigation, and data became available that could be incorporated into detailed models. Second, formal (which does not automatically mean unrealistic!) models have been used to demonstrate many phenomena that are interesting from the point of view of dynamic system theory, such as oscillation, multirhythmicity, bursting, chaos, excitability, and traveling waves. We will not elucidate the details (for a brief introduction, see Abbott 1994, and for a monograph on the foundations of cellular neurophysiology, see Johnston and Wu 1994) but will present the basic notions.

Neuronal Cable Equation To understand the electrical and electrochemical characterization of a neuron, the mechanism of the spatiotemporal change of its membrane potential must be clarified. The membrane potential of a cell at rest is approximately −70 mV, and may vary between roughly −80 mV and +50 mV in the active cell. The term *hyperpolarization* means that the membrane potential will be more negative, whereas *depolarization* denotes that the membrane potential moves in the positive direction. The spatiotemporal change of the membrane potential is described by the extended cable equation:

$$\tau \frac{\partial V}{\partial t} = \lambda \partial^2 V / \partial x^2 - \mathrm{R}(I_m + I_s). \tag{1}$$

Here V is the membrane potential, $\tau := \mathrm{RC}$ is the membrane time constant (R is the membrane resistance and C is the capacitance of the membrane), and λ is the cable length constant. I_m is the membrane current due to the transport of ions through the protein channels embedded in the membrane, and I_s is the synaptic current. Note that we have here left the realm of autonomous systems, with I_s providing the input that can affect the time course of the membrane potential.

The equation that contains the left-hand side and the first term of the right-hand side of equation 1 is the *cable equation* known from physics, whereas the last term comes from neurobiology. Extended cable theory (assuming that one-dimensional space is sufficient) was introduced by Rall (1962, 1977) to describe the passive properties of neurons. Boundary conditions must be specified to complete the statement of the problem. In many (but not all) cases, a cable with a sealed end is assumed. The steady-state and transient solutions have been summarized in Jack, Noble, and Tsien (1975) and Rall (1989). Before progressing further with the solution of the equations, the specific forms of I_m and I_s will be discussed.

Membrane Currents   Not a whole neuron but a part of it—namely, the giant axon of the squid—was studied by Hodgkin and Huxley (1952), who quantitatively described the electrogenesis of the action potential. They included two channels, a fast sodium channel and a delayed rectifier potassium channel. They took the total membrane current to be the sum of the individual currents transported through individual channels. Channels were assumed to be in either an open or closed state, and the probability of the transition between them was described by first-order kinetics, with voltage-dependent rate constants. Three elementary processes—namely, sodium activation, sodium inactivation, and potassium activation—were found, and therefore three (gating) variables—m, h, and n, respectively—were defined. Specifically, Hodgkin and Huxley modeled the sodium conductance using three gates of a type labeled m and one gate of type h. The potassium conductance is modeled with four identical n gates. The experiments were done under the so-called space-clamp method to eliminate the spatial variation of the membrane potential V. The mathematical consequence is that the partial differential equation is reduced to a four-dimensional system of ordinary differential equations in which the variables are the membrane potential and the three gating variables (see under Single-Cell Oscillators in sec. 4.2.2 for more details).

Axon membranes, even in the general case, can be described by the original Hodgkin-Huxley model. For somas and dendrites, further channel types should be taken into account. Dendrites were considered earlier to be passive elements; now their active properties are extensively studied (Johnston et al. 1996). The framework of the model, however, can be used even in such cases. The general form of the membrane current for each type of ion and channel is:

$$I_i(t) = \bar{g}_i P_i(V(t))(V(t) - E_i) \tag{2}$$

where $\bar{g}_i$ is the maximal conductance, P_i is the probability that the channel is open (which here depends on $V(t)$), and E_i is the equilibrium potential for the ion i. The channel kinetics depend on how the opening and closing is controlled by depolarization and hyperpolarization. A leakage current, I_L, which corrects the errors due to neglect of ions, is modeled by the assumption $P_L \equiv 1$. The delayed-rectifier potassium current is the prototype of currents that are called *noninactivating*: It opens with depolarization and closes with hyperpolarization. There are more complex channels to be described by taking into account two gates. One of them is noninactivating; the second behaves in the opposite way, closing with depolarization and opening with hyperpolarization. Fast sodium conductance is the best-known example for such a (transient or inactivating) current. The conductances just mentioned involve voltage-dependent channels. There are, however, channels that depend on other factors (e.g., calcium concentration; see Yamada, Koch, and Adams 1989; Johnston et al. 1994), so that P_i does not depend solely on $V(t)$.

The activation and inactivation kinetics are given formally by the same type of equation:

$$\frac{dx}{dt} = a_x - x/\tau_x \tag{3}$$

where x represents an activation or inactivation (i.e., the gating) variable, τ_x is the time constant, and $a_x \tau_x$ is the steady-state value of x. Through the time (or other) dependence of a_x and t_x, the kinetic equations for the channel activation and inactivation are coupled to equation 1.

Synaptic Currents   Most synaptic currents are due to channels activated by an extracellular transmitter. They can be expressed by

$$I_s(t) = \bar{g}_s s(V(t), t)(V_{post}(t) - E_s) \tag{4}$$

where $\bar{g}_s$ is the maximal synaptic conductance, V_{post} the membrane potential of the postsynaptic neuron, E_s the equilibrium potential, and s the probability of being open. Assuming a simple reversible mechanism for describing the opening and closing, equation 4 is supplemented with the kinetic equation

$$\frac{ds}{dt} = k_1 T V_{pre}(1 - s) - k_{2s} \tag{5}$$

where T is the transmitter concentration and V_{pre} is the membrane potential of the presynaptic neuron.

The most important excitatory synaptic currents are related to glutamate. Two types of glutamate receptors are the N-methyl-D-aspartate (NMDA) receptors and the (α-amino-3-hydroxyl-5-methyl-4-isoxazole-proprionic acid (AMPA) receptors, which are involved in the formation of so-called LTP (see sec. 4.5.1 and 6.3). The two most important inhibitory synaptic conductances are activated by γ-aminobutyric acid (GABA). $GABA_A$ receptors form fast responses, whereas $GABA_B$ receptors mediate slow responses.

Electric synapses (gap junctions) produce synaptic currents that are proportional to the difference of the pre- and postsynaptic potential.

Single-Compartment Models   The crucial assumption behind a single-compartment model is that the whole cell can be characterized by a single membrane potential. The model contains an equation for the temporal change of the membrane potential and a set of kinetic equations for the gating variables. The original Hodgkin-Huxley system and even its generalizations have been the subject of approximative reduction procedures for obtaining two-dimensional systems (e.g., FitzHugh 1961; Nagumo, Arimoto, and Yoshizawa 1962; Hindmarsh and Rose 1982; Kepler, Abbott, and Marder 1992). One advantage of two-dimensional systems is that they can easily be visualized and analyzed by applying phase-space techniques (Ermentrout 1995).

A few neurons containing many voltage-dependent conductances have been described by single-compartment models [e.g., the bullfrog sympathetic ganglion cell (Yamada, Koch, and Adams 1989); the stomatogastric ganglion neuron (Buchholtz et al. 1992; Golowasch et al. 1992); and neurons of the thalamocortical system, (see sec. 8.2)].

A popular, and highly simplified, single-compartment model characterizes the neuron by a single membrane potential, with the influence of neuron j on neuron i mediated by the "synaptic weight" w_{ij} of the synaptic weight matrix **W**. The membrane potential $a_i(t)$ then changes according to the differential equation

$$\tau \frac{da_i(t)}{dt} = -a_i(t) + \left(\sum_j w_{ij}(t)\phi(a_j(t)) + I_i(t) \right) \qquad (6)$$

where ϕ is some sigmoid function, τ is the time constant, and $\phi(a_j(t))$ is the instantaneous firing frequency. The term I_i corresponds to the sensory input and so is only nonzero for afferent neurons. The model defined by equation 6 is referred to as the *leaky integrator model*, because the activity level integrates its inputs with time

constant τ, save for the "leakage" given by the decay term $-a_i(t)$.

Multicompartment Models   Single-compartment models are not able to treat, for example, the effect of the location of the entering membrane and synaptic currents or the geometry of dendritic branching. Though some approximative analytical procedures exist (see Abbott 1994), the solution of the cable equation with nonlinear voltage-dependent membrane conductances and time-dependent synaptic conductances needs compartmentalization and numerical integration. Figure 4.2 shows how the branching patterns of a real hippocampal pyramidal cell are approximated by compartments (Traub et al. 1994b).

By assuming that each compartment is coupled to two neighbors—except for the compartments at the ends of dendritic branches, which have only one neighboring compartment—the discretized version of the cable equation takes the form

$$C_k \frac{dV_k}{dt} = g_{k-1,k}(V_{k-1} - V_k) + g_{k+1,k}(V_{k+1} - V_k) - I_{k,\text{total}}$$

$$(7)$$

where each compartment k has its own capacitance and membrane potential, and conductances are defined also between the neighboring compartments.

In a few cases, multicompartmental models based on data on the branching patterns and intrinsic electrophysiological properties have been solved. The NMDA-induced oscillatory properties of the neurons in the lamprey spinal cord were explained by the interaction of channels (Brodin et al. 1991). Pyramidal neurons in the hippocampus (Traub et al. 1991, 1994) and in the olfactory cortex (Wilson and Bower 1989), bursting cortical pyramidal neurons (Lytton and Sejnowski 1991), and Purkinje cells (De Schutter and Bower 1994a, b) have been simulated. Neural simulation systems such as NEURON (Hines 1984, 1993) and GENESIS (Wilson and Bower 1989; Bower and Beeman 1994) have been constructed to simplify the efficient simulation of branched neurons.

Whereas only deterministic models were considered earlier, the temporal firing patterns of single neurons can be treated as well with stochastic models (Gerstein and Mandelbrot 1964; Holden 1976; Lansky and Lanská 1987; Tuckwell 1988; Ricciardi 1994). The plausibility of this approach is justified in at least two ways. First, neural signals may be considered phenomenologically as the realizations of stochastic processes. Second, the kinetic mechanism of the channel-gating process is internally

A   B

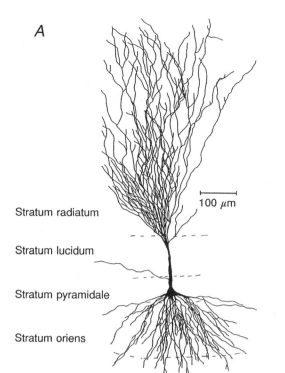

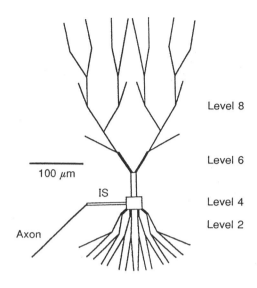

Stratum radiatum

Stratum lucidum

Stratum pyramidale

Stratum oriens

Figure 4.2
Structure of a hippocampal CA3 pyramidal neuron and the multi-compartmental approximation of its branching patterns. IS, initial segment. (Reprinted with permission from Traub et al. 1994b.)

stochastic (Sakmann and Neher 1983). In principle, the deterministic descriptions of such kinetic processes should be considered as an approximation of the stochastic model (Érdi and Tóth 1989).

The McCulloch-Pitts Neuron   In most models in this text, we usually will study either large multiregional networks in which each neuron is modeled as a leaky integrator neuron, or small networks in which each neuron is modeled by a multicompartment model. However, it is worth noting here the McCulloch-Pitts neuron both because of its historical importance and because of its use as a reference point for the neural models treated in sections 4.5.2. "Synaptic Matrix Models of Associative Memory" and 4.5.3. "Hopfield Networks". McCulloch and Pitts (1943) combined neurophysiology and mathematical logic to model the neuron as a binary discrete-time element. Their neuron operates on a discrete time scale ($t = 0, 1, 2, 3, \ldots$) in which the time unit is comparable to a refractory period, so that in each time period, which is on the order of 1 millisecond, at most one spike can be generated in the axon of a given neuron.

Let w_i be the strength or weight of the ith synapse onto a given neuron. We call a synapse *excitatory* if $w_i > 0$ and *inhibitory* if $w_i < 0$. McCulloch and Pitts also

associate a threshold θ with each neuron and assume exactly one unit of delay in the effect of all presynaptic inputs on the cell's output, so that a neuron fires (i.e., has value 1 on its output line) at time $t + 1$ just in case the weighted values of its inputs at time t is at least θ. Formally, if at time t the value of the ith input to a neuron is $x_i(t)$ and the output one time step later is $y(t + 1)$, then

$$y(t + 1) = 1 \text{ if and only if } \sum_i w_i x_i(t) \geqslant \theta$$

A slight generalization is to allow the state output to vary continuously from 0 to 1, so that the next state is computed by passing the weighted input sum through some suitable (e.g., sigmoid) function f to obtain the next state,

$$y(t + 1) = f\left(\sum_i w_i x_i(t)\right)$$

It is a standard exercise to choose weights and thresholds to obtain McCulloch-Pitts neurons that function as AND gates, OR gates and NOT gates, which can then be combined to form any boolean function (possibly with some delay). McCulloch-Pitts neurons thus are sufficient to build networks that can function as the control circuitry for a computer carrying out computations of arbitrary complexity. This discovery played a crucial role in the development of automata theory (see Arbib 1987b for a review) and in the study of learning machines.

Multilevel Models of Neural Networks

A rather large subset of brain models takes the form of networks of intricately connected neurons in which each neuron is modeled as a single-compartment unit whose state is characterized by a single membrane potential; anatomical, biophysical, and neurochemical details are neglected. Such neural network models are considered, at a certain level of description, as three-level dynamic systems:

$$\frac{da_i(t)}{dt} = f(a(t), \Theta(t), \mathbf{W}(t), I_i(t))$$

$$\frac{d\Theta(t)}{dt} = e(a(t)) \qquad (8)$$

$$\frac{dw_{ij}(t)}{dt} = g_{ij}(a(t), \mathbf{W}(t), u, R_{ij}(t))$$

Here a is the activity vector, Θ is the threshold vector, $\mathbf{W}$ is the matrix of synaptic efficacies, I is the sensory input, $R(t)$ is an additive noise term to simulate environmental noise, and u scales the time. The functions e, f, and g will be discussed soon. Because a noise term has been introduced, equation 10 is a system of stochastic differential equations, and its treatment needs a special stochastic calculus (e.g., Arnold 1973). One of the main difficulties of establishing a well-founded theory of neurodynamics is to define the functions e, f, and g. Equations 8 do not specify the general cases, since the change of state depends on the current values of a, $\mathbf{W}$, and θ only. Later we shall discuss cases where the past values of these quantities also influence the change of state.

Activity Level Activity dynamics often are identified with the membrane potential equation, and the potential change (i.e., the form of f_i) is determined by the rate of presynaptic information transfer and the spontaneous activity decay. It often is assumed that the activity dynamics are given by the leaky integrator model of equation 6.

Threshold Level The function e describes the time-dependent modification of the threshold due to adaptation. It usually is neglected (i.e., $e \equiv 0$ so that Θ is constant).

Synaptic Level The function g specifies the learning rule. Current learning theories generally assume that memory traces somehow are stored in the synaptic efficacies. The

celebrated Hebb rule (Hebb 1949) has been touted as a simple local rule for explaining synaptic strengthening based on the conjunction between pre- and postsynaptic activity. Qualms regarding the neurophysiological plausibility and some obvious mathematically unpleasant properties (such as unlimited growth, the lack of decreasing term) led to the introduction of a whole family of learning rules, which are discussed systematically in section 4.5.

Population Theories

The behavior of large networks of neurons may be studied by population theories. Just as collective phenomena emerging in physical systems made from a large number of elementary components (spins, molecules, etc.) are treated by statistical mechanics, so, analogously, have statistical dynamic theories of neural populations been established (Wilson and Cowan 1973; Amari 1974; Ventriglia 1974, 1994; Ingber 1982; Clark, Rafelski, and Winston 1985; Peretto 1984, 1992). Statistical theories work with distributions and averaged quantities. The future of population theories depends on how well knowledge about single neurons can be incorporated into the framework of such theories.

A step in this direction has been made by Gröbler and Barna (1996) who started from Ventriglia's kinetic theory. Ventriglia (1974, 1994) characterized neural population activity in terms of the probability density functions (pdfs) for the neurons and the spikes traveling between the neurons. The neural continuum has the following properties: The different excitatory and inhibitory neural populations have their own neural fields, and they can interact through the emission and absorption of spikes. The neurons are fixed in space, while spikes can travel freely among them. The change of subthreshold membrane potential of neurons is determined by the postsynaptic potentials caused by absorbed spikes. Gröbler and Barna (1996) also incorporated into the models the dependence on the different ionic currents. They defined a two-dimensional state space (both for neurons and spikes) that consists of a subthreshold membrane potential coordinate and an intracellular calcium concentration. Instead of having a mechanism based on channel kinetics, a dynamical threshold mechanism related to Na^+ was given (as a compromise between detailed description and the complete neglect of biophysical details) that determines the proportion of neurons that will fire. The pdf of neurons reflects the probability of the activity of a neuron in a fixed point and at a given time falling in an infinitesimal interval of membrane potential and calcium concentration. The pdf of spikes denotes the probable number of spikes in a given environment of a fixed point and moving into a direction given by an infinitesimal interval. The time evolution equations for the pdfs is basically a diffusion equation, which, under the present conditions, can be solved only by simulations. An elementary application of this model for hippocampal dynamics is mentioned in sec. 6.2.

Stochastic neurodynamics offer a compromise between models based on detailed single-cell-level descriptions and oversimplified networks of binary units: Large-scale neural activities are calculated (Cowan 1991). In one approach, a neuron is modeled as having three possible states, quiescent (q), activated (a), and refractory (r). Transition probabilities for elementary changes between subpopulations must be specified. For example, an elementary activation process $q \rightarrow a$ corresponds to the transition

$$(n_q, n_a, n_r) \rightarrow (n_q - 1, n_a + 1, n_r). \qquad (9a)$$

Assuming that the system is a time-homogenous, continuous-time, discrete state-space, markovian jump process, the evolution equation for the probability distribution of the states is

$$\frac{dPn(t)}{dt} = \mathbf{A}_{nn}P_n(t) \qquad (9b)$$

where $\mathbf{A}_{nn}$ is the (time-independent) interaction matrix. Equation 9b is a linear differential-difference equation. Introducing $a_{nn} \in \mathbf{A}_{nn}$ as the infinitesimal transition probability that gives the probability (per unit time) of the jump from the state n' to n, equation 9b can be rewritten as a gain-loss equation for the probability of each state n:

$$\frac{dP_n(t)}{dt} = \sum_{n'} [a_{nn'}P_{n'}(t) - a_{n'n}P_n(t)] \qquad (9c)$$

The first term of the right-hand side is the gain due to transition from all the other states n', and the second term is the loss due to jump to other states.

The stochastic dynamics of the transitions among the states of neurons is rather easily described and calculated under the assumptions just mentioned. More sophisticated techniques are necessary, however, if the transitions have "memory" or the state space has some more complex structure. Such anomalous stochastic models require special treatment (West 1985; Érdi and Tóth 1988).

Neurodynamical Problems

Having discussing the mathematical frameworks for the fundamental neural models, we turn to the basic neuro-

dynamical problems that can be treated within these frameworks. Many neurodynamical problems can be categorized into two groups, which we discuss briefly at this point and in more detail in later sections.

The first group of problems assumes *fixed wiring* (i.e., the matrix $\mathbf{S}$ is assumed to be constant over time. In this case, either the dynamics of activity spreading through the nodes of the network or the temporal change of specific activities a_i can be studied. In the latter case, the occurrence of regular (i.e., convergence to stable equilibrium point) or of exotic (oscillatory and chaotic) behavior is analyzed. The qualitative dynamic behavior of a network is determined strongly by the excitatory-inhibitory connectivity patterns in the network. To have an alternative formulation and to better understand the old structure-function problem of real networks (and to promote more efficient methods for designing artificial neural networks with given properties), the connections between (static) network architectures and (dynamic) functional behavior must be investigated.

In the cybernetic and biomathematical literature, there is a well-known, but many times misinterpreted, theorem on the connectivity-stability dilemma (Wigner 1959; May 1972; Érdi and Tóth 1990) that suggests that, at least for a class of randomly interconnected but deterministic networks, the degree of connectivity works against stability (see sec. 4.1.3 for more details). Developments in the theory of differential equations (Hirsch 1984, 1989) better illuminate the assumptions leading to regular dynamics. The immediate application of these results for neural networks makes it possible to see the relationship between the graph structure of neural networks and qualitative properties of the dynamic activity of the network. Based on this mathematics, we have a partial answer for the general question of what kinds of network architecture lead to stable equilibrium and what structural conditions make a network a rhythm or chaos generator (see sec. 4.2.2 and 4.3.4).

In the second group of problems, the existence of *modifiable synapses* is taken into consideration. Models based on the modification of synaptic efficacies are associated both with pattern formation, as in normal ontogenetic development and plastic rearrangement, and with learning as a network is tuned by experience (e.g., for successful pattern recognition). As discussed earlier, it is more or less accepted that embryonic and postnatal development are the result of pattern generation based on the interaction between genetically specified and environmental factors. For more details, see section 4.1.2 (Grossberg 1988) and our discussion of ocular dominance and orientation columns in chapter 8.

Concluding Remarks on the Brain as a Dynamical System

The brain, as a physical device, may be interpreted in terms of dynamical system theory and should be considered as a system of hierarchically arranged self-organizing structures. Self-organization is a mechanism for generating emergent neural structures. Neurodynamical phenomena, such as ontogeny, development, normal performance, learning, and plasticity, can be treated by the coherent concepts and formalism of neurodynamical system theory. Single-cell, multilevel, and population models may be set up to describe dynamic neural phenomena. Different qualitative dynamic phenomena, such as convergence to equilibrium, oscillation, and chaos, play an important role in implementing different neural functions.

4.1.3 Simple Dynamic Behavior and Network Architecture

The "simple" dynamic behavior studied in this section is convergence to equilibrium. We discuss qualitative constraints on networks (network architecture) that will ensure that a network's dynamics will be of only this simple kind. Sections 4.2 and 4.3 then advance our understanding of oscillatory and chaotic dynamics, respectively, in neural networks.

On the Structure-Function Problem

Studies on the connections between the structure of neural networks and the quantitative or qualitative properties of these networks dynamic behavior allow one to reinterpret the structure-function relationship. Synthesis and analysis of neural networks relies on the eventual existence of general relationships between the excitatory-inhibitory patterns of the network and the different types of temporal behavior, such as convergence to an equilibrium point, oscillation, or chaos. The dynamic behavior of autonomous systems is determined by three different factors: network structure, parameter values, and initial conditions. In particular, the quantitative and qualitative effects of parameter changes are studied by sensitivity analysis and bifurcation theory, respectively. The set of initial conditions is classified by the basins of the attractors (see sec. 4.5.4).

Sensitivity analysis is a mathematical tool for investigating the effect of parameter changes on the solution of dynamic systems. The intention of sensitivity analysis is to eliminate the less significant variables and processes from a model of a complex dynamic phenomenon. The mathematical, computational, and engineering aspects

of sensitivity analysis are well established (e.g., Frank 1978), and it is used extensively to reduce models of large chemical networks (Turányi 1990). The method would be useful to analyze neural networks, too, to remove those synapses from a model that do not make a significant contribution to the dynamic operation of the whole network.

Bifurcation theory is a mathematical method for studying the effect of parameter change on the quality ("topology") of the solution. For different values of parameters (which are time-independent, by definition), the behavior of the solutions can be very different qualitatively. Bifurcation theory studies the sudden change of the nature of attractors when a (control or bifurcation) parameter passes certain values (bifurcation points). Transition from a point equilibrium to small-amplitude periodic solutions (called the *Hopf bifurcation*) is a typical bifurcation phenomenon. Hopf bifurcation was found both in the standard Hodgkin-Huxley equations (see, for example, Holden, Hude, and Muhamed 1991) and in neural networks (e.g., Ermentrout and Cowan 1979; Borisyuk and Kirillov 1992).

Regarding the structural conditions of stability, periodicity, chaos, and so forth, we have to realize that the overwhelming majority of statements is conditional (i.e., system properties depend on the numerical values of parameters and initial conditions). Some properties (e.g., qualitative stability) depend only on the sign of parameters characterizing the strengths of connections.

The question to be studied here is what kinds of network architectures lead to stable equilibrium and what are the structural conditions that define whether a network may be a rhythmicity or a chaos generator (Érdi 1991, 1994).

The Connectivity-Stability Dilemma

The dynamic behavior of large networks has been the subject of many biomathematical investigations. Using neural terminology, we might ask: How might the establishment of new synaptic contacts within a set of neurons change the dynamics of the whole network? Chemical networks, immune networks, ecological food webs, and genetic networks, as well as neural networks, have been analyzed by applying the mathematical concepts to be discussed here. The common property of the networks *in the models discussed here* is that they are assembled apparently randomly but the system dynamics themselves are deterministic. Such random structures are apparently at odds with the modular architectonics principle discussed in chapter 2. Even if cortical organization exhibits randomness in small scale and structure in large scale (cf. Szentágothai 1978a), the following theory cannot be applied directly to the cortical networks. Nevertheless, the theory offers interesting results on structure-function relationships that point the way toward further investigation. The problem of the balance between determinism and randomnness in the nervous system is addressed in section 4.4.1.

Simulation experiments on randomly assembled deterministic systems (Gardner and Ashby 1970) suggested that to have a stable equilibrium point, a large system should not be strongly connected. A system loses its stability as the connectivity exceeds a certain threshold. Theoretical results for the connectivity-stability problem have been given within the framework of the Wigner-May theorem (Wigner 1959; May 1972) by analyzing the eigenvalues of certain matrices.

Let $\mathbf{B}_n$ be a random $n \times n$ matrix with connectivity c_n (i.e., $\mathbf{B}_n$ has $c_n n^2$ nonzero elements). The nonzero elements are chosen independently from a fixed symmetrical distribution of mean 0 and variance α^2. In the neural network context, α can be interpreted as the average synaptic strength. The trivial solution of the system of difference equations $x' = \mathbf{A}_n x$ with $\mathbf{A}_n = \mathbf{B}_n - I_n$ is, for large n, almost surely stable if $\alpha^2 n c_n < 1$ and almost surely unstable if $\alpha^2 n c_n > 1$. This implies that, at least in randomly connected networks of this type, the increase of (1) the synaptic strengths in a network with fixed wiring, (2) the number of neurons, and (3) the connectivity of synapses within a network all work against stability. The consequence of an increase of the synaptic strengths is that Hebbian learning may induce a transition from equilibrium to oscillation or between periodic and chaotic regimes. Such transitions have been demonstrated in a model of the olfactory bulb (see chapter 5). Such switching also may result from intrinsic changes in neural properties that are not included in the Wigner-May style of network model. For example, in the neural networks of the crustacean stomatogastric nervous system (Hooper and Moulins 1989; Meynerd, Simmers, and Moulins 1991), the same neuron can be part of different networks, and the switching of a neuron from one network to another can be triggered by sensory-induced changes in membrane properties.

The Wigner-May theorem usually is considered as a general statement on randomly assembled large deterministic systems, relating structural complexity and dynamic stability. Many misinterpretations of the theorem have appeared in the biomathematical literature due to the neglect of its very specific assumptions, as discussed in Érdi and Tóth (1990). For example, the immediate

consequence of assuming symmetrically distributed matrix elements with zero mean is that the expected numbers of positive and negative elements (i.e., of excitatory and inhibitory interactions) are the same. This biologically implausible condition is assumed also in the original Hopfield model (Hopfield 1982; see sec. 4.5.3) but was relaxed in later studies. Some remarks on the applications, and some hints on the extensions and limits of the Wigner-May theorem may be found in Érdi and Tóth (1990). To apply the theorem, it is necessary to check precisely all its assumptions or to delineate clearly its domain of validity. The assumption most often violated is that the ratio of positive and negative interactions is just one. Intuitively, it is not surprising that nonbalanced excitatory-inhibitory patterns might lead to instability. Furthermore, in certain situations, increase in connectivity may enhance stability.

The Qualitative Stability-Instability Problem

Many times we can make assumptions only for the sign and not for the numerical values of the strength of interactions. Consider an admissible system of nonlinear differential equations $dx(t)/dt = \mathbf{F}(x(t))$. We form a sign matrix from the jacobian matrix, $\mathbf{J}_{ij} = \partial \mathbf{F}_i / \partial x_j$, by writing "$+$" if $\mathbf{J}_{ij} > 0$ and "$-$" if $\mathbf{J}_{ij} < 0$, and say that two jacobians are *sign-equivalent* if they have the same sign matrix. It can be shown that $dx(t)/dt = \mathbf{F}(x(t))$ has at least one stable equilibrium point if its jacobian $\mathbf{J}$ is *qualitatively* stable, in the sense that every sign equivalent is stable. Qualitative stability (e.g., see Jeffries 1974 for proofs) is very restrictive, requiring many zeros in the jacobian ("sparse connections," in neural terminology). The lack of qualitative stability does not imply qualitative instability, however. A qualitative instability test has been given by Eisenfeld and DeLisi (1985). Qualitative stability implies convergence to a stable equilibrium point (regular behavior). The violation of the criteria of qualitative stability can (conditionally) lead to periodic and chaotic behavior. A more detailed analysis will be given in sections 4.3.2 and 4.4.4, which address the network architectures of possible rhythm and chaos generators.

In the light of newer mathematical results on the eigenvalues of random matrices (Juhász 1982, 1990, 1992), symmetric matrices around nonzero means and nonsymmetric block matrices can also be evaluated. The immediate consequence of these mathematical results is that conditions for the stability of much more complex networks can be established (Hogg, Huberman, and McGlade 1989; Hastings, Juhász, and Schreiber 1992).

4.2 Oscillatory Behavior in Neural Systems

In this section, we offer an initial perspective on the oscillations which, as we shall see in later chapters, provide a basic dynamical mode of activity in many brain regions. Oscillations may occur at the single-cell level due to intrinsic membrane properties or may be emergent network properties resulting from the pattern of connections between cells that are not themselves oscillators. In chapter 5, we will discuss oscillation and chaos in the olfactory bulb, rhythmical activity in the olfactory cortex, and cholinergic modulation of oscillations in pyriform cortex. Chapter 6 addresses a variety of electrical activity patterns in the hippocampus, including theta rhythms, irregular sharp waves, and epileptic seizures. In chapter 8, we look at thalamocortical oscillators, including intrinsic electrophysiological properties of thalamic neurons, spindle oscillations, delta oscillations, and slow-wave sleep oscillations.

4.2.1 Some Remarks on the Experimental Background

Single-Cell Oscillators

Though the spontaneous activity of single neurons often appears to have a generally random character, more regular autonomous (i.e., input-independent) time-ordered behavior, such as pacemaker oscillations, may occur in single neurons in consequence of their intrinsic electrophysiological properties (for a systematic study, see Llinás 1988). Neurons may behave not only as oscillators but also as resonators responding preferentially to certain frequencies. Single-cell oscillations occur in consequence of the interplay of a few currents (e.g., the low-threshold calcium conductance) and were demonstrated first mostly in invertebrates (Kandel 1976) but later even in mammalian neurons [inferior olivary cells, Purkinje cells, thalamocortical cells (see sec. 8.3), and cortical pyramidal cells]. A special type of single-neuron oscillations is ligand-induced (and may be voltage-dependent or voltage-independent). In particular, NMDA-induced oscillations have been demonstrated in the spinal cord of the lamprey (Grillner 1985) and of the rat (Hochman, Jordan, and MacDonald 1994), in rat ocular motoneurons (Durand 1993), and in medial vestibular nucleus neurons in the guinea pig (Serafin et al. 1992).

Neurons may show not only simple oscillatory behavior but also multirhythmicity (Jahnsen and Llinás 1984; see also sec. 8.3 on thalamocortical oscillations). *Multirhythmicity* means that the dynamic system can exhibit oscillations with more than one frequency. The

locally stable attractors associated with the different periodic behaviors coexist but are separated (by the "separatrix"). In mathematical terms, the initial conditions determine which rhythmicity among the coexisting stable oscillatory modes is selected. Transitions between different modes in single neurons can be generated by neuromodulators.

Conventionally, neuromodulators may induce parameter changes (Kaczmarek and Levitan 1987) but they also can play the role of the initial condition setter. Serotonin and dopamine serve as neuromodulators and select among the multiple oscillatory modes of activity in, for example, the neuron R15 in the abdominal ganglion of *Aplysia* (Canavier et al. 1994).

The existence of single-cell-level oscillation does not imply the generation of global oscillatory behavior. To avoid averaging due to irregular phase shifts, some synchronization mechanism should appear. Synchronization phenomena in different neural centers have been the subject of many recent investigations (Buzsáki et al. 1994; Gray 1994). The appearance of single-cell oscillation is, however, not a necessary condition for global oscillations, as the latter may arise as an emergent network property. This was suggested on the basis of combined physiological and pharmacological experiments in the thalamus (Buzsáki 1991) and also on the basis of theoretical studies concerning the connection between network structure and qualitative dynamic behavior (see sec. 4.2.2).

Central Pattern Generators

A *central pattern generator* (CPG) is a network of neurons that produces a pattern of behavior in the absence of sensory input. In many cases, this pattern is rhythmical in character. Relatively simple invertebrate systems, such as the crustacean stomatogastric ganglion, are capable of generating temporal patterns independently of peripheral reflex loops. The network structure (Selverston and Moulins 1987) and the transmitterology (Marder and Nusbaum 1989) of this system have already been thoroughly uncovered. The fundamental temporal patterns may be driven by single-cell oscillations or may reflect network oscillations induced by reciprocal inhibition between pairs of neurons together with postinhibitory rebound.

At a higher phylogenetic level, the locomotion of lower vertebrates, such as tadpoles and lampreys, has been studied. Motor patterns underlying locomotion are produced by a spinal circuit. Partial information now is available concerning neural circuitry, transmitters, and membrane properties (Grillner et al. 1991). Animal locomotion, even at a higher phylogenetic level, may be generated and controlled by a CPG. However, the total *motor pattern generator* (MPG) involves various feedback loops that use sensory input to adjust the motor pattern to current circumstances. Multilegged animals exhibit several distinct patterns of leg movements; the basic patterns are called *gaits* (e.g., walk, run, hop for humans; trot, canter, gallop for horses).

Synchronized Oscillatory Activity in Cortical and Cortexlike Structures

The ultimate source of neocortical rhythmicity appears to be the thalamus. The underlying thalamic oscillation is not generated by single pacemaker cells but seems to be a network property (Buzsáki 1991). Whereas thalamocortical relay cells can produce rhythms with a wide range of frequencies due to intracellular mechanisms, the reticular thalamic neurons (which innervate thalamocortical cells) show synchronized (so-called spindle; see sec. 8.3.3) rhythmic activity, most likely in consequence of inhibitory coupling (Destexhe et al. 1994; Golomb, Wang, and Rinzel 1994). There is a significant difference between the neural activity patterns in the aroused and sleeping brain; the transition from high-frequency rhythms to synchronized low-frequency activity is the physiological characteristic of the transition to sleep. The mechanisms for the genesis and control of sleep rhythms are reviewed in section 8.3.

The hippocampus, which is involved in memory trace formation, exhibits different kinds of temporal patterns. The rat hippocampus shows rhythmical slow (or theta) activity during exploratory behavior and awake mobility (e.g., Buzsáki 1989); irregular sharp waves occur during slow-wave sleep in humans. Whereas theta activities are believed to be generated extrahippocampally, the irregular sharp waves are formed intrahippocampally owing to a synchronization process mediated by recurrent excitatory synapses (see sec. 6.2). The machinery of the hippocampus is based in part on the neocortical-hippocampal-neocortical loop, and a complete cycle requires approximately 20–25 msec. Spindle oscillations have a 7- to 14-Hz frequency and are grouped in sequences that recur every 3–10 sec. Though the discovery of subcortical afferents that cause feedforward inhibition (Buzsáki 1984) and disinhibition (Freund and Antal 1988), and the demonstration of anatomical divergence of intrahippocampal projections (Amaral and Witter 1989), might significantly modify the scenario about the information flow (see sec. 6.1), it still seems rather likely that cyclical operations have a fundamental role in hippocampal information processing. Cortico-

hippocampal closed circuits may provide a mechanism for rapid consolidation of associations, and electrophysiological patterns play a crucial role in hippocampal memory formation (Buzsáki 1989, 1996; Buzsáki et al. 1994; see also sec. 6.2.).

Population oscillation seems to play an important role in both the olfactory bulb (Freeman and Skarda 1985) and the olfactory cortex (Wilson and Bower 1992) (see chap. 5). The occurrence of bulbar oscillation is the consequence of the interactions among excitatory mitral cell and inhibitory granule cell populations. The slow modification of some synaptic strengths due to the learning process results in switching the system from one dynamic regime to another (e.g., from limit cycle to chaos or vice versa). Oscillations in the olfactory bulb tend to be synchronized with cortical oscillations, but the latter may also be generated internally owing to the interaction between cortical excitatory and inhibitory cells (see sec. 5.2).

The finding of synchronized oscillation of multiunit activity in the visual cortex (Gray et al. 1989; Eckhorn et al. 1994) has generated much discussion. It seems remarkable, from a functional point of view, that rather remote columns oscillate in phase around 40 Hz (gamma oscillation). It has been suggested (Crick and Koch 1990) that phase- and frequency-locked oscillations are strongly connected to the neurobiological basis of visual awareness. This theory, though based on data from anesthetized(!) animals, recently was supported by similar findings in experiments in awake animals (Kreiter and Singer 1972; Murthy and Fetz 1992; Gray and Viana di Prisco 1993). The functional role of synchronous oscillation in visual processing has been questioned (Tovee and Rolls 1992) based on the incompatibility between the time required to establish synchrony and short recognition times. A subject for further study is whether synchronized cortical oscillations are the neural basis of binding different features (color, contour, orientation, velocity, etc.) of the same object by forming coherently firing cells into assemblies (von der Malsburg 1981) that code uniquely for the different stimuli.

There are complementary answers to the question "How the brain gets rhythm" (Schechter 1996). According to Gray and McCormick (1996) single cell oscillations are the base of synchronous cortical oscillations. They found a class of superficial pyramidal neurons termed *chattering cells*, which generate 20- to 70-Hz repetitive burst firing and exhibit membrane potential oscillation during visual stimulation. Traub et al. (1996), however, based on slice experiments and computer simulations, suggested a different mechanism for generation of long-range synchronous fast cortical oscillations. Their model network consists of pyramidal cells and interneurons; it predicts that when excitation of interneurons reaches a level sufficient to induce spike doublets, the network generates synchronized gamma oscillations.

4.2.2 Mathematical Techniques

Single-Cell Oscillators

When the spatial dependence of membrane potential can be neglected, the Hodgkin-Huxley model is a system of four-dimensional ordinary differential equations that describes the temporal change of the potential V and the three gating variables, m, n, and h. Taking into account the (constant) external current I, the form of the equation is

$$C\frac{dV}{dt} = g_l(E_l - V) + g_{Na}(E_{Na} - V_m) + g_K(E_K - V_m) + I$$
(10a)

where E_l, E_{Na}, and E_K are reversal potentials, and g_l, g_{Na}, and g_K are conductances. Conductance g_l is constant, but g_{Na}, and g_K are time-varying according to the equations

$$\left.\begin{aligned} g_{Na}(t) &= \bar{g}_{Na}m^3(t)h(t) \\ g_{Na}(t) &= \bar{g}_K n^4(t) \end{aligned}\right\}$$
(10b)

where m is an activation variable and n and h are inactivation variables, which themselves vary according to voltage-dependent equations:

$$\left.\begin{aligned} \frac{dm(t)}{dt} &= L_m(V)(m_\infty(V) - m(t)) \\ \frac{dn(t)}{dt} &= L_n(V)(n_\infty(V) - n(t)) \\ \frac{dh(t)}{dt} &= L_h(V)(h_\infty(V) - h(t)) \end{aligned}\right\}$$
(10c)

L_m, L_n, and L_h are voltage-dependent rate functions, $m_\infty(V)$ is a decreasing sigmoid function, and $n_\infty(V)$ and $h_\infty(V)$ are increasing sigmoid functions.

The four-dimensional Hodgkin-Huxley equation, and its reduced versions, have been the subject of (mostly, but not exclusively) numerical bifurcation analysis (see, for example, Holden, Hyde, and Muhamed 1991). In particular, Hopf bifurcation, (i.e., the transition from equilibrium point to small-amplitude oscillation) has been demonstrated analytically (Troy 1976) in the Fitz-Hugh-Nagumo model (a two-dimensional reduction of the Hodgkin-Huxley equation) considering the external current as the bifurcation parameter: Bifurcation takes place as the current passes through a critical value. Thorough numerical studies (Hassard 1978) showed that bifurcation may occur for current values taken from certain intervals. Other bifurcations (e.g., between equilibrium points, or from equilibrium point to large-amplitude oscillations) have been demonstrated by using two or three control parameters (e.g., the maximal potassium conductance, and the potassium equilibrium potential). The original Hodgkin-Huxley model does not show bifurcations between oscillations. Multirhythmicity can be explained either by taking into account more conductances or by adopting modified equations (Chay 1985; Chay and Rinzel 1985). These equations may even lead to chaos, as will be discussed in section 4.3.

Network Architecture of Possible Rhythm Generators

A way to obtain networks with oscillation dynamics is to study systems for which the conditions of convergence to equilibrium are violated. It was demonstrated by examples in the context of chemical instabilities (Tyson 1975) that two-dimensional models of chemical reactions might exhibit oscillatory behavior when some condition of qualitative stability does not hold. Once again, the matrix $\mathbf{J}$, the jacobian, expresses the sign and strength of interactions, as in sec. 4.1.3. The existence of self-excitation ($\mathbf{J}_{ii} > 0$), the occurrence of competition ($\mathbf{J}_{ij} > 0$ and $\mathbf{J}_{ji} > 0$) or of cooperation ($\mathbf{J}_{ij} > 0$ and $\mathbf{J}_{ji} > 0$), and the existence of positive feedback loops ($\mathbf{J}_{ij}\mathbf{J}_{jk}\ldots\mathbf{J}_{qi} > 0$) and of negative feedback loops ($\mathbf{J}_{ij}\mathbf{J}_{jk}\ldots\mathbf{J}_{qi} < 0$) all are possible sources of instabilities.

Results in the theory of differential equations attributable to Hirsch (1987, 1991, and references cited therein) established relationships between structural properties and the dynamics of the system. The structure of the jacobian matrix of five (not disjoint) important groups (though the definitions and statements are not restricted to three-dimensional systems) are as follows:

$$\begin{bmatrix} \searrow & - & - \\ - & \searrow & - \\ - & - & \searrow \end{bmatrix} \begin{bmatrix} \searrow & + & + \\ + & \searrow & + \\ + & + & \searrow \end{bmatrix} \begin{bmatrix} \searrow & * & [\\ * & \searrow & x \\ [& x & \searrow \end{bmatrix} \begin{bmatrix} \searrow & * & * \\ & \searrow & * \\ & & \searrow \end{bmatrix} \begin{bmatrix} + & & \\ & + & \\ & & + \end{bmatrix}$$

$$\quad(1)\qquad\quad(2)\qquad\quad(3)\qquad\quad(4)\qquad\quad(5)$$

Signs of the matrix elements are denoted by minus ($-$) and plus ($+$). The symbols $*$, $[$, and x are used to characterize the structure of the matrix: For example, in matrix 3, these symbols express that the symmetry condition holds.

There are some important statements on systems characterized by each one of these jacobian matrices, derived mostly from Hirsch (1984, 1987). Competitive systems (matrix 1, supplemented with proper negative elements) show convergence to equilibrium. Competitive systems can be transformed to cooperative ones (matrix 2), but the original system can have attracting period points. Sign-symmetrical systems (matrix 3) show convergence when the system has a feedback loop (matrix 4) and the even-loop property (i.e., the number of edges a negative sign is even) also holds. Self-excitation (also known as *positive feedback* or *autocatalysis* in different context; matrix 5) is believed to be an important source of periodicity.

The violation of the even-loop property leads to recurrent cyclical inhibitory networks (Székely 1965; Kling and Székely 1968; Adám 1968; Glass and Young 1979), which were assumed to be a possible source of rhythmical neural activity. The following small networks have been offered as substrates of oscillations:

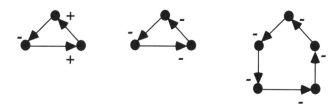

More generally, ring networks might exhibit oscillations (Atyia and Baldi 1989) if the number of inhibitory connections is odd and if the coupling between the neurons is sufficiently strong. The circulation of activation in a ring network was offered as the neural basis of simple locomotion (Székely, Czeh, and Vërös 1969). Atyia and Baldi (1989) extended their own analysis for certain classes of layered structures. It was assumed that all connections from one layer to the next had the same sign and therefore could be interpreted as being made of many ring structures. This kind of structure can exhibit oscillations.

The occurrence of oscillations in a field model of interacting excitatory and inhibitory populations was demonstrated by Ermentrout and Cowan (1979) in the case of a fully connected network.

Coupled Oscillators

We have seen that oscillators may result from membrane properties at the single-cell level and from qualitative patterns of coupling between cells that may not themselves be oscillators. In this section, we look at the question of what happens when many oscillators are coupled. Coupled oscillators play an important role in explaining the dynamics of CPGs as well as synchronized rhythmical cortical activity. Coupling may happen through both

gap junctions and chemical synapses. The first case is modeled by adding a term $\Delta V / R_{\text{gap}}$ to the membrane equation, where ΔV is the potential drop between the presynaptic and postsynaptic cells and R_{gap} is the resistance of the gap junctions. The treatment of the second case requires that synaptic currents be included (see equations 4 and 5). For further details, see Ermentrout (1994), who treats such special cases as coupling through slow, fast, and weak synapses.

The behavior of a population of oscillators can be studied by neglecting details of individual oscillators. Here we briefly examine studies motivated by the following observations on the CPG for swimming in the lamprey: First, even short, deafferented segments from the spinal cord of a lamprey can exhibit oscillations (fictive locomotion); and second, in a long segment, not only does each segment oscillate at the same frequency, but there is a constant phase lag between successive segments. [In section 6.3.2, we will discuss a more biologically detailed model: the analysis given by Träven et al. (1993) of the role of NMDA receptors in a network of interneurons conforming to experimentally identified cell types involved in the lamprey spinal locomotor pattern generator.]

Synchronizing a Chain of Oscillators Ermentrout and Kopell (1984; also Kopell 1988) studied a model

$$\dot{u}_k = F(u_k) + G^+(u_{k+1}, u_k) + G^-(u_{k-1}, u_k) \qquad (11)$$

with nearest neighbor coupling, where $F(u_k)$ specifies the free dynamics of the kth oscillator. To provide a general analytical study, they made hypotheses on the coupling functions G^+ and G^-.

• Only phase (i.e., the angle between 0 and 2π), which indicates progress around the limit cycle of each oscillator, is relevant. This is true provided that the coupling is not so strong as to overcome the power of attraction of the limit cycle.

• The coupling terms are replaced by their averages over each cycle. This assumption works always for the case of weak coupling only, and for strong coupling, if the oscillators communicate at phases distributed around the cycle.

• Coupling is synaptic (chemical and not electrical).

These assumptions reduce the equation to

$$\Phi_{k+1} = \omega_k + H_k^+(\Phi_{k-1} - \Phi_k) + H_k^-(\Phi_{k-1} - \Phi_k) \qquad (12)$$

where Φ_k is the phase of the kth oscillator, which has frequency ω_k. The H^* are 2π-periodic functions. In consequence of the assumptions made, the coupling terms depend on the phase differences alone. A further assumption is the *synaptic coupling hypothesis*, $H^*(0) \neq 0$, to ensure that synchrony is not a solution even if the oscillators are identical. For solving the equations, information about the spatial patterns of phase and frequency of the ensemble is obtained using the phase differences $\phi_k = \Phi_{k+1} - \Phi_k$.

As Kopell (1988) remarks, biologically it is more plausible to regard the chain of oscillators as coupled to many neighbors than to just nearest neighbors. By using a multicoupled structure, it is possible to explain that sometimes frequency differences do not imply a phase lag. (In other words, phase delays may emerge from a different mechanism and may not require frequency differences.)

In a further study, Kopell and Ermentrout (1990) reduced the complex dynamics of neurons in the spinal cord of a lamprey to chain of oscillators with constant amplitude and cooperative dynamics in the phases.

Networks of Limit-Cycle Oscillators with Local and Long-Range Coupling We now consider synchronization in networks in which individual oscillators are characterized by the phase variable Φ_i, oscillator i is driven by a random internal frequency ω_i taken from a distribution $g(\omega_i)$, and the interaction between oscillators i and k is homogenous (i.e., we no longer have a chain but rather a fully connected network) and depends only on the phase difference $\Delta\Phi_{ik} = \Phi_i - \Phi_k$ of the two oscillators. The interaction law $f(\Delta\Phi_{ik})$ should be continuous and periodic. To enable the system to synchronize itself, $f(0) = 0$ must be chosen (contrary to the synaptic coupling hypothesis in the lamprey model): That is, two synchronized oscillators ($\Delta\Phi_{ik} = 0$) do not drive each other but follow their internal driving force ω_i. Note the difference from the objective of Kopell and Ermentrout's lamprey model, wherein spatial patterns (such as traveling waves) and not a synchronized state of an oscillator chain is required to model the network behavior. Kuramoto (1984), Ermentrout (1986), and others have studied the following equation

$$\frac{d\Phi_i}{dt} = \omega_i - K \sum_{i;k \in N_i} \sin(\Phi_i - \Phi_k) + \xi_i, \qquad (13)$$

which expresses a generic choice for a limit-cycle system. Stochastic forces that act on the oscillator phases are described by the white-noise term ξ_i. N_i is the set of all oscillators that are connected to oscillator i. Thus, $N_i = \{i-1, i+1\}$ for a one-dimensional chain of limit-cycle oscillators, whereas $N_i = \{1, \dots, N\}$ for a fully connected network. A fully connected oscillator network

with dynamics as expressed in equation 13 exhibits a strong tendency to synchronize phases if the noise and the width of the distribution $g(\omega_i)$ are not too large and the global coupling parameter K is sufficiently strong (Sakaguchi 1988).

A special case of equation 13 is a network in which all oscillators exhibit the same internal frequency ω. The coordinate transformation $\psi := \Phi_i - \omega_o t$ reduces equation 13 to

$$\frac{d\Phi_i}{dt} = -\frac{\partial H}{\partial \Phi_i} + \xi_i \qquad (14)$$

with the energylike function $H = -K \sum_{i,k \in N_i} \cos(\Phi_i - \Phi_k)$.

This system of local nearest neighbor coupling in two dimensions has been studied extensively in physics, where it has been shown that phase synchronization is not a robust phenomenon. Any amount of noise, no matter how weak, will destroy a completely synchronized network state. Such a result indicates that the long-range synchronization observed in the visual cortex cannot be explained with a local connection scheme but requires long-range synapses. Indeed, long-range interconnections have been discovered in the first layer of the visual cortex of the cat (Gilbert and Wiesel 1983; Gilbert 1985, 1993; see chapter 8).

The generation of synchronized cortical oscillation has been the subject of a number of model studies (Buhmann 1989; Schuster and Wagner 1990a, b; Sompolinsky, Chrisanti, and Sommers 1990; Horn, Sagi, and Usher 1991; Horn and Usher 1991; König and Schillen 1991; Schillen and König 1991; Sporns et al. 1989; Sporns, Tononi, and Edelman 1991; Gerstner, Rita, and van Hemmen 1993; Ritz et al. 1994; Fukai 1994). These models explain different aspects of feature linking and pattern segmentation. Nonetheless, a biologically plausible and mathematically generic model still is missing.

Gait Transitions in Locomotion The general, model-independent properties of symmetrically coupled oscillators have also been studied by group-theoretical methods. In that venue, oscillators have been identified with locomotor CPGs. Six symmetrically coupled oscillators have been considered as models of CPGs in insects, and the transitions between the gaits were modeled as symmetry-breaking bifurcations (Collins and Stewart 1993a). In particular, the relationship between the different network structures of the symmetrically coupled oscillators and the possible rhythmical patterns (associated with gaits) that they can generate were derived and listed. The symmetries of quadrupedal animal gaits have also been analyzed (Schöner, Jiang, and Kelso 1990; Collins and Stewart 1993b, 1994). Such analysis showed that minor modification in the network structure may exert a significant effect on the resulting gait. It is not easy to localize CPGs. By making a symmetry analysis of animal gaits, information on the possible network structure of CPGs can be obtained. Because the same network may produce different rhythmical patterns, depending on the parameter values, the same locomotor CPG may produce and control very different gaits.

4.3 Chaotic Behavior in Neural Systems: Some Facts and Models

4.3.1 Conceptual Remarks on Chaos in Neural Systems

Chaos is a nonperiodic temporal behavior generated by deterministic mechanisms (in reality) and algorithms (in models). In a chaotic region, each trajectory is highly sensitive to initial conditions (i.e., even very small changes in initial condition eventually can yield large divergences in trajectory). Thus the long-term behavior of systems leading to chaos is unpredictable. It must be remarked, however, that only the individual trajectories—not the overall behavior of the system—are unpredictable. Analogously to stochastic processes, in which the probability distributions or density functions can be constructed from random individual realizations, the family of chaotic trajectories can also be analyzed, at least by statistical methods.

We will not discuss in detail here the general concepts and statements of chaos theory and the mathematical techniques of generating and detecting chaos (see Schuster 1984; Holden 1986; Gleick 1987), but we do provide a few introductory remarks. Analytical and numerical studies have revealed a few different mechanisms by which chaos can be generated, both in continuous systems described by differential equations and in discrete systems modeled by iterative maps. Chaotic phenomena lead to the so-called strange attractors, which a fractal structures and a topology characterized by fractal dimension. The definition of fractal structures and fractal dimension is beyond the scope of this book (see chapter 3 of Kaplan and Glass 1995 for an elementary introduction); however, the reader may think of trajectories in three-dimensional space that fill far more space than a limit cycle (hence, are more than one-dimensional) yet do not fill enough (in a certain technical sense) of any plane in the space to be considered two-dimensional.

The sensitivity to initial conditions, which is the fundamental property of chaotic systems, is quantified by the Lyapunov exponent. Consider trajectories of the finite dimensional system

$$x'(t) = F(x(t)), x(t) \in \mathcal{R}^d$$

starting near x_0. Prepare a small r-dimensional cube of side ε, which contains x_0, to represent the uncertainty in measurement of initial conditions. Let its volume be $V_r(x_0, \varepsilon)$. After time t, let $V_r(x(t), \varepsilon)$ be the volume of the smallest (hyper)parallelepiped that contains all the states obtained by system evolution from states in the initial cube. The volume at $x(t)$ divided by the volume at x_0 yields the local r-dimensional Lyapunov exponent by the formula

$$\Lambda_r(x_0, \varepsilon, t) = \frac{1}{t} \ln \frac{V_r(x(t), \varepsilon)}{V_r(x_0, \varepsilon)}.$$

Taking the limit as ε tends to 0 and t tends to infinity yields

$$\Lambda_r = \lim_{\substack{\varepsilon \to 0 \\ t \to \infty}} \Lambda_r(x_0, \varepsilon, t) = \lim_{\substack{\varepsilon \to 0 \\ t \to \infty}} \frac{1}{t} \ln \frac{V_r x(t)}{V_r(x_0)}.$$

Each such number is called a *Lyapunov exponent*. Consider $r = 1$. If the discrepancy $\delta(t)$ in initial conditions were reduced over time with an exponential decay $\delta(t) \approx \varepsilon \, e^{-\lambda t}$, we would have $\Lambda_1 = -\lambda$, whereas if $\delta(t)$ increased exponentially over time with $\delta(t) \approx \varepsilon \, e^{\lambda t}$, we would have $\Lambda_1 = \lambda$. Thus, the change of the distances in different directions between adjacent points during motion is characterized by a set of Lyapunov exponents. A single positive Lyapunov exponent indicates (but does not guarantee) chaos, whereas the presence of more than one positive exponent is associated with hyperchaotic systems (Rössler 1983).

Dimension analysis and the calculation of Lyapunov exponents serve as methods of detection of chaos, but they do not provide necessary and sufficient conditions for chaos. For example, an unstable equilibrium point also can yield positive Lyapunov exponents.

The structural conditions of chaos occur at different hierarchical levels of neural organization, and their eventual functional consequences are summarized in the following subsections. Both periodic and chaotic temporal patterns can be generated at the single-neuron level (sec. 4.3.2), at the multicellular network level owing to interactions among neurons (sec. 4.3.4), and at the global level in consequence of spatiotemporal integration (sec. 4.3.5). Neurochemical synaptic transmission also might produce chaotic signals (sec. 4.3.3). The diagnosis and the control of chaos associated with normal and pathological brain functions (sec. 4.3.6) and, more generally, the possible functional roles of chaos (sec. 4.3.7) also are discussed.

Overviews of chaotic neurodynamic systems include King (1991), Érdi (1993), and Elbert et al. (1994). Volumes on chaos and brain functioning include those by Basar (1990) and Dvořak and Holden (1991). In addition, two recent special issues of journals [*Integrative Physiological and Behavioral Science* 29(3), July–September 1994; *International Journal of Intelligent Systems* 10(1), 1995] are dedicated to chaotic neural systems.

4.3.2 Chaos in Neural Membranes

Experiments

Chaos can be generated both endogenously and by periodic forcing. A few chaotic phenomena have been demonstrated experimentally at the single-neuron level. Molluscan neurons have shown chaotic activity induced by K^+ blocking agents (Holden, Winlow, and Haydon 1982). Rapp et al. (1985) reported that spontaneous activity in the precentral and postcentral gyri of the squirrel monkey might be chaotic. The complex temporal pattern of spontaneous activity recorded from the molluscan pacemaker neuron was claimed to exhibit a chaotic time series (Mpitsos et al. 1988). The *Onchidium* pacemaker neuron can show regular beating, regular bursting, and irregular bursting discharges, depending on the current applied (Hayashi et al. 1982; Hayashi and Ishizuka 1992). The membrane potential of the squid giant axon demonstrates periodic and nonperiodic responses (Matsumoto et al. 1984). Hippocampal pyramidal cells also may be candidates for chaotic pattern generators (Hayashi and Ishizuka 1990).

Models

Holden (1985; Holden, Hyde, and Muhamed 1991) noted that chaotic behavior occurs in neurons (and model neurons) under rather restrictive conditions and only for small ranges of parameters. It was demonstrated that chaotic behavior can be found in the Hodgkin-Huxley equation in the case of a periodic input function but only for small ranges of forcing amplitudes and frequencies.

A model slightly different from the Hodgkin-Huxley equation was derived and studied to describe the dynamics of excitable membranes (Chay 1984, 1985; Chay and Rinzel 1985; Chay and Lee 1990; Fan and Chay 1994). The different endogenous rhythmical and arrhythmic activities of cardiac cells, β-cells of the pancreas, and neuronal somatic (rather than axonic, as in the Hodgkin-Huxley model) membranes were simulated. In the earlier versions, currents carried by sodium and calcium ions were treated by a single "mixed" effective conductance. In the later version (Chay and Lee 1990), the occurrence of two functionally distinct currents—namely, the slow and fast currents—is explicitly taken into account. The time dependence of the membrane potential is expressed by the equation

$$-C_m \frac{dV}{dt} = I_{\text{fast}} + I_{\text{slow}} + I_K + I_L \tag{15}$$

where I_{fast} is the fast inward current carried by either sodium or calcium ions, I_{slow} is a slow inward current carried by calcium ions, I_K is an outward current carried by potassium ions, and I_L is the leakage current. The equations for the four currents are:

$$I_{\text{fast}} = \bar{g}_{\text{fast}} m_\infty h (V - V_{\text{fast}}) \tag{16a}$$

$$I_{\text{slow}} = \bar{g}_{\text{slow}} \, df (V - V_C) \tag{16b}$$

$$I_K = \bar{g}_n (V - V_K) \tag{16c}$$

$$I_L = \bar{g}_L (V - V_L) \tag{16d}$$

where $\bar{g}_{\text{fast}}$, $\bar{g}_{\text{slow}}$, $\bar{g}$ and $\bar{g}_L$ are the maximal conductances of fast, slow, potassium, and leak currents, respectively, and m, h, d, f, and n are the voltage-dependent gating variables. In equation 16a, m is set at its equilibrium value $\tilde{m}$ due to rapid equilibrium. Equations 15 and 16 are supplemented with four kinetic equations (for the "slow" variables h, d, f, and n). Numerical simulations demonstrated that, by changing the time constant of the inactivation of I_{slow}, a series of complex patterned activities (simple slow oscillation, bursting, bursting-chaos, beating-chaos, and beating) were generated (figure 4.3).

Further studies of the emergence of chaos in single-neuron models include the following: Carpenter (1979) gave a rigorous mathematical classification of bursting in excitable systems (for the analysis of the different mechanisms of bursting, see Rinzel 1987). Mathematically simplified models (Lábos 1984; Aihara 1990) of neurons also may exhibit chaos. Bifurcations to periodic and chaotic behavior in the force-free, direct current–driven and alternating current–driven version of the FitzHugh-Nagumo equation, even in the control of chaos (see sec. 4.5) were systematically studied by Rajesekar and Lakshmanan (1994).

4.3.3 Transmitter Release: Random or Deterministic Mechanism?

Spontaneously occurring miniature end-plate potentials (MEPPs) were described first by Fatt and Katz (1952). MEPPs occur owing to spontaneous release of quanta of

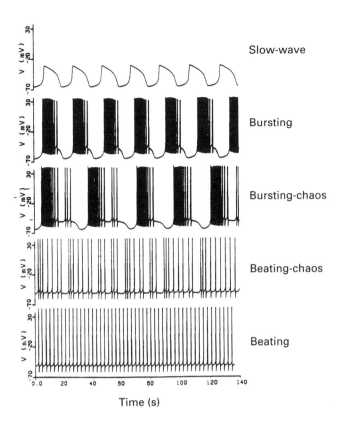

Figure 4.3
Complex oscillations to show how the I_{fast} inactivation kinetics give rise to chaos. Simple oscillation, regular bursts, bursting-chaos, beating-chaos, and repetitive beating are shown from top trace to bottom. (After Chan and Lee 1990.)

Slow-wave

Bursting

Bursting-chaos

Beating-chaos

Beating

Time (s)

transmitter molecules from the presynaptic terminal and were detected first at the frog neuromuscular junction. They are confined to the end-plate region of the muscle fiber, and the transmitter substance is acetylcholine. Statistical analyses of MEPPs seem to be in accordance with the vesicular hypothesis based on the morphological demonstration of synaptic vesicles (De Roberties and Bennett 1957). According to the classic, vesicular hypothesis (Del Castillo and Katz 1954), packets of transmitter molecules (quanta) are contained in synaptic vesicles and are released by exocytosis. The random character of the amplitude- and time-interval distributions of the MEPPs was explained by variable contents of the quanta.

Recently, Kriebel, Vautrin, and Holsapple (1990) offered an alternative hypothesis on the nature of transmitter release. The dripping faucet was suggested to be the proper model of the release process. The dripping faucet is a common example of the transition from periodicity to chaos (Crutchfield and et al. 1986). The main points of Kriebel and coworkers are that the packets are not preformed but are dynamically generated during

the release process and that MEPPs are not random but are deterministic chaotic signals (figure 4.4).

4.3.4 Network Structure and Chaos: Some Design Principles

Section 4.1.3 introduced qualitative conditions on connectivity of neural networks—the network architecture—that would guarantee convergence to a point equilibrium, while section 4.2.2 included a characterization of the network architecture of possible rhythm generators. We now look for a similar characterization of chaotic behavior. Methods of local analysis, such as linear stability analysis, are not appropriate methods for detecting chaos. Still, for three-dimensional systems without self-activation, King (1983) gave conditions under which jacobian matrix structures would be prone to chaos. Jacobians, as defined in section 4.1.3, are candidates for chaos only if their graphs are characterized by three conditions: (1) The graph is connected; (2) each node has at least one edge directed toward it and one edge directed away from it; and (3) there is a node with at least two edges directed toward it. The structures of the jacobian matrices satisfying these criteria are as follows:

$$
\begin{bmatrix} \searrow & & + \\ + & \searrow & \\ + & + & \searrow \end{bmatrix}
\begin{bmatrix} \searrow & + & \\ + & \searrow & + \\ & + & \searrow \end{bmatrix}
\begin{bmatrix} \searrow & & + \\ + & \searrow & + \\ + & + & \searrow \end{bmatrix}
\begin{bmatrix} - & + & + \\ + & \searrow & + \\ + & + & \searrow \end{bmatrix}
$$

Sompolinsky, Chrisanti, and Sommers (1988) considered fully connected large networks (in the limit of asymptotically infinite systems). Practically, the long time properties of a variant of the leaky integrator network of equation 6 has been studied by using the mean synaptic strength S^* as the control parameter. Two critical values ($S^*_{cr1} < S^*_{cr2}$) have been found. Structures with $S^* < S^*_{cr1}$ lead to a stable equilibrium point, those with $S^*_{cr1} < S^* < S^*_{cr2}$ exhibit a limit cycle, and those with $S^* > S^*_{cr2}$ might exhibit chaos. Because these networks are characterized by an "averaged parameter," networks other than those that are fully connected can be considered. Widely but weakly connected networks are implicitly (and biologically implausibly) suggested to be functionally equivalent to narrowly but strongly connected systems (the mean synaptic strength is rescaled by the relationship $S^* = c_n \alpha^2$).

4.3.5 Global Cortical Dynamics

The technique of recording the EEG has opened a window for measuring and understanding brain activity. Though the underlying biophysical mechanisms of EEG

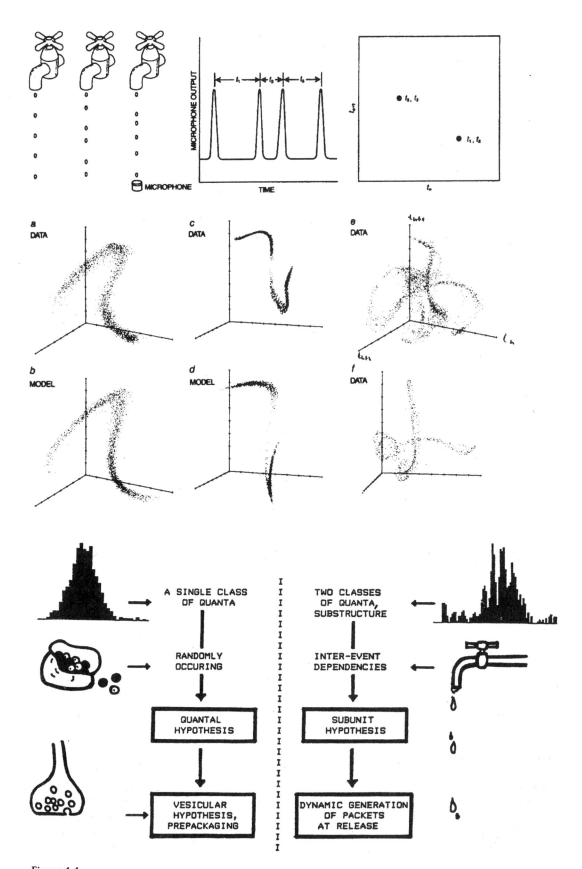

Figure 4.4

The dripping faucet can undergo a transition from regular to chaotic dripping. This has been considered as a model for release of neuro-transmitters. (Composite figure after Kriebel, Vautrin, and Holsapple 1990 and Crutchfield et al. 1986.)

signal generation are not clear, still the processing of EEG curves provides information about the structure-function relationship of the brain. According to the already classic approach, EEG records are treated as time series and considered as stationary stochastic processes, and their characteristic frequencies are determined by spectral analysis.

Nonlinear dynamic system theory offers a different conceptual approach to EEG signal processing (e.g., see Basar 1990; Dvorak and Holden 1991; Elbert et al. 1994; Skarda and Freeman 1987; Freeman 1992; Freeman and Barrie 1994). Time series, even irregular ones, are considered as deterministic phenomena generated by nonlinear differential equations. First, the phase space of the dynamic system is reconstructed; then its so-called embedding and correlation dimensions are calculated. Once again, the formal definition of these dimensions is beyond the scope of this book; rather, see Grassberger and Procaccia (1983) and chapter 6 of Kaplan and Glass (1995). Low (but larger than two) and fractal dimensions are associated with deterministic chaos, whereas it is difficult (if at all possible) to discriminate between high-dimensional chaos and a random process. Lyapunov exponents, as defined in section 4.3.1, measure the exponential divergence of nearby trajectories. (For an efficient algorithm, see Barna and Tsuda 1993.) The criterion of chaos (loosely speaking, the existence of at least one positive Lyapunov exponent) was reported to be fulfilled for the sleep cycle (Babloyantz, Salazar, and Nicolis 1985), epileptic petit-mal seizure (Babloyantz and Destexhe 1986), alpha rhythm (Soong and Stuart 1989), and Creutzfeldt-Jakob disease (Gallez and Babloyantz 1991).

Qualms regarding the usefulness of fractal dimensional analysis of neuronal activity have been mentioned by Prissl (1990) and Albano and Rapp (1993). Special attention is needed to evaluate both continuous-time signals (such as the membrane potential) and discrete-time processes (such as spike trains). Further research is expected to show whether the different proper discretization procedures of continuous signals lead to different fractal dimension. Recent opinions (e.g., Glass 1995; Lopes da Silva and Pijn 1995) also suggest that caution is needed to avoid overinterpreting the results of EEG signal analysis of by using dynamic system theory.

The first ten years of the dynamical analysis of biological data have been characterized by difficulties and disappointments, but much has been learned. The prospects for the application of improved measures to more realistically defined problems are encouraging... (Rapp 1994).

Wright the Liley (1996) have attempted to develop their own model for describing cortical eletrogenesis in the light of the results of some important previous modeling efforts (Freeman 1992). They gave a stochastic model for the generation of electrocortical activity. They have a principle, namely chaos in the small and stochasticity in the large (Érdi 1996b). Despite the existence of improved statistical methods to discriminate between noise and chaos, it is still hard to decide uniquely whether electrocortical recordings should be considered purely random or deterministic chaotic patterns.

4.3.6 Dynamical Disease and Controlling Chaos

A *dynamical disease* is defined as a disease that occurs in an intact physiological system yet leads to abnormal dynamics. For example, chaotic behavior has been found in a model of the central dopaminergic neuronal system and in association with schizophrenia (King, Barchas, and Huberman 1984).

Control of Cholinergic Synaptic Transmission

"Normal" and "abnormal" dynamic behaviors during cholinergic synaptic transmission arise from the metabolic processes during neurochemical transmission. Neurochemical studies suggest that synaptic-level rhythmic generation in the cholinergic system requires a fine-tuned neurochemical control system. Even mild impairment of the metabolism might imply "abnormal" dynamic synaptic activity.

Experimental evidence has accumulated to connect neural and mental disorders to disturbances of control of neurotransmitter synthesis. The hypoxia and hypoglycemia due to the failure of cholinergic metabolism leads to reduced acetylcholine (ACh) synthesis and neurological disorders (Gibson and Blass 1976a, b). Choline, a precursor of ACh, seemed to be useful in treating memory disorders associated with Alzheimer's disease and aging (Wurtman, Hefti, and Mclamed 1981), reinforcing the view that understanding the operation of the dynamic control systems of ACh metabolism could yield suggestions for new clinical treatments of such diseases.

Integrated synaptic activity (Dunant et al. 1977; Israel et al. 1977)—particularly the strong coupling between ACh release and synthesis (for a review, see MacIntosh and Collier 1976)—has been studied by a skeleton model of the transmitter-recycling hypothesis (Érdi 1983). In this model, the state of the system is characterized by four variables, and five subprocesses are defined (figure 4.5). The state variables are the ACh concentration in the cytoplasm (x) and at the postsynaptic

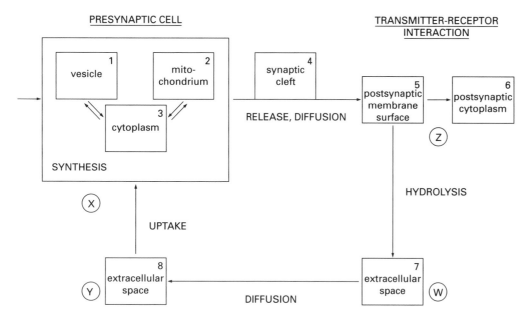

Figure 4.5
Skeleton model of integrated synaptic activity associated with the transmitter-recycling hypothesis. The eight-compartment system has been lumped into a four-variable system.

membrane surface (z), and the choline concentration near the presynaptic and postsynaptic cell (w and y, respectively). The subprocesses taken into account are: (1) transmitter release, cleft processes, and transmitter-receptor interaction; (2) ACh hydrolysis; (3) diffusion of metabolic products (mostly choline) in the vicinity of the presynaptic cell; (4) reuptake of choline; and (5) autocatalytic synthesis of ACh. It might be plausible to assume that rhythmical integrated activity is perturbed at least by another oscillator coupled to the ACh synthesis. ACh synthesis is controlled by sodium-dependent high-affinity choline uptake (Barker and Mittag 1975) and by the transport of acetyl groups (Jope 1979; Tucek 1983, 1993). Periodically added choline might lead to complex oscillatory behaviors. Under these assumptions, the lumped skeleton model is defined as follows:

$$\frac{dx(t)}{dt} = -k_1 x(t) + k_4 y(t) + k_5 x^2(t) y(t)$$

$$\frac{dz(t)}{dt} = k_1 x(t) - k_2 z(t)$$

$$\frac{dw(t)}{dt} = k_2 z(t) - k_3 w(t) \tag{17}$$

$$\frac{dy(t)}{dt} = k_3 w(t) - k_4 y(t) - k_5 x^2(t) y(t) + \alpha \cos(\omega t + \phi)$$

The unperturbed system ($\alpha = 0$) exhibits sustained oscillatory behavior. By fixing the "total mass" $M = x + y + w + z$ but changing the initial concentrations,

limit cycle behavior can be visualized (figure 4.6a). By changing M, a family of limit cycles (limit shells) can be derived (Tóth 1985; figure 4.6b). Extensive numerical studies (Érdi and Barna 1987; Barna and Érdi 1988) helped the discovery of many details of the fine structure of the amplitude-frequency phase space. Phase locking and also long-lived transient chaos have been demonstrated (figure 4.7)

The existence of rather long-lived transient arrhythmias and their abrupt decay to simple periodicity seems to be in accordance with the view that normal rhythmical dynamics are the result of the operation of a fine-tuned control system. The quantity and velocity of external choline uptake might control the ACh synthesis and can severely influence the course of certain neurological and mental disorders associated with ACh metabolism.

Not only the appearance of even transient chaos but other qualitative changes (e.g., emergence or loss of rhythms, appearance of altered or new periodicities) can be related to dynamic diseases (for temporal disorders in human oscillatory systems see Rensing, van der Heiden, and Mackey 1987).

Controlling Chaos: Different Strategies

The techniques of controlling chaos seem to offer "entirely new therapeutic and diagnostic tools for diseases ranging from heart disease to epilepsy" (Moss 1994).

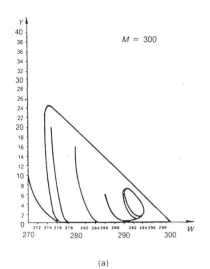

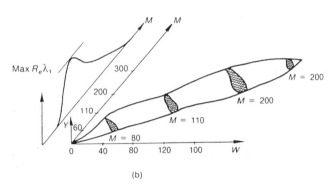

Figure 4.6

(a) The Y-versus-W selection curve seems to tend from outside to a stable limit cycle. (b) The relatively stable limit cycles are changed as a function of the total mass of the system. The system has limit cycles within a certain range of M. The shape and location of these closed curves vary as the constraint is varied. (After Érdi and Tóth 1989.)

There are several different strategies to control and suppress chaos. The similarities and differences of the approaches can be explained in terms of a few dichotomies, which we list here:

1. *Feedback versus feedforward control.* The processes can be controlled by some feedback mechanism: the controlling signal is determined by the deviation between the actual and the expected behavior. Alternatively, a predetermind strategy can be prescribed to influence the internal operation of the system by some feedforward mechanism.

2. *Model-based versus "data-only" control.* Control is possible with or without the knowledge of the model.

3. *Parameter versus input control.* A system may be controlled internally by adjusting some of its parameters or externally by adding some control function.

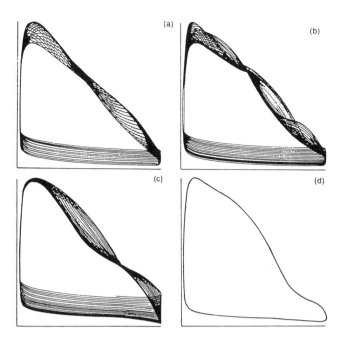

Figure 4.7

Phase plane diagram in different time regimens. (a) Approaching the transient attractor. (b, c) Intermediate regimens. (d) Near the true attractor. (Reprinted with permission from Barna and Érdi 1987.)

4. *Targeting versus control.* The prescribed goal of the control may or may not be prescribed. (The former case is called targeting.)

Interest in the control of chaos was reinforced by the presentation of Ott, Greborgi, and Yorke (1990) and Shinbrot, Greborgi, Ott, and Yorke (1993). They offered a feedback algorithm—now called the OGY algorithm—for stabilizing (not too fast) unstable periodic orbits embedded within a strange attractor which contains infinite number of unstable periodic orbits by making only small time-dependent perturbations in accessible system parameters. The OGY method can be extended to the case of a spatially distributed network of oscillators (Sepulchre and Babloyantz 1993).

The time-continuous control of chaos by self-controlling feedback (without and with delay) has been offered (Pyragas 1992; Pyragas and Tamasevicius 1993). The implication of continuous control is that even rapid periodic orbits could be stabilized, and the level of noise tolerance is also increased.

The adaptive control algorithm (ACA) starts from the model equations of the system exhibiting chaotic behavior

$$\frac{dx(t)}{dt} = F(x; p; t) \tag{18}$$

The system has chaotic solution with specific $p = $ const. values. The adaptive control algorithm (Huberman and Lumer 1990) is implemented by specifying the dynamics of the parameter change depending on the difference of the actual and desired states:

$$\frac{dp(t)}{dt} = \varepsilon G(x(t) - x_s) \qquad (19)$$

A class of problems of feedforward control (the term "open-loop" control is also used) has been formulated (Jackson 1991; Jackson and Kodogeorgiou 1991). Given a dynamic system $dx(t)/dt = F(x(t))$, where $x(t)$ can be a finite-dimensional vector, and prescribed goal dynamics $g(t)$, the problem is to choose an additive control function U to yield the "entrainment"

$$\lim_{t \to \infty} |x(t) - g(t_0)| = 0 \qquad (20)$$

for all initial values starting from the basin of the entrainment. In the simplest case (e.g., when the goal function is contained entirely in the convergent region of the phase space and some other technically restrictive conditions), the control function with the rather simple form

$$U(g(t), g'(t)) = g' - F(g(t)) \qquad (21)$$

provides the required control.

Another class of feedforward control strategies adopts the usually weak periodic perturbation of some parameter (for a general treatment, see Loskutov 1993). This method starts from equation 18 assuming that it exhibits chaotic dynamics in the range $p' < p < p''$. Substituting the constant p taken from the inside of the range with some periodic function $p + p \sin(\omega t)$, and giving some restrictive condition for p to force the systems to remain within the region of chaotic attractor, chaotic behavior can easily be suppressed. This method does not require that some prescribed goal be fixed, but the price to be paid is that no guess can be given as to which non-chaotic behavior will emerge as the result of the chaos suppression.

The efficacy of different controlling algorithms has been tested in the FitzHugh-Nagumo model (Rajesekar and Lakshmanan 1994.) Garfinkel et al. (1992) demonstrating the control of chaos in arrhythmic cardiac tissue, than the OGY method was applied to in vitro neural network, namely to spontaneously bursting hippocampal slices (Schiff et al. 1994). There is some hopes that similar techniques can be effective of such application as, for example, in vivo epileptic foci, visually guided motor activity (Gaál 1995), and the like.

Chaos, however, may be controlled not only "from outside" in the nervous system. The brain as a dynamic system obviously is extremely complex. Becaus even simple dynamical systems (e.g., the one-dimensional logistic map, May 1976) lead to chaotic behavior, the nervous system is not so chaotic as it might be expected from its structure (Holden 1985). Physiological parameters seem often to avoid those ranges of values that lead to chaos, and one may think that chaos is controlled "from inside."

4.3.7 Possible Functional Roles of Chaos

Structural conditions for the emergence of chaos in different hierarchical levels of neural organization have been studied extensively. In spite of much effort, however, we are still far from having a coherent view of the eventual functional roles of chaos (Tsuda 1992). Freeman suggested that an animal cannot memorize a new odor without chaos: Different periodic behaviors associated with known odors may emerge from a chaotic background. Freeman and Barrie (1994) also argue that neural chaos contributes not only passively to human information processing but also to the dynamic generation of meaning in the cerebral cortex. In other words, their view is that the brain is not only a passive transformer of the signals coming from the environment but also an information generator. However, "Freeman's claims that chaotic dynamics plays an essential role in cognitive functions and information processing must be viewed as hypothesis rather than established fact" (Glass 1995). Whether the hypothesis is correct is among the more interesting questions of neural information processing to be answered in the future.

There is no universal answer to the question of whether chaos can be associated with healthy or pathological behavior in a physiological context. The old, and many times well-operating, concept of homeostasis (Cannon 1929) suggests that a certain state of the internal medium (Bernard 1878) is totally maintained. It has been suggested (Iberall 1978; Yates 1980) that homeokinesis rather than homeostasis better captures the dynamics of control mechanisms for the self-maintenance of organisms. As a compromise between homeostasis and chaos, Tsuda, Iwanaga, and Takara (1992) suggested that biological organisms maintain a "homeochaotic" state to adapt dynamically to a variable nonstationary environment. Homeochaos may play a role in evolutionary processes: It was identified as the mechanism of evolution of symbiosis (Ikegami and Kaneko 1992). The strong instability in low-dimensional chaos is smoothed out, and dynamic stability is sustained in high-dimensional chaos. The beneficial role of chaos has been suggested by Goldberger and West (1986), who claimed that chaos provides the organism with an information-rich state. It appears obvious that analogous to periodic systems, which may be beneficial (e.g., in the case of many normal physiological rhythms at very different time scales), or indicators of malfunctions (e.g., tremor), another dynamic behavior—chaos—also may have positive as well as negative functional roles. Tsuda (1991) argued for the possible existence of three mechanisms for the emergence of chaos at a certain level:

1. Chaos might be the direct consequence of a lower-level chaos ("spatial cascade").

2. Chaos can be independent of lower levels and might be the product of coupling of oscillators.

3. Chaos might be the result of self-organized lower activities.

4.4 Self-Organization and the Development of the Nervous System

4.4.1 Self-Organization: Between Determinism and Randomness

The emergence of complexity through self-organizing mechanisms has been studied on both the ontogenetic and the phylogenetic time scale. Thinking in terms of dynamical concepts, ontogenetic development is associated with the temporal change of state due to interaction among the state variables (when these are considered to include the synaptic weights of our neural network), whereas phylogenetic evolution can be visualized as bifurcations in a parameter space that characterizes a whole range of evolutionary possibilities: Continuous changes in the control parameters may lead to a discontinuous change in the state space. Ontogenetic development and phylogenetic evolution are closely related as dynamic processes (Gould 1977). In particular, development of individuals of a population can explain elementary evolutionary changes, and individual life histories can be modified by certain "evolutionary feedback" mechanisms. In this chapter, we mostly analyze self-organizing mechanisms related to normal ontogenetic development and plastic behavior. Self-organization phenomena occurring at different hierarchical levels of the nervous system were mentioned in section 4.1.1. An important question here is the balance between *determinism* and *randomness* in the nervous system.

Whenever he is looking at any piece of neural tissue, the investigator becomes immediately confronted with the choice between two conflicting issues: the question of how intricate wiring of the neuropil is strictly predetermined by some genetically prescribed blueprint, and how much freedom is left to chance within some framework of statistical probabilities or some secondary mechanism of trial and error, or selecting connections according to necessities or the individual history of the animal. Even on brief reflection one has to arrive at the conclusion that the case may not rest on either extreme (Szentágothai 1978a; see also Szentágothai 1990).

Many examples from embryology, anatomy, and physiology suggest that the brain cannot be considered as a purely deterministic system, and probabilistic concepts have a role in our understanding of the formation and operation of some neural structures. A family of apparently random behavior has been identified with chaos and reduced to deterministic mechanisms, but irreducibly stochastic elements also are important both in neural signal analysis and in modeling neural ontogeny and performance.

A possible resolution of the determinism-randomness dilemma was based on the principle described as "randomness in the small and structure in the large" (Anninos et al. 1970; Harth et al. 1970). This principle accepts the existence of stochastic effects in the brain but allows averaging out of the fluctuations. Single-neuron activity can have a random character (Holden 1976; Ricciardi 1994), but the evolution equations at the population levels are deterministic ones. However, in the theory of dynamic systems, it turned out that in certain situations (mostly in the neighborhood of instability points), the effect of the fluctuations cannot be averaged out. On the contrary, they may cause drastic effects even at the macroscopic level. The theory of "noise-induced transitions" (Horsthemke and Lefever 1984) shows that fluctuations may operate as "organizing forces." Speaking somewhat more technically, noise may cause instability of the deterministic attractors, and a stochastic model might exhibit properties qualitatively different from those of the deterministic model. These phenomena are illustrated in modeling the ontogeny of ordered neural structures, both retinotectal connections (sec. 4.4.2) and ocular dominance columns (sec. 8.2.2).

4.4.2 Retinotectal Connections

In animals such as goldfish and frogs, the main visual center is the optic tectum. Retinotectal connections generate a topographical map that preserves visual information between subsequent layers of cells. Numerous mathematical models have been established to describe the mechanism of the formation of such ordered neural mappings (e.g., Willshaw and von der Malsburg 1976, 1979; Amari 1980, 1982, 1983; Gierer 1981; Whitelaw and Cowan 1981; Kohonen 1982; Overton and Arbib 1982a, b; Haussler and von der Malsburg 1983; Érdi and Barna 1984, 1985; Érdi and Szentágothai 1985; Bienenstock 1985; Cottrell and Fort 1986; Ritter and Schulten 1986; Obermayer, Sejnowski, and Blasdel 1995).

Some alternatives are available for setting up a mathematical model for the formation of retinotectal mappings. We briefly discuss some models within the framework of these alternatives.

Specificity Versus Plasticity

The main issue concerns the role of the tectum in the formation of the mapping. Sperry (1943a, b) asked whether the functional recovery after optic nerve transection is established by specific affinities between matching retinal and tectal cells or by functional sorting of largely random retinal regrowth. He made mismatch experiments by removing part of the retina, part of the tectum, or parts of both. Early experimental results at first suggested that, after a partial lesion, there was a strong tendency for retinal ganglion cells to grow back only to the same tectal cells they contacted originally. According to Sperry's classic idea, reinforced by Attardi and Sperry (1963), there is a specific point-to-point projection between retina and tectum. Sperry's chemoaffinity hypothesis suggests that order and orientation of the topographic map are derived uniquely from the interactions between presynaptic and postsynaptic cells. (For further study of the problems of neuronal specificity, see Székely 1990.)

The other extreme theoretical approach is based on the results of plasticity experiments which, in contrast to earlier findings, established that retinotopy (as opposed to the individual connections) is preserved when a whole retina projects onto a surgically formed half retina or when a half retina expands across a whole tectum (for a review of these experiments, see chapter 9 of Jacobson 1978). In the system-matching models (arrow model, Hope, Hammond, and Gaze 1976; branch arrow model, Overton and Arbib 1982a; and extended branch arrow model, Overton and Arbib 1982b) the information available for the individual retinal fibers is less specific than in other models.

The Willshaw and von der Malsburg (1979) model may be qualified as intermediate between the two extremes. The role of the postsynaptic tissue is less active than the strict chemoaffinity hypothesis suggests. The postsynaptic tissue provides only some rough polarity rules by which to orient the retinal projection. Érdi and Barna (1984, 1985) did not define a specific orientation rule, but the role of competition among the incoming fibers (fiber-fiber sorting procedures) was emphasized. Such a mechanism could strongly influence the structure of the final position of the synaptic contacts and determine the precision of the mapping.

Genetically Prespecified Versus Environmentally Controlled Wiring

As noted in section 4.1.1, it is more or less accepted that the postnatal ontogenetic development of the nervous system is determined by the interaction of the innate genetic program and environmental factors. Self-organizing mechanisms such as the selective stabilization hypothesis offer a compromise between strict genetic determinism and environmental control. Roughly speaking, it is not the connections between specific cells that are preprogrammed, but an algorithm is given genetically to select favorable (in some sense) system connections.

Marker Theories Versus Activity-Dependent Mechanisms

In the marker theories, growing axons are directed to the appropriate point with the aid of some guiding substance. In the original version of the chemoaffinity hypothesis, each retinal cell was labeled with a unique chemical marker, and the complementary marker on the tectal neuron was recognized by some molecular recognition mechanism. Modified versions of the model used considerably fewer markers: two molecules in orthogonal gradients in the retina and complementary molecular gradients in the tectum. Though several candidates have been described (Trisler 1982), no molecule has yet been demonstrated to have an obligatory role in coding for neural position. Gierer (1981) tried to provide a principle for growing of fibers in terms of markers: A correct final position may be characterized by a minimal value of potential functions. Edelman (1984, 1987) offered a highly selective dynamic pattern–forming system that did not possess a large range of different molecular specificities, the central issue being the cell-surface modulation of cell adhesion molecules that are responsible for determining the neural connectivity.

The Willshaw–von der Malsburg (1979) model also was based on the use of marker molecules. According to the learning rule used in this model, synaptic strength increases more when the composition vectors characterizing the presynaptic and postsynaptic sheets are closer to each other.

4 A Dynamical Overview

Many hypotheses and theories designed to explain neural development, learning, and conditioning are based on the modifiability of synapses by correlated electrical activity of presynaptic and postsynaptic cells. Model studies suggest that topographical mappings can be generated by activity-dependent self-organizing mechanisms (Willshaw and von der Malsburg 1976; Amari 1983; Kohonen 1984; Érdi and Barna 1984; Bienenstock 1985; Cottrell and Fort 1986; Ritter and Schulten 1986) in which retinal cells with correlated activity are more likely to project to nearby points of tectum than are those with uncorrelated activity. Shatz (1990) demonstrated the role of spontaneous retinal activity that arises even before eye opening.

The Whitelaw and Cowan (1981) model (see also Cowan and Friedman 1990, 1991) was an attempt to integrate marker- and activity-based algorithms, by combining a gradient of adhesive specificity with a synaptic updating rule used by Willshaw and von der Malsburg (1976). The model describes plasticity, mismatch, rotation, and compound eye experiments.

Decrease of Synaptic Strength by Normalization Rule Only or by Selective Mechanism

To avoid the unlimited growth of synaptic strength, a predetermined upper bound can be specified (see the discussion in sec. 4.5.1 later). A more realistic technique adopts the concept of the limited reinforcement signal, which helps avoid the saturation problem. The normalization procedure (von der Malsburg 1973) set up the constraint that the sum of the synaptic strengths on a cell should be constant. This constraint induces competition among synapses of the same cell. Qualms regarding the physiological reality of the normalization have been stated (Uttley 1975; Hirai 1980; Sutton and Barto 1981). Although it is acceptable, in certain measure, that normalization might be the result of the redistribution of a constant supply of receptor protein molecules, other mechanisms may be more plausible. The combination of a selective local learning rule and normalization rule has proved to be a proper compromise between biological plausibility and computational efficiency, at least in fiber-sorting procedures. (See section 4.5.1 for a systematic study of learning rules.)

Deterministic Versus Stochastic Models

In the spirit of the theory of noise-induced transitions, an additive random term was included in the learning rule by Érdi and Barna (1984, 1985), who demonstrated that a strict deterministic modification rule does not lead

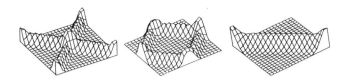

Figure 4.8
Visualization of the qualitative behavior of a self-organizing algorithm. Values of the synaptic strength are plotted. "Double-diagonal" and "craterlike" solutions are produced by deterministic learning rules. The "diagonal" attractor associated with topographic order emerged by including a small additive random term. (Reprinted from Érdi and Barna 1984 by permission of Springer Verlag.)

to globally ordered structures. Superimposed noise changes the qualitative behavior of the attractor by destabilizing temporary, metastable structures, and globally ordered structures can be generated, as is demonstrated in figure 4.8.

Sets of Discrete Nerve Cells Versus Continuous Neural Fields

Most of the models adopt a discrete neural network approach. In contrast, Amari (1980, 1983) used a continuous neural field description. The equilibrium solution of his field equation was identified with topographical connections. In the arrow model (Hope, Hammond, and Gaze 1976), retinal fibers must terminate at discrete points on a grid, whereas in the branch arrow model the tectum is considered a continuous field.

Positional Information: Yes or No?

Positional information (Wolpert 1969, 1971, 1981) implies the existence of a coordinate system within which cell position is specified. The general nature of positional information is not known. It might be a gradient of certain morphogens arising from a definite source and distributed through the cell population by diffusion (e.g., Crick 1970). Different versions of the chemo-affinity hypothesis adopt this view. Goodwin and Cohen (1969) attempted to describe developmental organization by traveling waves based on the phase differences between two signals. There is little experimental evidence for identifying the mechanism of positional information transfer. Map formation usually is explained not in terms of global organization principles but by local interactions.

Review of a Model

Let us review the choices made in a specific model, that of Érdi and Barna (1984):

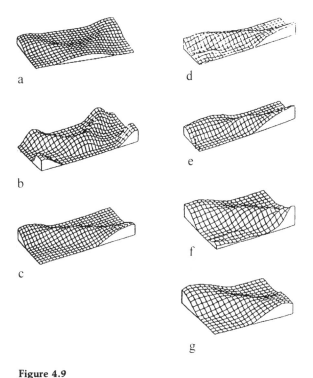

a

d

b

e

c

f

g

Figure 4.9
The formation and plasticity of retinotectal connections. (a and b) Deterministic simulation of normal development. (c) Ordered connection by taking into account the noise effect. (d) State during the reorganization process after partial retinal ablation. (e) Reorganized ordered conections after partial retinal ablation. (f) Reorganization after tectal ablation. (g) Reestablished ordered connections. (Reprinted from Érdi and Barna 1984 by permission of Springer Verlag.)

1. No specific orientation rule was defined; rather, the role of competition among incoming fibers was emphasized.

2. Connections between cells were not preprogrammed; rather, a genetically programmed algorithm was defined to select favorable system connections.

3. An activity-dependent mechanism used a Hebb rule that was supplemented by two types of decreasing factor.

4. The deterministic learning rule was supplemented with an additive random term.

5. A set of discrete nerve cells was assumed.

6. No particular condition for obtaining adequately positioned connections was postulated.

Simulation experiments showed that the model offers a common mechanism for normal ontogenetic development and plastic rearrangement of ordered neural connections. It was demonstrated that environmental noise is necessary in establishing globally ordered structures. Superimposed noise might (1) change the qualitative behavior of the deterministic system by destabilizing temporary, metastable states and (2) help accelerate the transient processes. Figure 4.9 (Érdi and Barna 1984)

illustrates the values of the matrix of topographic connections established by such a self-organizing algorithm.

4.5 Learning Rules

Learning in neural networks can be classified as supervised, reinforcement, or unsupervised learning (Hinton 1989). *Unsupervised learning*, in which a cell's connections change according to some built-in measure of performance (so that a measure of similarity acts as a fixed built-in supervisor) is distinguished from *supervised learning*, in which the environment-teacher specifies the correct classification and instructs the system by some error-correcting mechanism. In *reinforcement learning*, the learner does not receive complete teacher information but instead receives a reward/punishment, or reinforcement, signal depending on the quality of the output.

4.5.1 Hebbian Learning and Its Variations

The most celebrated suggestion for updating connection strength is Hebb's rule (Hebb 1949), expressing the conjunction among presynaptic and postsynaptic elements (using neurobiological terminology) or associative conditioning (in psychological terms). The underlying biophysical mechanisms and algorithms of even generalized Hebbian synaptic modification were reviewed by Brown, Kairiss, and Keenan (1990), and system-level computational models of the neural bases of learning and memory were summarized by Gluck and Granger (1993).

The generalized form of Hebb's idea is that the synaptic weight from neuron i to neuron j changes according to:

$$\frac{dw_{ij}(t)}{dt} = F(a_i, a_j) \tag{22}$$

where F is a functional, and a_j and a_i are presynaptic and postsynaptic activity functions (i.e., they may include activity levels over some period of time and not just the current activity values; see, for example, Sejnowski and Tesauro 1990). In Hebb's original learning rule, the functional F is reduced to $ka_i(t)\,a_j(t)$, a simple product of the actual states. This rule,

$$\frac{dw_{ij}(t)}{dt} = ka_i(t)a_j(t), \quad k > 0, \tag{23}$$

is local, interactive, and conjunctional, as we will now explain. To define other specific learning rules (e.g., the form of F) a few points should be clarified.

First, what are the assumptions about the form of the time-dependent activity functions? In the simplest case, only the actual activity values are involved. In somewhat more complex situations, short-term *averaged* activity values determine the synaptic change. More generally, the *history* of the activity values plays a role in the modification process.

Second, what are the assumptions about the locality of the modifying signal? In many cases, the modification of a synapse between neurons i and j depends on the state of these two cells alone (i.e., the mechanism is *local*). In this case, teacher or external reinforcement signals are not involved; local synapses are the bases of the unsupervised learning.

Third, how do the presynaptic and postsynaptic cells interact, if at all? Consider first the potential answers for the "if at all" part of the question. The modification can be interactive if both the presynaptic and postsynaptic cells are involved, and noninteractive if either the presynaptic or postsynaptic cell alone influences the modification. The mechanism of the interaction may be *conjunctional* or *correlational*. In the first case, the co-occurrence of the presynaptic and postsynaptic activity is sufficient to cause synaptic change, whereas in the second case the covariance of the two activities has to be taken into account. (From a formal point of view, additive interactions—for example, those given with the function $F(a_i \pm a_j)$—could have been defined, but they are considered noninteractive rules. In other words, not only an entire rule but even each term of the rule can be evaluated as interactive or noninteractive.)

An important and unfortunate property of Hebb's original rule (equation 23) is that the synaptic strengths are ever-increasing. There are a few slightly generalized versions of this rule that preserve this property:

$$\frac{dw_{ij}(t)}{dt} = k[x_i(t)][x_j(t)] \qquad (24)$$

where $[x_i(t)]$ and $[x_j(t)]$ denote the mean firing frequencies of the postsynaptic and presynaptic units (the average is taken for some short previous time period);

$$\frac{dw_{ij}(t)}{dt} = kg(a_i(t))h(a_j(t)) \qquad (25)$$

where g and h, functions of the actual activity, serve as some measure of the postsynaptic and presynaptic activity (i.e., $g, h > 0$); and

$$\frac{dw_{ij}(t)}{dt} = kg(a(\cdot))h(a_j(\cdot)) \qquad (26)$$

where g and h are now functionals of the activity function. A special case of equation 26 is

$$\frac{dw_{ij}(t)}{dt} = k \int a_i(t)dt \int a_j(t)dt, \qquad (27)$$

which takes into account the total activity history.

There is a particular time-dependent local and conjunctional rule that does not increase the synaptic weight. This is the case when the presynaptic and postsynaptic activities are correlated negatively:

$$\frac{dw_{ij}(t)}{dt} = ka_i(t)a_j(t), \quad \text{with } k < 0 \qquad (28)$$

This "anti-Hebbian" rule (a term that meets with some confusion in the literature) or "decorrelation" rule was suggested to describe features of pattern dissociations (Sutton and Barto 1981; Palm 1982; Barlow and Földiak 1989, Földiak 1990).

There are both brutal and sophisticated methods for eliminating the unpleasant property of ever-increasing weights which, unless compensated for, yield a network with saturated synaptic weights and thus no effective pattern discrimination. We adopt the term *brutal* for a situation in which some external constraint (somehow taking into account the finiteness of resources) is applied to the internal mechanism. First, a predetermined upper bound can be given, such as the maximal value of the synaptic strength. Second, the so-called normalization procedure (von der Malsburg 1973) imposes a zero-sum constraint on all synaptic strengths and can be interpreted as a competition of the presynaptic elements for postsynaptic resources (therefore violating locality). Such rules may explain some aspects of neural development (Artola and Singer 1987; Constantine-Paton, Cline, and Debski 1990).

More sophisticated methods decrease the synaptic strengths selectively. Brown, Kairiss, and Keenan (1990) use the expression *generalized Hebbian synaptic mechanism* for cases in which interactive synaptic increase is combined with activity-dependent synaptic depression. The underlying mechanism behind synaptic depression may be of interactive or noninteractive type.

Instead of a formal derivation of the rules capable of describing selective decrease, two important special cases are mentioned. First, the rule

$$\frac{dw_{ij}(t)}{dt} = kg(a_i(t))(h(a_j(t)) - \theta(t)) \qquad (29)$$

implements synaptic increase only if the $h(a_j(t))$ presynaptic activity is larger than the $\theta(t)$ modification threshold. If presynaptic activity is smaller than the threshold, the synaptic weight decreases. Second,

$$\frac{dw_{ij}(t)}{dt} = k(g(a_i(t)) - \theta(t))h(a_j(t)) \qquad (30)$$

implements a postsynaptic control mechanism on the modification process.

The learning rules represented by equations 29 and 30 can be written in the forms of $kgh - k\theta g$ and $kgh - k\theta h$, respectively. Each of these expressions may be interpreted as the sum of a Hebbian interactive term and a noninteractive term. In the first case, the decrease is due to the postsynaptic activity g and is called *heterosynaptic* depression, whereas in the second case the decrease depends on the presynaptic activity h and is called *homosynaptic* depression. Learning rules of the form in equation 29 were suggested by Bienenstock, Cooper and Munro (1982) and so sometimes are referred to as the *BCM theory*. These have been used by Bear, Cooper, and Ebner (1987) to model the plasticity of visual cortex: $\theta(t)$ was identified with a nonlinear function of the averaged postsynaptic activity:

$$\theta(t) = [ga(t)]^2 \qquad (31)$$

where $[\cdot]$ is the average taken for a period of time. The suggestion that the occurrence of either homosynaptic LTP or LTD depends on the strength of the depolarizing current induced by an NMDA blocker (which increases the modification threshold) in the visual cortex was based on the experiments of Singer's group (e.g., Kleinschmidt et al. 1987; Singer 1990; see also Stevens 1990). (LTP is discussed further in chapter 6 and LTD in chapter 9.)

The learning expression has also been described in the form $\phi(g, [g])h$, where the two-variable function ϕ depends on an actual value and an averaged quantity, so an underlying microscopic stochastic mechanism should exist behind the phenomenological and deterministic formalism.

Sejnowski (1977) offered the following equation to express a weaker form of the interactive rule (when correlational and not conjunctional interactions were assumed):

$$\frac{dw_{ij}(t)}{dt} = k(a_i(t) - [a_i(t)])(a_j(t) - [a_j(t)]) \qquad (32)$$

Depending on the sign of the correlation, the rule is capable of describing either synaptic enhancement or decrease. Covariance was suggested to induce associative LTD in the hippocampus (Stanton and Sejnowski 1989; see also Morris and Willshaw 1989, Willshaw and Dayan 1990).

Another way to describe the decrease of synaptic weights is to introduce a spontaneous decay (or "for-

getting") term. The original Hebbian rule (equation 23) supplemented with a decay term reads as follows:

$$\frac{dw_{ij}(t)}{dt} = -k_1 w_{ij}(t) + k_2 a_i(t)a_j(t) \qquad (33)$$

[Instead of first-order decay, a quadratic forgetting term was introduced and studied by Riedel and Schild (1992) to improve the stability properties of the learning rule.] If the decay is not spontaneous but is modulated with the postsynaptic activity, the rule has the following form:

$$\begin{aligned} \frac{dw_{ij}(t)}{dt} &= -k_1 w_{ij}(t)a_i(t) + k_2 a_i(t)a_j(t) \\ &\equiv a_i(t)\{k_2 a_j(t) - k_1 w_{ij}(t)\} \end{aligned} \qquad (34)$$

and describes the phenomenon called *competitive learning* (e.g., Grossberg 1976; Kohonen 1984). Postsynaptic neurons compete for incoming resources: The larger the postsynaptic activity, the larger is the measure of learning.

The conjunctional rule has been modified by replacing the activity values with their time derivatives:

$$\frac{dw_{ij}(t)}{dt} = k(d/dt)a_i(t)(d/dt)a_j(t) \qquad (35)$$

This rule is an example of differential learning mechanisms (Klopf 1986; Kosko 1986). The rate of change of activities obviously may be positive or negative; that is, both synaptic increase and decrease may occur. The differential competitive rule

$$\frac{dw_{ij}(t)}{dt} = (d/dt)a_i(t)\{k_2 a_j(t) - k_1 w_{ij}(t)\} \qquad (36)$$

implements the "learn only if change" principle (Kosko 1990).

In some cases, the time delay due to signal transmission is explicitly taken into account; consequently, earlier presynaptic activities, rather than current activities, are in conjunction:

$$\frac{dw_{ij}(t)}{dt} = ka_i a_j(t - \tau) \qquad (37)$$

This spirit of timing sensitivity is materialized in the rule

$$\frac{dw_{ij}(t)}{dt} = k_1(d/dt)a_i(t)[a_j(t)] \qquad (38)$$

used to describe conditioning (e.g., see Sejnowski and Tesauro 1990).

The experimental identification of learning rules found in real nervous systems is difficult. Increase and decrease of synaptic strengths (potentiation and depression, respectively) occur both in the short term and the long term. Section 4.5.5 and chapters 5, 6, 8, and 9 offer fuller treatments of this subject.

4.5.2 Synaptic Matrix Models of Associative Memory

Early Models

Here we review the early synaptic matrix models of associative memory (Arbib 1989, 8.2). We now apply simple learning rules to obtain general results on modeling associative memory that will be applied to the hippocampus in chapter 6. Many authors (beginning with, for example, Steinbuch 1961; Anderson 1968; Willshaw, Buneman, and Longuet-Higgins 1969; and Kohonen 1972) studied neural networks in which there are m input lines each forming synapses on the same n neurons, so that the state of learning of the net is described completely by the *synaptic matrix* (or *association matrix*) $\mathbf{W} = [w_{ij}]$, where w_{ij} is the weight of the synapse from input j to neuron i. Synaptic learning rules adjust these connections so that the matrix forms an associative memory that is distributed and thus resistant to localized damage. Some authors follow the McCulloch-Pitts convention in which neurons communicate via bits, 0 or 1, but we will look first at models in which the activity levels are real numbers in the range [−1, +1]. Many authors use a linear device so that, when the input vector for the synaptic matrix is $\mathbf{x}$, the output is the vector $\mathbf{Wx}$. Others follow this linear operation with some nonlinear output function. For now, we look at the linear system.

When viewing a neural network as an associative memory, we speak of the pattern on the input lines as the *key*, and the pattern on the output lines (the outputs of the neurons) as the *recollection*. In an *autoassociative* memory, learning is designed to make the key elicit the recollection of which it is a part, so that one has a content-addressable memory. In a *heteroassociative* memory, the key may be very different from the recollection. In either case, what is restored for an arbitrary input is a linear combination of what has been stored, weighted by the correlation of their keys with the current key.

We use the notation $\langle \mathbf{x}|\mathbf{y} \rangle$ for the scalar product of the two vectors $\mathbf{x}$ and $\mathbf{y}$, so that if $\mathbf{x}$ is the column vector with entries $(\mathbf{x}_1, \ldots, \mathbf{x}_n)$ and $\mathbf{y}$ is the column vector with entries $(\mathbf{y}_1, \ldots, \mathbf{y}_n)$, then

$$\langle \mathbf{x}|\mathbf{y} \rangle = \sum_{1 \leq i \leq n} \mathbf{x}_i \mathbf{y}_i = \mathbf{x}^T \mathbf{y}, \tag{39}$$

the matrix product of the row vector $\mathbf{x}^T$ ($\mathbf{x}$ transposed) with the column vector $\mathbf{y}$.

Suppose we had a single key f for which we desired the recollection g. Define $\mathbf{W}$ to be $\mathbf{gf}^T$, the matrix with $w_{ij} = g_i f_j$. Then note that if we supply the synaptic matrix $\mathbf{W}$ with key f, we have

$$\mathbf{Wf} = \mathbf{gf}^T \mathbf{f} \tag{40}$$

which is just the desired recollection g scaled up by $\langle \mathbf{f}|\mathbf{f} \rangle = \mathbf{f}^T \mathbf{f}$; and thus will be precisely g if $\mathbf{f}$ is a unit vector (i.e., if $\langle \mathbf{f}|\mathbf{f} \rangle = 1$).

More generally, given a set f_k of keys and g_k of corresponding recollections, define the synaptic matrix to be

$$\mathbf{W} = \sum_k g k^f k^T \tag{41}$$

which we may think of as obtained by adding up the "memory traces" $g_k f_k^T$ for each of the (f_k, g_k) pairings of key and recollection. This is similar to the basic Hebbian rule, wherein the input f_k is applied to the synaptic matrix and some "teacher" forces the neurons to fire according to the specified pattern g_k. Assuming that each f_j is a unit vector, we have

$$\mathbf{Wfj} = g_j + \sum_{k \neq j} g_k \langle f_k|f_j \rangle \tag{42}$$

which will equal g_j if the f_ks are orthonormal (i.e., $\langle f_k|f_j \rangle = \delta_{kj}$, the Kronecker delta, which is just the identity matrix (1 on the diagonal, 0 off the diagonal).

In such a memory, information is stored in a correlation matrix formed by the product of a vector of neurons representing the conditioned stimulus (axons) and a vector of neurons representing the unconditioned stimulus (dendrites). Many associations may be stored in this matrix by adding each product to the previously summed matrix contents. To recall an association, the conditioned stimulus is applied. The many biologically desirable properties of this type of information store include (1) recall of a complete stimulus from only a part; (2) generalization to similar stimuli on a novel presentation; (3) graceful degradation of response with increasing damage to cells; and (4) rapid performance (only one synaptic delay). The response of single neurons in such a matrix may be analyzed: A neuron may fire to a combination ranging from one to many of the conditioned stimuli. It is essential that each event be represented by an ensemble of neurons; however, such a network may show interference. To limit interference, the ensemble of stored patterns must be of limited size and distinctive in some sense such as that captured by orthogonality or, as we shall see in the next section, by some appropriate statistical distribution in pattern space.

Invariant Pattern Recognition and Dynamic Links

Understanding the mechanisms of invariant pattern recognition has been a great challenge. An object can be represented on the retina by highly different patterns. The brain has to organize the representation of objects, providing for invariance concerning size, position, and orientation. Two extreme solutions seemed conceivable, namely template matching and extraction of invariant features. To implement the former version, some pre-representation of the patterns to be recognized is necessary. The prototype of the latter is the perceptron (Rosenblatt 1962) and different versions of the cognitron and neocognitron model (Fukushima 1975, 1988, 1994). Rosenblatt applied a supervised learning rule. Fukushima suggested a multilayer network model with the unsupervised ability of rapid self-organization. In the newer version of the neocognitron (see Fukushima and Wake 1992), unsupervised and supervised learning rules have been combined. Repeatedly presented patterns that closely resemble one another yield the development of circuits responsible for extracting the parts of the patterns that overlap. Consequently, the neurons of even the deepest layer do not necessarily respond selectively to any particular pattern but often to two or more patterns. In the family of the cognitron models, however, the invariance is explicitly wired (as was remarked by Bienenstock 1985).

Invariant pattern formation has been treated by applying the concept of the dynamic link architecture (DLA; von der Malsburg 1981, 1985) to address the binding problem. The idea is to provide an algorithm (and, in the optimal case, even a neural mechanism) for synchronizing sets of neurons that are to be bound together into a higher-level symbol. Temporal signal binding can be realized by signal correlations (von der Malsburg 1981). It was suggested that such correlations truly may exist in the brain: Correlations between signals (actually $\approx$ 40-Hz oscillations) encode the binding of features into more comprehensive wholes in the visual cortex (Engel et al. 1992). Demonstration of the other important feature of DLA—namely, the existence of fast synapses—is not easy, though some indications have been offered (Zucker 1989). The DLA is able to detect pattern correspondences and to discriminate between objects composed largely of the same features, but in different spatial arrangements. It has been applied to invariant pattern recognition (Bienenstock and von der Malsburg 1987; Buhmann, Divko, and Schulten 1989), pattern segmentation (von der Malsburg and Buhmann 1992), and symmetry detection (Konen and von der Malsburg 1994).

The DLA offers an algorithm by which to teach a network relatively rapidly, from a few examples, by self-organization, and therefore it fulfills the two most important criteria of being realistic.

4.5.3 Hopfield Networks

Much recent work on neural networks has been motivated by the spin-glass analogy. Ising (1925) modeled magnets as a linear array of so-called Ising spins that could be in one of two states, up or down. Though many authors use +1 and −1 for these spins, we will employ the neural convention of using 1 and 0, respectively. The basic model associates with each point $k = (i, j)$ of a two-dimensional lattice a spin $s_k \varepsilon \{0, 1\}$. The dynamics of spins is stochastic. A spin tends to align with its neighbors, but the probability of doing so decreases toward 0.5 as the temperature T increases. The temperature dependence of the model reflects a basic discovery by Pierre Curie that there is a critical temperature, called the *Curie temperature* (T_C), such that the global magnetization induced by an external magnetic field will be retained if the material is below this temperature, whereas the thermal fluctuations will dominate the local interactions to demagnetize a magnet hotter than T_C. The Curie temperature thus marks a critical point at which the material makes a phase transition, from a phase in which it can hold magnetization to one in which it cannot. One-dimensional physical systems generally cannot exhibit phase transitions, but Onsager (1944) showed that a two-dimensional Ising model can. For example, if we allow spin k to be influenced by the spins in the set S_k of its four nearest neighbors in the two-dimensional lattice, we set spin k to 1 only if $h_k = \sum_{j \varepsilon S_k} s_j > 0$, and then only with probability

$$\text{prob}(s_k(t+1) = 1) = 1/(1 + e^{-h_k(t)/T}) \qquad (43)$$

which tends to 0.5 as T tends to infinity. In the deterministic case $T = 0$, this reduces to

$$s_k(t+1) = 1 \text{ if and only if } \sum_{j \varepsilon S_k} s_j > 0 \qquad (44)$$

which looks suspiciously like a special case of the McCulloch-Pitts rule:

$$y(t+1) = 1 \text{ if and only if } \sum_i w_i x_i(t) \geqslant \theta \qquad (45)$$

This analogy has been noted many times (e.g., Cragg and Temperley 1954, 1955; Little 1974). Little offered an Ising spin analogy of a neural network that introduced the "temperature" or statistical fluctuations directly and crucially into the firing equations. The model gave both static and cyclic behavior and had asymmetrical coefficients. However, Hopfield (1982) was the catalyst in attracting the attention of many physicists to this field of study. [Amit (1989) presents the fruits of the first 7 years of research by physicists studying neural networks.] Hopfield presented a model similar to that of Little but having symmetric connections and lacking statistical fluctuations. By introducing a discrete-time model with asynchronous firing, Hopfield obtained a dynamics that served to minimize a global energy measure. We use the familiar McCulloch-Pitts neuron, the output of which is 1 iff $h_i = \sum_{k=0}^{N} w_{ik}s_k \geqslant \theta_i$ and is otherwise 0, where s_k is the current value of the kth input and w_{ik} is the corresponding synaptic weight from unit k to unit i, the threshold of which is θ_i. Classically, a McCulloch-Pitts net uses the *parallel synchronous update scheme*, in which every neuron processes its inputs synchronously at each time step to determine a new output. By contrast, a *Hopfield net* (Hopfield 1982) is a net of such units with symmetric weights ($w_{ij} = w_{ji}$) that uses the *random asynchronous update scheme*, which operates as follows: "Pick a unit at random. If the sum of the weights on connections from other active units exceeds threshold, turn it on. Otherwise turn it off." The random choice of a neuron completely destroys all temporal correlations between neurons. Hopfield's contribution was to observe that, for a symmetrical network with the random asynchronous update scheme, the function

$$E = -\frac{1}{2} \sum_{i,k=1}^{N} s_i w_{ik} s_k + \sum_{i=1}^{N} s_i \theta_i, \qquad (46)$$

often called the *energy* of the neural system, decreases whenever the new activity state of a neuron differs from its previous state. This is not the physical energy of the neural net but, rather, a mathematical quantity that does for neural dynamics what potential energy does for a conservative newtonian system. In fact, exploiting the symmetry of w_{ik}, the decrease in energy (ΔE) can be rewritten as $|h_i - \theta_i|$ when neuron i changes its state. Because the function E is bounded from below, the network will reach a fixed point in finite time. Hence, the dynamics of the net tends to move E toward a minimum. We stress that different *local* minima may exist. Global minimization is not guaranteed!

The above expression for ΔE crucially depended on the symmetry condition. If $w_{ij} \neq w_{ji}$, the updating rule need not yield passage to a minimum of E but might instead yield a limit cycle or chaotic motion. In most vision algorithms, constraints can be formulated in terms of symmetrical weights, so that $w_{ij} = w_{ji}$ is appropriate. In a control problem, however, a link with w_{ij} might express the likelihood that the action represented by activation of neuron i should precede that represented by activation of neuron j, in which case $w_{ij} = w_{ji}$ is normally inappropriate.

Adopting the ideas of the synaptic matrix literature reviewed in the previous section, Hopfield (1982) specified the synapses w_{ik} in such a way that p predefined patterns $\{\xi^v = (\xi_1^v, \ldots, \xi_N^v); v = 1, \ldots, p\}$ are stable fixed points of the network. The novelty in his analysis is that it does not build on a specific set of patterns to be checked for, say, orthonormality, but rather is based on choosing random unbiased bit strings for the stored patterns (i.e., $\xi_i^v = 1$ has the same probability as $\xi_i^v = 0$) and then analyzing network properties with methods from statistical mechanics. Hopfield adopted a slight variant of equation 42 to devise the synaptic matrix

$$w_{ik} = \frac{1}{N} \sum_{v=1}^{P} (2\xi_i^v - 1)(2\xi_k^v - 1) \qquad (47)$$

for connecting the neurons to form an associative memory. The expression $(2\xi k^v - 1)$ is the *presynaptic factor* of the synaptic rule; $(2\xi_i^v - 1)$ is the *postsynaptic factor*. The symmetrical $N \times N$ matrix $\mathbf{w}_{ik}$ essentially stores the averaged correlations between neuron k and i with the average performed overall patterns.

If the neural network is to work as an associative memory, all pattern states $\{\xi^v; v = 1, \ldots, p\}$ must be stable fixed points of the dynamics or must at least be located close to attractor states. Otherwise, the network will not relax to the correct pattern and would not perform an associative completion of a corrupted input. Stability of a network state requires that the local fields h_i exceed the threshold θ_i whenever $V_i = 1$ and that h_i is smaller than θ_i if $V_i = 0$. This condition can be reformulated as $(h_i - \theta_i)(2V_i - 1) \geqslant 0$. We will now evaluate the stability of the pattern states of a network with the connectivity of equation 47. Assume, without loss of generality, that the network is in the first pattern state ξ^1. Then, the local fields take on the following values:

$$h_i = \sum_{k=0}^{N} w_{ik} \xi_k^1 = \frac{1}{N} \sum_{k=0}^{N} \sum_{v=1}^{p} (2\xi_i^v - 1)(2\xi_k^v - 1)\xi_k^1 \qquad (48)$$

The sum over all patterns $\{\xi^v; v = 1, \ldots p\}$ can be split into two parts, a signal part $(2\xi_i^1 - 1)(2\xi_k^1 - 1)\xi_k^1$ and a noise part $(2\xi_i^v - 1)(2\xi_k^v - 1)\xi_k^1$ with $v \neq 1$; that is,

$$h_i = h_i^s + h_i^n = \frac{1}{N}(2\xi_i^1 - 1)\sum_{k=0}^{N}(2\xi_k^1 - 1)\xi_k^1$$

$$+ \frac{1}{N}\sum_{k=0}^{N}\sum_{v=2}^{p}(2\xi_i^v - 1)(2\xi_k^v - 1)\xi_k^1. \qquad (49)$$

The noise term h_i^n is zero, on the average, for a finite number of patterns stored, because ξ_k^1 and $(2\xi_i^n - 1)$ are independent random variables. Its mean value is zero and its variance is of the order $\sqrt{p/N}$, which vanishes for finite p and very large numbers of neurons N. The noise part, however, limits the number of patterns that can be stored in a neural network in the interesting region of p proportional to N. The signal part h_i^s (first term in equation 5) stabilizes the pattern state ξ^1. To see that, we average over the variables ξ_k^v and calculate the expected value of

$$\left\langle \sum_{k=0}^{N}(2\xi_k^1 - 1)\xi_k^1 \right\rangle = \sum_{k=0}^{N}\langle(2\xi_k^1 - 1)\xi_k^1\rangle \approx N. \qquad (50)$$

Therefore, the signal term assumes the value 1 if $\xi_i^1 = 1$ and the value -1 if $\xi_i^1 = 0$. A threshold θ_1 between these two bounds will stabilize the pattern x^1 as a fixed-point attractor; $\theta_i = 0$ is a popular choice.

The dynamics of a Hopfield neural network can be visualized as a relaxation flow to a set of fixed points. The different stored patterns $\{\xi^v; v = 1, \ldots, p\}$ are surrounded by basins of attraction (bold lines). A network with an initial state located inside a basin of attraction will relax to the corresponding fixed point. If we initialize the network in a state far away from a prespecified attractor ξ^v, either it will flow to a dedicated state, which indicates failure of association, or it will relax to a spurious attractor. These spurious attractors are a nuisance for associative recall and can considerably degrade the capacity of an associative memory. For reliable associative recall, it is desirable to design a network with equally shaped basins of attraction and with no spurious states.

4.5.4 Computation with Attractors: Scope, Limits, and Extensions

Conventional Assumptions and Rules, Implications and Difficulties

The fact that neural computation became so popular among physicists, computer scientists, and theoretical neuroscientists is rather strongly related to the success of the notion of computation with attractors. A physical model and a computational algorithm were given to store memory traces and to recall them from their fragments.

Computation with attractors became a paradigm suggesting that dynamic systems theory is a proper conceptual framework for understanding computational mechanisms in such self-organizing structures as certain complex physical structures, computing devices, and living organisms (see, for example, Hopfield 1984; Hogg and Huberman 1985; Amit 1989; Serra and Zanarini 1990). Concentrating now on the continuous-time case, the underlying ideas are these:

1. The mathematical models of all these systems are equivalent in their essential properties to a system of first-order autonomous ordinary differential equations (ODE).

2. The specific structure of the ODE implies the existence of multiple attractors, and each attractor stores one memory trace.

3. The set of the initial values is classified based on the properties of the attractor-basin portrait. The elements of the subset of those initial values that are allocated in the same basin and therefore evolve toward the same attractor can recall the memory trace stored there. Figure 4.10 shows how a dynamic system is connected to its environment.

The recall dynamics is given in this special construction as

$$\frac{da(t)}{dt} = f(a(t), \mathbf{W}, I); \quad a(0) = a_0, \qquad (51)$$

where a (the only time-dependent variable in this scenario) is the activity vector that characterizes the state of the system, $\mathbf{W}$ is the connectivity matrix assumed to be constant during the recall process, and the input I also is constant (and not time-dependent). In case of specific f functions, the long-time behavior of the system can be characterized by a multiple attractor structure.

One of the main merits of the Hopfield model is that the architecture defined there implies the existence of such an attractor-basin portrait. According to the Hopfield model, which prescribes the already classic scenario of autoassociative memory:

1. The attractors are fixed points.

2. A separate learning stage precedes the recall process, and learning is described by a static "one-shot" rule.

3. The inputs, and particularly their temporal character, are neglected.

4. Furthermore, and most emphatically, the whole conceptual apparatus assumes that basically the mathematical objects to be classified are the static initial values of the generally rapidly varying activity variables. In neural

terms, it means that some rather arbitrary initial values of the rapid activity variables (and not, for example, the dynamic sensory inputs) are involved in the formation of associative memory.

Since the time when Hopfield constructed a particular artificial neural network with given properties, many explicit and implicit modifications of the classic scenario have been introduced. One sch modification holds that not only fixed points but limit cycle and strange attractors might be involved, as suggested by experimental neurophysiological results and theoretical considerations. Less specific architectures than the Hopfield nets may lead to oscillation or chaotic behavior (see secs. 4.2 and 4.3). Some structural conditions for the possible generation of rhythms and chaos, based on the notion of qualitative stability, have been given.

Activity equations in many network-theoretical models (e.g., Farmer 1990) are supplemented by dynamic equations for the connectivity (i.e., learning). Learning might cause distortion of the basin of attraction, which finally might lead to qualitative change even in the nature of the attractor.

Similarly, distortion of the basin, such as deepening of the valley, can be obtained by tuning the external input. A particular time sequence of input patterns was recognized by a special construction defining a time-dependent energy function (Tank and Hopfield 1987).

The behavior of autonomous systems, at least in regular cases, strongly depends on the initial values. Input variables were identified simply with initial values in a rather restrictive case studying a model of category learning in the olfactory system (Baird 1990). Based on the fact that violation of the Lipschitz condition eliminates this dependence, Zak (1988, 1990) suggested that nonlipschitzian neurodynamic models show much more flexible properties than conventional systems. Inputs, instead of initial states, can be the objects of classification. Constant inputs were classified by a few classes of network architectures: A symmetric, purely inhibitory network (Cohen and Grossberg 1983) and a class of right-hand side functions endowed with the property of contractiveness (Kelly 1990) were demonstrated to be stable encoders of constant input (i.e., the response states of the system did not depend on the initial values).

More generally, we might realize that the proper mathematical model of a dynamic system, open to continuous interaction with the environment, is a system of nonautonomous differential equations. The change of the system depends both on the internal state of the system and on the time-dependent sensory input.

Loosely speaking, an isolated system can be connected with the external world through different channels, as initial conditions, parameters, and external inputs (see figure 4.10). The parameters are associated with the geography of the attractor basin portrait ("categories"), whereas initial values and inputs are two different types of qualities to be classified.

Continuous-Learning, Dynamic Categories

According to the classic scenario discussed previously, the learning and recall stages are temporally separated, First, the elements of the connectivity matrix are adjusted by a static, one-shot rule; then the recall process given by equation 6 is executed (with fixed values of $\mathbf{W}$). In real neural systems, the dynamics of the modification of the connection strength usually is described by differential equations. The two-level dynamic system is:

$$\frac{da(t)}{dt} = f(a(t), \mathbf{W}(t), I)$$

$$\frac{dw_{ij}(t)}{dt} = g(a(t), \mathbf{W}(t)), \tag{52}$$

with the initial values $a(0) = a_0$ and $w_{ij}(0) = w_{ij0}$.

The geography of the attractor-basin portrait, which specifies the categories (by the local minima), is changing continuously during learning. Therefore, the classification of initial values cannot properly be formulated in this system, as permanent categories do not exist in this framework.

There is, however, a fundamental difference between fictive, infinitely slow learning and realistic continuous learning with finite velocity (figure 4.11). In the former case, to each fixed set of parameters a separate set of initial values can be reassigned, whereas in the latter case, there is only one initial value problem. In other words, in the first case the set to be classified can newly be tested with each attractor portrait, whereas in the second case, even in the regimen of the slowly varying geography, only one set of initial values can be (approximately) tested with dynamic categories. This interpretation gives an insight into the classic scenario and explain why it uses recall from networks with *frozen* connections.

Initial Values Versus Time-Variable Inputs: What to Learn?

At this point, we leave (at least temporarily) the world of autonomous systems. It is a truism that in autonomous systems, the state itself determines the change of state, whereas in nonautonomous (NA) systems the environ-

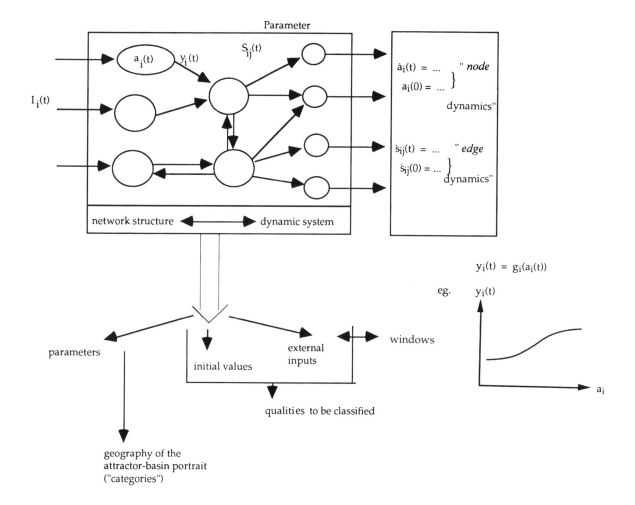

Parameter

$I_i(t)$

$a_i(t)$ $y_i(t)$ $S_{ij}(t)$

network structure ⟷ dynamic system

$$\dot{a}_i(t) = \ldots \quad \text{"} \textit{node}$$
$$a_i(0) = \ldots \left.\right\}$$
$$\text{dynamics"}$$

$$\dot{s}_{ij}(t) = \ldots \quad \text{"} \textit{edge}$$
$$\dot{s}_{ij}(0) = \ldots \left.\right\}$$
$$\text{dynamics"}$$

$$y_i(t) = g_i(a_i(t))$$

eg. $y_i(t)$

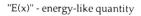

a_i

parameters

initial values

external inputs

windows

qualities to be classified

geography of the attractor-basin portrait ("categories")

"E(x)" - energy-like quantity

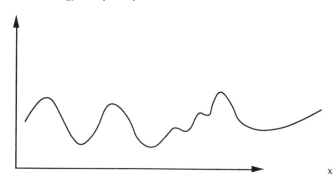

x

Figure 4.10
Dynamic networks have different "windows" to the external world:
initial values, parameters, and time-dependent inputs.

Infinite slow learning bifurcation

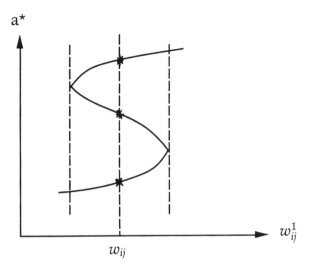

a*

w_{ij}

w_{ij}^1

Learning with finite (>0) velocity

* the classical interpretation of the activity
  dynamics can be preserved by using the
  notation of "dynamic categories"

* classical scenario: during recall process
  the connection strengths are frozen

Figure 4.11
The fundamental difference between fictive, infinitely slow learning and
realistic continuous learning with finite velocity.

ment has a direct influence on this change. There are two different sources of nonautonomy. First, we might think that the system parameters are not constant but explicitly depend on time. (Of course, setting a differential equation for the parameters, the nonautonomy can be eliminated in the cost of increasing the dimension of the state space. The new state space contains the old activity space together with the subspace of the time-variable parameter, which might imply difficulties in the interpretation.) Second, nonautonomy can be introduced as a time-dependent additive term (e.g., to take into account the continuously time-variable input).

Assuming an autonomous differential learning rule and an additive time-dependent input, the proper model in general form is

$$\frac{da(t)}{dt} = f(a(t), \mathbf{W}(t)) + I(t, \beta)$$

$$\frac{dw_{ij}(t)}{dt} = g(a(t), \mathbf{W}(t))$$

$$(53)$$

with the initial values $a(0) = a_0$ and $w_{ij}(0) = w_{ij0}$, where β denotes the parameters of the input function. (The difference between equations 51 and 52 is that in the former, the input is time-independent, whereas in the latter it is time-dependent.)

As in every classification problem, two questions can be raised. Which are the objects to be classified, and how does one define the classes or categories? As concerns the objects, in the general case the set of input functions should be classified. In a more specific case, the form of the input function is fixed, and the set of β parameters is the subject of classification. The problem of classes is much more difficult. An autonomous ODE generates a fixed number of "innate" categories associated to the number of local attractors, whereas in NA systems even the existence of the attractor is doubtful.

Storage of temporal sequences in the spinlike Hopfield network has been proposed by several authors (summarized by Amit 1989). In this paradigm, each pattern is stable over some time period, at the end of which a sharp transition occurs that leads to the next pattern, due to the stored transitions between consecutive patterns.

When an input changes its state continuously in time and in the state space, there is a serious difficulty of categorization:

[T]he phenomenon of "categorical perception" could generate internal discontinuities where there is external continuity. There is evidence that our perceptual system is able to segment a continuum, such as the color spectrum, into relatively discrete, bounded regions of categories. Physical differences of equal magnitude are more discriminable across the boundaries between these categories than within them. This boundary effect, both innate and learned, may play an important role in the representation of the elementary perceptual categories out of which the higher-order ones are built (Harnad 1987).

NA systems are qualified many times as being not very interesting, the claim being made that nonautonomy can be eliminated (in the cost of the increase of the dimension by one) by setting $\frac{dt}{dt} = 1$. A more proper transformation of NA systems to autonomous ones should convert the input parameters to initial values. Once this has been achieved, the classification of inputs [albeit in rather restrictive cases (Érdi, Grőbler, and Tóth 1992)] is reduced to the mathematical problem that arose in the classic scenario. In other cases (as will be illustrated in chapter 5), time-dependent inputs should be classified by using simulation methods. Time-dependent inputs exert control. More specifically, systems influenced by additive inputs are designated as *feedforward-controlled*.

$I(t)$ / $S_{ij}(t)$	CONSTANT	TIME-DEPENDENT
CONSTANT	classification of initial values, or almost constant I - . - 'classical' scenario	pattern classification ↙ ↘ e.g. oscillatory non-oscillatory - . - (Li - Hopfield olfactory bulb model)
TIME-DEPENDENT	'dynamic' categories 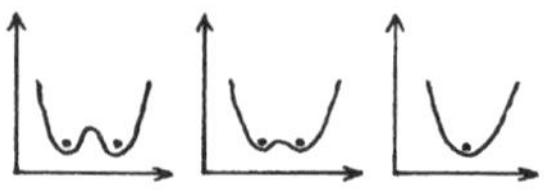 _____ synaptic modification induced transition _____ no real classification problems	nonautonomous ↓ autonomous _____ simulation methods classification or time-dependent inputs during learning

Figure 4.12
Basic model classes include constant connection strengths and time-variable connection strengths, each with constant inputs and time-varying inputs.

Rigid Versus Adaptive Learning: Reconsideration

Representation of the external world by dynamic systems is a popular issue (e.g., Hopfield 1984; Hogg and Huberman 1985; Nicolis 1986; Harnad 1987; Amit 1989; Atmanspacher 1992). Families of associative memory models based on dynamic systems can be classified according to the nature of input and of learning rules, as both of them can be static and dynamic. The following examples represent the basic model classes (see also figure 4.12):

I. Constant connection strengths

   A. Constant inputs: This is the classic scenario represented by the Hopfield model, in which the initial conditions are classified by fixed-point attractors.

   B. Time-variable inputs: With NA activity dynamics, the input patterns are classified by fixed-point or periodic attractors. A typical example is the Li and Hopfield (1989) model of the olfactory bulb (see chapter 5).

II. Time-variable connection strengths

   A. Constant inputs: Varying the connection strengths implies changes in the structure of the attractor-basin portrait. There is no real classification problem for this case.

   B. Time-variable inputs: The classification of time functions is difficult in the general case. It is possible, however, to classify parameters of the input function by transforming them into initial values, as was mentioned earlier. It is an easier problem to treat time-continuous inputs when the parameter space is discrete. A model for such a simple associative memory of the olfactory bulb will be demonstrated in chapter 5.

4.5.5 Varieties of Learning in the Brain

The study of learning rules can be explicitly expanded to include the relationship with LTP and LTD, explicit neurochemical mechanisms of synaptic plasticity that are reviewed briefly in section 6.3. We shall see that different brain regions appear to differ not only in the anatomy of cell types and circuitry but also in terms of their learning rules. In later chapters, we will link system-level study of the role of learning in different brain regions to the learning rules hypothesized to mediate this learning; we also will review a small portion of the data exploring the explicit biochemistry implementing synaptic plasticity. Models of hippocampus will include the role of LTP in associative memory (chapter 6). Models of cerebral cortex will include hebbian mechanisms in map formation and reinforcement learning in visuomotor conditioning (chapter 8). Models of the role of cerebellar cortex in motor learning will emphasize the efficacy of LTD in error-based learning and the notion of "eligibility" to bridge the time interval between command and error signal (chapter 9). Finally, our study of basal ganglia will suggest a form of reinforcement learning in which dopamine can "throw the switch" between hebbian and anti-hebbian forms of synaptic plasticity (chapter 10).

Part II

Interacting Systems of the Brain

Each of the next six chapters focuses on specific regions of the brain. However, as the title of this part, Interacting Systems of the Brain, emphasizes, our focus on one region at a time will be complemented by attempts (where appropriate) to place the region within the context of larger neural systems of which it is part, and to draw parallels between the focal region and others with which it has crucial similarities or differences. In chapter 11, we then will provide a retrospective view of the lessons on structural, functional, and dynamical organization offered by the preceding chapters, and then suggest how these lessons may be applied in the future development of cognitive neuroscience.

The Olfactory System

In this chapter, we begin by describing the anatomical structure of the olfactory bulb and cortex. In the remainder of the chapter, we discuss rhythmic activity and learning and memory in the olfactory system. Thus, the focus is on the dynamics of the olfactory system. The only explicitly functional issue is the role of the olfactory system as an associative memory for odor inputs. In the next chapter, we will make explicit important parallels between the olfactory system and the hippocampus.

Section 5.1.1 traces three stages of odor information processing: The first takes place in the receptor neurons of the olfactory epithelium. The second takes place in and around the glomeruli of the olfactory bulb, where the receptor cells synapse with the dendrites of mitral and tufted cells and with the periglomerular cells. The third is composed of the bulbar layers containing the mitral and tufted cells and the granule cells. Reciprocal dendrodendritic synapses between these cells play a role in spatiotemporal pattern formation. The layers, cell types, and synaptic organization of the olfactory bulb are reviewed in more detail in section 5.1.2 and, in section 5.1.3, the story continues into the olfactory cortex, with emphasis on how its laminar structure relates to the afferent fibers from the olfactory bulb (those in the lateral olfactory tract [LOT]), reexcitatory connections that may be the anatomical substrate for olfactory associative memory, commissural fiber systems connecting the two halves of the cortex, and neurochemically varied centrifugal inputs from different brain areas.

Section 5.2 is focused on the dynamics of activity in the olfactory system. In section 5.2.1, we provide the experimental background for the study of rhythmic activity, contrasting slow oscillations (~ 5 Hz), which may be imposed on the olfactory bulb by the respiratory nuclei, with fast oscillations (frequencies of 35–90 Hz in different parts of the olfactory bulb). Rhythmic activity in the olfactory cortex may occur as a consequence of bulbar oscillation, in response to stimulation of the lateral olfactory tract, or due to intrinsic interactions between cortical excitatory and inhibitory populations. These data are addressed in section 5.2.2, using the methods of our dynamical overview to model oscillation and chaos in the olfactory bulb, with a bifurcation analysis of a simple network model (including single-compartment models of the neurons) using the parameter c, which controls the strength of lateral connections in the mitral layer as control parameter. As c increases from 0, the dynamics passes through five stages: I, fixed point; II, limit cycle; III, strange attractor; IV, coexistence of limit cycle and strange attractor; and V, coexistence of fixed point and strange attractor. As c decreases from 0 (lateral inhibition), the attractor regions are VI, fixed point; VII, limit cycle; and VIII, fixed point. Thus, in this model, lateral excitation is necessary to obtain chaotic activity.

In section 5.2.3, we model rhythmic activity in the olfactory cortex. The Wilson-Bower model of temporal patterns in the piriform cortex uses a five-compartment design for each pyramidal cell and explicit delays for transmission and axonal activity in a network model designed to clarify the assumptions leading to near-40-Hz cortical oscillations. Oscillatory activity did not occur when a strong "shock input" was applied but was found for a weak shock input and for "natural" LOT inputs. In contrast, the Liljenström-Hasselmo model is designed to simulate modulatory cholinergic effects. This network is built from relatively simple units, whose output depends on a factor Q designed to represent the level of acetylcholine. Depending on the values of Q, the system may exhibit convergence to a fixed point, limit-cycle oscillation, or at least transient chaotic behavior. Moreover, the strengths of the synaptic connections also can drastically influence the dynamic behavior.

Our study moves up a level in section 5.3, from neural activity to synaptic dynamics. Some biology of learning and plasticity in the olfactory bulb is reviewed, and two views of learning in the olfactory bulb are described (rhythmic activity and associative memory). The chapter closes with models of learning and plasticity in the olfactory cortex. After a brief review of experimental literature (sec. 5.3.1), we turn to models of learning and memory in the olfactory bulb (sec. 5.3.2) and olfactory cortex (sec. 5.3.3). Building on the relation of different attractor regions to different lateral connection strengths (addressed in sec. 5.2.2), we show how synaptic modification can induce transitions among these regions. The ensuing study of the olfactory bulb models associative memory and shows that incomplete input patterns due to lower odor concentrations can also be identified as proper stimuli if a suitable learning rule is used to modify the lateral connections between mitral cells.

In section 5.3.2, we present two scenarios for learning and memory in the olfactory cortex. The Granger-Lynch scenario is based on the observation that the "sniffing

rhythm" of 5 Hz may be optimal for inducing long-term potentiation (LTP) in olfactory cortex. The associated model describes a hierarchical clustering of input stimuli based on the assumptions that olfactory bulb projections into olfactory cortex are sparse, that olfactory cortex projects back into the inhibitory cells of the olfactory bulb via the anterior olfactory nucleus (AON), and that afferent connections are modifiable by a competitive learning rule leading to "winner-take-all" interactions. The Haberly-Bower-Hasselmo scenario is based on the argument that the mechanism of object recognition in the olfactory cortex is close to those offered by abstract associative memory models. The attendant model emphasizes the observations that the incoming (bulbar) information has a complex, distributed representation, that afferent projections from the olfactory bulb are extensive and diffuse, and that intrinsic excitatory connections between pyramidal cells are spatially extensive, overlapping, and modifiable.

5.1 Anatomical Organization

Nasochemosensory systems are indispensable devices of communication at all phylogenetic levels, from bacteria to humans. The human nose is capable of discriminating thousands of different odor substances, but this achievement is modest compared with the performance of other organisms. During odor information processing, the information carried by chemical molecules of the external world is transformed into electrical patterns of brain activity. Many different aspects of olfaction, such as the nature of stimuli, mechanisms of reception and central processing, olfactory coding, learning, and memory, have been studied in detail. Although the olfactory pathway of mammals is well-known, the mechanisms of odor perception and processing remain subjects of extensive research.

5.1.1 The Stages of Odor Information Processing

Sensory information is processed in several stages of the olfactory pathway (Shepherd 1991; Buck 1996).

Stage 1

The first stage takes place in the receptor neurons of the olfactory epithelium, where a selective odor image is constructed. The very first step is ligand-receptor interaction. The olfactory receptors were found to be members of the so-called G-protein-coupled seven-transmembrane-domain protein family (Buck and Axel 1991). (G-proteins are guanosine triphosphate–binding proteins.) The transduction between receptor molecules and conductance channel molecules is mediated by a second-messenger system. The role of cyclic adenosine monophosphate (cAMP) as a secondary messenger system, first verified in the photoreceptors of the visual system, has been demonstrated in modulating olfactory ciliary membrane conductance (for a review, see Lancet 1992). Different types of odors are believed to activate different regions of the olfactory epithelium, as was suggested by Adrian (1950). Most receptor cells appear broadly tuned but respond with individual profiles to test odors. It seems likely that odors may establish (i.e., they are encoded in) spatio-temporal activity patterns even in this stage of olfactory information processing. The dependence of the firing frequency of receptor neurons on the concentration of the oderant molecules was the subject of many experimental (e.g., Getchell and Shepherd 1978) and model (e.g., Lánský and Rospars 1993) studies.

Stage 2

The second stage of olfactory information processing takes place in and around the glomeruli of the olfactory bulb, where the receptor cells make synapses with the dendrites of mitral and tufted cells and with the periglomerular cells. The glomeruli do not contain cell bodies; their mass is made up of olfactory nerve terminals and dendrites of neurons whose somata are located outside the glomerular layer. There is a strong convergence of receptors onto a single glomerulus, with ratios of up to 25,000 : 1. The projection of the receptor sheet to the glomeruli exhibits a broad topography (much more patch-to-patch than point-to-point mapping), but apparently haphazardly arranged fibers also occur. The degree of topographical order seems to be sufficient at least to preserve the molecular image formed in the epithelium. Another fact, interesting from the functional point of view, is that the estimated number of receptor types ($\sim 10,000$) is of the same order as the number of glomeruli ($\sim 2,000$). Though much evidence has accumulated to support the view that the glomerulus serves as a functional unit, it is remarkably true (Hudson and Distel 1987; Risser and Slotnick 1987) that a rather large lesion in the glomerular layer does not imply functional loss.

Stage 3

The third stage of representation is composed of the bulbar layers containing the second-order cells (mitral and tufted cells) and the granule cells. The mitral and tufted cells provide the only output of the bulb, the axons of which form the LOT. There is a divergence from the glomeruli to mitral and tufted (M/T) cells, but its degree is smaller than the convergence from the epithelium to the glomerulus). The M/T cells are excitatory and interact with the inhibitory, axonless, granular cells (~ 200 per mitral cell) via their basal dendrites and also via collaterals. These reciprocal dendrodendritic synapses play a role in spatiotemporal pattern formation (Freeman 1975, 1978) and are considered to be functional building blocks of the bulbar information-processing apparatus. It is interesting to note that the recognition of reciprocal dendrodendritic synapses (an important feature of olfactory architecture, discussed in later sections) came from the theoretical reconstruction of field potentials in the olfactory bulb (Rall and Shepherd 1968). Granule cells also are the targets of centrifugal afferents arriving from cortical and subcortical structures, which modulate the output of the bulb.

Stage 4

The M/T cells of the olfactory bulb make synapses on the distal dendrites of the pyramidal cells of the olfactory cortex (fourth stage). These projections show some regional specificity but, within a region, there is considerable divergence and convergence from a single M/T cell to pyramidal cells. Such reexcitatory connections may be the anatomical substrate of the associative memory systems found in the olfactory cortex (Haberly and Bower 1989).

5.1.2 The Olfactory Bulb

The olfactory bulb is the first relay center of the olfactory system, the site of the first synaptic interactions (Scott and Harrison 1987; Halász 1990). It is a highly layered structure, with synaptic contacts between particular neurons precisely localized in individual layers. The main histological layers and main cell types were described in the classic works of Golgi (1875) and Ramón y Cajal (1911).

Layers and Cell Types

The major layers and cell types of the olfactory bulb are illustrated in figure 5.1. The olfactory nerve layer (ONL) is formed by the nasal epithelial afferents (i.e., the unmyelinated axons of the olfactory receptor neurons). The most characteristic structures of the olfactory bulb are the glomeruli located in the glomerular layer (GL). The glomeruli are roughly spherical structures surrounded by glial sheaths separating each glomerulus from surround-

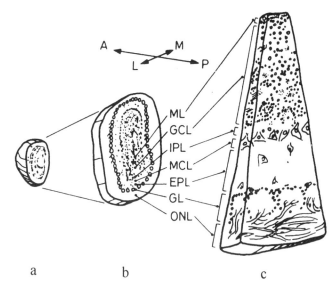

A M
L P

ML
GCL
IPL
MCL
EPL
GL
ONL

a   b   c

Figure 5.1
(a) Characteristic layers of the olfactory bulb in frontal view, as revealed by light microscopy of sections cut through the medial portion
of the rodent olfactory bulb. (b) The glomerular and the inner cellular
strata are apparent already at low magnification. (c) Other details can
be resolved with regular staining and microscopical techniques. ML,
medullary layer; GCL, granule cell layer; IPL, internal plexiform layer;
MCL, mitral cell layer; EPL, external plexiform layer; GL, glomerular
layer; ONL, olfactory nerve layer; A, anterior; L, lateral; M, medial;
P, posterior. (Reprinted with permission from Halász 1990a, p 46.)

ing groups of neuronal somata. The periglomerular region—the upper part of the GL in figure 5.1, not shown
as a separate layer—contains at least two types of interneurons, the periglomerular (PG) cells and superficial
short-axon (SSA) cells. The borderline between the PG
region and the external plexiform layer is not clearly defined. The main components of the external plexiform
layer are the basal dendrites of the M/T cells and the
peripheral processes of the granule cells, which lie more
deeply than the M/T neurons.

The mitral cells and their subtype, the tufted cells,
which are the main output neurons of the olfactory bulb,
form the mitral cell layer (MCL). The apical (primary)
dendrites are directed toward the glomeruli, whereas
secondary dendrites and axons are directed toward
deeper layers. In many adult vertebrates there exists a
thin, relatively cell-free region between the MCL and the
granule layer, called the *internal plexiform layer*. The cell
bodies of the most numerous local interneurons, namely
of the granule (GR) cells, are located in the deep granule
cell layer (GCL). [Perhaps it is better to say that the
granule cells do not form a distinct layer but are grouped
into islands (Reyher et al. 1991)]. GR cells do not have
axons (they seem, rather, to be involved in dendrodendritic interactions), but the GCL does contain deep short-

axon (DSA) cells. Large populations of GR cells are
organized in a very specific way, as their extended dendritic trees have a parallel orientation. In the GCL, the
myelinated axons of the output neurons are gathered to
form the olfactory tracts.

Synaptic Organization

The synaptic organization of the olfactory bulb is summarized in figure 5.2 (based on Halász 1990b, but modified based on Halász, personal communication). The first
level of synaptic connections is arranged in the GL. The
most characteristic synapses, arranged within the glomeruli, are those formed between the olfactory nerve
terminals and the primary dendritic branches of the M/T
cells. Olfactory nerve, however, may also establish contact on local neurons, mostly on PG cells. Reciprocal
dendrodendritic connections between PG neurons and
intraglomerular apical dendrites of M/T cells may be
observed. These synapses, together with synapses of
the olfactory nerve, constitute the most important intraglomerular connections. At least two cell types are
involved in forming connections between discrete
glomeruli—and SSA cells—both of which contribute to
the interglomerular loop. SSA cells innervate PG cells,
though inputs to the SSA cells can derive from different
sources (PG cells, central afferents, and collateral fibers
of the M/T cells) but not from the olfactory nerve. It
appears likely that SSA cells may inhibit the activity of
the (inhibitory) PG cells, resulting in disinhibitory effects
on the output neurons.

At the second level of bulbar synaptic organization,
there are reciprocal synapses between the dendrites of
the deep primary interneurons (i.e., the GR cells) and the
secondary dendrites of the mitral cells. DSA cells form
inhibitory synapses on GR cells, but the latter do not innervate DSA cells. Central afferents and axon collaterals
of the output cells may excite GR cells. There is some
uncertainty concerning the existence of synapses on
DSA cells from central afferents and from collaterals of
output neurons.

Chemical Neuroanatomy of the Olfactory Bulb

The olfactory bulb, particularly its neurochemical characterization, is one of the most extensively studied neural
structures. Though many data have been accumulated to
substantiate the presence of neuroactive substances such
as transmitters, neurohormones, and regulatory peptides,
(for an excellent review, see Halász 1990), the question of the bulb's neurochemical constituents is still
controversial.

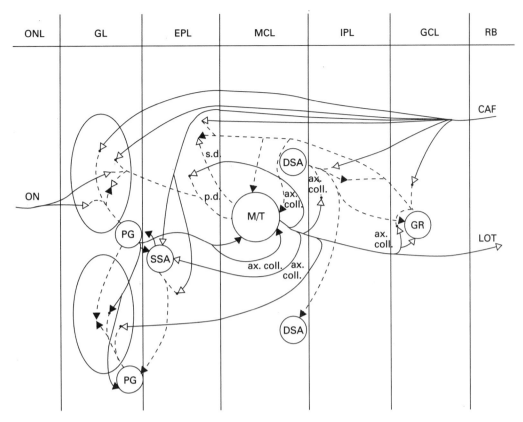

Figure 5.2
Scheme of the main synaptic contacts in the vertebrate olfactory bulb. Arrows show polarity of synapses and indicate the most likely post-synaptic effects (dotted lines, dendrites; solid lines, axons; open arrows, activation; closed arrows, inhibition). ONL, olfactory nerve layer; GL, glomerular layer; EPL, external plexiform layer; MCL, mitral cell layer; IPL, internal plexiform layer; GCL, granule cell layer; RBA, retrobulbar area; CAF, central afferents; DSA, deep short-axon cells; GR, granule cells; LOT, lateral olfactory tract; M/T, mitral or tufted cells; PG, periglomerular cells; ON, olfactory nerve; SSA, superficial short-axon cells. (Modified from Halász 1990b.)

As concerns the functioning of the olfactory bulb, odor-induced activity patterns of the output are controlled by local inhibitory circuits, as in cortical structures in general. The mitral cells are subject to GABAergic control exerted by both PG and GR cell populations (Duchamp-Viret and Duchamp 1993; Duchamp-Viret, Duchamp, and Chaput 1993). The partial blockade of GABAergic interactions has been implicated as having a major role in the formation of hippocampal epileptic seizures and will be studied in chapter 7.

5.1.3 The Olfactory Cortex

Primary olfactory cortical areas are defined as regions directly innervated by inputs coming from the olfactory bulb. Though different primary areas may be distinguished, the most remarkable is the *piriform cortex*, which is so called because it contains pear-shaped (piriform) cells. Confusingly, these cells also are called *pyramidal cells*, in accordance with the terminology for the principal cells of other areas of cerebral cortex. The piriform cortex's structure appears similar to other olfactory cortical areas, such as the AON. Results referring to the structure of the piriform cortex are believed to be applicable to other cortical areas (Haberly 1985).

Lamination Patterns

The piriform cortex has a trilaminar structure (fig. 5.3). Layer I (i.e., the most superficial, or *plexiform*, layer) contains (1) dendrites of cells having their somas in deeper layers, (2) fiber systems, and (3) a few nonpyramidal cells. Layer I is subdivided into two sublaminae. Whereas the afferent fibers originating from the olfactory bulb (those in the LOT) terminate in superficial layer Ia, the association fibers connecting cortical pyramidal cells terminate in layer Ib. Layer II is a compact region containing cell bodies. Layer III is less compact than layer II and contains cell bodies as well as axonal and dendritic elements.

The most characteristic input carrying olfactory information to the piriform cortex is the LOT, which is

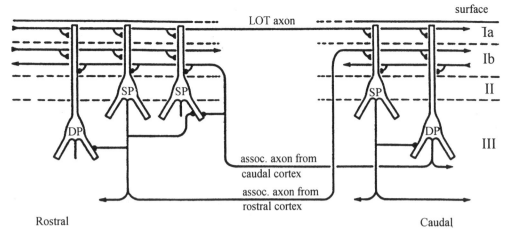

Figure 5.3
Scheme for excitatory inputs to pyramidal cells in piriform cortex. Excitatory events are postulated to occur in four different dendritic segments of both superficial (SP) and deep (DP) pyramidal cells in layers II and III, respectively. Afferent fibers in the lateral olfactory tract (LOT) excite distal apical segments in layer Ia. Local axon collaterals of pyramidal cells excite nearby pyramidal cells via their basal dendrites in layer III. Association fibers from the rostral part of the cortex excite distant pyramidal cells via intermediate apical segments in the outer part of layer Ib. Association fibers from the caudal piriform cortex excite pyramidal cells via their proximalmost apical segments in the deep part of layer Ib and also probably via basal dendrites. (Modified after Haberly 1985.)

derived from the olfactory bulb and terminates in layer Ia, innervating distal apical segments of pyramidal cells. The M/T cells of the olfactory bulb make synapses on the distal dendrites of the pyramidal cells of the olfactory cortex. These projections show some regional specificity but, within a region, there is considerable divergence and convergence from single M/T cells to pyramidal cells. Pyramidal cells are innervated not only by these afferent fibers but also by association fibers originating from other pyramidal cells. Such reexcitatory connections may be the anatomical substrate for the associative memory systems found in olfactory cortex (Haberly and Bower 1989).

There seems to be a remarkable difference in the vertical and horizontal organization of the afferent fiber system. In vertical organization (i.e., the segregation into layers shown in figure 5.3), there is a rather precise ordering, whereas the horizontal organization (i.e., across each layer) does not demonstrate topographical order.

In addition to the afferent fibers originating in the olfactory bulb, there are commissural fiber systems connecting the two halves of the piriform cortex, and there are centrifugal inputs from different brain areas, such as brainstem, thalamus, hypothalamus, and basal forebrain. Centrifugal inputs are neurochemically varied: Noradrenergic, serotoninergic, cholinergic, and dopaminergic fibers exist.

There are intrinsic association fiber systems within the piriform cortex that make connections between cortical pyramidal cells. The vertical-horizontal organization of this fiber system is similar to that of the afferent fiber system. Different association fibers make synapses lamina-specifically on different postsynaptic targets in layers Ib and III. Innervation seems even to be sublamina-specific: Fibers originating in the anterior piriform cortex terminate mostly in the superficial part of layer Ib, whereas neurons in the posterior piriform cortex project to the deeper sublaminae of layer Ib and also to layer III.

Olfactory cortical areas send their outputs to different neural centers responsible for further processing of olfactory information. The most important of these centers are the deep amygdaloid nuclei, hypothalamus, thalamus, neocortex, and hippocampal formation. Though the existence of a few different projections from the olfactory cortex to the mediodorsal and submedial nuclei of the thalamus has been demonstrated, there also are direct projections to the orbital and insular cortex. (The nuclei mentioned are in reciprocal connection with the orbital and insular cortex.) Furthermore, based on the number and location of the projecting cells, it seems likely that olfactory information is conveyed mostly by the direct projections, and the transthalamic links are less dominating. The functional role of the triangular relationship is discussed by Price et al. (1991).

As for other cortical areas, the principal cells of the piriform cortex are the pyramidal cells. Semilunar cells show some common features with pyramidal cells, but lack some of the processes necessary to perform integrating functions. Other classes of non-pyramidal cells most likely mediate inhibition.

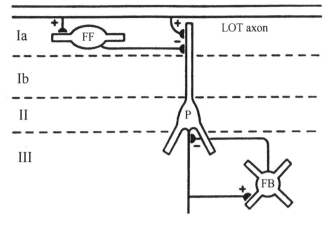

surface

Figure 5.4
Summary of hypotheses for inhibitory processes in pyramidal cells in piriform cortex. Feedforward inhibition is mediated via interneurons (FF) that are excited directly by afferent fibers. Feedback inhibition is mediated via interneurons (FB) that are excited by local axon collaterals of pyramidal cells. Several types of feedforward and feedback interneurons probably are present. The locations indicated for inhibitory synapses from the two populations of interneurons are arbitrary. (Modified after Haberly 1985.)

Pyramidal Cells

Cell bodies of pyramidal cells are located in layers II and III (superficial and deep pyramidal cells, respectively). Their apical dendrites, originating near the layer I–II border, are directed toward the brain surface; basal dendrites are concentrated in the upper part of layer III and are directed toward the deep pole of the cortex. Pyramidal (myelinated) axons forming association fibers make primarily long-distance contacts on the initial portion of the apical dendrites. Proximal collaterals, making connection with nearby pyramidal cells, however, form synapses mainly on basal dendrites.

Inhibitory Cells

Although from a strictly morphological point of view at least eight types of nonpyramidal cells have been described, only three of them have thus far been shown to have clear functional relevance. First, the large multipolar neurons concentrated in the deep part of layer III (*FB* in figure 5.4) are excited by local axon collaterals of pyramidal cells and send strong GABAergic feedback inhibition to pyramidal cells. Second, large fusiform cells (*FF* in figure 5.4) located in layer I, also mediate GABAergic inhibition. They get their inputs from the afferent fibers in layer Ia and send their feed-forward inhibition to pyramidal cells. Third, neurogliaform cells (not shown in fig. 5.4), which also seem to mediate

GABAergic inhibition, occur in all layers. Their processes are restricted spatially. Generally, their effect is confined to single sublayers or specific parts of a neuron.

5.2 Electrical Patterns in the Olfactory Bulb and Olfactory Cortex

5.2.1 Rhythmic Activity: Experimental Background

The demonstration of oscillatory activity in olfactory systems (Adrian 1942, 1950) was one of the first experiments to illustrate stimulus-induced activity in the mammalian central nervous system.

Phenomenologically, there are two main types of rhythmic activity in the olfactory system: slow and fast oscillations. Slow oscillations (~ 5 Hz) may be imposed on the olfactory bulb by the respiratory nuclei (Freeman 1991) or may be induced in the olfactory cortex by cholinergic antagonists (Biedenbech 1966; for further details, see sec. 5.2.3). The "respiratory wave" in the olfactory bulb is generated by the GR cells in response to input from the receptors through the PG and M/T cells. It can be detected in the mucosa by volume conduction. The slow background activity is phase-locked with the respiratory wave, and it is identified with the *sniff cycle*. A sniff cycle is composed of an inhalation and exhalation stage, and its duration is 200–500 msec for rabbits. A slow potential evoked by odorants (Ottoson 1959) appeared also in the electro-olfactogram, a receptor potential recorded in the nasal mucosa, which can spread through the brain by volume conduction.

Both the respiratory wave and the slow potential depend on receptor activation by odorants drawn into the nose by inhalation, which is driven by the respiratory nuclei in the medulla. The output of the mitral cells from the olfactory bulb causes waves to appear successively in the AON, in the prepiriform, periamygdaloid, and entorhinal cortices, and then in the different regions of the hippocampus, each wave having progressively lower amplitudes and longer delays (Freeman, personal communication).

Electroencephalogram patterns also show fast oscillations (35–90 Hz) in different parts of the olfactory bulb (Freeman 1978; Freeman and Schneider 1982). (The terminology here is: slow, ~ 1 Hz; intermediate, ~ 10 Hz; and fast, ~ 40 Hz.) It was suggested by Freeman's pioneering work (1975) that the spatiotemporal activity patterns of the olfactory bulb can be interpreted within the framework of dynamical system theory. Later, it was suggested (e.g., Skarda and Freeman 1987) that sensory information was encoded in *spatiotemporal periodic and chaotic patterns.* Generally, field potentials do not provide sufficient information about the underlying neural mechanisms. Still, one important message of Freeman's experimental and theoretical work is that rhythmic-arrhythmic bulbar activity is the result of the interactions between excitatory (mitral) and inhibitory (granule) cell populations. The situation, however, might be more complex. Odor-induced (mitral cell) activity is under GABAergic control (Duchamp-Viret, Duchamp, and Chaput 1993). Even in the case of blockade of the $GABA_A$-mediated inhibitory effect of the GR cells, oscillatory bulbar activity may occur as a consequence of recurrent excitatory connections.

Rhythmical activity in the olfactory cortex may occur as a consequence of bulbar oscillation, in response to electrical or chemical stimulation of the LOT, and as natural oscillation due to interaction between cortical excitatory and inhibitory populations (Bressler 1987a, b; Bower 1990). Model studies (see sec. 5.2.3) give specific information about the role of timing in the formation of different temporal patterns. Some population studies are based on single-compartment models in which single-cell activity is characterized by an internal state defined by the intracellular membrane potential and by an output expressed as a *firing frequency.* The behaviors of neural populations are observed either with multiunit recordings or with extracellular recordings of field potentials. Field potentials might be either evoked or spontaneous. The macroscopic activities of cell populations can be interpreted in terms of time-ensemble or spatial-ensemble averages of single cell-activities. The investigations of the single-cell responses (Kauer et al. 1991) should contribute to the understanding of population patterns.

In section 6.2.5 we will compare the hippocampus with the olfactory system, starting with the comparative phenomenology of electrical patterns and structural analogies and discussing the functional role of rhythms in hippocampal and olfactory information processing and the styles of modeling efforts devoted to their study.

5.2.2 Oscillation and Chaos in the Olfactory Bulb: Modeling

Modeling studies, based on relatively simple units, illustrate how the interactions among excitatory and inhibitory populations may generate oscillatory and more complex temporal patterns (Li and Hopfield 1989, Érdi et al. 1993; Aradi et al. 1995). Recently, both mitral and granule cells have been the subject of detailed single-

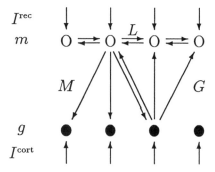

Figure 5.5
Model structure of olfactory bulb. The two layers of excitatory mitral cells (open circles, *m*) and inhibitory granule cells (filled circles, *g*) interact through the synaptic connections M and G. Here, L denotes modifiable lateral synaptic connections in the mitral layer.

neuron modeling. The mitral cells, for example, were subdivided into six regions (Bhalla and Bower 1993), and six channel kinetics were taken into account. The effects of small structural differences and of channel distributions have been demonstrated. Detailed parameter sensitivity analysis appears to be very time-consuming. Aradi and Érdi (1996a, b) made further simulations of the mitral and granuled cells and also studied the effects of the synaptic connections. A reasonable compromise between "reality" and "efficiency" is necessary to analyze large-scale network simulations, at least for the time being (White et al. 1992; Linster and Gervais 1996).

Population Studies

Structural Aspects A skeleton model (figure 5.5) consists of two layers of neurons: the layer of excitatory mitral cells (*m*) and the layer of inhibitory granule cells (*g*). The rather significant difference between the numbers of cells in these two layers of the olfactory bulb is neglected here, and both layers are assumed to contain N units. The model neurons are arranged in a one-dimensional ring (the Nth and the first neurons are considered neighbors) in order to avoid edge effects.

Each unit has an internal state corresponding to the membrane potential of the cell, which is converted by a static nonlinear transfer function to yield the cell's output (the leaky integrator model of sec. 4.1.2). This output can be interpreted as the firing rate of the cell. Each mitral cell excites the three nearest granule cells. The physiological nature of lateral connections within the MCL is not specified here: Both excitatory and inhibitory connections are investigated, and their different effects on the qualitative dynamics of the model are discussed. In these simulations, nearest-neighbor connections are studied, whereas full lateral interconnection is assumed when modeling associative memory.

The sensory input to the system is provided by the input I^{rec} from the receptors to the mitral cells. Granule cells receive constant input corresponding to the modulatory effect I^{cort} of cortical regions and other higher centers. The granule-to-mitral synapses are inhibitory. No lateral connections are assumed in the granule cell layer.

Activity Dynamics Membrane potentials of mitral and granule cells at time t are expressed, respectively, by the following vectors:

$$m(t) = \{m_1(t), m_2(t), \ldots, m_N(t)\}$$

$$g(t) = \{g_1(t), g_2(t), \ldots, g_N(t)\}$$

Their transfer functions are denoted by f_m and f_g. The form of these functions is taken from Li and Hopfield (1989), though the experimentally measured curves (Freeman 1979) significantly depart from those used by Li and Hopfield.

$$f_m(m_i) = \begin{cases} S'_m + S'_m \tanh\left(\dfrac{m_i - \theta}{S'_m}\right) & \text{if } m_i < \theta; \quad S'_x = 0.14 \\ S'_m + S_m \tanh\left(\dfrac{m_i - \theta}{S_m}\right) & \text{if } m_i \geqslant \theta; \quad S_x = 1.4 \end{cases}$$
(1a)

$$f_g(g_i) = \begin{cases} S'_g + S'_g \tanh\left(\dfrac{g_i - \theta}{S'_g}\right) & \text{if } g_i < \theta; \quad S'_y = 0.29 \\ S'_g + S_g \tanh\left(\dfrac{g_i - \theta}{S_g}\right) & \text{if } g_i \geqslant \theta; \quad S'_y = 0.29; \quad \theta = 1 \end{cases}$$
(1b)

The time evolution equations governing the activity dynamics are specified by the following set of coupled, nonautonomous, nonlinear, first-order ordinary differential equations (ODEs):

$$\dot{m}_i(t) = -a \cdot m_i(t) - b \sum_{j=1}^{N} G_{ij} \phi_g(g_j(t)) + c \sum_{j=1}^{N} L_{ij} \phi_m(m_j(t))$$
$$+ I_i^{rec}(t)$$

$$\dot{g}_i(t) = -d \cdot g_i(t) + e \sum_{j=1}^{N} M_{ij} \phi_m(m_j(t)) + I_i^{cort} \quad (2)$$

where $i = 1, 2, \ldots, N$, and a, b, d, and e are positive constants; c can be positive or negative depending on whether lateral excitation or lateral inhibition is assumed. The only source of nonlinearity is the form of the transfer functions. Nonautonomy is due to the temporal character of the input. The synaptic matrices $\mathbf{M}$, $\mathbf{G}$, and $\mathbf{L}$

correspond to the mitral-to-granule, granule-to-mitral, and lateral (mitral-to-mitral) connections, respectively. In this model, the lateral connections are modifiable so that $\mathbf{L}$ may be a function of time, but $\mathbf{M}$ and $\mathbf{G}$ are fixed. I^{cort} and $I^{rec}(t)$ denote the cortical and receptor inputs, respectively, and

$$I^{rec}(t) = \alpha I^{odor}(t) + I^{backgr} \quad (3)$$

where α scales the input intensities. $I^{odor}(t)$ contains information about the quality and intensity of odors; it represents the "sniff cycle" with a characteristic period of 400 milliseconds for rabbits, and 1 second for humans, and is described by a linear inhalation and an exponential exhalation stage. The background I^{backgr} is assumed to be constant over time.

Bifurcation Analysis Given the model structure and the related set of ODEs, the first question to be answered here is what qualitative dynamical behavior emerges in the parameter space. The nature of attractors, the parameter windows belonging to them, and the bifurcation sequences are determined through systematic (numerical) studies.

To study the inherent bulbar dynamics, the time dependence of external inputs is omitted here (i.e., $I_i^{odor}(t) =$ constant for any cell i). While all elements of the modulatory cortical input I^{cort} and the receptor background input I^{backgr} vectors have the same values, odor patterns are taken into account by assigning randomly chosen values to the different elements of I_i^{odor}. Then the free parameters in equation 2 are a, b, c, d, e, and the input vectors I^{backgr} and I^{cort}.

Li and Hopfield (1989) did not systematically analyze the effect of lateral connections. Because of the lack of firm data on the physiological nature of the lateral interactions in the mitral layer, the potential effects of both inhibition and excitation on dynamic behavior were studied. It therefore was particularly important to study the different (positive and negative) values of the parameter c, which controls the sign and strength of lateral connections in the mitral layer, while the synaptic matrices are fixed. The main questions are which values of the parameter c imply stationary, oscillatory, or chaotic behavior, and what kinds of bifurcation phenomena can be observed between the different parameter regions. To complete the analysis, experiments with the other parameters have also been made.

Simulations have shown that, for either sign of c, the parameters previously listed can be classified into two groups: Systematic change of $|c|$, d, and I^{rec} generates the same bifurcation sequence (recall sec. 4.2.2), although the

Table 5.1
Parameters in the olfactory bulb model

Parameter	Value		
N	11	11	11
S'_m	0.14	0.14	0.14
S_m	1.4	1.4	1.4
S'_g	0.29	0.29	0.29
S_g	2.9	2.9	2.9
θ	1.0	1.0	1.0
a	0.1	0.1	0.1
b	1.0	1.0	1.0
c	−5.0–5.0	1.0	1.0
d	0.2	0.2	0.2
e	1.2	1.2	1.2
α	1.0	1.0	0.32
I^{odor}	1.0*	1.0*	**
I^{backgr}	0	0	0.02
I^{cort}	0.1	0.1	0.1
M_{ij}			
$\quad i = j$	1.0	1.0	1.0
$\quad |i - j| = 1$	0.5	0.5	0.5
$\quad |i - j| > 1$	0	0	0
G_{ij}			
$\quad i = j$	1.0	1.0	1.0
$\quad |i - j| = 1$	0.5	0.5	0.5
$\quad |i - j| > 1$	0	0	0
L_{ij}			
$\quad i = j$	0	0	0
$\quad |i - j| = 1$	1.0	†	†
$\quad |i - j| > 1$	0	0	†
T	—	—	400 msec
τ	—	—	33 msec
k_1	—	0.0005	10^{-5}
k_2	—	0.035	0.1
k_3	—	0.005	0.1
P^2	—	—	6
p^2	—	—	4

*Expectation of a gaussian distribution.

†The parameter is a function of time (see text for details).

size of the parameter windows may be different. All these parameters act in the direction of mitral cell excitation (or disinhibition). The change of the other group of parameters (i.e., a, b, e, and I^{cort}) has just the opposite effect (mitral cell inhibition or granule cell excitation) and thus the same bifurcation sequence appears in reverse order. Note that this phenomenon was observed in the case of positive parameter values except for c, which could be either positive or negative.

A bifurcation diagram can be constructed by representing each attractor region in the space of the bifurcation parameters. For the reasons just cited, however, results are presented here only in terms of one parameter, the lateral connection strength c. Values of the other parameters are fixed (table 5.1).

Figure 5.6a shows the different attractor types with a characteristic phase diagram in each region. The activity of an arbitrary mitral-granule pair is chosen for the two-dimensional representation of phase portraits. The largest Lyapunov exponent λ is plotted against the bifurcation parameter c in figure 5.6b. It can be observed that leaps of the largest Lyapunov exponent occur *exactly at the bifurcation points* where the qualitative attractor picture changes. Negative values of the largest Lyapunov exponent correspond to fixed-point attractors, positive values support the existence of chaos, and values approximating zero belong to limit cycles.

At $c = 0$, the trajectories converge into a stable focus (i.e., into a fixed point). When lateral excitation is considered ($c > 0$), the following attractor regions can be observed in figure 5.6a as c increases:

Region I: fixed point (stable focus)

Region II: limit cycle

Region III: strange attractor

Region IV: coexistence of limit cycle and strange attractor

Region V: coexistence of fixed point (stable node) and strange attractor

For negative values of c (lateral inhibition), the attractor regions are (as $|c|$ increases) as follows:

Region VI: fixed point (stable focus)

Region VII: limit cycle

Region VIII: fixed point (stable focus)

These results show that chaos can be found only when $c > 0$ so, in our model, lateral excitation (as distinct from lateral inhibition) is necessary to obtain chaotic activity. It has also been observed that all neurons oscillate in phase in each periodic region (and also during damping oscillation to a stable focus), and no wave phenomena have been detected in the parameter range studied here.

To complete the analysis, not only the nature of attractors but also the different types of bifurcations between them were identified.

At small values of $|c|$, the first bifurcation is a Hopf bifurcation in the case of both lateral excitation and inhibition (between regions I–II and VI–VII in figure 5.6a). The fine structure of this type of bifurcation is shown in figure 5.7. At somewhat larger values of $|c|$, the amplitude of the limit cycle continuously increases. The bifurcation between regions II and III is a period-doubling bifurcation (figure 5.8).

There is a coexistence phenomenon in regions IV and V. While the strange attractor remains stable over regions III, IV, and V, a stable limit cycle also appears in

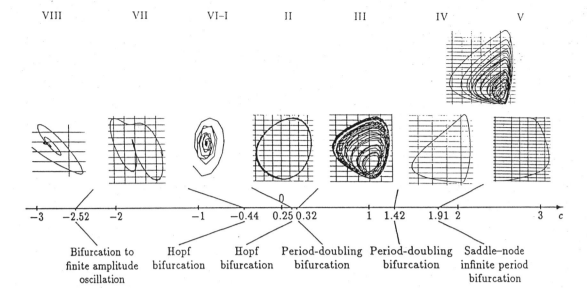

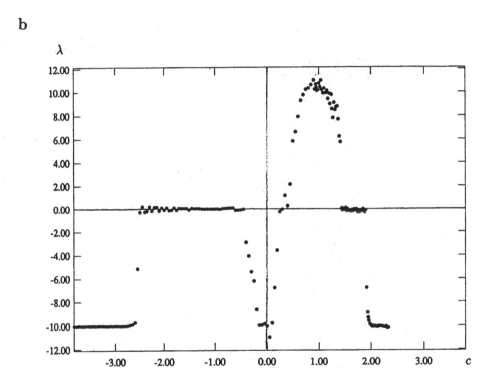

Figure 5.6

(a) Attractor regions in terms of the bifurcation parameter c in the range $(-3, 3)$. In each region, a characteristic phase diagram is shown. Bifurcation types between the regions also are indicated. (b) The largest Lyapunov exponent λ is plotted against the bifurcation parameter c.

Leaps of the largest Lyapunov exponent occur exactly at the bifurcation points where the qualitative attractor picture changes in (a). (a reprinted with permission from Érdi et al. 1993; b reprinted with permission from Érdi et al. 1995.)

region IV. Further increasing c, the period of this limit cycle begins to grow, and large plateaus appear (figure 5.9a–d). Finally, as the period of the oscillation becomes infinitely large (figure 5.9e), the limit cycle disappears and a stable node emerges. This is characteristic to the so-called saddle-node infinite period bifurcation (Keener 1981).

For negative values of c, the bifurcation between the regions VI and VII has already been mentioned. The bifurcation between the regions VII and VIII is different in that the limit cycle has a finite amplitude at the bifurcation point.

The effects on dynamic behavior of the eventual lateral inhibition and excitation in the MCL have been studied. The results of computer simulations have shown

that chaotic activity can be found only if lateral excitation is assumed, in accordance with the assumption of Skarda and Freeman (1987).

Multicompartmental Studies

Ionic Currents and Channel Kinetics The mitral cell model (Bhalla and Bower 1993) has been assumed to contain six channel types, such as fast sodium (Na), fast delayed rectifier (K_f), slow delayed rectifier (K_s), transient outward potassium current (K_A), voltage- and calcium-dependent potassium current (K_{Ca}), and L-type calcium current (L-Ca). The GR cell model included five channel types: sodium (similar to, but different from, the sodium current of the mitral cells), K_f, K_s, K_A, and non-inactivating muscarinic potassium current (K_M). The channel kinetic data were taken from Bhalla and Bower (1993).

Signal Generation and Propagation Four types of problems have been studied (Aradi and Érdi 1996b):

1. The effects of the individual currents and their role in the generation and suppression of action potentials and in the control of firing frequencies (intracompartmental studies)

2. Signal propagation through the compartments of both the mitral and GR cells, which has been simulated, and the effects of both orthodromic and antidromic stimulation

3. The excitatory-inhibitory coupling between the mitral and GR cells through dendrodendritic synapses and the effects of the (partial) blockade of the GABAergic inhibition

a **b**

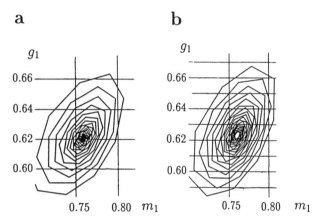

Figure 5.7
Typical scheme of Hopf bifurcation. (a) stable focus with long oscillatory transient at $c = 0.23$. (b) The periodic attractor emerging at $c = 0.25$ with very small amplitude. (Reprinted with permission from Érdi et al. 1993.)

a **b** **c**

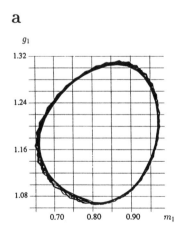 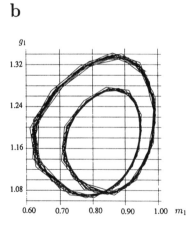 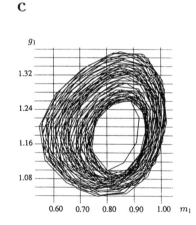

Figure 5.8
Period-doubling bifurcation. (a) Periodic attractor at $c = 0.3$. (b) Biperiodic attractor at $c = 0.32$. (c) Strange attractor at $c = 0.34$. (Reprinted with permission from Érdi et al. 1993.)

5 The Olfactory System

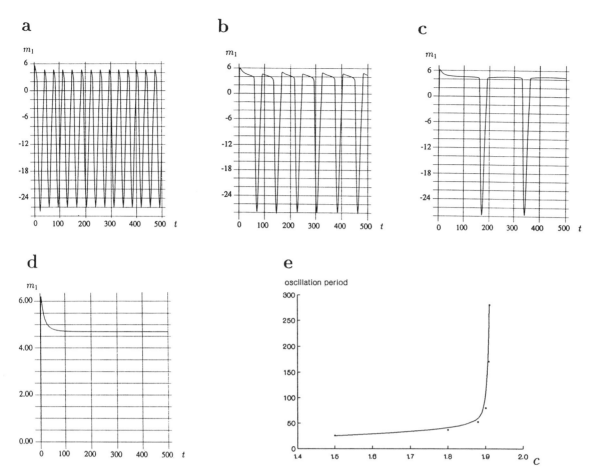

Figure 5.9
Saddle-node infinite period bifurcation. oscillations at $c = 1.80$ (a), 1.90 (b), 1.908 (c), and stable node at $c = 1.91$ (d). Time curves instead of phase portraits are plotted directly to visualize period differences.

The period of oscillations in terms of the bifurcation parameter c is shown in (e). (Reprinted with permission from Érdi et al. 1993.)

4. Dynamic behavior of a skeleton network of the bulbar circuitry, taking into account even the periglomerular cells

Intracompartmental Studies The interactions among the different conductances were studied within a single (mostly somatic) compartment. A compartment can be composed of several segments. The distributions of channel densities were uniform within the entire compartment, but the potential values have been calculated in each segment. The approximately proper values of the maximal conductances either were taken from Bhalla and Bower 1993 or were determined by some parameter estimation technique. The response of the mitral and GR cells for different inputs—that is, for a short square impulse—and for a constant stimulus have been simulated. The simulation results were compared with experimental data to find the proper, but experimentally unknown, spatial density of each included channel class. The par-

ticular effect of the different ionic currents have been demonstrated by a series of simulation experiments (Aradi and Érdi 1996a, b; Érdi, Aradi, and Gröbler 1997). These simulations are in accordance with experiments in which specific channel-blocking agents were applied. Tetrodotoxin (TTX) and tetraethylammonium (TEA) block the Na^+ and K^+ currents, respectively, and they are taken into account in the model by reducing the numerical value of the maximal conductances.

Signal Propagation Through the Compartments Detailed geometric data on the mitral and granule cells were taken into account by adopting multicompartmental computer simulation technique. Six compartments were considered, such as the soma, primary dendrite (or trunk), glomerular tuft, proximal secondary dendrite, distal secondary dendrite, and axon (Bhalla and Bower 1993). As usual, the channel densities were distributed uniformly within these compartments, and each compartment was divided into several segments to compute the membrane potential. The effects of both orthodromic and antidromic stimulation of mitral cells have been simulated to describe the synaptic activation due to external input coming from the olfactory nerve and due to the processes within the LOT, respectively.

Elementary Synaptic Interactions In a relatively simply organized region such as the olfactory bulb, it has been possible to combine the results of anatomical, physiological, neurochemical, and computational studies into a basic circuit (Shepherd 1991). The basic circuit is a key concept for computational neuroscience, as it defines the irreducible minimum of neural components that must be incorporated into neuronal and network models in order to capture the neural basis of the functions carried out by that region. Synaptic interactions are taken into account by the synaptic current, given as

$$I_{syn}(t) = g_{syn}(t)(V - E_{syn}). \tag{4}$$

Here g_{syn} is the synaptic conductance, and E_{syn} is the synaptic reversal potential. The excitatory nature of the mitral-to-granule and the inhibitory character of the granule-to-mitral synaptic connections have been specified by the alpha function (Rall 1967):

$$g_{syn}(t) := g_{max} \cdot (t/t_p) \cdot \exp(1 - t/t_p) \tag{5}$$

Here, the function g_{syn} increases to its maximum of g_{max} at $t = t_p$. A synapse is strong if g_{max} is large, and slow if t_p is relatively large.

Three types of microcircuits can be distinguished within the olfactory bulb:

1. Excitatory-inhibitory coupling between the mitral and granule cells.

2. Excitatory-excitatory interaction: Its prototype is self-excitation of mitral cells established by their axon collaterals (Halász 1990b).

3. Inhibitory-inhibitory coupling: An example is the synaptic contacts among PG cells. Additionally, there are some indications that self-inhibition exists even between granule cells.

The excitatory-inhibitory coupling between the mitral and granule cells through dendrodendritic synapses (see figure 5.10A) and the effects of the (partial) blockade of GABAergic inhibition have been shown by Aradi and Érdi (1996b). The behavior of a small network of three mitral and three granule cells also was simulated. Isolated trains of spikes have been generated, whereas, by increasing the inhibitory effect, the amplitude of the externally stimulated mitral cell exhibits a waning and

waxing amplitude structure, reminiscent of the spindle rhythms known in the thalamocortical system (Steriade, McCormick, and Sejnowski 1993).

The self-excitation between mitral cells also was studied. GABA antagonists produce prolonged depolarization in the mitral cells (Nowycky, Mori, and Shepherd 1981; Nicoll and Jahr 1982), and the reentrant excitation in the mitral layer may be associated with a particular mode of bulbar rhythmogenesis. In the case of two mitral cells connected by mutual excitatory couplings, synchronized burst activity may appear (figure 5.10B). These simulation results are in accordance with the physiological findings and the suggestion that the blockage of GABAergic inhibiton controls the odor-induced activity (Duchamp-Viret 1993). According to our simulation experiments, both the mitral-granule feedback loop and the self-excitation in the MCL may provide the anatomical substrate of bulbar rhythmogenesis.

Not only excitatory but also inhibitory coupling (van Vreeswijk, Abbot, and Ermentrout 1994) may lead to synchronized oscillation, as happens, for example, in the reticular nucleus of the thalamus (Steriade, McCormick, and Sejnowski 1993). According to the anatomical findings, synaptic connections between inhibitory cells, such as between PG cells and deep short axon-to-granule cells (Halász 1990a), can be found in the olfactory bulb. Self-sustained sychronized oscillatory behavior in case of mutual inhibitory coupling of granule cells has been simulated (figure 5.10C).

Skeleton Network Studies

The effects of the other two cell types—namely, the PG and DSA cells—short axon cells have been taken into account in more complicated network models. Figure 5.11 shows the skeleton network of the olfactory bulb. The structure of this model network is based on anatomical findings (Halász 1990b). Four major cell types have included: the excitatory mitral cell and the inhibitory granule, PG, and DSA cells. Sensory input comes through the olfactory nerve to the PG and mitral cells; there are excitatory-inhibitory interactions among the mitral and PG cells and among the mitral and granule cells. The axons of mitral cells constitute the LOT, which projects sensory information toward the olfactory cortex. The central afferents come back to the bulbar DSA cells, and these inhibitory interneurons make synaptic contacts with the granule cells. This neural circuit constitutes the anatomical basis for our simulations to describe the dynamic behavior of individual neurons. Emergent behavior results from the interplay of intraneuronal and

A

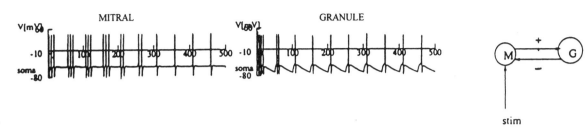

B

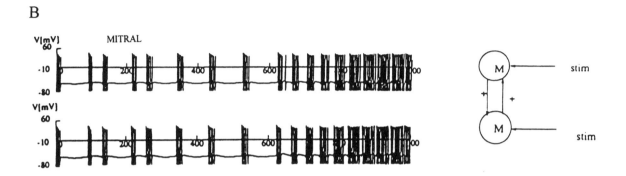

C

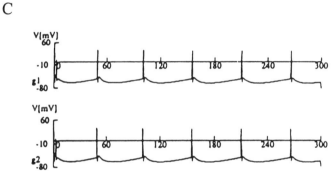
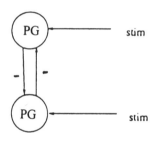

Figure 5.10
(A) Dynamics of the excitatory-inhibitory loop between a mitral (M) and a granule (G) cell. (B) Sychronized oscillation due to self-excitation as a response for a sustained stimulus. (C) Synchronized oscillation due to self-inhibition. PG, periglomerular cell. (Reprinted with permission from Aradi and Érdi 1996b.)

interneuronal effects. Simulations of single-cell recordings have been done to model the contribution of these newly introduced inhibitory cell types to rhythmogenesis of the olfactory bulb.

Experimental data are available for identifying several types of granule and PG cells (Wellis and Scott 1990). These intracellular recordings were made during electrical and odor stimulation of the ONL and the LOT. Three types of granule cells can be distinguished according to the experiments. Figure 5.12 shows the responses of these identified classes of granule cells during electrical stimulation of LOT, and our simulations for each class can be seen also. The only difference between the

first two simulated classes (see figure 5.12A,B) is in the maximal synaptic conductance describing the excitatory effect of the mitral cell on the granule cell. The third type of granule cell responding to the stimulation is a result of the geometrical differences of the deeply localized granule cells; in our simulations, we had to enlarge the electrotonic length of this type of neuron (see figure 5.12C). Network effects are demonstrated more explicitly in figure 5.13. In accordance with the electrophysiological findings of Wellis and Scott (1990), long-duration hyperpolarization of the granule cell is due to the inhibition that results from the DSA cells and cannot be considered an intrinsic cell property.

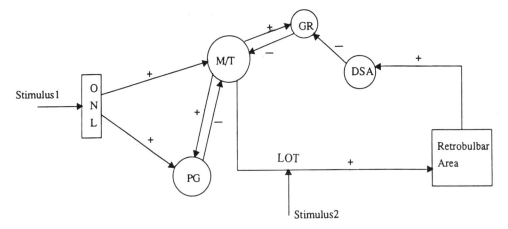

Figure 5.11
Skeleton circuit of the olfactory bulb. Arrows show polarity of synapses, and the postsynaptic effects are indicated (+, activation, −, inhibition). ONL, olfactory nerve layer; M/T, mitral or tufted cells; PG, periglomerular cells; GR, granule cells; DSA, deep short-axon cells; LOT, lateral olfactory tract.

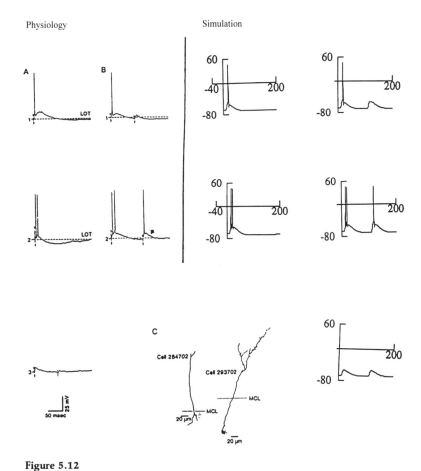

Figure 5.12
Comparison of the measured (modified after Wellis and Scott 1990) and simulated responses of granule cells to electrical stimulation. Three classes of granule cells were distinguished owing to their responses to single-pulse (A) and paired stimulation (B) of the lateral olfactory tract (LOT). (A1) Responses of a granule cell to single-pulse stimulation of the LOT; (A2) the EPSP evoked two spikes at suprathreshold stimuli; (B1) the second stimulus of a pair evoked a diminished EPSP, which did not reach threshold for a spike; (B2) the second stimulus evoked an EPSP that evoked on a single spike; (B3) no spike was produced. (C) Reconstruction of granule cells located near the mitral cell layer.

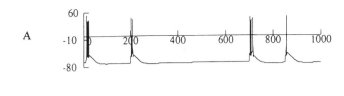

A

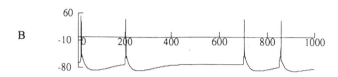

B

Figure 5.13
Response of modeled granule cells. (A) GABAergic inhibition resulting from blocking deep short-axon cells (hyperpolarization did not occur). (B) Inhibition from deep short-axon cell is necessary for the emergence of long-duration hyperpolarization.

The response of PG cells to ONL stimulation was studied both experimentally and computationally (figure 5.14). In our simulations, after adjustment of the proper values of maximal conductances for each channel type, we varied only the maximal value of synaptic conductance, which characterizes the amplitude of the excitatory postsynaptic potentials coming from the axon terminals of the receptor cells.

5.2.3 Rhythmic Activity in the Olfactory Cortex: Modeling

Oscillations in the olfactory cortex have been modeled by adopting different strategies. Wilson and Bower (1989, 1992) built a network using both a single-compartment and a five-compartment model for each pyramidal cell. They also provided a simpler treatment by substituting detailed channel kinetics with a less complicated spiking algorithm. Liljenström (1991) reproduced the essential results of these simulation experiments by using a single-compartment model. Barkai and Hasselmo (1994) and Barkai et al. (1994) reported on a more detailed single-cell model to describe the role of some ionic conductances in the frequency adaptation.

Temporal Patterns in the Piriform Cortex

The Wilson-Bower model offers a bottom-up description of the temporal patterns in the piriform cortex. Specifically, Wilson and Bower's intention was to clarify the assumptions leading to near-40-Hz cortical oscillations. Though it contains strong simplifications in the structural assumptions (e.g., the pyramidal cells were assumed to be fully interconnected), the model did serve to integrate cellular and network properties. The mathemat-

Physiology   Simulation

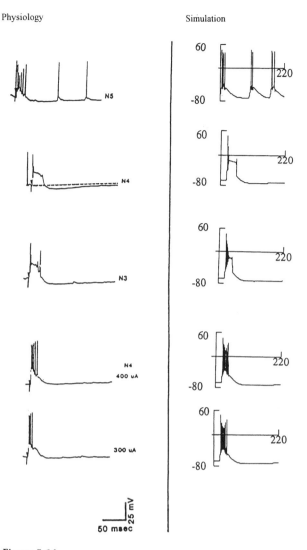

Figure 5.14
Comparison of the measured (after Wellis and Scott 1990) and simulated responses of periglomerular cells to electrical stimulation of the olfactory nerve layer.

ical framework presented here is the single compartment model with n_c channels, and the time dependence of the membrane potential V_j is given by

$$\frac{dV_j}{dt} = 1/c_m \sum_{k=0}^{n_c} [E_k - V_j(t)]g_{jk}(t) + I_{ext}(t) \qquad (6)$$

where $I_{ext}(t)$ denotes the external current injection, c_m is the membrane capacitance, and E_k is the equilibrium potential for channel type k. Instead of giving a detailed single-cell model based on channel kinetics of membrane and synaptic currents, the output of a single neuron is characterized by a binary variable $S_i(t)$.

$$S_i(t) = \begin{cases} 1, & \text{if } V_i(t) \geq T_i, \text{ and } t > t_{\text{last firing}} + t_r \\ 0 & \text{otherwise} \end{cases} \qquad (7)$$

Here V_i is the membrane potential of the cell i, T_i is the threshold, and t_r is the refractory period. An action potential is generated when the membrane potential crosses the threshold, and the cell has not fired in the refractory period.

The transmission time delay from cell i to cell j along fiber q is assumed to satisfy:

$$t_{t(ijq)} = t_{p(ijq)} + t_{s(ijq)} \qquad (8)$$

where the first term of the right-hand side (i.e., the propagation delay) depends on the distance between the two cells and the velocity along the connecting fiber. The second term corresponds to the time lag between the arrival of the presynaptic signal and the generation of the postsynaptic response.

Chemical transmission implies a net conductance change of the particular ion channels. The net conductance in channel k of cell j due to input from cell i along fiber q is

$$g^*(t)_{ijkq} = \int_0^{t-t_{t(ijq)}} G_{jk}(\lambda) S_i(t - \lambda - t_{t(ijq)}) W_{ijq}(t)\, d\lambda \qquad (9)$$

where G denotes the postsynaptic activation function and W_{ijq} is the synaptic strength. The form of the $G(t)$ function often is assumed to be $G(t) = t \exp(-t/\tau)$ (the alpha function), or

$$G(t) = \frac{\tau_1 \tau_2}{\tau_1 - \tau_2} (\exp(-t/\tau_1) - \exp(-t/\tau_2)) \qquad (10)$$

(the dual exponential). The time constants t, τ_1, and τ_2 can be estimated by making assumptions about the underlying mechanism of the transmitter-receptor interaction at the postsynaptic membrane surface.

The total conductance change $g_{jk}(t)$ is calculated by summing over all synaptic inputs to that channel:

$$g_{jk}(t) = \sum_{i=1}^{n \text{ cells}} \sum_{q=1}^{n \text{ fibers}} g^*(t)_{ijkq} \qquad (11)$$

This relatively simple algorithm for calculating conductance changes should be replaced by a detailed model of channel kinetics to describe the different kinds (weak and strong) of firing adaptation (Barkai and Hasselmo 1994).

In the multicompartmental case (see also Wilson and Bower 1992), each compartment is coupled to its immediate neighbors with an axial resistance. Two kinds of currents are taken into account: the axial (I_a) and the transmembrane (I_m) currents. The latter consists of the passive leakage term and the synaptic currents. The formal equation for the dynamics of the membrane potential of each compartment is given by

$$\frac{dV}{dt} = (1/c_m)(I_a(t) + I_m(t)). \qquad (12)$$

Extracellular field potentials are considered as a linear superposition of fields generated by current sources. A current source is identified with a transmembrane current in a compartment calculated from the multicompartment model and lumping it to a point. The field potential V_f is estimated as

$$V_f(x', y', z'; t) = \text{const } x \sum_j^{n \text{ cells}} \sum_k^{n \text{ compartments}} I_{m(jk)}(t)/r_{jk}. \qquad (13)$$

where the coordinates (x', y', z') denote the recording site, r_{jk} is the distance between compartment k in cell j and the recording site, and $I_{m(jk)}(t)$ is the total membrane current in the k compartment of the cell j.

Depending on the strength of the natural input from LOT, cortical activity exhibits different behavior. Oscillatory activity did not occur when the "shock input" (which takes the form of 2-msec square pulses) was strong but was found for weak input (figure 5.15). Though the details of the transition have not been published, the qualitative differences pinpoint the role of timing.

Natural inputs (as opposed to an overall shock to LOT) lead to oscillatory behavior. Rhythmical cortical activity was found not only in the case of periodic bulbar input but also in response to continuous random input. The role of timing seems to be significant even in this case. The high-frequency (~ 40-Hz) component is produced by the fast feedback inhibitory neurons, whereas the low-frequency (~ 5-Hz) component is generated owing to the slow feed-forward inhibition.

Cholinergic Modulation of Cortical Oscillation

Acetylcholine and cholinergic agonists seem to control the dynamics of olfactory cortex by several different mechanisms. First, they can suppress the neuronal adaptation of pyramidal cells by shutting down the postsynaptic voltage-dependent potassium currents (Constanti and Sim 1987). Second, acetylcholine appears to suppress excitatory synapses. According to Hasselmo and Bower (1992), in the olfactory cortex this suppression is selective for intrinsic fiber synaptic transmission (and has little effect on synaptic transmission via afferent fibers). Third, it may suppress even inhibitory synapses, as might analogously be expected based on experiments made on hippocampal slices (Pitler and Alger 1992).

The different effects of cholinergic neuromodulation have been take into account in the Liljenström-Hasselmo

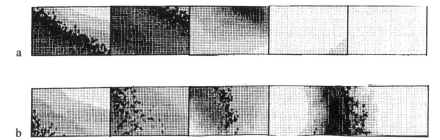

Figure 5.15
Comparison of the effects of (a) strong and (b) weak shock strength for the Wilson-Bower simulation. The level of activity distributed over the networks is shown at five different time steps. The shock inputs originate in the lower left corner. Waves of activity move from left (rostral) to right (caudal) in the networks. Reactivation of the "rostral cortex" occurs for weak shocks only. Whereas (a) shows the decay of the spatiotemporal activity, in (b) temporal periodicity is demonstrated. (Based on Wilson and Bower 1992.)

model built from relatively simple units (Liljenström and Hasselmo 1993; Barkai et al. 1994; Barkai and Hasselmo 1994; Wu and Liljenström 1994; Liljenström and Hasselmo 1995). A network unit represents a (sub)population of neurons characterized by a mean membrane potential, u. The activity equation is:

$$\frac{du_i}{dt} = -u_i/\tau + \sum_{j=1}^{N} w_{ij} g_j[u_j(t - \delta_{ij})] + I_i(t) \qquad (14)$$

where τ characterizes the spontaneous decay, w_{ij} is the synaptic weight, δ denotes the specific axonal transmission delay, and I_i is the afferent input. The input-output relationship of a population of neurons in the piriform cortex was determined by recording evoked potentials. This relationship can be fit by the sigmoidal function

$$g_i(u_i) = CQ\{1 - \exp[-\exp(u_i) - 1/Q]\} \qquad (15)$$

where Q is the only parameter, and C is a normalization constant. (Q is assumed to correspond to the level of acetylcholine.) This model can be supplemented by taking into account neuronal adaptation. By way of a simple description, the output function is multiplied by an exponential decay proportional to the time average of the previous unit output over the last time period. The adapted output value is calculated as

$$h_i[u_i(t+1)] = g[u_i(t+1)] \exp\{-[ag[u_i(t)]_{t-T}]^2\} \qquad (16)$$

where a is a constant expressing the strength of adaptation, and T is the "last" time period.

The modulatory cholinergic effects can almost trivially be implemented within the framework of this model. The suppression of neuronal adaptation can be taken into account by decreasing the value of the adaptation parameter. The cholinergic suppression of synaptic transmission can be represented by decreasing the strength of the different synaptic transmissions: The synaptic strength of the intrinsic (but not the afferent) connections decreases, whereas both types of inhibitory synaptic transmission decrease.

Simulation studies (Wu and Liljenström 1994) showed that, depending on the values of the (control) parameter Q, the system may exhibit convergence to a fixed point, limit-cycle oscillation, or (at least transient) chaotic behavior.

The strengths of the synaptic connections also can drastically influence the dynamic behavior. If the fast feedback inhibitory synapses are the strongest, the system dominantly shows oscillatory behavior approximate 40 Hz. When the slow feedforward inhibitory synapses are the strongest, the model shows oscillatory behavior near the theta frequency. When both types of synapses are in the same range, oscillatory behavior with an intermediate frequency may occur. Because the oscillatory behavior depends strongly on the relative strength of the two types of inhibition, further studies should clarify the selective modulatory effects of the cholinergic agents on the individual inhibitory processes. Furthermore, the suppression of intrinsic fiber synaptic transmission appears to decrease the relative contribution of the 40-Hz component to that of the theta rhythm. (Cholinergic modulation may have an important functional role in learning and memory; see sec. 5.3.) The behavior of the model is close to experimental data obtained by electroencephalography (Bressler 1984) and evoked potentials (Bressler and Freeman 1980).

5.3 Development, Learning, and Memory in the Olfactory System

5.3.1 Plasticity, Learning, and Memory: A Few Examples

Behavioral studies (mostly on rats and rabbits) suggest that the developing olfactory system shows a remarkable plasticity (Hudson, Distel, and Zippel 1991, Leon, Wilson, and Guthrie, 1991). Three different kinds of plasticity in the developing olfactory bulb have been demonstrated. First, compensatory mechanisms respond to early odor deprivation. Second, partial damage of the olfactory bulb is compensated to preserve olfactory function. A possible mechanism for this plasticity is that new receptor neurons might innervate the bulb. Third, olfactory preference conditioning also may evoke neural plasticity. This preference learning begins in utero and continues postnatally to enable the neonate to become attracted by maternal odors.

It was shown (Brennan, Kaba, and Keverne 1990) that the female mouse has a simple olfactory memory system by which to recognize pheromones of the male with whom she mates. (The term *pheromone* denotes chemical signals produced by the animals themselves that generally cannot be replaced by initially neutral odors through learning.) This memory prevents pregnancy loss, whereas pheromones from strange male mice causes pregnancy block. Memory formation established during (and a few hours after) mating persists for the reproductive life of the female. The neural substrate involved in this memory system is the accessory olfactory bulb. The structure of the accessory olfactory bulb is similar to, but simpler than, that of the main olfactory bulb. It seems likely that memory formation is established by an activity-dependent synapse-modifying learning mechanism. Specifically, the reciprocal dendrodendritic mitral-granule synapses seem to be modifiable (Brennan and Keverne 1989; Trombley and Shepherd 1991).

5.3.2 Learning and Memory in the Olfactory Bulb

Synaptic Modification–Induced Transitions

Having determined different attractor regions in terms of lateral connection strengths (sec. 5.2.2), it now is natural to ask how synaptic modification can induce transitions between these regions. It is expected that slowly varying the synaptic strengths can result in dramatic and instantaneous changes of qualitative dynamic behavior. A learning process is materialized via synaptic modifications. Specifically, Skarda and Freeman (1987) have suggested that transitions between oscillatory and chaotic states may occur due to learning . It is assumed in the simulations presented here that only the lateral excitatory connections between mitral cells can be modified.

The set 2 of ODEs is supplemented with differential equations for the matrix elements L_{ij}. The increase of synaptic strengths can easily be formalized in the spirit of Hebb's (1949) rule:

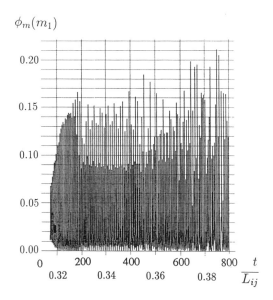

Figure 5.16
Synaptic modification induced bifurcation. Both the time scale and the corresponding values of the average lateral synaptic strength are indicated on the horizontal axis. Vertical axis represents output of an arbitrarily chosen mitral cell. The full learning process shows oscillation with increasing amplitude, then period doubling, and later the emergence of chaos. (Reprinted with permission from Érdi et al. 1993.)

$$\dot{L}_{ij}(t) = k \cdot \phi_m(m_i(t)) \cdot \phi_m(m_j(t)) \qquad (17)$$

where the constant k controls the rate of learning. The calculation is stopped before "explosion" (see figure 5.16) as chaotic activity can be obtained even at moderate value of L_{ij}. Hence, it is not necessary to supplement the rule 17 with other terms. Only nearest-neighbor connections are taken into account here (i.e., $j = i - 1$, or $j = i + 1$).

The randomly chosen vector elements I_i^{rec} (as in sec. 5.2.2) ensure that the values $m_i(t)$ are different for different is, and thus different matrix elements L_{ij} are modified differently.

The initial states $[L(0)]$ determine the attractor region where the learning process begins. To study a transition between two physiologically plausible attractors, from oscillation to chaos, region II in figure 5.6 was chosen as a starting point.

In the series of simulations we now present, $c = 1$ was chosen for convenience as L_{ij} now is the variable. Thus, the uniform initial values $L_{ij}(0) = 0.3$ for all neighbors i, j corresponded to the state $c = 0.3$ of the previous section, which was inside the periodic region II of figure 5.16. The value $k = 0.015$ of the learning rate was found to be sufficiently large to induce transition to region III within reasonable time and sufficiently small not to destroy the patterns obtained without learning. The values of all other parameters were set as given in the middle column of table 5.1.

Because the phase-space technique cannot be applied to temporally changing qualitative dynamics, the output of one mitral cell over time was directly plotted here, and the average inward synaptic strength, as an independent variable, also was monitored.

In the early phase of learning, the amplitude of the oscillation of the periodic region is increasing gradually. Later, transition to biperiodicity can be observed. After an intermediate multiperiodic stage, the emergence of chaos can be seen. Because of the low speed of learning, the process stopped when the average synaptic strength reached 0.4, which was inside the chaotic region.

The oscillations of all neurons remained synchronized even in the multiperiodic stage, and the transitions also occurred simultaneously, although the rate of synaptic modification was different from cell to cell owing to the randomly chosen input. This result shows that the inherent synchronous activity is a robust property of the model.

Associative Memory: Recognition of Incomplete Odor Patterns

The problem of associative memory is a particularly difficult issue in sensory systems wherein continuous interaction with the environment is explicitly taken into account. The task to be solved here is a special case of odor recognition with time-continuous input.

Our aim is to show that incomplete input patterns due to lower odor concentrations can also be identified as proper stimuli if a suitable learning rule is used to modify the lateral connections between mitral cells. A difficulty of this approach is the existence of very restrictive additional constraints for the periodic temporal patterns emerging when the odor input is present.

Let an odor pattern be denoted by the vector $P = \{P_1, P_2, \ldots, P_N\}$ with P_i being 0 or 1. The size of the pattern (i.e., the number of active cells in it) is taken as the squared length of the vector P. A vector p is called an *incomplete part* of the pattern P if $p_i < P_i$ for all i.

The odor input $I^{\text{odor}}(t)$ is given only to the active cells of the input pattern, whereas other cells receive only the constant background input I^{backgr}. $I^{\text{odor}}(t)$ follows the sniff cycle and carries a sequence $s = 1, 2, \ldots$ of different incomplete parts $p^{(s)}$ of the odor pattern P. One sniff cycle consists of a linear increase and an exponential, and the period for rabbits is approximately 400 milliseconds. Its form is adopted from Li and Hopfield (1989):

$$I_i^{\text{odor}}(t) = \begin{cases} p_i^{(s)} \cdot (t - t^{inh})/(t^{exh} - t^{inh}) & \text{if } t^{inh} \leqslant t < t^{exh} \\ p_i^{(s)} \cdot \exp\left(-\frac{1}{\tau}(t - t^{exh})\right) & \text{if } t \geqslant t^{exh} \end{cases}$$

(18)

where $p_i^{(s)}$ is 0 or 1, t^{inh} and t^{exh} are the onset times for inhalation and exhalation, respectively, and t is the exhalation time constant.

The lateral connection matrix L is fully interconnected here, but self-excitation is excluded (i.e., $L_{ij} > 0$ if $i \neq j$ and $L_{ii} = 0$ for all i). The learning rule consists of three terms. First, a second-order decay term controls the upper bound of the increase of connection strengths. A similar nonlinear forgetting term has been introduced by Riedel and Schild (1992). Second, a Hebbian term is responsible for the strengthening of connections between simultaneously firing cells. Finally, the third term is introduced to decrease selectively the synaptic strength between active and inactive cells:

$$\dot{L}_{ij}(t) = -k_1 \cdot L_{ij}^2(t) + k_2 \cdot \varphi_m(m_i(t)) \cdot \varphi_m(m_j(t)) - k_3 \cdot L_{ij}(t)$$
$$\cdot [\varphi_m(m_i(t)) - \varphi_m(m_j(t))]^2$$

(19)

where k_1, k_2, and k_3 are positive constants. This learning rule is local (i.e., the change of a synaptic weight depends only on its value and the activity of the pre- and postsynaptic neurons). The learning task is to modify the initially randomly distributed synaptic weights so that the incomplete input patterns $p^{(s)}$ evoke the mitral response characteristic of the odor pattern P.

The initial values $L_{ij}(0)$ of the synaptic strengths were taken from the gaussian distribution $\mathcal{N}(0.12, 0.06)$. The values of the learning constants are given in the last column of table 5.1. The time was scaled so that with $T = 400$ msec the average spike frequency was 40–60 Hz. During learning, the different incomplete parts of the same odor pattern were presented randomly. The specifically constructed learning rule with proper parameter values ensured the separation of synaptic weights without violating their boundedness and sign-preserving property. The decreasing connection strengths converged to zero, whereas the increasing ones remained between 0.15 and 0.25 in the long run, so that there was no need to "switch off" the learning process.

Figure 5.17 shows the outputs of the 11 mitral cells during one sniff cycle before learning (a) and after 60 cycles of learning (b). Before learning (figure 5.17a), only the four cells receiving the incomplete input pattern produced relevant but still very low output because the weak lateral connections did not transmit their low activities to the other cells. In contrast, figure 5.17b shows

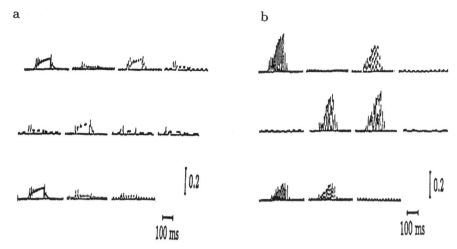

a　　　　　　　　　　b

Figure 5.17

Outputs of the $N = 11$ mitral cells before (a) and after (b) learning. The incomplete patterns {i.e., those that contain four 1s [(1 0 1 0 0 1 0 0 1 0 0) and (1 0 1 0 0 1 1 0 0 0 0), respectively} were presented as input.

The complete odor pattern, which contains six 1s, was (1 0 1 0 0 1 1 0 1 1 0).

that all six cells belonging to the complete odor pattern exhibited large-amplitude, high-frequency firing bursts, although only four of them received the odor input. The oscillations of different cells were synchronized, with a frequency of approximately 60 Hz. It can be concluded that the learning rule 17 leads to the recognition of incomplete odor patterns, preserving physiologically justified oscillatory burst activities (see Li and Hopfield 1989) at the same time.

5.3.3　Learning and Memory in the Olfactory Cortex

Behavioral studies also suggest that rats exhibit very rapid learning and retain learning during olfactory discrimination tasks. (Here, *very rapid* means approximately five trials, and the duration of retention may be more than 1 year; Slotnick and Katz 1974; Staubli et al. 1987). It seems likely that olfactory learning behavior has a physiological correlate—namely, synchronized, slow oscillation approximately 5 Hz. On the basis of the finding that this rhythm may be optimal for inducing LTP in olfactory cortex as well as in hippocampus (Larson and Lynch 1986; see also Roman, Staubli, and Lynch 1987), it was strongly suggested (Otto et al. 1991; see also Gluck and Granger 1993) that there is a dependence among synchronized rhythmical activity, behavioral learning, and synaptic plasticity. (LTP is a possible correlate of hebbian learning; see sec. 6.3 for details.) The computational model (Ambros-Ingerson Granger, and Lynch 1990) within this framework (what we call the *Granger-Lynch scenario*; see Granger, Ambros-Ingerson, and

Lynch 1989; Granger et al. 1991) describes a hierarchical clustering of input stimuli based on the assumptions that (1) olfactory bulb projections into olfactory cortex are sparse; (2) olfactory cortex projects back into the inhibitory cells of the olfactory bulb, via the AON; and (3) the afferent connections are modifiable by a competitive learning rule leading to winner-take-all (WTA; see sec. 4.5.1) interactions.

On the basis of these assumptions, a combined olfactory bulb–olfactory cortex model was established. Briefly, feedforward bulbar inputs are processed by the cortex, the cortical feedback to bulb inhibits a portion of the input, the feedforward remainder from bulb then is processed by the cortex, and the process iterates, successively removing portions of the input and then processing them.

There is an alternative view (what we call the *Haberly-Bower-Hasselmo scenario*) of the structural basis, physiological mechanisms, and computational algorithms of information processing in the olfactory cortex. Emphasizing the remarkable similarities between the architectures and operation of anatomical and formal networks, several investigators suggested (Haberly 1985; Haberly and Bower 1989; Bower 1991; Hasselmo and Bower 1992) that the mechanism of object recognition in the olfactory cortex is close to those offered by abstract associative memory models (reviewed earlier in secs. 4.5.2 and 4.5.3). According to this line of argument, the olfactory cortex is appropriate for implementing an associative memory system, because (1) the incoming (bulbar) information has a complex, distributed representation;

(2) the afferent projections from the olfactory bulb are extensive and diffuse; and (3) the intrinsic excitatory connections between pyramidal cells are spatially extensive, overlapping, and modifiable.

The Granger-Lynch Scenario

As we shall now show, simulations of the olfactory cortex reciprocally connected to the olfactory bulb within the framework of the Granger-Lynch scenario showed hierarchical clustering of the learned odor cues. According to the calculations, distinct output responses are generated to individual stimuli to encode different levels of information about a stimulus. The repetitive sampling and the modifiability of the afferent fibers via LTP (see sec. 6.3 for details of long-term potentiation) are the key features of the mechanism posited to connect synaptic plasticity to behavioral learning.

An important structural assumption is that pyramidal cells are innervated randomly and sparsely by the axons of the LOT. Many fewer inhibitory than excitatory cells are assumed, and the former have a short arborization radius. It is assumed that each inhibitory interneuron affects a "patch" within the radius of reach of its axon terminals. In the simulations, pyramidal cells were arranged in patches containing one inhibitory cell and approximately 8–12 pyramidal cells. Adjacent patches overlap, typically by two to three pyramidal cells.

There are two physiological forms of input activity from the LOT: single pulses with a 40-Hz frequency and a series of short, high-frequency (100-Hz) bursts occurring at 5 Hz. Neurons receiving the most input activation would be the first to reach spiking threshold. (In the simulation experiments, this threshold was set to 0.5 mV, whereas each active input line transmits 0.1 mV.) Specifically, those postsynaptic cells have the highest probability of becoming active that get the most connections from the input lines activated by the particular input cue. Similar inputs will select similar patterns of output cells. This similarity is, however, not sufficient to perform input clustering. "Difference making" also is necessary (i.e., similar input should select similar, but not identical, output patterns). To complete the similarity-based cluster formation, a competitive, "winner-take-all" learning algorithm was incorporated.

Before discussing the learning rule applied, we remark that the model operates in two distinct modes: learning mode and nonlearning (performance) mode, each characterized by the frequency of the rhythmic input patterns. When receiving input of approximately 40 Hz, the network is sampling stimuli but not learning; when the in-

put is around the theta rhythm, the network is learning. Correlation between olfactory learning and the theta algorithm has indeed been found (Kumisaruk 1970; Macrides 1975; Macrides et al. 1987) and, on the basis of these findings, it was suggested (Pavlides et al. 1980; Larson and Lynch 1986) that theta is optimal for inducing LTP in the olfactory cortex and even in the hippocampus (see chap. 6; Otto et al. 1991).

An algorithm is given to update the $P \times N$ connectivity matrix W, where P is the number of cells in the network patch and N is the number of input lines. The network is trained on a sequence of input binary vectors $A^1, A^2, \ldots$ The updating rule is as follows:

$$W_{ij}^{t+1} = \begin{cases} \min\{W_{ij}^t + \varepsilon, w_2\} & \text{if the conditions i, ii,} \\ & \text{and iii are fulfilled} \\ W_{ij}^t & \text{otherwise} \end{cases} \quad (20)$$

Let $\hat{W}$ be a binary matrix indicating the location of synapses in the initial connectivity matrix W^0, whose elements are either 0 or w_1—that is,

$$\hat{W}_{ij} := \begin{cases} 1, & \text{if } W_{ij}^0 \neq 0 \\ 0 & \text{otherwise} \end{cases} \quad (21)$$

and $\hat{W}_{(i)}$ is the ith column of $\hat{W}$, $L > 0$ is the minimal number of active synapses needed for a "winner" cell to potentiate, $\varepsilon > 0$ is the incremental change in the synaptic weight, w_2 is the saturation value of the synaptic weight, and * denotes the inner product. The conditions are

1. $\hat{W}_{(i)} * A^t \geqslant \hat{W}_{(k)} * A^t$ for $0 < k \leqslant P$,

2. $\hat{W}_{(i)} * A^t \geqslant L$ and   (22)

3. $\hat{W}_{ij} A_i^t \neq 0$ otherwise.

It can be seen that (1) synapses with strength 0 do not change; (2) synaptic strengths cannot be decreased; and (3) synaptic modification occurs when both presynaptic and postsynaptic cells are active, the presynaptic cell receives sufficient activation to exceed the learning threshold, the synaptic strength is lower than a prefixed maximal value, the input vector is novel, and each novel input vector in a category is relatively distinct from the others. Increase in the synaptic strength occurs if and only if burst inputs arrive at theta rhythm; during the first burst, those neurons that receive the strongest input are activated, and these inhibit the excitatory neurons, which receive less input. Then the active neurons become refractory, and neurons slightly less activated become active. Excitatory cells are activated in subsequent stages, and the summed activation can exceed the learning threshold to simulate the behavior of the voltage-dependent N-methyl-D-aspartate channels associated with LTP.

Simulation experiments reinforce the hypothesis that each patch of cortical cells constitutes a subspace into which the input is decomposed and that the sequence of outputs (over several sniffs) produces a hierarchical decomposition of the input. The first "sniff" corresponds to a broad class of the input stimulus; later sniffs correspond to the subdivision of these broad categories. An important prediction of the model has been tested and verified experimentally (Granger et al. 1991): Rats spontaneously encoded and used similarity-based categories.

The Haberly-Bower-Hasselmo Scenario

The associative memory function of olfactory cortex has also been studied with a family of models by combining bottom-up techniques based on anatomical and physiological data and abstract computational algorithms of associative memory. The associative memory character of the olfactory cortex was simulated by Wilson and Bower (1988). In a specific model, even the cholinergic modulation of cortical associative memory function was taken into account (Hasselmo, Anderson, and Bower 1992; Barkai et al. 1994; Barkai and Hasselmo 1994). Oscillatory activity, however, does not appear in this model.

The most important structural elements of the model are the pyramidal cells, which form a tightly packed layer with their cell bodies in layer II. These cells are represented by a one-dimensional array of n units, and their state is characterized by the (continuous) membrane potential vector $a = (a_1, a_2, \ldots a_n)$. The resting membrane potential of a cell is represented by $a_i = 0$; $a_i > 0$ expresses depolarization, and $a_i < 0$ represents hyperpolarization. The output of a neuron (i.e., the number of action potentials fired by each pyramidal cell per unit time) is determined by the g output function:

$$g[a_i - \mu] = \tanh[a_i - \mu]$$

with threshold μ.

The (broadly distributed, excitatory) bulbar input arriving along the LOT and synapsing on the distal dendrites of the pyramidal cells in layer Ia is represented by the binary vector $A = (A_1, A_2, \ldots, A_n)$. Different odors are represented by different A^j vectors.

The effect of the (broadly distributed, excitatory) intrinsic connections on the activation level of each neuron i has been taken into account through the synaptic connectivity matrix B_{ij}. Local inhibitory effects have been represented by the connectivity matrix H_{ij}. The local

character is modeled by setting the off-diagonal elements to zero out to a particular radius.

The cholinergic suppression of intrinsic-fiber synaptic transmission is modeled by homogeneously reducing the connectivity matrix **B**. A multiplier constant $0 \leqslant c_{sup} \leqslant 1$ describes the suppression. Another cholinergic effect is the postsynaptic increase in excitability of pyramidal cells. This effect is represented by shifting the threshold of the output function to lower values by a parameter $0 \leqslant c_{exc} \leqslant 1$.

By combining all these effects, the (discrete time) activity dynamics is given according to the equation

$$a_i(t+1) = A_i + \sum_{j=1}^{n} (c_{sup}) B_{ij} g[a_j(t) - c_{exc}\mu]$$
$$- \sum_{j=1}^{n} H_{ij} g[a_j(t) - c_{exc}\mu]. \qquad (23)$$

It is assumed that only the intrinsic excitatory connections (i.e., the elements of the **B** matrix) are modifiable. The model operates in a learning and a recall stage. In the learning stage, the network is trained by a set of input patterns A^j. An input pattern contains six active elements ($A_i = 1$). A training period consists of two cycles. After synchronous modification of the activity values, the B_{ij} connectivities are modified. To limit the strength of the connections, a sigmoid-type function was applied to the hebbian-type modification. The latter depends on the presynaptic output and the presynaptic activation reduced by a threshold

$$\Delta W_{ij} = zg[a_j(t) - c_{exc}\mu][a_i(t) - \phi]. \qquad (24)$$

Here z is a learning constant and ϕ is a threshold, and

$$\Delta B_{ij} = \psi(1 - \exp - (\Delta W_{ij})). \qquad (25)$$

This function exhibits saturation at ψ.

Learning was interrupted at regular intervals, and the network was tested by degraded versions of the input patterns. During this recall stage, the cholinergic modulation was not taken into account, and the synaptic connectivities were fixed.

The model is capable of storing a single input pattern and recalling it even from its degraded form. There is a possibility for storing nonoverlapping patterns. The storage of overlapping inputs can be improved by cholinergic suppression of intrinsic fibers. The best memory performance was obtained when this suppression was combined with the increase in cell excitability.

It has also been suggested (Hasselmo 1994) that the exponential ("runaway") increase of synaptic modification may be at the root of the initiation and progression of cortical neuronal degeneration found in Alzheimer's disease. Suppression of synaptic transmission during learning works against the strengthening of undesired connections.

5.3.4 Conclusion

In conclusion, we quote Shepherd (1991):

Computational models such as these are component-based, and thus have the merit of generating network properties that reflect real neural architectures... When combined with computational models of earlier stages in the olfactory pathway, they will permit simulation of the entire sequence of processing of molecular information from the olfactory molecule to its cortical representation. The olfactory pathway is thus a prime target for simulation by a new generation of more realistic neural networks. This will contribute toward a definitive understanding of the nature of olfactory processing. It should also lead to the development of devices, with practical applications in many fields of scientific and industrial interest, for detecting, discrimination, analysis, and representation of molecular information.

Hippocampus

The hippocampus has been studied on different levels and by different methods. This chapter comprises a study of the following:

1. The anatomical organization of the hippocampus, including its afferent and efferent systems and the local circuitry of its components (sec. 6.1)

2. The electrical activity patterns related to global brain states (sec. 6.2)

3. The cellular synaptic plasticity that occurs during long-term potentiation (sec. 6.3)

4. The role of the hippocampus in rats learning a spatial environment (sec. 6.4)

5. The function of hippocampus in human memory (sec. 6.5)

The hippocampus is an excellent candidate for unifying functional, dynamic, and structural aspects of the brain. Our challenge is to provide a coherent view of the structure and function of the hippocampus by integrating anatomical, physiological, and behavioral data. Though to a great extent we will review these different aspects in separate sections, this chapter will exemplify the book as a whole, both for the integration we achieve and for the many problems that remain open for future research.

Section 6.1 provides the structural view of the hippocampus, and we treat the intrinsic organization of its cells and circuits (sec. 6.1.1), its afferents and efferents (both cortical and subcortical, sec. 6.1.2), and basic quantitative data on cell numbers and on the convergence and divergence of connections (sec. 6.1.3). Section 6.2 then builds on this structural analysis to provide a dynamical analysis of electrical activity patterns, addressing data (reviewed in secs. 6.2.1–6.2.3) pertaining to the normal electrical activity patterns known as *theta rhythms* and *sharp waves* and to the abnormal electrical activity exhibited in epileptic seizures. In section 6.2.4, we present multicompartmental neuron models of pyramidal cells and interneurons as a basis for a large model of the CA3 network, which allows us to see how variations in key parameters can switch the network between normal and epileptiform activity. Section 6.2.5 is a comparison of the hippocampus with the olfactory system, with special attention paid to the neural mechanisms of rhythm generation and synchronization.

Section 6.3 contains a look at one of the best-studied forms of dynamics at the synaptic level: long-term potentiation (LTP), showing its implication in experimental studies of hebbian synaptic modification (sec. 6.3.1) and analyzing models of potentiation based on alpha-methyl proprionic acids (AMPA) and N-methyl-D-aspartate (NMDA) receptors. Section 6.3.3 forms a link back to dynamics at the activity level by studying the role of NMDA receptors in the generation of oscillations at the cellular level. Section 6.3.4 is a return to the hebbian theme wherein we discuss the need for long-term depression (LTD) in hebbian synapses; this leads into the discussion (sec. 6.3.5) of the relation of LTP and LTD to the learning rules of the various brain regions that we will study in later chapters.

Section 6.4 combines a functional view of the hippocampus—its role in the cognitive maps underlying navigation and spatial behavior in rats—with a dynamical view of synaptic plasticity. We show how hebbianlike plasticity (of the kind studied in section 6.3) may enable hippocampal cells to learn to encode different "places" in a cognitive map. Sections 6.4.1–6.4.3 provide a general framework for the study of spatial representation and cognitive maps in rats, including the general idea of world graphs as cognitive maps for motivated behavior. Section 6.4.4 presents a review of the neurophysiology of spatial representation, with special emphasis on the "place cells" of the regions CA3 and CA1 of hippocampus. In section 6.4.5, we offer two contrasting systems views of the role of the hippocampus in navigation, in each case emphasizing that the representation of current place in CA3 and CA1 is insufficient for a cognitive map underlying navigation. Sections 6.4.6 and 6.4.7 contain reviews of various neural network models of place cell training, allocentric location, and navigation. In one of the models, we pay special attention to data that relate place cell activity to the theta rhythm studied in section 6.2.

Section 6.5 encompasses the role of hippocampal function in human memory, with an introduction in section 6.5.1 of the crucial dichotomies of procedural versus declarative memory and of skill versus episodic learning. The data suggest that the hippocampus is involved in declarative rather than in procedural memory and in episodic rather than skill learning; section 6.5.2 presents a look at data suggesting that hippocampus may form but not store memories. Section 6.5.3 contains an examination of the role of orbitofrontal cortex, amygdala, hippo-

campus, and lateral septum in motivational processes and contains major new data on longitudinal organization in the hippocampus. We close the chapter in section 6.5.4 with comparisons of hippocampal function in humans and rats, seeking to address the challenging and very much open question: Is there a commonality of process and mechanism in the two main functions attributed to the hippocampus, cognitive mapping in rats and declarative memory in humans?

6.1 Anatomical Organization

Most of us are guilty of it. Hippocampologists have preached for decades that the hippocampus is a relatively simple structure and thus an ideal region for studying the relationship between structure and function. And it is! But one potentially misleading implication of the "hippocampus is simple" message is that the anatomical organization of the structure is thoroughly understood. It is certainly true that the basic organizational scheme of hippocampal anatomy has been well established through the classical Golgi studies of Ramón y Cajal (1893), and Lorente de Nó (1934), and the more recent experimental studies such as those conducted for the last 40 years by Blackstad and his colleagues (e.g., Blackstad 1956). However, as the computational modelers and physiologists ask the anatomists for detailed information concerning the network characteristics of the hippocampal formation, it becomes painfully apparent that there are still gaping holes in our understanding of hippocampal circuitry, even at a descriptive level. And when quantitative questions are raised concerning hippocampal neurons or circuitry, these are more often met with shrugs than with answers . . . (Amaral et al. 1990).

The hippocampal formation is a cortical structure located in the temporal lobe. It is called *archicortex* for its evolutionary precedence over neocortex and is relatively simple compared to neocortical structures. It has an elongated C-shaped form and looks like a tube oriented perpendicular to the corpus callosum. A slice orthogonal to the longitudinal axis reveals the basic neural connectivity (figure 6.1). Some of the excitatory connections between hippocampal subfields are restricted highly in the longitudinal axis, giving rise to the notion of a predominantly transverse or "lamellar" organization of hippocampal circuitry, but extensive longitudinal excitatory connections exist, and the intrinsic inhibitory circuits also have considerable longitudinal spread. Strangely enough, prior to 1996 there were virtually no data on variation in lamellar specificity as position changed along the longitudinal axis. This changed dramatically with the

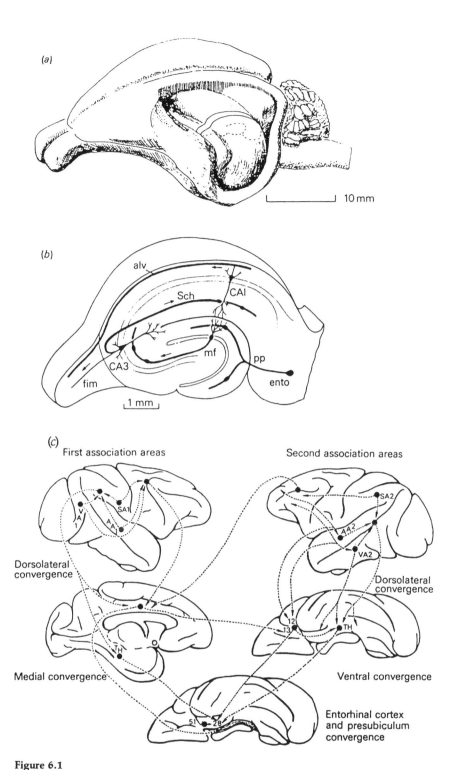

Figure 6.1
(a) Lateral view of the rabbit brain with the parietal and temporal neocortex removed to expose the hippocampal formation. The hippocampus has an elongated C-shaped form; a slice orthogonal to the longitudinal axis reveals the basic neural connectivity. (b) A lamellar slice showing the basic circuitry of hippocampus. alv, alveus; ento, entorhinal cortex; fim, fimbria; mf, mossy fiber; pp, perforant path; Sch, Schaffer collateral. (From Andersen et al. 1971). (c) Convergence of afferent information onto the entorhinal cortex from primary (SA$_1$, AA$_1$, VA$_1$) and secondary (SA$_2$, AA$_2$, VA$_2$) association areas of the neocortex in the monkey. (Reprinted with permission from G. W. Van Hoesen, D. N. Pandya, and N. Butters, Cortical efferents to the entorhinal cortex of the rhesus monkey. *Science* 1972; 175:1471–1473.)

work of Risold and Swanson (1996). We examine their findings in section 6.5.3.

Hippocampal slice preparations (which contain nearly 20,000 cells for the longitudinal CA3 slices used in most experiments) preserve many important properties of the in vivo circuitry; therefore, many physiological properties of hippocampal neurons are expressed in the slice. Furthermore, slices can be the subject of pharmacological treatment by the application of drugs that block specific receptors or ion channels, and the ionic milieu of the bathing medium also can be altered. As a result, slice preparations can be used to study the biophysics and pharmacology of synaptic effects, but because some of the axons and dendrites are transected in vitro (Gulyás et al. 1993; Li et al. 1994), the intact brain seems more advantageous for investigating the emergent properties of large networks.

Structurally, the hippocampus is the simplest form of cortex, but this simplicity is in stark contrast with its role in processing information from the external world through the sensory systems and from the "internal world" conveyed by subcortical inputs (Buzsáki et al. 1994). Whereas primary visual cortex, for example, is specialized for processing a single modality, functionally the hippocampus is one of the most complex supramodal association areas, containing many routes to many cortical areas. Polymodal association areas converge directly or indirectly on the entorhinal cortex, which in turn forms the principal source of afferents to hippocampus. The hippocampus receives refined information from virtually all sensory modalities, both exteroceptive and interoceptive, via entorhinal cortex (Amaral 1987; Swanson, Köhler, and Björklund 1987). It is thought to prepare information for long-term storage elsewhere in cortex, with the return projections from hippocampus possibly providing cells in polymodal cortex with a "condensed sketch" of the overall context in which their unimodal input occurred (McNaughton 1989). The hippocampus has an important role in learning and memory processes. Alzheimer's disease, epilepsy, and the ischemia associated with learning and memory impairment are accompanied by selective neuronal death or characteristic changes in hippocampal circuitry.

6.1.1 Intrinsic Organization of the Hippocampus

The hippocampus is a part of the hippocampal formation, which includes the dentate gyrus (DG), the hippocampus proper [called Ammons' horn—cornu Ammonis, CA)—after Ammon, the Egyptian god with the head of a ram], the subicular complex, and the entorhinal cortex. The term *hippocampus* is used to designate the DG and the hippocampus proper (figure 2.18, after Ramón y Cajal). According to Lorente de Nó (1934), the hippocampus proper contains the CA1–CA4 regions, but CA4 now is not considered as a separate region, and the boundaries of the small transitional field CA2 also are not clear. Thus, we usually refer to hippocampus as comprising DG, CA1, and CA3. At least 90% of all extrinsic afferents of the hippocampus are provided by the perforant path, which comprises the projection of entorhinal cortex (ENT) to hippocampus.

Though the hippocampus has only one layer (compared to the six layers of the neocortex), both the dentate gyrus and the hippocampus proper contain sublayers (strata).

The dentate gyrus contains (1) an outermost sublayer called *stratum moleculare*, wherein the dendrites of its principal cells—the granule cells—arborize, (2) the stratum granulosum, where the granule cell bodies are located, and (3) the polymorphic sublayer (also called the *hilus*) in which the polymorphic cells are located.

The innermost sublayer of the hippocampus proper (CA regions) is the stratum lacunosum-moleculare, followed by the stratum radiatum, stratum pyramidale (in which the cell bodies of the pyramidal cells are located), and the stratum oriens. Furthermore, CA3 contains the stratum lucidum, in which the main afferents from the dentate gyrus (i.e., the mossy fibers) terminate.

Principal Cells

The principal cells of the dentate gyrus, the granule cells, generally do not have basal dendrites but have only spiny apical dendrites. Their axons form the mossy fibers, which pass through the hilus (the area contained within the C formed by DG) before terminating on the dendrites of the CA3 pyramidal cells. The granule-cell axons are considered to form excitatory synapses; the most likely neurotransmitter is glutamate. The hilus itself contains polymorphic cells (i.e., cells of varied morphology).

The principal cells of the hippocampus proper, the pyramidal cells, have thick apical dendrites extending through the stratum radiatum up to the stratum lacunosum-moleculare and have shorter and thinner basal dendrites that arborize in the stratum oriens. The thick, myelinated main axons of the CA3 pyramidal cells arising from the soma and terminating in the stratum radiatum and oriens of the CA1 region are the Schaffer collaterals. Furthermore, CA3 pyramidal cells have recurrent collaterals terminating in the CA3 region itself. Axons of the CA1 pyramidal cells are thin and provide part of the hippocampal output, projecting mostly to subiculum and sometimes straight to the entorhinal cortex. Both CA3 and CA1 pyramidal cells also have collaterals that descend to the septal area via the fimbria. For most pyramidal neurons, glutamate is the (excitatory) neurotransmitter, which binds to (at least) three different receptor subtypes: metabotropic, AMPA, and NMDA. Recently, metabotropic excitatory amino acid receptors also have been taken into account (Miller 1991). (The interactions among these receptors play a major role in memory formation; see sec. 6.3.)

Nonprincipal Cells

Nonprincipal cells have relatively short axons, and therefore are generally (but not exclusively) considered as local interneurons—although interneurons with extensive axonal arborization have also been demonstrated (e.g., Buchmaster and Schwartzkroin 1995). In later sections, we will rely only on the most basic properties of inhibitory neurons in our modeling, but we here note that the classification of nonprincipal cells based on their morphology, chemical content, and electrophysiological properties has been the subject of intensive study in recent years (e.g., Gulyás et al. 1991, 1992; Katsumaru 1988; Kosaka et al. 1987; Miettinen et al. 1992; Nunzi et al. 1985; Ribak et al. 1990; Tóth and Freund 1992; Buhl et al. 1994; Sik et al. 1995; Turner et al. 1995).

Morphological Characterization Three main cell types can be discriminated morphologically on the basis of their specific target. Both in the hippocampus proper and in the dentate gyrus, the most studied interneurons are the basket cells, terminating on the soma and proximal dendrites of the principal cells (Gulyás et al. 1993a). Axo-axonic cells, found first in the cerebral cortex and called *chandelier cells* (see sec. 8.1), making contacts exclusively on the axon initial segments of the principal cells, occur in different regions of the hippocampus (Somogyi et al. 1983b). A third, rather heterogeneous group of cells makes synapses in the distal regions of the principal cells. The search for newer cell types is an unfinished project. For example, very recently three additional types of interneurons were revealed in the dentate gyrus (Han et al. 1993; Halasy and Somogyi 1993a,b). Hilar cells with axon associated with the commissural association pathway (HICAP cells), hilar cells with axon associated with the perforant pathway (HIPP cells), and molecular layer cells with axon associated with the perforant pathway (MOPP cells) were found, and their local inhibitory characters were also established.

Neurochemical Characterization Nonpyramidal cells can be classified neurochemically, based on their content of different neuroactive substances, such as neurotransmit-

ters, calcium-binding proteins and neuropeptides. Most of the interneurons contain γ-aminobutyric acid (GABA) as the neurotransmitter. The most important non-GABAergic nonpyramidal cells were thought to be the mossy cells (Amaral 1978; Ribak et al. 1985) located in the polymorphic sublayer of the dentate gyrus. Current debates (Li et al. 1994) suggest, however, that at least some of them may be interpreted as modified CA3 pyramidal cells.

Three types of calcium-binding proteins—parvalbumin (PV), calbindin D28k (CaBP) and calretinin (CR)—and a few types of neuropeptides, such as somatostatin (SOM), neuropeptide Y (NPY), vasoactive intestinal polypeptide (VIP), cholecystokinin (CCK), and enkephalin have been identified in nonprincipal cells. Some important relationships have been found between morphological and neurochemical characterizations. PV cells correspond to basket and chandelier cells (Kosaka et al. 1987; Katsumaru et al. 1988), whereas cells that make synapses on the distal dendrites of pyramidal cells contain CaBP or SOM (Gulyás et al. 1991; Seress et al. 1991). The subpopulations containing PV, CaBP, and CCK are nonoverlapping. CR cells have two classes. The spiny CR cells can be found in the regions innervated by the mossy fibers and get synaptic inputs almost entirely from granule cells. CR cells with smooth dendrites are located uniformly in the hippocampus, and their axons arborize in the dendritic region of the principal cells. For the numerical distribution of these neurochemically characterized neurons, see figure 6.2 (Gulyás 1993). Though the functional consequences of the discriminability of interneurons on the basis of their neurochemical characterization has not yet been clearly clarified, some results are mentioned after the discussion of electophysiological characterization and of the circuitry, although they lie beyond the scope of current modeling.

Electrophysiological Characterization There is no clear picture at present of the different mechanisms of inhibition. Inhibitory mechanisms were thought to be classified either as feedback and feedforward or as $GABA_A$ or $GABA_B$ receptor–mediated inhibition (Alger and Nicoll 1982). Feedback inhibition occurs when the recurrent collaterals of the principal cells activate interneurons that inhibit principal cells in the same subregion. If the local inhibitory cells are driven by afferents originating outside the subfields, they implement feedforward inhibition (Buzsáki 1984). $GABA_A$ receptors mediate a chloride-dependent fast inhibitory postsynaptic potential (IPSP), whereas a potassium-dependent slow IPSP is mediated by $GABA_B$ receptors. The hippocampal basket and chandelier cells (which, as was mentioned, contain PV and

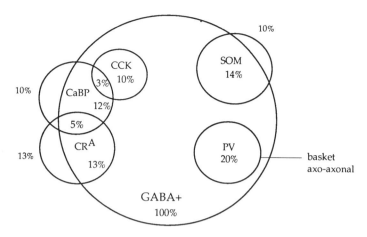

Figure 6.2
Numerical distribution of these neurochemically characterized inter-neurons. CCK, cholecystokinin; CaBP, calbindin D28k; CR, calretinin; SOM, somatostatin; PV, parvalbumin. (Based on Gulyás 1993.)

establish perisomatic inhibition) mediate their effect through GABA$_A$ receptors and participate both in feed-back and feedforward inhibition. Earlier, it was specu-lated that the inhibitory cells, which mediate their effects by GABA$_B$ receptors and establish dendritic inhibition, are neurochemically heterogeneous and take part mostly in feedforward inhibition. GABA release from basket and axo-axonic cells seems to be modulated by presynaptic GABA$_B$ receptors, and the postsynaptic effect is medi-ated by GABA$_A$ receptors (Buhl et al. 1994). The debate on the mediation of slow IPSP is not ended. It was sug-gested that postsynaptic GABA$_B$ receptors mediate the slow IPSP through the activation of a G-protein-coupled potassium conductance (e.g., Newberry and Nicholl 1985; Andrade, Malenka, and Nicholl 1986; Pitler and Alger 1994; Sodickson and Bean 1996). However, both fast, perisomatic IPSPs and even slow, dendritic IPSPs can be mediated by GABA$_A$ receptors, because both GABA$_A$ responses have been found (Pearce 1993), at least in the CA1 region.

Figure 6.3 is a schematic drawing of the innervation of different regions of a pyramidal cell (distal dendrites, soma, and axon initial segment) by different nonprincipal cells containing different substances. The characteristics of the established types of inhibition also are illustrated (based on Gulyás 1993).

Functional Differences Fine division of labor among in-hibitory neurons, even within a small family, has been found (Buhl et al. 1994). Basket and axo-axonic cells containing PV, as well as bistratified cells, elicit GABA$_A$-mediated, short-latency IPSPs, but they have different kinetic characteristic and synapse on different domains of the postsynaptic target. The anatomical segregation of

the release sites and differences in the time course of in-hibition may have specific functional consequences. Due to their divergence, basket cells may play a role in the synchronization of principal cells (see Nicoll 1994). Bi-stratified cells may provide a pathway-specific control of excitatory inputs, because their GABAergic axon is co-aligned with the glutamatergic Schaffer collateral input to the dendrites of CA1 pyramidal cells, so that dendritic inhibition may reduce the EPSPs.

Circuits

To understand the internal organization of the hippo-campal circuitry, we start from the idealized picture of the three main subregions—the DG, the CA3, and the CA1 fields—as quasi-independent structural units con-nected by excitatory synapses. The mossy fibers (axons of the granule cells of DG) project to the proximal part of the CA3 pyramidal cell dendrites, and the Schaffer collaterals (axon collaterals of the CA3 pyramidal cells) innervate the apical and basal dendrites of the CA1 py-ramidal cells.

For each of these units, the interactions among prin-cipal cells and different local interneuron populations (especially the feedback and feedforward character of the inhibition) must be clarified and are the subject of ex-tensive current investigations. Mossy fibers of granule cells of DG innervate CA3 and the "polymorphic" cells of the hilus. Polymorphic neurons project bilaterally to the granule cells.

CA3 pyramidal cells have extensive recurrent col-laterals that make synapses with other pyramidal cells and with CA3 inhibitory neurons (Gulyás et al. 1993; Sík et al. 1993). Some collaterals leave the hippocampus an-

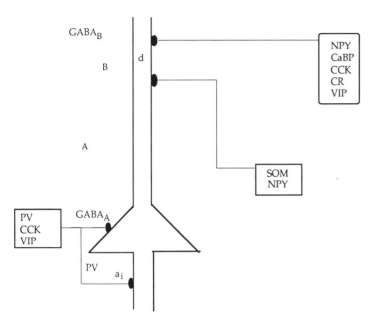

Figure 6.3

A schematic drawing of the innervation of different regions of a pyramidal cell by different nonprincipal cells containing different substances. The characters of the inhibition established also are illustrated. *d*, distal dendrites; *a_i*, axon initial segment; PV, parvalbumin; NPY, neu-

ropeptide Y; CaBP, calbindin D28k; CCK, cholecystokinin; CR, calretinin; VIP, vasoactive intestinal polypeptide; SOM, somatostatin. (Based on Gulyás 1993.)

teriorly to innervate the lateral septum and basal forebrain. Others ramify extensively within CA3 to form a dense commissural-associational plexus that extends into CA1. These Schaffer collaterals provide the only hippocampal input to the pyramidal cells of CA1. Recently, it was also found (Li et al. 1994) that CA3 pyramidal cells send some projections back to the hilus and also onto granule cells of DG. CA1 does not possess a commissural-associational plexus of its own but seems dominated by CA3. The majority of axons of CA1 pyramidal cells terminate in the subiculum and deep layers of ENT, linking CA3 with the retrohippocampal cortex (Swanson et al. 1981). CA1 also sends a small projection anteriorly into the lateral septum and basal forebrain. Recent studies (Han et al. 1993; Halasy and Somogyi 1993a,b) suggest that in the DG, the granule cells are spatially and selectively innervated by at least five distinct types of dentate neurons. It seems to be most likely (Somogyi 1991) that, in cortical structures generally, local interneurons may be highly selective for their postysynaptic targets, or at least for the laminae in which they form synapses.

6.1.2 Hippocampal Afferents and Efferents

Cortical Connections

The ENT hippocampus-ENT loop It is well established that the major input (the perforant path) to the hippo-

campus arises from layer II of ENT. The ENT itself is considered as a relay for information coming from multimodal association areas in the temporal, prefrontal, cingulate, and insular regions. It seems likely that olfactory information is relayed through the lateral ENT, whereas the medial ENT conveys visual information. The former terminates in the outer third of the molecular layer, the postsynaptic targets being the distal dendritic field of the granule cells. The latter terminates on the middle third of the molecular layer.

One important output field of the hippocampus is the subiculum; other projections exist to the presubiculum, parasubiculum, and the ENT. The subicular efferents to the deep layers of the ENT close the multisynaptic ENT-hippocampus-ENT loop. Subiculum also generates a massive projection that travels in the fornix to the anterior thalamic nuclei and the mammilary bodies lying at the posterior edge of the hypothalamus (Swanson and Cowan, 1975, 1977). Deep layers of ENT are innervated by the hippocampus and project to neocortex, especially to zones neighboring ENT and to the medial frontal areas (Swanson and Kohler 1986).

In the classic scenario (Andersen, Bliss, and Strede 1971), the excitatory connections in the hippocampus are organized in transverse lamellae, with DG, CA3, and CA1 arranged in series. At least two major classes of observations modified the scenario. First, the DG and also the CA3 and CA1 regions are innervated by fibers originating in the ENT (Steward 1976; Witter et al. 1988). Yeckel and Berger (1990) showed physiologically that ENT is the source of a powerful excitatory input to the pyramidal cells of CA1 and CA3. Second, the intra-hippocampal pathways generally cannot be considered topographic projections, because the perforant path shows convergence, whereas the Schaffer collaterals and the fibers from the subicular complex to the ENT exhibit divergence (Berger, Semple-Rowland, and Bassett 1981). There are extensive lateral interactions, at least within DG and CA3. In DG, lateral interactions are mediated by relatively few large excitatory interneurons located in the hilar region just below the granular layer. CA3 pyramidal cells have direct lateral interactions. As a result, it was suggested (Amaral and Witter 1989; Ishizuka, Webber, and Amaral 1990) that the hippocampus should be considered as a three-dimensional cortical structure, where both transverse and longitudinal information transfer takes place, rather than as a structure where the information is preserved within each two-dimensional lamella.

Commissural Connections Some hippocampal cells—CA3 pyramidal cells, some nonpyramidal cells, and cells located in the hilus—to some extent form commissural projections (Amaral 1978; Swanson, Köhler, and Björklund 1987). Both pyramidal and nonpyramidal cells may be targets of commissural connections (Frotscher and Zimmer 1983). In ENT (both lateral olfactory and medial nonolfactory), layer II cells, which form the lateral perforant path projecting to DG, also generate a commissural associational system. There are also direct projections from CA1 to prefrontal cortex and amygdala.

Subcortical Connections

The hippocampal formation also receives sparse cholinergic inputs from medial septal nucleus, catecholaminergic and serotoninergic fibers from the brainstem, and small projections from hypothalamus and thalamus. Septum and brainstem inputs seem targeted for the interneurons and polymorphic cells of the hilus.

Septal Area An important input to hippocampus arises from the medial septum. The septohippocampal pathway has two main components. One type of fiber, presumably being cholinergic (Amaral and Kurz 1985), does not show target-selective innervation. Another type of fiber was found to be GABAergic: Fibers of this type selectively innervate inhibitory interneurons of the hippocampus proper (Freund and Antal 1988; Gulyás, Görcs,

and Freund 1990). Because the interneurons contain mostly GABA as transmitter substance, the GABA-GABAergic interaction implements the phenomenon called *disinhibition.* There are some backprojections from the hippocampus to the septal area, both from the pyramidal cells of the CA3–CA1 regions (Alonso and Frotscher 1989) and from nonpyramidal (Tóth and Freund 1992) and GABAergic (Tóth, Borhegyi, and Freund 1993) cells. The eventual functional consequences of the existence of topographic projections from hippocampal areas to the lateral septal nucleus was analyzed by Risold and Swanson (1996; see sec. 6.5.3).

Midbrain The raphé nuclei of the midbrain area innervate the hippocampus. The main neurotransmitter of the raphé-hippocampal projections is serotonin (Kohler and Steinbusch 1982). Specifically, the median raphé projections selectively innervate a subclass of interneurons in the CA regions (Freund et al. 1990), namely, those containing calbindin.

Other Subcortical Areas There are a few other subcortical inputs to the hippocampus. Afferents arising from the brainstem originate mostly from the locus coerulus, which is the major nonadrenergic nucleus. Thalamic and hypothalamic afferents to different hippocampal regions also have been found (e.g., Swanson, Köhler, and Björklund 1987).

6.1.3 Quantitative Data: Cell Numbers, Convergence, and Divergence

The qualitative picture of cellular and network organization is supplemented with quantitative data on cell numbers and on the divergence and convergence of projections. Divergence is the number of target cells innervated by a presynaptic cell. Convergence shows the number of cells projecting to one target cell. Though there are many uncertainties in the data, "quantitative assessment of the hippocampal neuronal machinery is tractable" (Amaral, Ishizuka, and Claiborne 1990).

The number of pyramidal cells in the rat ENT projecting to the DG is approximately 200,000, whereas the number of granule cells in DG is of the order of 1 million, a roughly fivefold increase in the number of principal cells. Each granule cell receives approximately 6,000 weak excitatory inputs from ENT, of which 5%–10% must be active to fire the cell. There appears to be a much smaller subset of inputs the synaptic efficacy of which is significantly greater (McNaughton, Barnes, and Andersen 1981). Each granule cell in the DG projects to as few as 15 pyramidal cells in CA3 (Claiborne, Amaral,

ENT: 100,000 cells	ENT → DG	1 : 100,000; 10,000 : 1 (moderate spread)
DG: 1,000,000 cells	DG → CA3	1 : 10; 100 : 1 (little spread)
CA3: 100,000 cells	CA3 → CA3	1 : 5,000; 5,000 : 1 (broad spread)
	CA3 → CA1	1 : 10,000; 10,000 : 1 (broad spread)
	ENT → CA3	1 : 5,000; 5,000 : 1
CA1: 100,000 cells	CA1 → association cortex	

and Cowan 1986) via contacts that are relatively powerful and have a unique morphology. Each CA3 pyramidal cell (there are approximately 300,000) receives as many as 16,000 other modifiable excitatory contacts, approximately a third from ENT, the rest from other CA3 pyramidal cells. Pyramidal cells in the CA3 region project to the pyramidal cells in the CA1 region ($\sim$ 400,000), which in turn project to subiculum ($\sim$ 100,000 pyramidal cells). Both the divergence and convergence of the projections of CA3 and CA1 pyramidal cells is quite large, each cell projecting to, and receiving from, many thousands of cells.

There are far fewer inhibitory than excitatory cells (the ratio is approximately 1 : 10), but they are essential to normal function; moreover, blocking them produces epileptic seizures. Approximately 40% of the inhibitory cells are perisomatic, and 60% are dendritic. One pyramidal cell (receiving $\sim$ 15,000 boutons) innervates approximately 300 PV-containing cells, whereas the convergence to one inhibitory cell is approximately 1,000 (Sík, Tamamaki, and Freund 1993). An inhibitory cell may innervate 600–4,000 pyramidal cells, whereas based on a rough estimation (Gulyás 1993), the convergence is approximately 400–500. Not very much is known about the interaction between the inhibitory populations; the probability of the existence of synapses from slow inhibitory cells (with $GABA_B$ receptors) to fast inhibitory cells (with $GABA_A$ receptors) is larger than in the opposite direction.

6.2 Electrical Activity Patterns

6.2.1 Global Brain States and Behavioral States

Global brain states, in both normal and pathological situations, may be associated with spontaneous activities of large populations of neurons. Experimentally, these activities may be detected by recording both from large neural assemblies, as in the electroencephalograph (EEG) or from a single neuron of the cell population. Generally, behavioral correlates can be defined for electrophysiologically global brain states.

Two main, normally occurring global hippocampal states are known: the rhythmical slow activity, called the *theta rhythm* (Green and Arduini 1954), and the irregular *sharp waves* (SPW) (Buzsáki, Leung, and Vanderwolf 1983; Buzsáki 1986, 1989). A pathological brain state associated with epileptic seizures, the epileptiform patterns, is also characteristic of the hippocampus. More precisely, a set of different types of collective neural behaviors are called "seizures" (Traub and Miles 1991, p. 29). Both normal brain states (see sec. 6.2.2) and epileptic states (sec. 6.2.3) are related to some not clearly defined synchronous activity. Though a certain degree of synchronization is characteristic of normal rhythmic activity, highly synchronized cellular activity is more characteristic of clinical disorders. Other oscillations, such as a fast (40- to 100-Hz) gamma oscillation found mostly in the hilus, and transient high-frequency (200-Hz) oscillation in the CA1 region also have been reported (Buzsáki et al. 1992, 1994; Bragin et al. 1995).

6.2.2 Normal Electrical Activity Patterns: Theta Rhythms and SPWs

Theta Rhythms

The theta rhythm is a population oscillation with large ($\sim$ 1 mV) amplitude and with 4- to 12-Hz frequency. Originally, the theta rhythm was found to occur whenever an animal engages in such behaviors as walking, exploration, sensory scanning and occurs in rapid eye movement (REM) sleep (Vanderwolf 1969). O'Keefe and Nadel (1978) suggested that displacement movements (but not stationary voluntary movements, such as bar pressing at low speeds) in the rat coincide with theta; moreover, the frequency of theta has been found to correlate with speed of movement (O'Keefe and Recce 1993). It can also be phase-locked to sensory stimuli (Buzsáki et al. 1979).

Single-cell physiological studies showed different relations between the behavior of individual cells and the theta rhythm. Granule cells fire rhythmically during theta waves, with a fivefold to eightfold increase in frequency relative to nontheta states (Buzsáki, Leung, and

Vanderwolf 1983). For a thorough study of the intracellular correlates of theta rhythm in identified pyramidal, granule, and basket cells, see Ylinen et al. (1995b). Pyramidal cells in the hippocampus proper generally discharge with a very low frequency (0.01–0.5 Hz), although spatially sensitive "place cells" show firing at 4–8 Hz when the rat is in its place field (sec. 6.4.4), and the position of the animal within a cell's place field may be correlated with the phase of its firing relative to the theta rhythm.

Generally, theta rhythm is thought to depend on septal input (Petsche, Stumph, and Gogolak 1962): Medial septal lesions eliminate theta in the hippocampus (Vanderwolf and Leung 1983). The septo-hippocampal pathway has a cholinergic component (Buzsáki, Leung, and Vanderwolf 1983), but it is not the only one to contribute to the generation of theta rhythm. Atropin, a muscarinic antagonist of ACh, does not abolish the rhythmic slow activity entirely (Stewart and Fox 1989; Smythe, Colom, and Bland 1992). The GABAergic component of the septal afferents modifies the activity of the principal cells by disinhibition (Freund and Antal 1988) and also is involved in the generation of theta rhythm.

Population oscillation at the theta frequency can be induced by charbachol in hippocampal slices (Konopacki et al. 1987; MacVicar and Tse 1989). (Charbacol, similarly to ACh, can activate the muscarinic type ACh receptor but is resistant to the enzymes that degrade and so terminate actions of ACh molecules.) On the basis of these findings, it was suggested that theta rhythms may be generated not extrahippocampally but mostly by the intrinsic properties of the neurons of the CA3 region. Traub et al. (1992) analyzed the underlying single-cell firing patterns during both in vitro carbachol-induced oscillation and in vivo theta waves and found that even though the two oscillations occur with the same frequency, they are still different. For example, during carbachol-induced oscillation, the pyramidal cells fire at a much higher frequency than is seen in vivo.

One of the most important theoretical questions related to neural oscillators is whether and how a population of neurons can generate oscillations detectable in the extracellular field potential activity but not apparent in the activity of individual neurons. This problem was studied by Traub and Miles (1991), who built network models by using very detailed single-cell models (discussed in sec. 6.3). A very different and abstract aspect of a related problem (i.e., the relationship between neural architectures and the possibility of oscillatory behavior) was studied in section 4.2.2.

Buzsáki et al. (1994) speculated on the double functional role of hippocampal theta rhythm. First, a large-scale oscillation in the entorhinal-hippocampal network induced by the septum is maintained by phase-locking. Second, because the majority of the pyramidal cells are silent during theta and their membrane voltage is kept close to (but below) the threshold, relatively few excitatory synapses are sufficient to discharge them. In addition, the relationship between theta rhythm and LTP in the olfactory system and the hippocampus was already mentioned in section 5.3.3.

Irregular SPWs

SPWs have a very large amplitude (up to 3.5 mV), their duration is 40–120 msec, and their frequency can be between 0.2 and 5 Hz (Suzuki and Smith 1988). Though maximal SPW frequencies do overlap theta frequencies, theta waves are much more regular than are SPWs. SPWs also have behavioral correlates: They occur during awake immobility, drinking, eating, face washing, grooming, and slow-wave sleep. During SPWs, pyramidal and inhibitory cells fire with increased frequency. Furthermore, there is a partial synchronous cellular activity of both pyramidal and inhibitory neurons. However, the degree of synchrony is under the threshold for induction of epileptic seizure.

The amplitude and frequency of SPWs can be increased by high-frequency stimulation of the commissural system and the Schaffer collaterals (Buzsáki 1984), suggesting that such stimulation enhances the efficacy of the excitatory synapses. This suggests a relation of SPWs to memory (addressed in sec. 6.3). The activity of neurons in the deep layers of ENT (the main output cells of ENT) also are correlated with SPWs (Buzsáki et al. 1994).

Both "normal" SPWs and epileptiform SPWs can occur. The latter are characterized by an amplitude larger than 4 mV, or their pattern is less irregular, or they correlate with behavior normally associated with theta waves. Their duration is shorter than during normal SPWs.

Though theta rhythms depend on septal input, SPWs are formed by internal processes. One important precondition for SPW generation is the occurrence of a population burst in a small set of CA3 pyramidal cells. Their synchronization is mediated by excitatory synaptic connections. It is interesting to note that Whittington, Traus, and Jefferys (1995) found partially synchronous 40-Hz activity in networks of inhibitory neurons in hippocampal and cortical slices. Furthermore, mathematical studies (van Vreeswijk, Abbott, and Ermentrout 1992) showed that inhibition (and not excitation) synchronizes neural firing in simple networks built from Hodgkin-Huxley type and "integrate-and-fire models."

Traub and Miles (1991, p. 119) have formulated a series of questions:

Under what conditions does population firing become syn-chronized? What factors regulate the extent of synchronization? At one extreme, all cells might fire nearly simultaneously (complete synchrony), or alternatively small subsets of neu-rons might discharge at the same time (partial synchrony). How can one cell or a small group of cells, influence the rest of the population? If synchronization is partial, rather than com-plete, what factors determine which selected cells participate?

Answers obtained by their model studies are summarized briefly in section 6.2.4.

CA3 pyramidal cells have recurrent excitatory connections that terminate within the CA3 region. The autoexcitation due to these connections produces large excitatory postsynaptic potentials (EPSPs) that are propagated to the CA1 region through the Schaffer collaterals. Inhibitory connections control the population activity in both region. Though SPWs were found in rat hippo-campus during consummatory behaviors and slow-wave sleep, there is a normal human EEG phenomenon called *small sharp spikes* (SSS), which is thought to be analogous to SPWs, because it also results from partial synchronous cell firing.

6.2.3 Epileptic Seizures

Epileptic activity occurs in a population of neurons when the membrane potentials of the neurons are synchron-ized "abnormally." As we already know, a certain degree of synchrony is necessary for normal theta and SPW be-havior, and the transition between normal and abnormal degrees of synchrony is not clear. Rather arbitrarily, activity has been considered epileptic if more than 25% of the cells fire during 100 msec (Traub et al. 1992). In vitro models of epilepsy (Traub, Wong, and Miles 1987; Traub and Miles 1991; Traub and Miles 1992; Traub et al. 1992; Traub and Jefferys 1994) offer a means to study the cellular mechanisms of the different types of epileptic phenomena by combined physiological and simulation methods (see sec. 6.2.4 for further details).

There are a few different epileptic phenomena found in vitro: synchronized bursts, synchronized multiple bursts, and seizurelike events. Synchronized bursts, last 50–100 msec, and interburst intervals generally are longer than 1 sec. They are analogous to the so-called interictal (i.e., "between seizures") event found in vivo and can be elicited by applying a localized $GABA_A$ blocking agent (e.g., picrotoxin, bicucullin, penicillin). Synchronized multiple bursts are characterized by a series of up to approximately 10 synchronized bursts occurring at 65- to 75-msec intervals. The intervals be-tween the complex events are greater than 10 seconds.

This phenomenon also can be generated by applying $GABA_A$ blocker. Seizurelike events can be generated both with and without the aid of chemical synapses. The latter possibility was demonstrated in slices with low $[Ca^{2+}]_o$ solutions. Low $[Ca^{2+}]_o$ blocks spike-dependent synaptic transmission, yet spontaneous bursts of pop-ulation spikes ("field bursts") with underlying high fre-quency firing of pyramidal cells still are evoked (Taylor and Dudek 1982; Jefferys and Haas 1982).

The elevated-potassium model of epilepsy (Traynelis and Dingledine 1988; McBain, Traynelis, and Dingledine 1993; McBain 1994) suggests that a modest elevation of the extracellular potassium ion concentration produces hypersynchronous epileptiform activity. One important element of the epileptogenesis may be related to the attenuation of the inhibitory synaptic inputs to pyrami-dal cells during high-potassium seizures.

Both experiments and theoretical studies suggest the existence of a general synchronization mechanism in the hippocampal CA3 region. Synaptic inhibition regulates the spread of pyramidal neuron firing. Inhibition may be reduced by applying drugs to block mostly $GABA_A$ re-ceptors. If inhibition falls below a critical level, complete synchrony occurs. Collective network properties have been studied successfully by Traub and Miles (1991).

6.2.4 The Traub-Miles Approach

Traub and Miles (1991) simulated hippocampal, mostly CA3 population activity by building bottom-up models from data on anatomical connectivities, ionic conduc-tances, and synaptic properties. In most of their simula-tions, the aim was to reproduce the results of physiological measurements made on hippocampal slices. Physiologi-cal measurements (both intracellular recording from one cell or, mostly, from a pair of cells and field potential re-cording from a localized cell population) and simulations under various circumstances contribute to discovering the mechanism of both normal and pathological phe-nomena (e.g., epileptogenesis).

Single-Cell Model

Neurons in the Traub-Miles networks are modeled with a Hodgkin-Huxley formulation that has been modified in numerous ways.

• Structural details of a neuron are taken into account to represent passive properties of the dendrites.

• The model includes the spike-generating sodium- and potassium-active channels and calcium channels, calcium-dependent potassium channels, and potassium channels.

• The nonuniform distribution of channels is taken into account.

• The kinetics and densities of Na and K channels are altered to describe the spiking patterns of the pyramidal cells.

Two types of action potentials can be generated in the CA3 pyramidal cell: fast, sodium-mediated potentials localized mostly to the soma and slow, calcium-mediated potentials mostly in the apical dendrite. Roughly speaking, the role of the potassium channels is repolarization.

The response of CA3 pyramidal cells to injected currents—the intrinsic burst discharges—are reproduced by the model. The frequency and even the regularity of the action potentials depends on the strength of the applied current. A burst consists of a series of fast spikes at intervals of 5–10 msec, terminating in one or more slower action potentials. The burst is *called* intrinsic, because isolated neurons can produce it. Some characteristic features of the physiological responses were reproduced: (1) an intrinsic burst followed by a long after-hyperpolarization (AHP), (2) the dependence of bursting on the resting potential, (3) summation of spike after-depolarization to produce a depolarizing envelope; and (4) the ability to prevent full burst generation by properly timed hyperpolarizing input.

The complete formal model will not be recapitulated here, but remarks on specific terms (*membrane currents* and *synaptic currents*) will be made. In the simplest version of the model, the membrane current I_m is composed as

$$I_m = I_{Na} + I_K + I_{Ca} + I_{K[Ca]} \tag{1}$$

where

$$I_{Na} = \bar{g}_{Na} m^3 h (V(t) - V_{Na})$$

$$I_K = \bar{g}_K n^4 y (V(t) - V_K)$$

$$I_{Ca} = \bar{g}_{Ca} s^5 r (V(t) - V)$$

$$I_{K[Ca]} = \bar{g}_{K[Ca]} q (V(t) - V_K).$$

(c_{Ca} does not occur in the equation for $I_{K[Ca]}$ because only the rate constants for the gating of q are Ca concentration-dependent.) The kinetic equations for the gating variables m, h, n, y, s, r, and q have the standard form, whereas the internal calcium concentration c is governed by an equation of the form

$$\frac{dc_{Ca}(t)}{dt} = -k_1 I_{Ca}(t) - k_2 c_{Ca}(t) \tag{2}$$

To model synaptic currents, both quickly relaxing AMPA and slowly relaxing NMDA receptors were in-

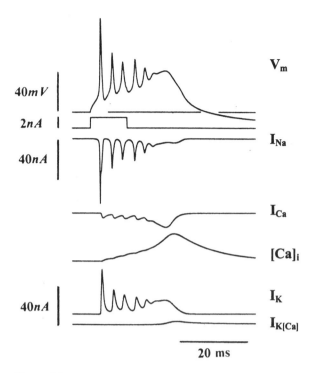

Figure 6.4
Membrane ionic currents and $[Ca^{2+}]_i$ during a current-induced simulated burst. Note the relatively slow kinetics of I_{Ca} compared to I_{Na}. (From Traub and Miles 1991 by permission.)

cluded. They are assumed to be localized in the dendritic regions. (The role of these receptors in LTP is discussed in section 6.3.) A single Ca^{2+}-dependent K^+ current is used. This current has some voltage dependence but is controlled mainly by a threshold-dependent process triggered by an increase in intracellular Ca^{2+} concentration. Once activated, the current is independent of Ca^{2+}.

Multicompartmental models of hippocampal pyramidal cells (Traub and Wong 1982; Traub et al. 1991, 1994) discriminate between somatic compartments and apical and basal dendritic compartments. Each neuron consists of 19 compartments, but for simulating a network of approximately 1,000 neurons, only seven compartments were taken into consideration (Traub and Jefferys 1994; see figure 4.2).

A typical behavior of the model is illustrated by figure 6.4 (Traub and Miles 1991; figure 4.3), which shows the time dependence of the membrane potential and the calcium concentration and of the four ionic currents. An intrinsic burst was generated in response to current injection. The calcium current shows much slower kinetics than does the sodium current. The model also was able to show how a small hyperpolarizing current injected at the correct time can prevent the development of a full burst. Interneurons were simulated with almost the same model as that used for the pyramidal cell, calcium, and calcium-dependent currents, and voltage-dependent inactivation of the potassium current was neglected to avoid intrinsic burst generation.

Model Reduction

The 19-compartment model has been reduced to a two-compartment model by Pinsky and Rinzel (1994). In this model, there is one compartment for the soma and proximal dendrites and another for the distal dendrites. The currents are segregated into these two compartments; fast currents are assumed to be in the somalike compartment, whereas slow currents are localized in the dendritelike compartment. The coupling conductance between the two compartments is an important electrotonic parameter. This reduced model (1) was capable of qualitatively reproducing the salient stimulus-response characteristics of the Traub-Miles single-cell model, (2) was useful for studying the effect of intercompartmental coupling on the responses generated, and (3) proved to be a computationally effective unit for network simulations. Some might argue that such reduction procedures lead only to a model of a model. We think that there is no predetermined optimally complex model. The modeler must (and can) select the proper level of description only in the knowledge of the very specific problem. One of the pioneers of computational neuroscience, Wilfrid Rall, voted for building models of intermediate level of complexity but with the smallest number of compartments that reproduce the proper behavior. Speaking of the Rinzel-Pinker model, he said

[A] single lumped compartment, with all of the ion channels in parallel, could not produce the same behavior, especially the rhythm which basically involves an alternating flow of current between the two coupled compartments. A special advantage of the reduced neuron model is that much simpler computations can explore how much the interesting behavior depends on the values of key parameters, especially the parameter which defines the tightness of coupling between the two compartments. Also, the behavior of very large networks can be explored more efficiently using such a reduced neuron model. Further study may show that the two compartment model cannot match the fuller model in certain important tests, but, in any case, these findings, so far, represent a very satisfying example that illustrates the thesis of this essay [stated earlier in the article as follows:] ... I freely state my bias for the more realistic neuron models. I do not choose the most complex, in the sense of including all known anatomical and physiological details; I favor an intermediate level of complexity, which preserves the most significant distinctions between regions (soma, proximal dendritic, distal dendritic,

different trees) especially when further justified by nonuniform distributions of synapses and ion channels (Rall 1995).

Model of the CA3 Network

Each network model must specify the types, number, and geometrical arrangement of cells, the mechanisms of intercellular communication between cells, and the structure and connectivity of the network (see also Traub, Miles, and Wong 1989).

Three basic cell types—pyramidal cells (i.e., excitatory or *e* cells) and two types of inhibitory cells (i_1 and i_2 cells) were assumed. The postsynaptic effect of the i_1 cells is mediated by perisomatic GABA$_A$ receptors, whereas the inhibition of the i_2 cells is mediated by the dendritic GABA$_B$ receptors (as it was believed at that time, but as mentioned in the subsection, Electrophysiological Characterization, the change in the interpretation does not affect the essence of the simulation results). The ratio of excitatory and inhibitory cells is set as 10 : 1, though it is assumed rather arbitrarily that the number of i_1 cells is equal to the number of i_2 cells. The simulated network contained up to 10,000 cells (i.e., approximately half of the slice was modeled). In a typical simulation, 9000 excitatory and 900 (450 + 450) inhibitory cells were specified. A network of such size proved to be sufficiently large to study population phenomena (e.g., synchronization).

The model of synaptic action had to take into account both the transduction of soma potential into axonal output and the axon conduction delay. Four types of synapses were considered: (1) the excitatory synapses between pyramidal cells, (2) the excitatory synapses between pyramidal cells and both types of inhibitory cells, (3) the fast, GABA$_A$-mediated inhibitory synapses from the i_1 cells on both excitatory and inhibitory cells, and (4) the slow inhibition (from i_2) on both excitatory and inhibitory cells. The unitary conductance for each synapse was described by the "alpha function" (Rall 1967; Jack, Noble, and Tsien 1975) just as in the model of activity of the olfactory cortex (reviewed in sec. 5.2.3).

Instead of giving detailed wiring, the strategy for specifying synapses in this model was to define the statistical properties of the topology of the neural structures. On the basis of data from dual intracellular recordings, it was estimated that all cell types receive 20 excitatory and 20 inhibitory inputs on average. To put it another way, an *i* cell has, on average, 220 outputs: 200 to *e* cells and 20 to *i* cells. An excitatory cell has an average of 22 outputs, 20 to *e* cells and 2 to *i* cells. Traub and Miles (1989) defined both globally and locally random networks. The probabilities of synaptic connections for a given type of cell pair is constant in the former case and decreases with distance in the latter one. [This construction is very similar to that introduced by Braitenberg (1978), Palm and Braitenberg (1979) and Braitenberg and Schüz (1991) for the synapses between cortical pyramidal cells. Palm and Braitenberg used the terms *ametric* and *metric* for the long-range and local connections, respectively.] Traub and Miles used globally random organization for small ($\sim 1,000$-neuron) networks and used locally random structures for larger networks. The $p(M,L)$ probability of the connection between cells L and M was given by

$$p(M,L)\alpha \exp(-d(L,M)/\lambda).$$

Here $d(L,M)$ is the distance between the cells L and M, and λ defines how localized the connections will be. Depending on whether the presynaptic cell is excitatory or inhibitory, the typical value for λ was 30 or 6, respectively.

Synchronization   Different epileptic phenomena found in vitro were listed in section 6.2.3. The network model outlined previously is an appropriate tool for simulating synchronized population activity associated with epilepsy. Synchronization is an emergent property of the network, a collective phenomenon generated in consequence of mostly local cellular interactions. (We have to add the restrictive qualification *mostly* because global field effects also may occur.) From a formal point of view, synchronized activity in the CA3 region is similar to that described by the physicists' percolation theory (see Schulman's appendix in Traub and Miles 1991). Percolation theory describes such phenomena as the generation of a forest fire after a single tree has caught fire, or the spreading of epidemics. Depending on the conditions of interaction among the elements of a population, synchronization may be complete or partial (i.e., localized in size). In extreme cases, when the first "activated" element is isolated sufficiently from the others, the chain reaction is inhibited, and the activation does not spread at all.

Fully and Partially Synchronized Bursts   Fully synchronized bursts in hippocampal slices can be induced by blocking the GABA synapses, as was mentioned earlier. The total suppression of inhibition leads to fully synchronized population activity in consequence of the excitatory interactions between pyramidal cells, as comparative experiments and simulations with networks also demonstrate (see Traub and Miles 1991, figures 6.4, 6.5). The degree of synchrony critically depends on the

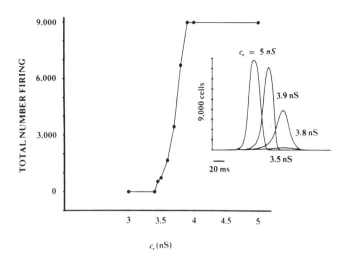

Figure 6.5
The extent of synchronization in the disinhibited model network, regulated by the strength of the excitatory synapses. The inflection is sharp and reflects two factors: the ability of bursting to propagate from cell to cell at all and bursting must propagate fast enough to "outrun" delayed inhibition. This latter effect explains why the inflection in this curve does not begin until 3.5 nsec and why it does not have a perfectly sharp corner. Note that increasing c_e shortens the population latency, as expected (inset). The stimulus was to one cell. What is plotted is the total number of e cells that fire at all, not the total number that fire at any one time. (From Traub and Miles 1991 by permission.)

strength of excitatory synapses. If it is zero (i.e., totally blocked), synchronized activity disappears (though the individual cells still show bursts). Furthermore, the propagation should be faster than the effect of slow delayed (GABA$_B$-mediated) inhibition (see figure 6.5, after Traub and Miles 1991, and figure 6.6).

Partial synchronization is associated with normal hippocampal activities such as theta waves and irregular SPWs in vivo and synchronized synaptic potentials (SSPs) in vitro. The partial blockade of inhibition may be established by careful addition of drugs that block GABA$_A$ receptors or GABA$_A$-activated chloride channels. (The disinhibition phenomena, produced by septal GABAergic fibers inhibiting interneurons, implements partial blockade of inhibition in the intact brain.) The degree of synchrony critically depends also on the measure of the inhibition blockade, as simulation studies support (see figure 6.6, after Traub and Miles 1991).

Synchronization can occur in the presence of inhibition if excitatory synapses are made powerful enough (Traub, Jefferys, and Miles 1994a). This possibility proved to be the basis of epileptogenesis established in low-magnesium media or by adding 4-aminopyridine (4-AP). Both these forms of epileptogenesis were reported to be reproduced by simulations (Traub, Jefferys, and Miles 1994a).

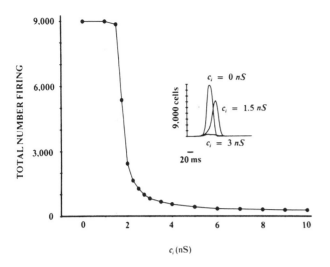

Figure 6.6
How inhibition regulates the influence that one cell can exert on a large neuronal population. One simulated pyramidal cell was excited by using different values of the unitary $GABA_A$ conductance (c_i), and the total number of e cells firing was counted (ordinate). When $GABA_A$ synapses are sufficiently effective, varying c_i has little effect. Between 4 and 2 nsec, small changes in c_i produce major changes in the population response. Below approximately 2 nsec, there is an abrupt transition, so that stimulation of a single cell is able to excite the entire population. Inset shows sample simulations (number of cells firing as a function of time). Note that c_i affects both the latency and the amplitude of the response. Interesting questions arise: Is the brain itself able to regulate the effectiveness of recurrent inhibition within a local population? How is it accomplished? (From Traub and Miles by permission.)

Multiple Bursts: Afterdischarge Single and even multiple bursts also can be synchronized. Epileptic events sometimes may be associated with the phenomenon called *afterdischarge* (AD): A relatively long initial burst is followed by a series of so-called secondary bursts (*secondary* meaning nonprimary, thus possibly tertiary and the like as well). The entire event is followed by a prolonged AHP. Secondary bursts also can be synchronized in CA3 tissue containing approximately 1,000 cells. Synchronized AD can be elicited by different methods (blockade of $GABA_A$ receptors, bathing solution with low-magnesium concentration, administration of 4-AP, and the like).

To reproduce the formation of AD by simulation, both the growth phase and the steady-state phase have to be described. During the growth phase and after the stimulation of a single cell, a large set of cells becomes involved. This activity can be achieved by chain reactions (as supported by simulation studies) if the synapses between pyramidal cells are assumed to be sufficiently strong. During the steady-state phase, the synchronized population activity is organized in the form of a series of bursts. Why? It was found (and simulations partially supported these findings) that AD can be elicited by

three different causes, but two common principles seem to be shared between the different experimental epilepsies (Traub, Jefferys, and Miles 1994): Recurrent excitatory synaptic connections yield sustained dendritic excitation, and this dendritic excitation induces rhythmical dendritic bursts.

Oscillatory and Chaotic Population Activity Synchronous rhythmic activities have been found in various parts of the nervous system, such as the olfactory system, visual cortex, hippocampus, and somatomotor cortex, and the mechanism of their genesis and their eventual functions have been reviewed by Gray (1994).

Synchronized population oscillations (i.e., repeated SSPs) have been recorded in hippocampal slices. SSPs are considered to be the in vitro analog of the irregular SPWs found in vivo. As Traub and Miles (1991) remark, population rhythms may denote not only regular but even chaotic rhythmic activity.

The origin of the population oscillation found in slices has been explained by model studies (Traub, Miles, and Wong 1989). The operation of a few spontaneously bursting, and many silent, cells is self-organized into an autonomous population oscillation by the propagation of activity through the excitatory connections. It was found by simulation experiments made in a broad regime of parameters that population oscillation was much faster than the rhythmic activity of any individual cells. The features of the oscillation have been influenced by a few factors, the most important of which are mentioned here:

• *Fast inhibition:* Progressive blockade of fast inhibition increases the amplitude and decreases the frequency of the excitatory SSPs.

• *Recurrent excitation:* Increased excitatory synaptic strengths also contribute to the increase of the amplitude and the decrease of the frequency of the partially synchronized oscillation.

• *Cellular excitability:* Diminished excitability of the pyramidal cells reduces the number of spontaneously bursting cells and decreases the effect of excitatory synapses in activity propagation.

6.2.5 Comparing the Hippocampus with the Olfactory System

The Comparative Phenomenology of Electrical Patterns

Both the hippocampus and the olfactory system exhibit complex dynamic behavior: They generate rhythmic temporal patterns with different frequencies and with variable spatial coherence. Both systems also were suggested to be candidates for chaos generators. Global electrical patterns measured by EEG have behavioral correlates and have crucial roles in learning and memory formation, and these functions can be subject to cholinergic modulation.

Specifically, oscillations with theta (around 7 Hz) and gamma (around 40 Hz) frequency were found in both systems. Though hippocampal theta rhythm seems most likely to have a septal origin, it appears to be synchronized with the sniff cycle both in the olfactory bulb (Freeman 1978) and in the olfactory cortex (Macrides, Eichenbaum, and Forbes 1982). A 40-Hz brain oscillation was found first in the olfactory system and now seems to be a rather general phenomenon in different cortical and cortexlike structures. However, even if the phenomenon is common, the generating mechanism can be different in different regions. Whereas the Freeman experiments suggested the interaction of excitatory and inhibitory populations as the source of 40-Hz oscillation in the olfactory system, Whittington, Traus, and Jefferys (1995) demonstrated that in the hippocampal CA1 region, a network formed by pure (GABAergic) inhibitory synapses produces this rhythm; oscillations in the pyramidal cells are the consequence of entrainment by this oscillation. If the pyramidal cells show intrinsic oscillation, the entrainment is more robust. The abstract analysis of network architectures leading to oscillations (sec. 4.2.2) allows the occurrence of both mechanisms. As mentioned, SPWs and high-frequency oscillations, however, seem to be characteristic of the hippocampus alone.

Structural Analogies

Though similar phenomena may be generated even by different mechanisms and the hippocampal and the olfactory 40-Hz oscillation may show differences in their origins, it is also reasonable to speculate about the existence of striking structural analogies and their functional consequences. In particular, Hasselmo and Schnell (1994) argued that both the hippocampal CA1 region and the olfactory cortex show a laminar segregation of excitatory synapses. The modifiability of the memory performance of the two systems (but not their rhythms) was explained by using this analogy.

The Hippocampus as an Olfactory Center

Hippocampus participates in processing olfactory information. The ENT gets a sparse projection from the olfactory bulb and from layer II of the piriform cortex. (The olfactory cortex has parallel efferents to other structures as well: to the olfactory tubercle and peri-amygdaloid cortex and also to frontal cortex, both monosynaptically and via the mediodorsal thalamic nucleus; Lynch and Granger 1991; Eichenbaum et al. 1991.) Theta-bursting patterns [i.e., a series of short (30-millisecond) high-frequency bursts separated by 100–200 milliseconds, the period of theta] was found to characterize hippocampal single-cell activity during the performance of an olfactory discrimination task (Eichenbaum et al 1987). This theta burst pattern seems to be optimal for LTP induction (see Larson et al. 1988; Pavlides et al. 1988; Huerta and Lisman 1993; and Diamond, Dunwiddie, and Rose 1988 for further details).

Neural Mechanisms of Rhythm Generation and Synchronization

Though it cannot be excluded that some elementary rhythmicity occurs even at the single-cell level in the mitral cells and more likely in pyramidal cells both in the olfactory cortex and in the hippocampus (owing to the interaction of inward and outward currents), the oscillations are dominantly emergent network properties. Long-range synaptic interactions are thought to be the anatomical substrate of synchronization. As for the olfactory bulb, it is not known clearly whether the axon collaterals or rather the branching dendrites of the mitral cells make the major contribution to the synchronization. In the olfactory cortex, the excitatory axon collaterals of the layer II and layer III pyramidal cells promotes the establishment of synchrony (and also associative memory). It seems to be plausible that in the hippocampus, different rhythms cohabitate (such rhythms as single-cell oscillations, network oscillations due to the interaction of excitatory and inhibitory synapses, and oscillations due to purely inhibitory interactions). Recurrent axon collaterals of the pyramidal cells in the CA3 region may have a crucial role in synchronization.

The Functional Role of Rhythms in Hippocampal and Olfactory Information Processing

Synchronized rhythmic activities now are thought to be a general property of neuronal systems (Gray 1994). Their functional significance is perhaps more clearly understood in the olfactory system and the hippocampus than in other areas (visual cortex, somatomotor cortex). Coherent rhythmic states may provide the substrates for synaptic modifications and storage of information. The details of the relationship between physiological patterns and synaptic plasticity in both systems is the subject of other ongoing projects (Buzsáki and Chrobak 1995).

Styles of Modeling

Though the hippocampus has been the subject of bottom-up modeling efforts (sec. 6.2.4), the olfactory system was described first by less-detailed network models (secs. 5.2.2 and 5.2.3). Data for the voltage-dependent kinetics are more readily available for hippocampal pyramidal cells than for, say, the mitral cells of the olfactory bulb (at least for the time being). There seem to be two tendencies for present and near-future model studies of the hippocampus and the olfactory system: to establish detailed multicompartmental models for the single cells and to try to simulate the dynamic behavior of networks built from this model's neurons, and to increase the biological plausibility of present population models by building scaling-invariant kinetic models (Gröbler and Barna 1996) and by incorporating the bursting properties of the single cells and the specific intra- and interregional connectivities.

6.3 Brain States and LTP

LTP was discovered first in the hippocampus and is very prominent there (Bliss and Lømo 1973). LTP is an increase in synaptic strength that can be induced rapidly by brief periods of synaptic stimulation and that has been reported to last for hours in vitro and for days and weeks in vivo (Baudry and Davis 1991). This time course may be insufficient to sustain long-term memory, but there appear to be multiple LTP mechanisms; one dependent on protein synthesis might serve long-term memory: Protein synthesis inhibition disrupts the maintenance of LTP but leaves its induction relatively or totally intact. Maren and Baudry (1995) relate properties and mechanisms of long-term synaptic plasticity in the mammalian brain to learning and memory.

6.3.1 Hebbian Synaptic Modification

There is evidence for both homosynaptic and heterosynaptic LTP in area CA1 of the hippocampus, and an associative form of LTP has been reported in hippocampal CA1 and dentate gyrus.

Hebbian synaptic modification depends on the co-occurrence of pre- and postsynaptic activity, and this effect was found in the form of LTP occurring in the Schaffer collateral–commissural synaptic input to the pyramidal neurons of hippocampal CA1 (Bliss and Collingridge 1993; Brown et al., 1988; Brown, Kairiss, and Keenan 1990). Tetanic stimulation of either a "weak" pathway (i.e., unable to induce potentiation on its own) or "strong" pathway (i.e., capable of inducing potentiation on its own) *alone* failed to induce LTP in the weak input, but temporally overlapping pairing of the two inputs produced associative LTP. Moreover, such LTP occurs even if there is a temporal gap of up to 40 milliseconds (see Brown, Kairiss, and Keenan 1990, for a review).

As mentioned earlier, the hippocampal excitatory transmitter glutamate exerts its action through at least two major classes of receptors, NMDA receptors and AMPA receptors (selectively activated by NMDA and α-amino-3-hydroxy-5-methyl-4-isoxazole, respectively). [A second non-NMDA receptor, the metabotropic receptor (a second messenger-coupled receptor), will not be discussed further here.] The fast component of the excitatory postsynaptic current at the Schaffer collateral–commissural synapse in CA1 is mediated primarily via the AMPA receptors, whereas the slow component is mediated by NMDA receptors. The fast AMPA receptor component lasts a few milliseconds, it has a fast rise time, and its duration is limited by the time constant of the cell membrane. The postsynaptic potentials mediated by the AMPA receptors are caused by an increase in the conductances mainly of Na^+ and K^+. The NMDA receptor mediates a relatively slow EPSP and is 10 times more permeable to Ca^{2+} ions than to Na^+ or K^+. However, NMDA activation requires not only the binding of an agonist (i.e., a compound that mimics the effect of glutamate) to the receptor site but also sufficient depolarization of the postsynaptic membrane to remove the voltage-dependent blockade of the channel that normally is mediated by Mg^{2+} ions (Bliss and Collingridge 1993).

This particular form of Hebbian synapse found in CA1 thus rests on the conjunction of presynaptic activity to cause glutamate release to the NMDA receptor and on a sufficient amount of postsynaptic depolarization to AMPA receptors to relieve the channel block and to allow Ca^{2+} influx into the postsynaptic cell. The influx of Ca^{2+} ions through the NMDA receptor channel triggers a cascade of molecular processes that leads to various forms of synaptic plasticity, including short-term potentiation (STP), LTP, and LTD. In particular, the induction of the associative LTP in CA1 is controlled by the NMDA receptor; the Ca^{2+} influx through the NMDA receptor–gated channel and the resultant increase in postsynaptic Ca^{2+} are partly responsible for triggering the induction of LTP. The LTP observed at the mossy fiber synapse in area CA3 of the hippocampus has properties that are fundamentally different from that found in CA1 and DG (Johnston et al. 1992).

Nevertheless, mossy fiber LTP depends on activation of postsynaptic voltage-dependent Ca^{2+} channels *and* high-frequency presynaptic activity, seemingly providing a different Hebbian mechanism. See Zalutsky and Nicoll (1990) and Staubli, Larson, and Lynch (1990) for more information on CA3 LTP.

We saw in section 6.2.2 that the amplitude and frequency of SPWs can be increased by high-frequency stimulation of the commissural system and the Schaffer collaterals (Buzsáki 1984), suggesting a relation of SPWs to memory. Buzsáki (1989) hypothesized that LTP can be induced by SPW bursts, although Buzsáki (1994) notes, "To date, no direct evidence is available to support the view that SPW population bursts in the awake rat do indeed result in long-term modification of synapses." Furthermore, disinhibition induced by subcortical afferents may facilitate the formation of LTP.

Buzsáki et al. (1994, p. 168) argue that the sequential potentiation mechanisms

ensure that discharge of a given set of entorhinal neurons during subsequent visits to the same part of [a] maze (recall) will reactivate the same subsets of neurons in CA3 and CA1. The hierarchy of neuronal firing during the SPW-associated bursts, therefore, is precisely determined by the recent past of the neural network. The rules of burst initiation and reconvergent excitation, subserved by the anatomical-physiological organization of the CA3 region, ensure that the synchronized events during consummatory behaviors and slow wave sleep carry biologically meaningful information.

6.3.2 Compartmental Models of Potentiation

Liaw, Berger, and Baudry (1995) review kinetic models of the NMDA receptor. Here, we examine compartmental models that include a detailed analysis of LTP.

Pongrácz et al. (1992) studied short-term changes in pyramidal neuron excitability in the hippocampal CA1 field by using a compartmental model having five compartments each for the apical and basal dendrites, a compartment for the soma, and a layer representing extracellular K^+ concentration. The model included intrinsic membrane conductances and excitatory (NMDA and AMPA) and inhibitory (GABA$_A$ and GABA$_B$) synaptic conductances distributed in the compartments of the apical dendrite. The voltage dependence of the NMDA receptor (due to Mg^{2+} blockade) resulted in a weak conductance for a single stimulation, but the conductance increased with increasing number and intensity of repeated stimulation, yielding frequency-dependent EPSP potentiation, a form of short-term plasticity.

Holmes and Levy (1990) developed a compartmental model of a DG granule cell to study LTP. An 11-compartment model was constructed to represent a spine and a small patch of the neighboring dendrite. Calcium dynamics, including Ca^{2+} influx, buffering, pumping, and diffusion were computed over this domain. One glutamate binding site and the voltage-dependent Mg^{2+} block were included in the NMDA receptor kinetics. When few synapses were activated, Ca^{2+} influx was small, even with high-input frequency. When a large number of synapses were activated at the same time, a steep rise in Ca^{2+} influx was seen, with increasing frequency due to the voltage dependency of the NMDA-mediated conductance. However, total Ca^{2+} influx never increased by more than fourfold, which is too small to account for the selective induction of LTP, if the amplitude of peak intracellular free Ca^{2+} concentration is regarded as the indicator of the induction of LTP. The 3- to 4-fold increase could be amplified 20- to 30-fold by transient saturation of the fast Ca^{2+} buffering system. When a weak input was paired with a strong one, the largest increase in peak $[Ca^{2+}]_i$ was seen in cases in which the weak stimulation preceded the strong input by 1–8 msec because of the slow rate constant of NMDA receptor kinetics.

The Holmes-Levy model was extended by De Schutter and Bower (1993) to evaluate the effect of Ca^{2+} permeability of the NMDA receptor channel. Maximum amplification of $[Ca^{2+}]_i$ was obtained at permeability close to values reported in the literature and decreased significantly when permeability was reduced by more than 50%. Similar issues were studied in a microscopical model for the Schaffer collateral–commissural synapse (see Zador, Koch, and Brown 1990), wherein the trigger for synaptic enhancement was assumed to be Ca^{2+} influx through NMDA receptor–gated channels that are located on the dendritic spine head. In this model, the peak transient increase in intracellular Ca^{2+} is localized within the dendritic spine, the spine amplifies the local change in intracellular Ca^{2+}, and the relationship between the peak transient increase in Ca^{2+} and the amount of LTP is nonlinear. Calcium buffering and extrusion mechanisms are posited for the spine head and neck, with longitudinal calcium diffusion between the spine and the dendrite. Voltage-gated Ca^{2+} channels in this model were assumed to be located only on the dendritic shaft. More subtle experiments have called this model into question, leading to new models (Jaffe, Fisher, and Brown 1994; Brown and Chattarji 1994; see Brown and Chattarji 1995 for a brief review).

6.3.3 NMDA Receptors and Oscillations

As noted in section 6.2.4, NMDA receptors also play an important role in oscillations. In the Traub, Miles, and Jefferys (1993) model of the hippocampal CA3 region, each pyramidal neuron was connected randomly to 20 other pyramidal neurons via excitatory (NMDA and AMPA) receptors and to 20 interneurons via inhibitory (GABA$_A$ and GABA$_B$) receptors. The computation of the NMDA receptor–mediated current involved a scaling factor, a synaptic conductance term with a slow-decay time constant, and a term representing the voltage-dependent Mg^{2+} blockade. The NMDA receptor conductance was not necessary for the population oscillation. The model generated synchronized population bursts that resemble those in experimental data obtained from hippocampal slices perfused with a GABA$_A$ receptor blocker. The synchronized firing was blocked in the absence of AMPA receptor conductance but persisted without NMDA receptor current. Introduction of GABA inhibition (most significantly, GABA$_A$ IPSP) suppressed the synchronized bursts. The model predicted that dendritic calcium spikes would occur during each secondary burst generated by the AMPA receptor current. However, with sufficiently high NMDA receptor conductance, synchronized bursts could occur in the absence of AMPA receptor current.

NMDA receptors also play a role in "functional" oscillations. For example, Trävén et al. (1993) constructed a network of interneurons conforming to experimentally identified cell types so as to simulate the spinal locomotor pattern generation in lamprey (contrast the more abstract analysis given in section 4.2.2). Excitatory synapses displayed both NMDA and AMPA receptors, whereas the inhibitory synaptic transmission was glycinergic and mediated by chloride. The NMDA receptor current was modeled as a product of channel conductance, the difference of the membrane potential and the equilibrium potential, and a state variable that accounted for the voltage-dependent Mg^{2+} block of the channel. Oscillatory bursts could be evoked in a postsynaptic cell driven by NMDA receptor–mediated synaptic current, but the presynaptic neuron had little effect on oscillation frequency. The presynaptic control of oscillation frequency increased when non-NMDA receptors were added. A continuous range of burst rates of the network could be produced by the NMDA receptor–mediated and non–NMDA receptor–mediated conductances. The simulations suggest that the spinal locomotor network could be modulated by controlling the balance between NMDA receptor–mediated and AMPA receptor–mediated synaptic input. The NMDA receptor–containing synapses mainly served to stabilize the rhythmic motor output, whereas the non–NMDA receptor–containing synapses provided direct phasic control of the burst pattern.

6.3.4 The Need for Reversal of LTP in Hebbian Synapses

As noted in section 4.5.1, synapses that can only increase in efficacy have serious deficiencies. Among other approaches to this problem, we noted Sejnowski's (1977) *covariance rule* that makes the change in strength of a plastic synapse proportional to the covariance between presynaptic and postsynaptic firing:

$$\frac{dw_{ij}(t)}{dt} = k(a_i(t) - [a_i(t)])(a_j(t) - [a_j(t)]) \tag{3}$$

where the $[a_j(t)]$ are the average firing rates of the output neurons and $[a_i(t)]$ are the average firing rates of the input neurons. Thus, the strength of the synapse should increase if the firing of the presynaptic and postsynaptic elements are correlated positively, decrease if they are correlated negatively, and remain unchanged if they are uncorrelated. Taking a time average of the change in synaptic weight in equation 3, we have

$$[\Delta w_{ij}] = \kappa([a_i(t)a_j(t)] - [a_i(t)][a_j(t)]) \tag{4}$$

The first term on the right hand side has the same form as the simple hebbian synapse. The second term is a learning threshold that varies with the product of the time-averaged pre- and postsynaptic activity levels. This learning threshold ensures that no change in synaptic strength should occur if the average correlation between the pre- and postsynaptic activities is at chance level (i.e., when there is no net covariance). As we saw also in section 4.5.1, the BCM rule of synaptic plasticity (Bienenstock, Cooper, and Munro 1982; see Intrator and Cooper 1995 for a current review)

$$\frac{dw_{ij}(t)}{dt} = k(g(a_i(t)) - \theta(t))h(a_j(t)) \tag{5}$$

implements a postsynaptic control mechanism on the modification process which strengthens the synapse when the average postsynaptic activity exceeds a threshold and weakens the synapse when the activity falls below the threshold level for potentiation, as in the covariance rule. This threshold for depression gives the network model desirable stability properties.

On the empirical front, O'Dell and Kandel (1994) showed that low-frequency stimulation erases LTP through an NMDA receptor–mediated activation of protein phosphatases; Staubli and Lynch (1987, 1990) found stable depression of potentiated synaptic responses in the hippocampus with 1- to 5-Hz stimulation, whereas Larson, Xiao, and Lynch (1993) demonstrated reversal of LTP by theta frequency stimulation. For a recent review on LTD in hippocampus, see Bear and Abraham 1996.

6.3.5 The Relation of LTP and LTD to the Learning Rules of Various Brain Regions

Here, we discuss the relation of LTP and LTD to the learning rules used in later chapters, complementing our current discussion of LTP and hippocampus (see Lynch and Granger 1991 for more regarding CA3 LTP and learning rules).

Cerebral Cortex

Without discussing its relation to LTP, in section 8.4.2 we shall consider a model of reinforcement learning. In the experimental setup, positive reinforcement is given when the monkey exhibits a correct response, but not otherwise. Similarly, in the model, a scalar quantity called *reinforcement* is set by the critic to +1 if the selected motor program is correct, and to −1 otherwise. When positive reinforcement is given, the weights leading into the active feature detector units are adjusted so that the feature detector more clearly recognizes the current sensory input (a hebbian adjustment is made). In the case of negative reinforcement, the weights of active units are adjusted in the opposite direction so that the current input is recognized to an even lesser degree (an antihebbian adjustment). Note that this reinforcement depends on whether the overall system response was correct, not on the output of any individual motor selection column. The learning equation contains a normalization term. As a result, the weights are self-regulating, forcing unneeded or undesirable weights to a value near zero. If a unit continues to receive negative reinforcement (as a result of being involved in an incorrect response), it becomes insensitive to the current stimulus and is reallocated to recognizing other stimuli. Note that in this scheme, all the active units are punished or rewarded as a whole, depending on the strength of their activity. Thus, a unit whose activity is "incorrect" still will be rewarded as long as the entire network chose the correct output. In general, this method works because this "incorrect unit" either will always be active in conjunction with "correct units" that override it or will be involved in wrong decisions sufficiently often to be adjusted toward a correct response.

There is increasing evidence for similarities in properties of LTD in cortical regions besides that of hippocampus. Bear, Cooper, and Ebner (1987) proposed that the BCM modification threshold is related to the membrane potential at which the NMDA receptor–dependent Ca^{2+} flux reached the threshold for inducing LTP. In support of the hypothesis that NMDA receptors play a role in plasticity in visual cortex, Bear, Press, and Connors (1992) have found that the pharmacological blockade of NMDA receptors with the competitive antagonist AP5 disrupts the plastic changes in striate cortex normally resulting from monocular deprivation. Dudek and Bear (1992) electrically stimulated the Schaffer collateral projection to CA1 in rat hippocampal slices at frequencies ranging from 0.5 to 50 Hz. In agreement with assumptions of the BCM theory, presenting 900 pulses at 1–3 Hz yielded a depression of the CA1 population EPSP that persisted without signs of recovery for at least 1 hour following cessation of the conditioning stimulation. This LTD was specific to the conditioned input and could be prevented by application of NMDA receptor antagonists. Of course, this work was performed in hippocampus, whereas the BCM theory was developed for visual cortex. However, Kirkwood et al. (1993) found that very similar forms of plasticity (LTP and LTD) are evoked with precisely the same types of stimulation in adult rat hippocampal field CA1 and in adult rat and immature cat visual cortical layer III. Further, in all three preparations, both LTP and LTD depend on activation of NMDA receptors. These data suggest that a common principle may govern experience-dependent synaptic plasticity in CA1 and (at least) the superficial layers of sensory neocortex.

Cerebellum

Purkinje cells, the output cells of the cerebellar cortex, receive two distinct types of excitatory input: one from parallel fibers, axons of cortical granule cells, and the other from climbing fibers, axons of inferior olivary neurons. When signals reach a Purkinje cell through the two inputs in approximate synchrony, synaptic transmission from parallel fibers is depressed (rather than being facilitated as in LTP), and this depression lasts a long time; thus, this form of plasticity is called *long-term depression* (Ito 1989). We will later look at models in which function depends on paying very careful attention to the phrase *approximate synchrony*.

The molecular mechanisms of LTD generation have been studied extensively (see Crepel and Audinat 1991 for a review). Inflow of Ca^{2+} ions evoked by climbing fiber signals is an important step of LTD, and LTD essentially is due to desensitization of glutamate receptors that mediate parallel fiber–Purkinje cell synapses (Ito 1989). Ito and Karachot (1990) have demonstrated a chain of reaction linking the Ca^{2+} inflow to the receptor desensitization. The enhanced Ca^{2+} stimulates nitric oxide synthase, which requires Ca^{2+}-activated calmodulin. In turn, nitric oxide (NO) so produced stimulates guanylate cyclase and consequently enhances production of cyclic guanosine monophosphate (cGMP). Thence, cGMP-dependent protein kinase (PKG) would be activated to modify responsiveness of glutamate receptors through phosphorylation. The glutamate receptors involved in LTD have been identified as a subtype preferring AMPA. Also, it has been shown that intracellular Ca^{2+} concentration is enhanced not only by entry through voltage-dependent ion channels but also by release from intracellular Ca^{2+} stores. LTD now can be manipulated by certain pharmacological agents that affect these chain reactions.

Further insight into the role of NO has come from studies of the role of the flocculus (a region of the cerebellum) in adaptation of the vestibulo-ocular reflex (VOR) (sec. 9.3.5). Hemoglobin, which absorbs NO, has been found to block LTD effectively. Accordingly, the adaptive changes of VOR in rabbits and a monkey was abolished when 5 M hemoglobin was injected subdurally onto the floccular surface (Nagao and Ito 1990).

The most fully developed hypothesis concerning the role of the cerebellum (chap. 9) is twofold: The Purkinje cells provide inhibitory modulation of cells in the cerebellar nuclei, and these modulate MPGs to yield motor activity that is both adapted to changing conditions and well coordinated. It is postulated that parallel fibers carry contextual, sensory, and internal-state information to the Purkinje cells, whereas climbing fibers carry error information. This returns us to the issue of approximate synchrony: If parallel fibers are continually active and a climbing fiber error signal depends on the result of earlier parallel fiber activity (i.e., Purkinje cell modulation precedes action, and action precedes the evaluation of error), how does LTD affect only the "relevant" synapses?

To address these temporal problems, a number of our chapter 9 models assume synapse *eligibility* (Klopf 1982; Sutton and Barto 1981; Houk, Keifer, and Barto 1993). The form postulated by Houk et al. is that activation of a dendritic spine by a parallel fiber leads to the release of a chemical called a *second messenger* in the spine, where its concentration acts as a short-term memory. We say that the synapse is eligible if the concentration is above some threshold. It is posited that if an error signal is provided

to the whole cell by the climbing fiber, the resulting increase in Ca^{2+} in the cell will only affect the eligible synapses; therefore, only the efficacies of eligible synapses are changed. If a parallel fiber–Purkinje cell synapse participates in synaptic transmission, it becomes eligible to be weakened by LTD if a climbing fiber signal is sent somewhat later. Schweighofer, Arbib, and Dominey (1996a,b) add to this view of eligibility the requirement that, when the error signal arrives, the concentration of the messenger should tend to be largest for synapses involved in the initial saccade. Therefore, we introduced the concept of a time window of eligibility. In our model, concentration rises then falls over time, having the response of a second-order system for the concentration [2nd] of the messenger (although, alternatively, we can imagine a second messenger following a first-order equation but with a significant delay). Ideally, peak concentration matches in time the occurrence of the error signal and the concentration decays relatively rapidly to ensure a minimum of interference with the next saccade.

In the model, there are weight vectors w_{ltd}, one for each Purkinje cell, representing parallel fiber synaptic contacts with the Purkinje cell. With the assumption that the rise in calcium concentration is rapid compared to the second-messenger dynamics, the weight update rule representing LTD at each time step is, for the ith synapse and for each Purkinje cell,

$$\Delta w_{ltd_i} = -\alpha IO[2nd]_i$$

which enforces depression of an eligible synapse (i.e., one for which parallel fiber activity has left a positive eligibility trace, $[2nd]_i > 0$) when the climbing fiber is active. Here, α is the learning coefficient, IO the binary climbing fiber error signal, and $w_{max} > w_{ltd_i} \geqslant 0$. However, if this equation alone were operative, all the weights would tend to zero. Thus, Schweighofer et al. (1996a,b) implemented a weight normalization that can be thought of as providing nonspecific LTP of synaptic strength, so as to keep constant the sum of synaptic weights for each Purkinje cell.

Basal Ganglia

Observations of reward-related dopamine (DA) release during learning and the impairment of learning with DA depletion suggest that DA plays an important role in long-term synaptic changes in the basal ganglia required for learning stimulus-response habits. Ljungberg, Apicella, and Schultz (1991) found that during learning of a delayed alternation task, dopamine-producing cells projecting from the substantia nigra pars compacta (SNc) to the striatum (part of the basal ganglia) are activated by the reward and by cues associated with the reward. They found also that these responses are preserved qualitatively during conditioning, postconditioning, and overtraining. On error trials, a depression of activity was seen at the time in which a reward would have been given (Ljungberg, Apicella, and Schultz 1991). Moreover, depletion of dopamine from the dorsal striatum in rodents impairs their ability to learn a cued-choice task (Robins et al. 1990) similar to our cued-saccade task (chapter 10). The relatively high level of NMDA receptors in striatum (Monaghan and Cotman 1985) and the observation that striatal NMDA receptor density varies inversely with striatal DA levels in PD patients (Weilhmuller et al. 1992) suggest a relation between DA and learning-related corticostriatal plasticity.

Thus, it appears that phasic, reward-related DA activity participates in long-term modification of corticostriatal synapses that link contextual sensory inputs with striatal cells involved in producing the correct behavior. Both LTP and LTD have been observed in the striatum, and at least LTD has been observed to require specifically the presence of dopamine (Calabresi et al. 1992a). Repetitive activation of cortical inputs produces LTD in striatal cells wherein NMDA channels are inactive and LTP in those wherein NMDA channels are active—effects that can be observed readily by manipulating the Mg^{2+} NMDA block (Calabresi et al. 1992b; Walsh and Dunia, in press). We can simplify this by saying that sufficient depolarization (which removes the Mg^{2+} block of the NMDA receptors) in striatal cells makes these cells candidates for LTP in the presence of additional cortical input, whereas insufficiently depolarized cells will be candidates for LTD. The role of dopamine in reinforcement is related intimately to studies of its role in addiction (Dichiara 1995; Self and Nestler 1995).

In chapter 10, we consider a model in which reinforcement is used to adjust the strengths of synapses from the inferotemporal cortex (IT, part of the visual system) to the caudate nucleus (CD, part of the striatum). If the monkey is correct in a visual-motor task, it is rewarded with a squirt of juice. Our hypothesis is that the effect of reward is such that dopamine is released by SNc to serve as the reinforcement term in a learning rule that describes the plasticity of the IT → CD synapses. The rule says that at active CD cells, when dopamine is released, synapses from active IT cells will be strengthened (LTP), whereas those for other IT cells will be weakened (LTD) to yield a normalization effect with overall synaptic strength remaining the same.

The formal model is expressed by the equations:

$$\mathbf{w}_{ij}(t+1) := \mathbf{w}_{ij}(t) + DA\_Modulation *$$

$$(RewardContingency - 1) * C1 * F_i * F_j \quad (6)$$

$$\mathbf{w}_{ij}(t+1) := \mathbf{w}_{ij}(t+1) * \frac{\sum_j \mathbf{w}_{ij}(t)}{\sum_j \mathbf{w}_{ij}(t+1)} \quad (7)$$

where the ":=" denotes assignment rather than equality. F_i and F_j are the firing rates of the IT and caudate cells, respectively, and $\mathbf{w}_{ij}$ is the strength of the synapse connecting IT cell i to caudate cell j. (The term $DA\_Modulation$ expresses a role of dopamine complementary to its role in learning [see sec. 10.5.1].)

We simulate the reward-related modulation (which we regard as mediated by dopamine release from SNc) by the term $RewardContingency$, which is 1.5 for correct trials, 0.5 for incorrect trials, and 1 when no reward or punishment is applied, corresponding to the increases and decreases in SNc activity for reward and error trials, respectively (Schultz 1989). The term $(DA\_Modulation * (RewardContingency - 1))$ will be positive on rewarded trials and negative on error trials. C1 is a constant that specifies the learning rate and is set to $2.5e^{-5}$.

Weight normalization conserves the total synaptic weight that each IT cell can distribute to its striatal synapses (equation 7). If, after learning has occurred, one synapse from cell i to cell j was increased then, since the total synaptic weight from cell i is conserved, the result of this increase is a small decrease in all other synapses from i. Similarly, when a weight is decreased owing to an incorrect response, the other synapses from i are increased. Via this normalization, postsynaptic cells compete for influence from presynaptic cells, producing cue discrimination. Especially in the case of rewarded trials, equations 6 and 7 approximate how LTP may occur in the most active postsynaptic cells (via equation 6), and LTD in the others (via normalization, equation 7).

6.4 Hippocampal Function and Cognitive Maps

6.4.1 Spatial Representation and Cognitive Maps in Rats

Rats are highly exploratory. In a new environment, they tend first to explore outward from some base, then to shift to other bases until they become highly adept at navigating from one place to another, visiting sites where food has been taken and returning to inaccessible hiding places (figure 6.7). Rats entering one arm of a T-

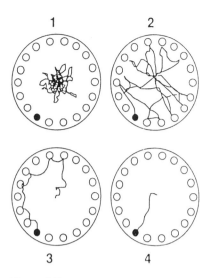

Figure 6.7
Schematic illustration of the typical sequence of behavioral patterns observed on successive days of training at one trial per day on a circular platform apparatus used to assess spatial memory ability in rats. The animals are released from a false-bottomed start chamber onto the center of a brightly illuminated white circular platform around which is placed an array of visual cues. Beneath one of 18 peripherally located holes is a dark tunnel into which the naturally photophobic rats are motivated highly to escape. The maze surface is rotated randomly from trial to trial, but with the tunnel fixed relative to the corotating visual cue array. (From McNaughton and Nadel 1990.)

maze will tend to choose the other arm on the next exposure ("spontaneous alternation"). A landmark is not merely a stimulus to be approached for a reward; rats remember headings relative to the landmark and can use the position of a number of objects toward which to navigate (e.g., a food source or hiding place). In the water maze (Morris 1981), a rat can use such cues to swim to a platform located beneath opaque water.

Rats exhibit a working memory structured by a "map" of their environment. For example, a rat can remember with considerable accuracy which of 17 arms in a radial maze have been visited recently (Olton and Samuelson 1976) if it takes food that is not replaced on visiting each arm. Kesner and Novak (1981) forced rats to collect food in a random order from the eight arms of a radial maze. Subsequently, the animals were rewarded for choosing between the earliest visited of the eight arms. Normal rats could choose successfully the first arm in preference to the second and the seventh in preference to the eighth. They could not distinguish between the third and fourth arms visited. Rats with hippocampal lesions could distinguish between the more recent of the seventh or eighth arms but not between the first and second. This finding supports the idea that there is a rather coarse temporal dimension to the spatial map.

O'Keefe and Conway (1980) trained rats to find food in one arm of a plus-shaped maze, the arm defined by its position relative to visual cues external to the maze. Having learned this, the animal would choose the correct arm even if started from a novel starting point. This counters Hull's view (1943) that navigation is achieved exclusively by following a list of stimulus-response-stimulus steps but (see next section) does not preclude the notion that the animal may use remembered motor sequences in some circumstances.

Collett, Cartwright, and Smith (1986) taught gerbils to find buried food. If they learned that food was buried equidistant between two landmarks and these landmarks then were placed farther apart, the gerbils tended to search at two points each near the original distance from one of the two landmarks, suggesting that the animal encodes the vectors linking the goal to each landmark. If the vectors agree, the correct location is searched. If conditions change, a subset of vectors (perhaps supplemented by heading information) may determine a set of search sites. However, this hypothesis is silent on the nature of these vectors. The preceding data suggest that the components of the vector specifying a given place include the size and placement of visual cues for salient objects in the vicinity of that place. Not only can rodents locate themselves by visual cues for object size and placement; they also can update this estimate of location as they move. Mittelstaedt and Mittelstaedt (1980) showed that rodents can combine vestibular input and "efference copy" to integrate a complex search path so that a direct return path could be taken in darkness (i.e., in the absence of spatial cues).

All these findings suggest that rats have associative memory for complex stimulus configurations, can encode the spatial effect of their own movements, and are able to form sequences of actions to go from a starting location to a goal. In other words, rats have a *cognitive map*. To understand this notion (introduced by Tolman 1932, 1948 to explain place learning in rats, including the rat's ability to perform shortcuts), first we must distinguish *egocentric* representations from *allocentric* representations. The former, based on the organism's current view of the world, are appropriate for looking, reaching, grasping, and locomotion with respect to directly visible features of the landscape. The latter can be understood in terms of a road map used by the driver of a car. Such a map is not drawn from the viewpoint of any driver but nonetheless sets out the spatial relations between different places and the roads that link them. To go from this familiar type of map to a cognitive map we must augment the map with the processes needed to use it. To use a road map, we must be able to locate the representations of where we are and where we want to go on the map and then find on the map a path that we can use as we navigate toward our goal.

In sum, the ingredients of a cognitive map are (1) an allocentric spatial framework, (2) a mechanism for the animal to locate itself and places of interest (e.g., goals) in that framework, and (3) the means to combine current location and intended movement so as to infer new location (or current location and desired location to infer movement). We shall discuss in some detail the hippocampal "place" cells that fire when the animal is in a certain place in its environment and shall see that these cells may be activated when the animal views an arrangement of cues normally seen from that position—an apparently egocentric representation. How does this square with item (1)? As so often happens, the distinction between the two concepts is not clear-cut. A piece of paper is not a useful map without indicators of what point corresponds to what. Imagine a map like the car-driver uses, but with a view of the scene as one drives past a place in a specific direction rather than the name of the nearest town to label the point that represents the place and side of the highway on which one traverses it. Place cells seem to lie on the path from visual input to activation of the region of the map that represents the given location.

Because all this discussion must serve motivated exploration, we are interested in two related issues: how a cognitive map is used and (the learning issue) how it is acquired and updated. In the next section we look at a general answer to these questions (provided by Arbib and Lieblich 1977; Lieblich and Arbib 1982). Then, we turn to data pertinent to the question, "Does the hippocampus provide a cognitive map?" The answer will be that it provides elements of such a map, and we will assess a number of system models and neural network models of this functionality.

6.4.2 World Graphs as Cognitive Maps for Motivated Behavior

The Lieblich-Arbib (L&A) approach to building a cognitive map is based on building a "world graph", i.e., a set of nodes connected by a set of edges, wherein the nodes represent recognized places or situations, and the links represent ways of moving from one situation to another.

A node is created whenever the animal recognizes a distinctive place or situation, and it is coupled with a perceptual schema for that place or situation. A crucial point is that a single place might be encountered in different circumstances and thus be represented by several distinct nodes; these nodes may be merged, drastically restructuring the world graph, on discovery of the fact that the nodes correspond to the same place. In this regard, it is interesting to note that place cells seem to be direction-specific for places in a maze but not for places in an open field. In a neural network model, where would the linking of views to places be carried out? The linkage of views by "just turn around" offers one solution, with subgraphs of related nodes becoming "super nodes."

Tagging the Node with a Motivational Valence

A "place" becomes a "goal": Nodes can be formed during random exploration for any place that is distinctive. However, the schema for a node is not restricted to a perceptual schema but also includes relevant information, such as "a place to eat," "a place to drink," or "a place to get an electric shock." As a result, a node can become a place to approach or avoid but with approach behavior dependent on the drive-state of the animal.

Linking Places

Exploratory behavior not only leads to creation of nodes but to creation of links characterized by motor schemas for getting from one place to another. Thus, the world graph is posited to represent the information necessary for goal-directed behavior: the movement from the current position to some currently desirable goal.

Behavior

L&A use animal data to compare different strategies whereby the animal might choose a path through a maze to reach a currently relevant goal while avoiding known aversive stimuli. As we saw earlier, a rat can remember not to search for food in places where recently it has eaten the available store; thus, the L&A model needs extension to include working memory information, and stable perceptual and motor schemas and goal information at world graph nodes.

6.4.3 Does the Hippocampus Provide a Cognitive Map?

Rats with damage to the hippocampal system still can learn many tasks, including those that normally would be classified as spatial. This capability has led some to conclude that the hippocampus is not a spatial system (e.g., Olton, Becker, and Handelmann 1979a). To clarify this difference, O'Keefe and Nadel (1978; see also O'Keefe 1991) distinguished between two paradigms for navigation—one based on routes and the other based on maps—and proposed that independent neural systems exist in the brain to support these two types of navigation. They called these systems the *taxon (behavioral orientation) system* for route navigation (*taxis* is the biological term for an organism's response to a stimulus by movement in a particular direction) and the *locale system* for map-based navigation, and they proposed that the locale system resides in the hippocampus. Later, we will qualify the latter assertion, showing how the hippocampus may function as *part* of a locale navigation system (i.e., cognitive map).

O'Keefe and Nadel (1978) take the map to be an explicit euclidean description of the environment in a coordinate system based on the world; they propose further that the map is a complete and homogeneous representation for an environment rather than being a collection of independent fragments or sets of associations between movements and local views. However, anyone who has used a subway map knows that it is neither euclidean nor complete, though it must contain sufficient information to plan a reasonably short route from one station to another. Again, a map need not be homogeneous, we may know a route very well from one side of town to another and yet know little of the placement of individual houses save in our immediate neighborhood. Thus, the inclusion of landmarks is based on some combination of need and familiarity rather than on some homogeneous criterion for representation. We suspect that this must be true of the rat's cognitive map, too.

Evidence for a nonhippocampal taxon system includes the observation that both normal and hippocampal-lesioned rats can learn to solve a simple T-maze in the absence of any consistent environmental cues except its T shape. If anything, the lesioned animals learn this problem faster than do normals (O'Keefe 1991). After criterion was reached, probe trials with an eight-arm radial maze were interspersed with the usual T-trials. Animals from both groups consistently chose the side to which they were trained on the T-maze. However, many did not choose the 90-degree arm but preferred either the 45- or the 135-degree arm, suggesting that the rats had solved the T-maze by learning to rotate within an egocentric orientation system at the choice point through *approximately* 90 degrees. This finding leads to the hypothesis that an orientation vector is stored in the animal's brain, with the actual turn depending on environmental cues to determine the appropriate movement most consonant with the encoded orientation.

With the short (approximately 1-minute) intertrial intervals used in this study, well-trained lesioned rats readily learn to reverse the T-maze habit. During reversal, every third trial was a probe with the eight-arm radial maze to assess the position of the orientation vector at that stage of learning. Fornix-lesioned animals show a steady, incremental shift in the direction of the orientation vector, from the original quadrant straight ahead and into the new reversal quadrant, with the shift from one arm to the other in the binary-choice T-maze occurring at approximately the point at which the continuous sweep of the vector crosses the midline.

Such behavioral data do not tell us where or how the orientation vector is stored. One possible model would employ coarse coding in a linear array of cells, coded for turns from −180 degrees to +180 degrees. The animal's turn then would be to the available direction closest to that encoded by the "center of mass" of the neural activity in this array. From the behavior, one might expect that only the cells close to the preferred behavioral direction are excited and that learning "marches" this peak from the old to the new preferred direction. However, it requires a simpler learning scheme to "unlearn" −90 degrees, say, by reducing the peak there, while at the same time building a new peak at the new direction of +90 degrees. If the old peak has mass $p(t)$ and the new peak has mass $q(t)$, then as $p(t)$ declines toward 0 while $q(t)$ increases steadily from 0, the center of mass

$$\frac{(-90)p(t) + 90q(t)}{p(t) + q(t)} \tag{8}$$

will progress from −90 to +90, fitting the behavioral data. Note that because actual behavior involves choice of the arm nearest to this intended direction, the representation provides constraints and biases on the distance and direction of movement rather than on exact prediction or control.

The determination of movement direction is modeled easily by a reinterpretation of the Arbib and House (1987) model of frog detour behavior (sec. 3.2.2). In it, prey were represented by excitation coarsely coded across a neural population, whereas barriers to movement were encoded by inhibition whose extent was closely linked to the retinotopic extent of each barrier. The resultant sum of excitation was passed through a winner-take-all circuit (WTA; see sec. 3.2.1) to yield the choice of movement direction. In many cases, the result was that the direction of the gap closest to the prey, rather than the direction of the prey itself, was chosen for the frog's initial movement. We may use exactly the same model for the behavioral orientation system once we replace the direction of the prey (for the frog) by the direction of the orientation vector (for the rat), while the barriers correspond to directions in which no arm of the maze is visible. Here, an imprecise specification of the direction of movement is refined by current sensory data regarding the environment so as to yield an appropriate course of action.

During reversal training, control rats show a large increase in latency in the early trials of reversal, though this is not seen in the lesioned rats. Another difference was that the underlying orientation vector of the group did not shift in a smooth fashion but jumped around. Examination of the individual curves failed to reveal any systematic shifts. All these results suggest that without hippocampus, the rat uses a pure orientation cue, whereas with hippocampus, there is competition and cooperation of the orientation cue with a "view" cue of the kind to be analyzed in our discussion of place cells in the next section. Latency shifts may be measuring slowed dynamics of convergence in the necessary WTA circuitry when conflict increases or data are equivocal.

6.4.4 Neurophysiology of Spatial Representation

Place Cells

The primary neurophysiological evidence for the cognitive map view of rat hippocampus is provided by the most common type of cell encountered in the CA3 and CA1 fields of the hippocampus in the freely moving rat. These *place cells* (O'Keefe and Dostrovsky 1971), mentioned briefly in section 6.2.2, are pyramidal cells that fire when the rat moves to a particular place in the environment. The *place field* of a place cell usually is one contiguous region, but the place field is not homogeneous and is characterized by a gradient of firing. Field firing can be nondirectional when the rat is moving through an open area, but when the animal is moving down an arm of a maze (like, say, a human highway driver), the firing usually depends both on where the animal is and the direction in which it is facing (McNaughton, Barnes, and O'Keefe 1983; Bostock, Muller, and Kubie 1991; O'Keefe and Recce 1993; see figure 6.8). The firing properties of place cells can be manipulated by changing the rat's environment; rotating the major cues in an environment can cause the place fields to move accordingly (O'Keefe and Conway 1978), and increasing the environment's size can cause some of the place fields to expand correspondingly (Muller and Kubie 1987). Place cells also have been identified in primates (Ono et al. 1991).

Thus, the cells are related to view rather than to any euclidean description of space. A cell responds to place with respect to landmarks, so that the cell's view field rotates with the array of landmarks if this array has been

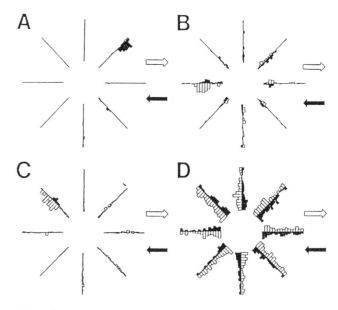

Figure 6.8
Response of hippocampal cells as a rat moves through an eight arm radial maze. The histograms show the average firing rate of a cell at each place in the maze and for each direction of travel. (A, B, C) Pyramidal place-view cells, showing great specificity for place and direction of travel. (D) Inhibitory interneurons, showing no such specificity. (From McNaughton and Nadel 1990.)

rotated. Spatial memory appears dependent on the spatial arrangement of perceptual cues; location (rather than the body turns required) is remembered for goal acquisition; shifts can occur. If the rats first are required to make a detour into one or more nongoal arms instead of being allowed to run directly to the goal, they still choose the goal as defined by its relation to the external world. However, place fields appear to be no more affected by the location of the goal than by the location of any other cues (Speakman and O'Keefe 1990).

Activation of a small percentage of the total synapses onto a dentate granule cell (McNaughton, Barnes, and Andersen 1981) or CA1 pyramidal cell (Andersen et al. 1980) is sufficient to fire the cell. If the perforant path input represents environmental information, each cell would be potentially capable of responding to a large number of combinations of environmental cues. Simultaneous activation of a small percentage of these would increase the potency of each and might explain the finding that some place cells can be activated in the place field by any two of four extramaze cues (O'Keefe and Conway 1978).

The spatial arrangement of the registration cues is important. When the cues are spread around the environment, memory formation is rapid. The same cues bunched behind the goal do not support memory (O'Keefe and Conway 1980; O'Keefe, Conway, and Schenk 1983). It appears that the former cue arrangement lends itself to place learning, whereas the latter is learned most easily by using a taxon hypothesis (i.e., orienting toward the specific cue constellation). Consistent with the taxon hypothesis, fornix lesions disrupt performance on the former but not the latter.

O'Keefe and Recce (1993) found firing of place cells to have a systematic phase relationship to the local EEG. When a rat on a linear track runs through a place field, the place cell fires in a burst, with each successive burst occurring at an earlier phase of the theta cycle. (A cell that fires at phase 360 degrees when the rat enters the place field may fire as much as 355 degrees earlier in the theta cycle when exiting the field). Turning from mechanism to function, McNaughton and Nadel (1990) speculated that the theta rhythm is a mechanism that periodically shuts down the network globally to terminate the previous recall operation and so prepare the system for arrival of the next input. Mizumori et al. (1989) injected procaine hydrochloride (Novocaine) into the medial septal nucleus, the source of subcortical modulatory afferents to hippocampus, and found that during the 15–20 minutes when the theta rhythm was abolished, the animal's memory capacity was impaired severely, whereas spatial selectivity of place cells was impaired highly in CA3 but not in CA1.

When a rat traverses the eight arms of a radial maze (both inward and outward), many hippocampal cells may fire moderately in a number of such places but have a locus and direction wherein activity is strongest, whereas inhibitory neurons have been observed to fire for all places and in both directions (fig. 6.9D). It is important to stress that a given pyramidal cell will have a place field in a highly familiar environment with up to 70% probability. This suggests that place cells do *not* provide a map of the rat's entire world but rather seem to represent a somewhat limited environment. Of course, it may be that a wild rat able to roam freely over a large territory would have a much more varied set of place cells. However, it might also be that the hippocampus is tuned more dynamically to one "chart" of the current locale, thus acting as a chart table rather than as the complete atlas of the rat's world (an idea to which we shall return later).

Wilson and McNaughton (1993) used multielectrode recording in CA1 to demonstrate rapid changes in hippocampal ensemble codes for space during exposure to a novel environment. Three rats were trained for 10 days to forage for small chocolate pellets in half of a rectangular box (A); during this period, the other half of the box (B) was shut off by a partition. The CA1 place representation was found to be sparse: From 30% to 40% of pyramidal cells sampled in each rat showed firing significantly correlated with place in box A; the remaining such cells were silent. It was found that a population code extracted from the population could predict position with reasonable accuracy. By extrapolation from the more limited number of cells actually observed, it appeared that 380 cells would suffice to achieve 1-cm accuracy in the 0.1-sec period of the theta rhythm.

After 10 minutes of exploration in A (phase 1), the partition was removed; 20 minutes (divided into phases 2 and 3) then were allowed for exploration of A + B, prior to 10 minutes in A with the partition restored (phase 4). During phases 2 and 3, the cells that were active for places in A during phase 1 had place-dependent activity highly correlated with that exhibited during phase 1, and the population code for positions in A was unimpaired. However, relatively few cells were active for places in B during phase 2, and the positional code was correspondingly innacurate. In phase 3, the number of cells with place fields in B increased, and the error in the positional code decreased. The average correlation of spatial firing distributions between phases 2 and 3 was low; thus, place fields were initially unstable in B. Spatial firing was correlated highly for phases 1 and 4, showing that the novel experience in B did not affect substantially the representation of A. However, note that place fields of hippocampal neurons can be highly selective to particular environments (Thompson and Best 1989), with spatial codings in general unrelated across different environments and different behavioral paradigms performed in the same environment.

The rapid emergence of cells with place fields for places in B suggests a role for rapid synaptic modification. During phase 2, there was a marked suppresion (up to 70%) of 10 of the 15 inhibitory neurons recorded. This occurred abruptly as the animal entered B; normal firing resumed when the rat crossed back into A. Because inhibition by neurons containing GABA can regulate the extent to which an excitatory input can activate NMDA receptor–based synaptic enhancement (Diamond, Dunwiddie, and Rose 1988), Wilson and McNaughton (1993) suggest that the suppression of inhibitory interneurons may facilitate the synaptic modification necessary to encode new spatial information.

Place cells fire much more frequently when a rat is moving actively in space than when it is passive in one position. Foster, Castro, and McNaughton (1988) trained a rat to remain still when confined in a handtowel, with its head free to look and sniff. Place cells were recorded first while the animal was free to move about a platform and secondly while it was restrained and moved by the experimenter. Under restraint, almost all place-selective activity in hippocampus was abolished. Normal activity returned once the rat was free to move, even if it was not moving, suggesting that motor set is a fundamental determinant of the spatial activity in hippocampus.

Though it would seem more accurate to rename place cells *view cells*, this terminology also is misleading, because these cells are not responsive only to a specific view of the landmarks. Because the converging information that activates the cell comes from multiple modalities and seems to embody a short-term memory, a label such as *context* might be more appropriate. Nonetheless, the term *place cell* is established firmly.

The rat's spatial behaviors are not disrupted by removal of subsets of the dominant spatial cues, and the same is true for the firing of place cells. In the memory task variant of a task with four spatial cues, O'Keefe, Conway, and Schenk (1983) presented the cues for 30 sec while the rat was confined to the start arm. Then cues were removed, and the animal was allowed to make its choice, forcing it to remember the cues' location on that trial. This is a delayed-response task wherein the animal had to remember the places rather than the cues. Many of the animals found this new task rather simple. In one experiment, 12 rats that required a median of 13 trials to learn the perceptual task required only an additional 5 trials (median) to learn the memory task, and there was good retention of the location of the goal for periods of up to 30 min after a 30-sec presentation of the cues.

In this memory task, in which all the cues are removed once the animal has "located" itself, when the rat continues to run on the + maze, the cells fire for the place occupied by the animal as long as the animal made the correct choices. When errors were made, the place fields tended to shift according to where the rat "thought" it was in relation to the cue array. Cues set up the pattern but are not necessary to drive it and can be overridden so that the animal errs. There is also multimodality of place fields: Traversing an arm in the dark, the rat can use tactile cues to determine where it is in the arm (but not in which arm it is), leading to firing of some place cells corresponding to that position on different arms, though failing to reach threshold for other place cells.

All these considerations show that place cell activation depends on pattern completion (i.e., a place cell can be activated by a subset of its multimodal cues) and on updating of working memory (i.e., in the absence of visual cues, the animal can use efference copy to update its estimate of its position).

The latter requirement—updating of working memory—is related to the Dominey and Arbib (1992) model of working memory and dynamic updating for saccades (sec. 8.4.2), but here bodily movements replace eye movements, and "views" replace retinotopic points. Moreover, as in the L&A model, a graph of landmarks replaces the retinal "continuum."

Where is the Goal?

Forming a map requires the joining of disparate environmental cues, which activity presumably takes place during exploration. The nature of place cell firing thus raises immediate problems for their use in navigation, because navigation requires having access to information about the location of the goal; a representation of the rat's own position in space is not enough. Although Ranck (1973) reported that some hippocampal complex spike cells fired when the rat drank water or approached water sources, O'Keefe and Conway (1978) did not find the role of food or water to be markedly different from other cues that identify the location of a place field. This finding suggests that coding for the reward or incentive value of places within an environment takes place elsewhere (e.g., in amygdala and orbitofrontal cortex).

Unfortunately, there are scant reports to date of the existence of the postulated destination cells; access to the firing of a place cell can be gained only by the rat's visiting (or "believing" it is visiting) that place. Although the background activity recorded from the place cells outside their place field may reflect connections between the place cells, perhaps via axon collaterals (see Kubie and Ranck 1983), this possibility does not provide any mechanism for choosing a movement toward a goal nor for updating the place representation with movement (see the earlier discussion of Wilson and McNaughton 1993). This finding suggests that to obtain a cognitive map, the hippocampus must be embedded in a larger system (a theme to which we return in sec. 6.4.5).

We have seen that hippocampal cellular activity is associated with an animal's position within an environment during a place task. In addition (Wiener et al. 1989), the firing rate may depend also on the rat's speed, direction, and turning angle as it passes through the cell's place field. However, hippocampal cells may exhibit quite different activity in different tasks. Eichenbaum et al. (1986) found that in a simultaneous-cue, odor-discrimination task, most cells fired as the rat sampled discriminative cues or when it executed specific, task-relevant approach movements. They observed cue-sampling cells that fire after onset of odor-cue sampling and goal-approach cells that fired prior to arrival at either an odor-sampling port or a reward cup. Wiener et al. (1989) further noted that many cells with distinctive place fields in a place task did not show peak firing in the same place during the odor-discrimination task.

Environmental alterations that change the rat's judgment about the environment result in dramatic and unpredictable effects on the hippocampal spatial representation (Muller and Kubie 1987; Breese et al. 1989; Bostock, Muller, and Kubie 1991). For example, after a stable spatial representation was observed in an environment, a subtle stimulus change at first produced no alteration in the spatial representation but, after multiple comparisons between the original and changed environment were permitted, a new and unpredictable spatial representation appeared for the changed environment (Bostock, Muller, and Kubie 1991). This result is to be contrasted with the findings of Wilson and McNaughton (1993) regarding extending an environment. Their findings raise three points.

First, there is still no evidence that the hippocampus proper (DG and CA) simultaneously can encode the rat's current location and the goal of current navigation. In other words, it may provide a map's "you-are-here" function but not the "this-is-where-you-are-going" and "this-is-how-to-get-there" functions, which thus must depend on a larger system of which hippocampus proper is but one part.

Second, to the extent that is part of a cognitive map, the hippocampus proper seems (to return to an earlier metaphor) more like a chart table than like a complete atlas in the sense that its cells are not linked to fixed places in the entire world but rather to places in the current map of the current environment—and this map may be specific to the current task.

Finally, this consideration suggests at least two alternatives: (1) The different charts are stored elsewhere and must be reinstalled in hippocampus as dictated by the current task and environment, or (2) the cells of hippocampus receive task- and environment-encoding inputs that determine how sensory cues are used to activate a neural representation of the animal's locale.

In either case, we see that these charts are highly labile. Even if we accept position (2), we must note the importance of parietal systems in representing the personal space of humans (see the brief review of neurological data pertaining to parietal function relating to cognitive maps in section 6.4.5). Thus, we must seek to understand cognitive maps in a cooperative computation framework embracing (at least) the parietal cortex and the hippocampus.

Other Cells Related to Spatial Behavior

It is possible to summarize data on a number of other cells related to spatial behavior and found in presubiculum, parietal cortex, and CA1.

Head Direction Cells in Presubiculum Presubiculum contains a significant population of head direction cells (Taube, Muller, and Ranck 1987, 1990) that fire only when an animal's head is pointed in a certain direction, regardless of where the animal is in its environment. If the landmark array is visible, the activity fields of head direction rotate with the landmark array. Such cells could form the basis of an inertial direction sense that computes head orientation and could serve as the basis for computing a novel trajectory to a hidden goal on the basis of knowledge of its relation to a single distal landmark. As such, it might be compared with the "neural integrator" for eye movements (sec. 3.3.1) posited to update the tonic neuron activity that keeps the eye pointing in a given direction and (thus) also serving to provide an "efference copy" that neurally encodes that direction.

CA1 Movement Cells CA1 contains high-frequency cells with small action potentials, coding for movement. When a rat sits quietly, there is little firing and random EEG. When the rat runs, cells burst in synchrony with theta activity in the EEG. These are the interneurons. It has been speculated that the amplitude and phase relations code for movement vectors.

Posterior Parietal Cortex McNaughton, Leonard, and Chen (1989) found a few cells in rat posterior parietal cortex with location specificity and dependent on visual input for their activation. Forty percent of the cells had responses discriminating whether the animal was turning left, turning right, or moving forward (figure 6.9). Some cells required a conjunction of movement and location (e.g., one parietal cell fired more for a right turn at the western arm of a cross-maze than for a right turn at the eastern arm, and these firings were far greater than for all left turns). Another parietal cell fired for left turns at the center of the maze but not for left turns at the ends of the arms or for any right turns. Turn-direction information was varied, with a given cell responding to a particular subset of vestibular input, neck and trunk proprioception, visual field motion, and (possibly) efference copy from motor commands. However, note that in general this location information is more generic than that provided by the place cells; in the next section, we suggest an alternative interpretation to the notion of place-movement cells.

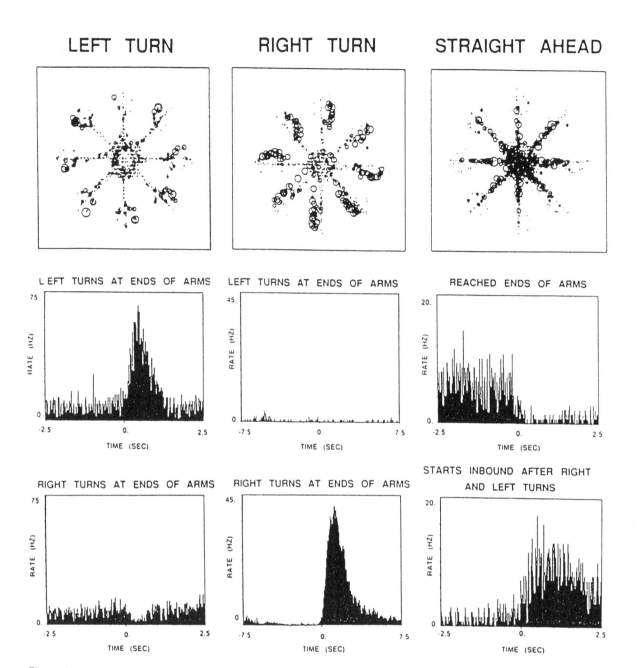

Figure 6.9
Single neurons in the parietal cortex of the rat. Many neurons appear to provide a robust representation of the type of movement of the animal, irrespective of location as it runs an eight-arm radial maze. The cells shown fire most vigorously when the animal is executing a left turn or a right turn or is moving along an arm of the maze, respectively. (From McNaughton 1989.)

6.4.5 Systems Views of the Role of the Hippocampus in Navigation

McNaughton and Nadel (1990; see also McNaughton 1989) provided a systems view of the role of the hippocampus in navigation, providing a transition matrix in which stored representations of local views of the world are linked together by representations of the elementary movements that connect them. The system has four components (figure 6.10a):

1. B provides a spatiosensory input (which may be visual, tactile, or other).

2. A, posited to be in hippocampus, provides a place (local view) representation.

3. L has as output a movement representation and is posited to be in parietal cortex.

4. AL provides a compound place-movement representation and also is posited to be parietal.

However, the parietal cells observed by McNaughton, Leonard, and Chen (1989) are *not* place-movement cells in the sense of *place* in *place cells*. Examples of such a cell's place-movement field are "left turn at end of arm" or "move ahead along arm." To proceed, we must pursue some analogies with the parietal cortex of the monkey. They will lead us to hypotheses about the parietal cortex of rat taking us beyond the data of McNaughton et al. (1989) and suggesting new experiments for behavioral and neurophysiological investigation.

In our discussion of reaching to grasp (sec. 8.4.3), we suggest that the IT of monkey (and by inference, of human) provides at best generic information about how to grasp an object. Also, we suggest that this information can be refined by posterior parietal (PP) cortex that can extract from the visual input a representation of the object's precise *affordances* (Gibson's term for parameters for motor interactions signalled by sensory cues). However, we shall see also that the parietal cortex has areas specialized for a variety of sensory-motor functions, including saccadic eye movements, ocular fixation, and grasping. Other parts of parietal cortex are involved in more purely visual functions, such as shape extraction and (most relevant here) motion extraction (Andersen, Snowden, and Graziao 1991; Graziao, Andersen, and Snowden 1991, 1994; Sakata et al. 1994; Assad and Maunsell, 1995). For example, Andersen et al. (1991) studied the functional properties of rotation-sensitive (RS) neurons of the posterior parietal association cortex in detail. These neurons were localized in the postero-lateral part of parietal cortex, on the anterior bank of the caudal superior temporal sulcus (STS), in the region partly overlapping the medial superior temporal (MST) area. Unlike MST neurons, which seem specific for rotation in a frontoparallel plane, here the neurons were mostly sensitive to rotation in depth. The authors concluded that continuous change of direction of movement was the most important cue for RS neurons to respond selectively to rotary movement in contrast to linear translational movement. Such cells may be the primate analog of cells like those in figure 6.9, which thus may be tuned for patterns of visual movement, without any encoding of place in the sense defined in earlier sections.

These monkey data are complemented by the neurological data on parietal function in relation to human cognitive maps [returning to the territory of the work of Head and Holmes (1911) that brought the term *schema* into the neurological literature (see sec. 3.1.1)]. Bilateral parietal lobe damage often yields global spatial disorientation (Kase et al. 1977). Despite normal language and intellect, these patients have randomly wandering eye movements, they fail to track slow-moving objects with their eyes, and are unable to touch or grasp objects reliably with either hand, overshooting, undershooting, or veering to left or right. In addition, there can be associated disorders of topographical learning and memory; such patients may fail to find their way from corridor to ward and, on being guided to the bed, may be quite unable to orient themselves into a reasonable position for lying down (despite adequate object recognition). Some of these deficits can be seen in relatively "pure" isolated form. Defective localization of stimuli in peripheral vision can be dissociated from generalized visual disorientation (Ratcliff and Davies-Jones 1972), whereas deficits in visually guided maze learning (wherein maze and patient are in a fixed relationship) can be dissociated from locomotor map following, wherein the patient's orientation relative to the environment changes (Ratcliff and Newcombe 1973).

Bilateral parietal lobe patients may be unable to perceive visually more than one object at a time, but this inability to perceive two objects simultaneously (*simultanagnosia*) can coexist with good ability to recognize single objects after bilateral occipitoparietal injury (Luria 1959). In the VISIONS system for visual scene recognition (sec. 3.1.5), the creation of the working memory (short-term memory, STM) not only required the activation of perceptual schema instances with activity level representing the confidence that the corresponding object was present in the environment; it also required that the various schema instances be embedded in a network that indicated where the putative objects were in space. We saw that relative position could provide powerful contextual cues in the competition and cooperation between schema instances. In the same vein, we may note the importance to the animal in the cognitive map studies of the *relative position* of visual cues.

Left-neglect, wherein the patient with right-posterior damage behaves as if the space contralateral to the lesion does not exist, can present in a variety of forms and further fractionates into disorders of extrapersonal and personal space (Bisiach et al. 1986). With respect to personal space, very selective autotopagnosias (difficulty with pointing to the body parts on command) have been reported after left parietal damage (Ogden 1985) in non-aphasic patients.

The fact that visuospatial deficits can be fractionated in humans does not exclude combinations of such impairments after large lesions, nor would it exclude possible selective input disorders after smaller deafferentation lesions earlier in the visual system than parietal cortex. The crucial point here is that the parietal cortex is a

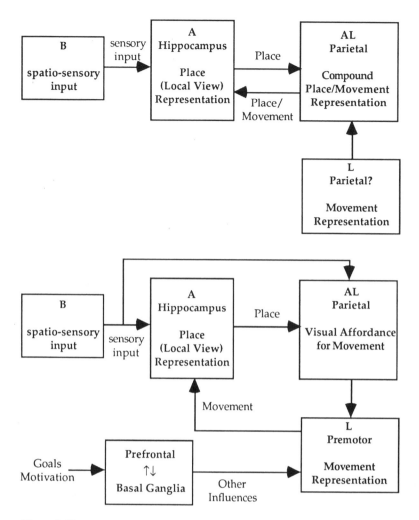

Figure 6.10
(a) A systems view of the role of hippocampus in spatially guided navigation. (Adapted from McNaughton and Nadel 1990.) (b) A recasting of the systems view, making explicit that parietal cortex provides "affordances" rather than explicit place information. See text for further explanation.

complex system involved in a great diversity of subfunctions. With this background, we can return to our critique of figure 6.10a. For McNaughton and Nadel (1990), A not only transforms visual input from B into place cell activity; it also responds to input from AL by transforming the input code of (prior place, movement) into the neural code for the place in which the rat will be after the movement. In the terminology of the next section, these authors model A as a heteroassociative synaptic matrix wherein forcing input (from B) and corresponding output represent spatial locations, whereas the AL output serves as nonforcing input to A, so that prior place-movement pairs become associated with current place.

However, this model becomes untenable if, as we have suggested, the McNaughton-Leonard-Chen cells in parietal cortex are measuring state of motion on the basis of,

say, optic flow. We believe that these cells monitor an animal's progress against its expectations so that the animal can correct its actions or internal representations when discrepancies arise. However, the model in figure 6.10a is meant to be a model of *creating* expectations, not of testing them. Thus, we hypothesize (for future experimental testing) that the parietal cortex of the rat *also* contains affordance cells for locomotion and navigation (akin to those documented in the monkey for reaching and grasping). Our systems level model (see figure 6.10b) thus has the cells in area AL (parietal cortex in both versions of figure 6.10) code for affordances rather than place-movement pairs. (The McNaughton-Leonard-Chen cells would be part of a supplementary circuit, not shown here, for checking expectations.)

We also take further note of ideas developed in sec. 8.4.3. It has been found that the grip affordance cells in

the anterior intraparietal sulcus (AIP) project to grip premotor cells in region F5 of premotor cortex (area 6).
Rizzolatti et al. (1988) described various classes of F5
neurons, each of which discharge during specific hand
movements (e.g., grasping, holding, tearing, manipulating). Thus, whereas figure 6.10a tags the movement representation area as possibly parietal and projecting to
AL, in figure 6.10b it is tagged as premotor and driven
by AL (though we believe there is a return path for
corollary discharge). Once again, the current place is
encoded by the state of A, and we posit that through
training, movement information from L can enable A to
compute the correct transformation from current place to
next place. Note the difference:

The response of A in figure 6.10a to input from AL
does not depend on its internal state; its response to AL
input [place(t), movement(t)] is place ($t + 1$).

In figure 6.10b, the response of A to input from L *does*
depend on its internal state: Its response to L-input
movement(t) when its internal state currently represents
place(t) is place ($t + 1$).

Thus, whereas the McNaughton-Nadel model has A
learn to function as an input-output map $X \rightarrow Y$, our
model has A learn how to function as an automaton
$Q \times X \rightarrow Q$ in the sense of our quasi-formal overview of
schema theory (sec. 3.1.2).

Note that in either model, the loop via AL can, in
absence of sensory input, update the place representation
in A, with the cycle continuing until errors in this *expectation* accumulate excessively (e.g., with respect to pattern correction provided by tactile cues). What neither
model explains is how the rat's brain can choose its next
movement on the basis of its current position relative to
its goal. The resolution may involve some form of planning based on a potential field approach that integrates
view of obstacles and other environmental affordances
(the Arbib and House model of sec. 3.2.2) with world
graph constraints (the L&A model of sec. 6.4.2). The
world graph provides a model for motivation-dependent
transition from local view to movement to next local
view to next movement, and so on. This model is supported by two facts presented earlier: In some situations,
place cell firing depends on the rat's direction (and therefore its local view); and place cells can continue to fire
in the correct places after all the salient cues in an environment have been removed (or the lights have been
switched off). The model shows how a route (possibly of
many steps) may be chosen and lead to the desired goal,
how short cuts may be chosen, and why (through its
account of node merging) in open fields place cell firing
does not seem to depend on direction. A neurally real-

ized updating of the model must take into account that
hippocampectomised rats are capable of simple route-
following strategies.

The CRAWL model (Touretzky and Redish 1996)
illustrates interactions among navigational subsystems,
namely the place code, the head direction system, and
the path integrator. Visual perception provides the type,
range, and bearing (T_i, r_i, ϕ_i) of each landmark. The local
view system computes allocentric bearings ϕ_i by adding
in the current head direction Φ_i, available from the head
direction system. The retinal angle, or bearing difference,
between pairs of landmarks $\alpha_{ij} = \theta_i - \theta_j$ also is computed
as part of the local view. Position $\langle x^*, y^* \rangle$ is maintained
by the path integrator in cartesian coordinates, though
polar coordinates seem more plausible (though in either
case, once a plausible neural population code is found,
the choice of a pair of coordinates may or may not make
computational sense). The path integrator refers to Φ_i to
update its position estimate. CRAWL is assumed to receive information about an animal's movements via an
efference copy of motor commands, but it also may use
vestibular sensations or visual cues, such as optic flow,
to estimate the magnitude of movements.

In CRAWL, the place code is realized as a set of place
units wherein activity levels are products of gaussian
response functions tuned to $\langle r_i, \phi_i \rangle$ values, retinal angles
α_{ij}, and path integrator coordinates $\langle x^*, y^* \rangle$. Because
these units are tuned to enough visuospatial parameters
to localize a point in space, they exhibit visually controlled place fields. A critique of this coordinate-based
model must point out the *gradual* emergence of place
fields when the animal enters a new territory, suggesting
that hippocampus (HC) is not necessary for path integration. In fact, one might imagine that this non-HC
place signal helps train HC place cells by rewarding the
association of views associated with a given place as
determined by the path integrator. Another issue is the
resetting of the integrator when a new base of exploration is established. In general, we may use both a set of
landmarks and a path integration appropriate to a few of
these landmarks.

A major question that CRAWL does not address is,
"How is the place code learned?" The model requires
that a code exist with a sufficient number of place units
associated with each location in the environment. The
simulations use an iterative procedure to construct a
place code. At each step, it picks a random location in
the arena and initializes the path integrator to those
coordinates. Then it calculates the local view from that
location and activates the current population of place
units by using both landmarks and path integrator input.

If too few units become active, it recruits a new unit, sets its path integrator coordinates to the current location, and picks a pair of currently visible landmarks at random to generate the distance, bearing, and retinal angle features. Then the process repeats until no new unit has been recruited for 20 successive steps, indicating that the set of place cells it has constructed is sufficient to cover the environment.

In the study, CRAWL is shown to replicate several behavioral and physiological results. For example, the model explains place cells firing in the dark. CRAWL also is explicit about interactions of multiple spatial representations but does not provide an explicit behavior. In a typical simulation, a rat is placed at a random position of the environment. Then it is allowed to localize itself and predict the goal location. This process is repeated 100 times, and the main simulation results are given as histograms of the goal predictions.

Finally, Touretsky and Redish (1996) made a series of predictions on the basis of the simulation results provided by CRAWL. They consider two to be the most important.

On reintroduction into a familiar environment, the place code will be initially inconsistent. After some (short) time, the place code will return to being consistent. In ambiguous environments, place cells should show a multimodal distribution of activity during the transitory initial period.

Additionally, the place code will shift before the animal changes goal locations.

6.4.6 Synaptic Matrix Models of Hippocampus

In section 4.5.2, we presented a number of general results on the use of synaptic matrices as associative memories. In this section, we review a number of models of hippocampal circuitry based on synaptic matrices. Figure 6.11 motivates this notion: Rolls (1987) sees hippocampus as comprising several synaptic matrices.

First, the granule cells of the DG receive perforant path input from ENT (which in turn receives input from neocortex via the parahippocampal gyrus). Rolls views this synaptic matrix as a *competitive learning network* enabling selection of a sparse set of DG cells to represent each pattern entering on the perforant pathway.

Further, the CA3 pyramids receive sparse inputs from DG and perforant path input. Recirculation of CA3 on itself may serve an autoassociative memory allowing efficient completion of patterns in, say, three iterations (which seems to be the time allowed). One may consider CA3 as having three input types: contextual, noncontextual, and reentrant. Rolls believes that recurrent col-

laterals in CA3 of hippocampus are crucial to episodic memory. CA3 recurrent collaterals have Hebb synapses.

The CA1 neurons are driven by CA3 output. Recently, Liao, Hessler, and Malinow 1995 demonstrated activation of postsynaptically silent synapses during pairing-induced LTP in CA1 in a hippocampal slice, suggesting that training may recruit synapses wherein initial weight effectively is zero.

Finally, subiculum cells receive input from CA1 and project to entorihinal cortex and thence to the parahippocampal gyrus and on to neocortex. There are cells that require complex inputs (e.g., visual and parietal input in certain combinations).

Events are encoded as patterns of firing across a population of neurons. As we have seen, distributed information processing has advantages: completion of an incomplete pattern, generalization, graceful degradation after the system is damaged, and speed. However, it is possible to form associations in distributed matrix memory systems only if the neuronal representations of the stimuli have been orthogonalized at least partly to minimize interference.

Marr (1971) proposed a theory stating how the hippocampus could provide a memory function. The general form of synaptic matrix (figure 6.12) employed by Marr was also used in his models of cerebellum and cerebral cortex, though with different neurophysiological correlates. In the cerebellar theory (Marr 1969; see sec. 9.3.2), each Purkinje cell (the output unit of the cerebellar cortex considered as a *synaptic matrix*) receives input from 200,000 parallel fibers and 1 climbing fiber. The climbing fiber is viewed as the teacher for learning patterns presented on the parallel fibers to the Purkinje cells (see Willshaw and Buckingham 1990 for a critique). This approach uses a modified form of synaptic matrix in which the inputs $\mathbf{x}$ and outputs $\mathbf{y}$ are binary vectors, and the neurons have "floating" threshold $\langle \mathbf{x} | \mathbf{x} \rangle$.

A set of principal cells (PCs), whose output is to convey the desired response, each receives input pattern $\mathbf{x}$ on a set of parallel fibers. Another set of fibers, one per PC (see the relation of climbing fibers to Purkinje cells [also PC] in the cerebellum) carry the vector $\mathbf{y}$ via detonator synapses that force cell P_i to fire if input $\mathbf{y}_i$ is active. This yields a hebbian "print now" that sets the jth synaptic weight $\mathbf{w}_{ij}$ on P_i to 1 if both $\mathbf{y}_i$ and $\mathbf{x}_j$ are equal to 1, and is otherwise 0. Thus, the synaptic matrix is defined by the vector product $\mathbf{x}^T\mathbf{y}$ (see equation 38 of sec. 4.5.2).

A third input comes from a single inhibitory neuron (corresponding to a Golgi cell in the cerebellar theory) that divides the activation parameter of each PC by a

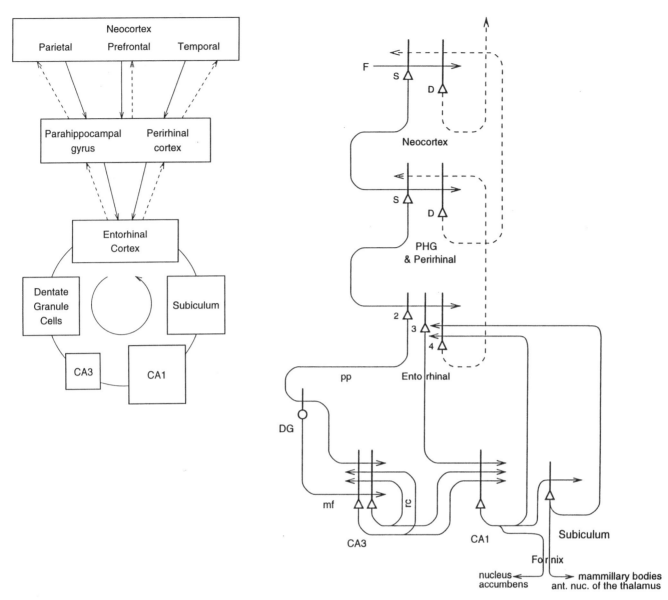

Figure 6.11
Schematic diagram of hippocampal connections. This simplified view of the pathways diagrammed in figure 6.3 preserves those explicitly considered in synaptic matrix models of the hippocampus. CA3, CA1, pyramidal cells. PHG, parahippocampal gyrus; DG, dentate gyrus; mf, mossy fiber; rc, recurrent fibers. Reprinted with permission from E. T. Rolls, A theory of hippocampal function in memory. *Hippocampus*, in press.

term equal to the number of elements of the modifiable input pathway that were active during an event, namely $\langle \mathbf{x} | \mathbf{x} \rangle$ because $\mathbf{x}$ is a binary vector. To ensure proper timing of learning, we must assume that the delay for the PCs to generate output is substantially greater than that required for the inhibitory cells, so that the output indeed will be normalized properly. The model requires *divisive* inhibition, not subtractive inhibition. (Other tasks may require different interneurons playing a subtractive role.) If each PC has unit threshold,

$$\mathbf{y}_i = 1 \text{ if } \sum \mathbf{w}_{ij}\mathbf{x}_j \geqslant \langle \mathbf{x} | \mathbf{x} \rangle, \text{ and is otherwise } 0 \qquad (9)$$

If $\mathbf{W}$ has been trained only with $\mathbf{x}$ and $\mathbf{y}$ so that $\mathbf{W} = \mathbf{x}^T\mathbf{y}$, "input" $\mathbf{z}$ yields output $\mathbf{y}\mathbf{x}^T\mathbf{z}/\langle \mathbf{z} | \mathbf{z} \rangle$, and this equals $\mathbf{y}$ when $\mathbf{z} = \mathbf{x}$, because $\mathbf{x}^T\mathbf{x} = \langle \mathbf{x} | \mathbf{x} \rangle$. Thus, for input $\mathbf{x}$, $\mathbf{y}$ indeed is the correct output. Suppose the input pattern $\mathbf{z}$ is a subpattern of $\mathbf{x}$ (in the sense that if $\mathbf{z}_i = 1$, $\mathbf{x}_i = 1$); then $\mathbf{x}^T\mathbf{z} = \langle \mathbf{z} | \mathbf{z} \rangle$ and the net retrieves $\mathbf{y}$. This is called *pattern completion*.

More generally, several patterns are stored in this manner:

$$\mathbf{W} = \sum_k \mathbf{y}_k \mathbf{x}_k^T \qquad (10)$$

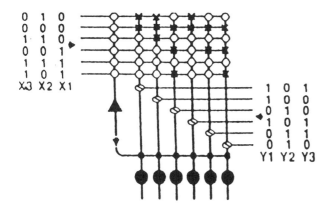

● PRINCIPAL NEURONS

▲ INHIBITORY (DIVISION) NEURONS

Y1 X1 etc INPUT PATTERNS

○ FUNCTIONAL (ENHANCED) SYNAPSE

✕ NONFUNCTIONAL SYNAPSE

⊘ DETONATOR SYNAPSE

■ INHIBITORY SYNAPSE

Figure 6.12
Marr's network model of how associative memory might be implemented in hippocampal circuitry. In addition to the principal cells, sets of powerful, point-to-point inputs (detonators) impose on the network the pattern to be stored. A set of extensively connected inputs with modifiable synapses encode the contexts in which particular principal cells learn to fire. Inhibitory interneurons set the criterion for output on the principal cells. (From McNaughton and Morris 1987.)

and then the output vector corresponding to input $\mathbf{x}_m$ is

$$\mathbf{y}_m + \sum_{k \neq m} (\langle \mathbf{x}_k | \mathbf{x}_m \rangle / \langle \mathbf{x}_m | \mathbf{x}_m \rangle) \mathbf{y}_k \qquad (11)$$

Note that recall will be perfect if each $\langle \mathbf{x}_k | \mathbf{x}_m \rangle$ is close to 0 for $k \neq m$. We say that the net is *saturated* if it has been trained with patterns for which at least one $\langle \mathbf{x}_k | \mathbf{x}_m \rangle$ is not close to 0.

More generally, note that if we insert a pattern $\mathbf{x}$ for which $\langle \mathbf{x}_k | \mathbf{x} \rangle \approx 1$ while $\langle \mathbf{x}_m | \mathbf{x} \rangle \ll 1$ for $m \neq k$, $\mathbf{x}$ will retrieve $\mathbf{y}_m$. This is the sense of similarity that makes the network an associative memory.

We follow McNaughton and Nadel's 1990 application of the preceding type of synaptic matrix, which they call a *Hebb-Marr network*, to the analysis of hippocampus. They view the hippocampus as a matrix memory, wherein cascades of stages run orthogonally across dendrites, creating modifiable synapses with a low probability. Recurrent collaterals are used to generate LTP by running the output of some stages back as input to other stages. CA3 pyramidal cells are used for processing the

input to the memory, and CA1 pyramidal cells accept the outputs of CA3 cells to bring all the processing together to a final result. Schaffer collaterals from CA3 thus provide CA1 cells with a sparse matrix of synapses, which may form an associative net.

What, then, is the evidence for detonator cells, excitatory cells strong enough to coerce another cell to fire, and for inhibitory division by interneurons? The evidence that in the radial maze, inhibitory neurons fire for all places and in both directions is consistent with the notion that inhibitory cells should not be place-coded because they only signal overall level of activity. In this regard, note that it is primarily the inhibitory neurons that are modulated by a variety of subcortical inputs from systems wherein the main function appears to be an involvement in the mediation of attention and arousal. McNaughton and Nadel (1990) claim that at least one major class of inhibitory synapses in hippocampus is divisory. The equilibrium potential for the chloride-conducting, GABA$_A$-mediated, inhibitory synapses is near to the resting potential of most hippocampus neurons recorded in vitro. Thus, these actions shunt (short circuit) the membrane of the cell at its spike trigger zone, so that any excitatory current crossing this membrane will generate a voltage change that is roughly inversely proportional to the strength of the inhibitory input. Antidromic activation of granule cells in DG (McNaughton 1989) results in massive activation of the inhibitory neurons via the recurrent collateral of the granule cell axon. This activity causes a complete inhibition of the evoked discharge of the granule cells when the perforant path is stimulated some tens of milliseconds later. However, there is no effect on the size of the synaptic field potential, as there should be if the inhibition were acting in a subtractive manner. Other evidence supports the claim that inhibitory cells in the pyramidal layers of hippocampus respond sooner than do principal cells to afferent activation. DG has 10^6 granule cells (output cells) and 10^4 basket cells (inhibitory interneurons) per hemisphere in the rat. A double stimulus (25-msec separation) to the perforant path afferent fibers yields a first response, with a sharp negative component reflecting the postsynaptic discharge of the granule cells, but the "population spike" is abolished on the second response because of the inhibition set up by the first stimulus. Single-cell recording shows that cells firing at the time of the population spike (putative granule cells) do not fire to the second stimulus, whereas those firing before the spike (putative inhibitory interneurons) do. However, it is not clear that this evidence is

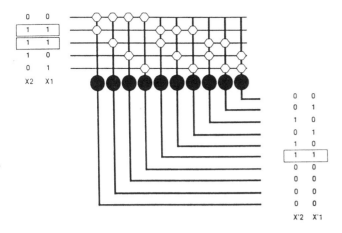

Figure 6.13
The principal underlying orthogonalization of representation vectors, using Marr's codon expansion. Two input patterns that overlap considerably are projected onto a larger system. The resulting output patterns overlap less than do the inputs. (From McNaughton and Nadel 1990.)

sufficient to show that the inhibition in this system does perform the necessary division in the form required by a Hebb-Marr network.

We now turn to the key problem of avoiding saturation in the associative memory, finding an efficient recoding to orthogonalize the representation so that different vectors will have small overlap and yield the desired result that $\langle \mathbf{x}_k | \mathbf{x}_m \rangle$ is close to 0 for $k \neq m$. Marr's technique of codon expansion is to project the representations from one set of neurons to a larger set, with the number of active elements the same in both codings, but with the connections so arranged that the proportion of shared elements is smaller in the second population. To this end, note that ENT has $\approx 100,000$ neurons, whereas DG has $\approx 1,000,000$ neurons, which certainly provides a possibility for sparse recoding.

The principal underlying orthogonalization of representation vectors by using Marr's codon expansion is shown in figure 6.13. In this simple example, two input patterns that overlap considerably are projected onto a larger system, each of whose elements responds to subsets of size 2 of the input. The resulting output patterns overlap less than do the inputs (i.e., they are more orthogonal). There is a drawback to this simple solution: To preserve this orthogonality, the higher dimension of the expanded representation vector must be maintained in subsequent processing; this may become biologically expensive. The table in section 6.1.3 summarized the approximate numerical convergence and divergence relations of the main hippocampal circuitry and the anatomical topography of these interconnections. Both Rolls (1987) and McNaughton and Nadel (1990) argued that

the large expansion and divergence that occurs from ENT to DG implements the codon expansion of figure 6.12A. The corresponding compression from DG to CA3 may result in an orthogonalized representation of the same dimensionality as the original entorhinal input, thanks to the highly restricted divergence and parallel geometry of the DG $\rightarrow$ CA3 projection. Thus, the well-known "lamellar" organization of the granule cell projection to CA3 may reflect a mechanism for increasing the difference between the representations of two initially similar events without changing the final size of the neuronal population used to code these events.

6.4.7 Other Neural Net Models

Place Cells as View Cells

Zipser (1986) models the firing rate of a place cell as a function of the sensory input from cues around the edge of a rat's environment by using a simple pattern recognition network. The idea is that, from a particular place in the environment, a cue will project on the retina with a specific size. Input cells are designed to respond to the size on the rat's retina of a particular cue, with a unimodal response peaking at a particular value of retinal size. A place cell's response then is posited to be a linear threshold function of these inputs. The model predicts the characteristic shape of a place cell's firing rate map rather well, including the scaling of place field size with environment size observed in some cells in some environmental set-ups (Muller and Kubie 1987). However, a model place cell would fire equally well even if the cues were moved around, as long as the size of each cue was preserved, and so lacks the crucial property that firing may vary with the animal's orientation. The model offers no ways for cells that code different places to be linked in a way that can serve navigation.

Sharp (1991) addresses the first problem (orientation-dependence) by having two types of cells in the input layer: A type 1 cell is like the inputs in Zipser's model, firing if a particular cue is at a given distance from the rat, but type 2 cells respond only to a particular cue if it is within a certain range of angle from the rat's head; thus, type 2 firing depends on the orientation of the rat. The input layer drives two layers of cells governed by competitive learning dynamics (von der Malsburg 1973; Rumelhart and Zipser 1986); that is, cells are arranged in groups, and only the cell with the greatest net excitatory input in each group fires. In hebbian fashion, whenever both the pre- and postsynaptic cells fire, the synaptic weight is increased; after each time step, the sum of the synaptic weights onto each cell is normalized (see discussion of the need for reversal of LTP in hebbian synapses in sec. 6.3.4). As the simulated rat moves around its environment, competitive learning leads to unsupervised clustering of the input vectors; a cell learns to fire in a portion of the environment in which the inputs (i.e., the distances and angles of cues) are similar. Cells in the same group will fire in different places; cells from different groups can have overlapping firing fields. The size of place fields scales with the size of the environment. Interestingly, if the simulated exploration is restricted to movements consistent with being on an eight-arm radial maze, place cell firing tends to be correlated much more strongly with the orientation of the rat than in the case of unrestricted exploration. However, note that this model still cannot explain the role of place cells in navigation, including their ability to fire in the dark according to where the rat "thinks" it is; we argue that this requires embedding of the place cell circuitry in a more comprehensive system, such as that posited in figure 6.10b.

A Model of Allocentric Location

O'Keefe (1991) argued that the hippocampus uses egocentric information provided by the views that activate place cells to get two types of allocentric information: the centroid of the landmarks and the eccentricity. The centroid is calculated as the average of the vectors (orientation and distance) to the spatial cues, whereas the slope is calculated as the vector difference between pairs of cues. These parameters can be used as the origin and 0 degrees direction of a polar coordinate framework. O'Keefe suggested that the place cell firing represented the vector average of a small number of environment cues (minicentroids), whereas the head direction cells of the dorsal presubiculum represent the cue-pair slopes. He suggested further that two-dimensional vectors could be represented by the activity of single cells as a phasor in which both phase (relative to the theta rhythm) and amplitude would code information. More specifically, if each cycle of theta rhythm is considered as a clock cycle, the amplitude of firing would code for distance, and the phase relative to the clock cycle would code for angle of direction.

In this formalism, summing the output of several neurons performs vector addition, and subtraction is equivalent to a phase inversion of one vector followed by addition. Thus, for example, the rat's place cells could provide a vector $\mathbf{v}(t)$ continually pointing to the centroid of the environment; then, if the "goal" was encountered at time t_g, storing $\mathbf{v}(t_g)$ somewhere outside the

hippocampus would enable the translation vector from the rat to the goal [i.e., $\mathbf{v}(t) - \mathbf{v}(t_g)$] to be calculated by the rat whenever it wanted to go to the goal.

The suggested calculation of the environmental centroid by averaging the centroids of small subsets of cues (minicentroids) gives a plausible interpretation of place cell firing, each responding to a different subset of cues such that its firing rate codes for the proximity of the minicentroid and its phase codes for the angle α between the rat's direction of travel and the direction of the minicentroid. If we assume that phase of firing with respect to theta is given specifically by 360 degrees $- 2^*\alpha$, the model is consistent with the phase shift data on linear tracks (O'Keefe and Recce 1993). Assuming that place field center (i.e., minicentroid) lies slightly off the track, the phase of firing starts at 360 degrees (late in the cycle) and fires progressively earlier, firing as early as phase 0 degrees by the time the rat exits the field.

Models of Navigation

The simplest map-based strategies (as opposed to route-following strategies; see O'Keefe 1991) are based on defining an evaluation surface over the whole environment, on which, assuming "higher is better," gradient ascent leads to the goal (e.g., see Barto and Sutton 1981). These tend to have the problems: (1) To build up this surface, the goal must be reached many times, from different points in the environment; (2) a new surface must be computed if the goal is moved; and (3) the system must perform latent learning (i.e., exploring an environment in the absence of goals in such a way as to improve subsequent performance when searching for a goal).

Already we have noted the head-direction cells of Taube, Muller, and Ranck (1990) and experiments suggesting that goal location seems to be stored in terms of distance and direction from one or more cues (Collett, Cartwright, and Smith 1986) and that animals are capable of homing on the basis of an internal sense of direction rather than on external cues (Mittelstaedt and Mittelstaedt 1980). Some aspects of this are captured by a model of dead-reckoning (McNaughton et al. 1995), in which the hippocampus is invoked to correct cumulative errors in direction by associating the local views at different locations with heading direction.

Muller et al. (1991) posited a functional role for the CA3 recurrent collaterals (each place cell contacting approximately 5% of the others) distinct from being part of an associative memory. Consider a Hebbian mechanism in which pre- and postsynaptic firing within a short interval leads to a small increase in synaptic efficacy, or strength. This activity yields a model of CA3 in which, as a result of place cell firing as the rat moves around, the synaptic strength of a connection between two place cells comes to be proportionately larger as the corresponding place fields are closer. Further development of the model will benefit from an analysis of the eligibility of synapses (see chapter 9) that modifies the Hebbian learning rule. Instead of requiring that presynaptic activity x_i and postsynaptic activity y_j must be coincident for learning to occur, the revised model uses a term $x_i(t)e_j(t - \tau)$, where τ is the last time of activation of the postsynaptic cell, and the eligibility function rises from 0 to its maximum in, say, 150 msec, and then decays back to 0 again. Clearly, then the synaptic strength established between two place cells is greater for cells that encode places relatively near to each other but varies with both distance between the places and the rat's speed of traversal. But how could this information be used to guide navigation? It is attractive to postulate that activation of place cells for both current position and a goal would activate the place cells corresponding to places along the shortest path to the goal. However, as already noted earlier, such activation has not been seen in single unit recordings. Another problem is that if the eligibility interval is relatively short, the range of linkages also would be very short. (For a further discussion of this model, see Traub et al. 1992.)

Clearly, the assumptions made as to the form of the output of the hippocampal system play a crucial role in determining a model. Burgess, O'Keefe, and Recce (1993) base their model of navigation on a population vector coding of direction inspired, for example, by the work of Georgopoulos, Kettner, and Schwartz (1988) who studied cells in motor cortex of monkeys reaching toward a target. Georgopoulos et al. (1988) studied a population of neurons each with a preferred direction in that the neuron fires maximally when the monkey reaches in that direction. The population vector (i.e., the vector sum of cells' preferred directions weighted by the extent to which their firing rates exceed the resting level) approximates the direction of reaching of the monkey (though this correlation does not prove that the cells *encode* the direction of movement rather than simply correlating with them).

Burgess, O'Keefe, and Recce (1993) suggested how the firing of CA1 place cells could be used to create a directional representation for the position of interesting objects (e.g., goals) encountered by a rat during exploration. If the rat uses a group of neurons whose population vector continually points toward the goal, there are two possibilities: a population vector indicating the absolute direction of the goal from the rat (e.g., north) or one indicating the direction of the goal relative to the rat's orientation (e.g., left). The model applies only to open fields in that place cell firing is assumed to be nondirectional and that the rat cannot distinguish between different environments. Their model (figure 6.14) relies on four assumptions:

1. The phase of firing of a place cell with respect to hippocampal theta shifts from late in the cycle (when a rat enters the place field) to early in the cycle (when it leaves the field).

2. Synaptic increment occurs only late in the cycle (i.e., when the rat just enters the field).

3. As for place cells, each goal cell is assumed to fire maximally when the rat traverses a specific goal in a specific direction. The rat performs local exploration of any goals that it finds, crossing its location in many different directions.

4. When the rat crosses a goal location, the goal cell for that goal and direction fires maximally so that synaptic increment occurs in the connections to it.

Between the input layer of CA1 cells and the output goal cells, there is a layer of "subicular" cells. There is a sparse projection from the CA1 to the subicular layer and a dense projection from the subicular layer to the goal cells. All synaptic connections are modeled as *on* or *off*; most connections are initialized to be off and are switched on whenever the presynaptic cell is active and the postsynaptic cell is firing maximally (within the same time step—0.02 sec).

The middle layer of cells in the model are called *subicular* because the subiculum seems a likely site for them, given single-unit recordings (Barnes et al., 1990) showing spatially consistent firing over large parts of the environment. These subicular cells are divided into groups; at each time step, the cells with the strongest excitatory input in each group fire a number of spikes, depending on that input. Overall, the dynamics resemble competitive learning, but the connections stabilize more rapidly and avoid the global normalization of synaptic weights. Importantly, there is no difference in cell and synapse dynamics between exploration and searching.

The firing of place cells is simulated so that whenever a rat is within a place field, the corresponding place cell fires a number of spikes, depending on its proximity to the place field center. As the rat moves about, previous assumption (2) means that place cells active late in a theta cycle tend to have place fields centered ahead of the rat. After brief (random) exploration of an environ-

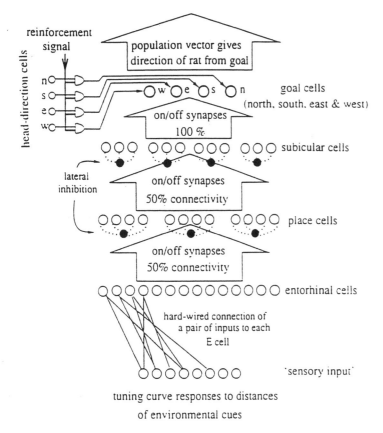

reinforcement signal

head-direction cells

population vector gives direction of rat from goal

n
s
e
w

goal cells
(north, south, east & west)

on/off synapses
100 %

subicular cells

lateral inhibition

on/off synapses
50% connectivity

place cells

on/off synapses
50% connectivity

entorhinal cells

hard-wired connection of a pair of inputs to each E cell

'sensory input'

tuning curve responses to distances
of environmental cues

Figure 6.14
Neural network model of the role of the hippocampus in navigation. Entorhinal input encodes the position of a rat relative to cues placed around the environment. The subicular output provides a population vector that determines the direction in which the rat should move to reach the goal. (From Burgess, Recce, and O'Keefe 1994.)

ment (e.g., 60 sec for 1 sq m), subicular cell firing fields come to resemble the superposition of many place fields (owing to connections from CA1 switching on). The effect of this activity is to overcome the problem of local access of information: The net firing rate map of all the subicular cells active late in a theta cycle resembles a cone, again centered ahead of the rat and covering the entire environment.

The switching on of synaptic connections to goal cells according to preceding assumptions (3) and (4) results in populations of goal cells coding for the position of each interesting object encountered. Each goal cell has a conical firing rate map covering the environment, the peak of which is displaced from the goal position in a particular direction. If we consider the preferred direction of each cell to be the direction from the peak in its firing field to the goal, the population vector of the goal cells gives the absolute direction from the rat to the goal during its subsequent movements throughout the environment. A bonus of this particular representation is that the net firing of the goal cells increases with proximity

to the goal and can be used to estimate how far away it is.

This representation of the direction and distance of interesting objects could be thought of as the output of a map and allows the simulated rat to navigate, returning to previously encountered goal sites. Thus, we have a biologically fairly plausible model of how place cells could be used for navigation; learning is relatively fast and occurs during exploration in the absence of goals (latent learning), and the rat can cover novel parts of the environment on its way to the goal (figure 6.15).

6.5 Hippocampal Function and Human Memory

6.5.1 Procedural Versus Declarative Memory

Bilateral removal of the hippocampus (and nearby structures of the medial temporal lobes) to control severe epileptic seizures in a patient (referred to as HM) yielded a profound retrograde and anterograde amnesia and an apparent inability to form new memories (Scoville and

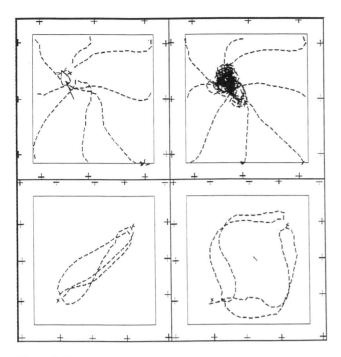

Figure 6.15
Trajectories taken by a simulated rat controlled by the network shown in figure 6.14. (Top) Navigation from eight starting positions toward the goal (x) after the goal has been encountered (left) and subsequent navigation after goal removal, showing localization of search (right). (Bottom) Navigation between two goals (left) and when an obstacle (/) is interposed (right). (From Burgess, Recce, and O'Keefe 1994.)

Milner 1957). However, the picture became more subtle when Milner (1962) observed that HM could learn motor skills. HM also learned mirror tracing though having no recall of having seen the task before. More generally, Squire (1986) argued that amnesics can learn not only motor skills but a larger domain of *procedural* skills or habits (but with no conscious knowledge of having done so) perhaps in the same way in which normal subjects can learn a skill (e.g., a tennis stroke) without conscious recall of the particular plays used to acquire the skill. According to Squire (1986), what HM's amnesia affects is *declarative* learning, the memory of specific events, and this needs hippocampus and mamillary bodies, whereas skill memory does not.

Priming

In studies that helped establish the procedural versus declarative dichotomy for memory, Cohen and Squire 1980 (see also Squire, Cohen, and Zouzounis 1984) showed that amnesics matched normals in their acquisition and retention curves for the skill of mirror-reading complex words but did not recall having learned this skill. Simple classical conditioning and priming also are spared in amnesic patients. In one priming task, a subject is shown a list of words in each of which the first three letters can occur as the prefix of many different words. Shown such a prefix and asked to give (within 2 hours) a word that completes it, the subject will offer the previously exhibited word with 50% chance, even though there would be only a 10% chance of choosing the word without priming. Both amnesics and normals exhibit this skill, but if asked why the word was chosen, a normal will say, "Because you showed it to me," whereas the amnesic's response is, "Oh, it just popped into my head."

Priming involves early-stage processing systems in posterior neocortex. Priming can last over a period of days, rather than for seconds or minutes. Priming by a visual word fragment may be increased if the prime and the test present the fragment in the same case and font. Similarly, using the same voice may enhance auditory priming. Yet, these procedures do not enhance the performance on declarative memory tasks.

Skill Versus Episodic Learning

Episodic memory is based on "one-shot" learning—LTM *without* external rehearsal—wherein training signals presumably cause large changes in synaptic activity. However, note that episodic memory is richer than just forming a "neural snapshot" of the event itself: One also must place it in a temporal context before and after other separable events. In humans this can be enhanced by the ability to check date and time explicitly, 2 PM rather than "just after lunch." Clearly (although some would deny this), we do not have episodic memory for every episode we experience. Drives and emotions can affect what is encoded. Specific details of scene, state of mind, time of day, place, smells, colors, people, outside events—any piece—can evoke the whole. Memory must bind salient details to the episode; then it can retrieve the whole from few details. Here we are reminded of the completion property of associative memory: Synaptic matrix models have the ability to reconstruct recollections on the basis of partial cues, as long as these cues do not interfere. However, the fact that human memories are structured richly by different relationships between different segments of memory poses the earlier binding problem with even greater urgency.

In psychology, it is common to distinguish short-term memory STM from LTM. In the terminology of chapter 3, we view STM (in the sense of what we have called earlier *working memory*) as comprising an assemblage of schema instances both serving as an adaptable structure and being linked to an entire network of knowledge.

STM, then, is not so much a set of recently acquired items as it is a short-term model, a compilation of knowledge of current relevance to the subject. A patient with hippocampal amnesia still can exhibit short-term retention of information and normal social and language skills and memories of the distant past. "Old" schemas still may be instantiated and used, but recently formed schema assemblages are lost (i.e., in retrograde amnesia), and new ones cannot be formed (as in anterograde amnesia). However, this latter assertion has proved to be too simplistic.

One important form of working memory is obtained by holding a particular pattern of firing during a delay task. Such neurons have been found in dorsolateral prefrontal cortex as well as in hippocampus. What distinguishes these two systems? The answer to that question still is far from clear (but see Guigon and Burnod 1995 for a review of relevant models). The usual definition of declarative memory requires that the human be able *consciously to declare* knowledge of related episodes, but must this involve the same relational representation that rats exhibit? Rather, portions of the hippocampus must have co-evolved with those portions of the cortex involved in language so as to coordinate the relational representations of these hippocampal regions with the semantic and syntactic structure of language. [cf. sec. 8.3 of Arbib (1989) for the point that an account of consciousness seems to be a necessary part of any satisfactory account of procedural memory.] In schema-theoretic terms, the perception of a situation or the carrying out of a particular action requires the construction of a particular schema assemblage (*assimilation*, in Piaget's terms); to the extent that the perception or action is problematic, the schemas may become modified to increase the chance of success in similar situations in future (accommodation). We learn both by storing schema assemblages (memory of a specific situation and course of behavior) and by tuning extant schemas. However, it is too facile to say that the former corresponds to fact memory and the latter to skill memory, because skill memory also partakes of some aspects of assemblage formation. That is because skills are tuned versions of programs constructed from prior instructions rather than being only tuning of single previously extant schemas, or single instructions. The fact that a schema may be activated without conscious awareness emphasizes the notion that different neural processes must be involved in monitoring the use of a schema as distinct from the use per se of the schema. The parietal "what" versus IT "how" distinction between visual areas (reviewed in sec. 8.4.3)—one patient may be able to declare the size of an object yet not be able to preshape the hand appropriately to grasp it, whereas another patient may exhibit the opposite behavior—shows that some schemas are instantiated on paths to conscious awareness and others are not. Moreover, at least some of the working memory systems of prefrontal cortex are coupled tightly to specialized areas of parietal cortex and thus are integrated tightly into the procedural "how" system rather than into the conscious-declarative "what" system. Therefore, the loop of explanation must be closed back from the theory of consciousness. This notion is consistent with Rozin's (1976) view that procedural learning may be phylogenetically old, having developed as a collection of encapsulated special-purpose abilities of specific neural systems to register cumulative changes in their functioning. By contrast, the capacity for declarative learning reaches its full development only with the elaboration of medial temporal areas in mammals, especially the hippocampus and related cortical areas. However, earlier we reviewed neurological data regarding parietal function in relation to cognitive maps and suggested that we must seek to understand cognitive maps in a cooperative computation framework embracing at least the parietal cortex and the hippocampus. The hippocampus may mediate updating of the map; then changes may be installed in parietal cortex but on a far slower time scale, as suggested by the data pertaining to consolidation (sec. 6.5.2). One disturbing point for future clarification remains: Our discussion of the "what" and "how" systems (sec. 8.4.3) suggests that the parietal system is nondeclarative as compared to the IT system when it involves discussing the size and orientation of objects. How is this to be reconciled with the view that the hippocampus is involved primarily in human declarative, rather than procedural, memory?

6.5.2 Hippocampus: Forming But Not Storing Memories?

Another property of memory storage is consolidation: Memories are not fixed immediately but rather stabilize over a long period of time. In fact, this process may continue for several years. Patients in whom a seizure has been induced by electroconvulsive therapy behave like amnesiacs after recovering from the seizure. In a test of the effects of electroconvulsive therapy on the ability to remember television programs, Squire, Slater and Chace (1975) found that one hour after the fifth treatment, memory was impaired selectively for programs broadcast one to two years previously, although memory for older programs was normal. Thus, there is both gradual forgetting and a parallel increase in resistance to disruption of the memories that remain.

Because amnesiacs with damage to the medial temporal region can answer questions about their remote life, hippocampus seems unnecessary for retrieval processes or for maintained storage. However, given our repeated stress on cooperative computation, we do *not* claim (as some authors seem to do) that hippocampus has no normal role in these processes. In any case, there must be storage sites other than hippocampus. One hypothesis is that memory is stored in the very neural systems that make use of this stored information. Hippocampus receives input via ENT from many cortical areas and projects back to them in turn. It is one of the few areas to receive input from cortical areas in all modalities. The hippocampus allows data from many parts of cerebral cortex to become associated. External input from different cortical areas provide context.

Mishkin (1982) proposed that the IT is both a site of higher-order visual processes and the site of visual memories resulting from these processes. In our terms, this would say that certain perceptual schemas are instantiated in IT and that the schemas themselves are stored there. We have seen that Rolls (1987) modelled hippocampus as a cascade of associative networks that evaluate the importance of inputs funneling in from cerebral cortex. Further, he uses backprojections (not backpropagation) to signal to cortical areas when the patterns they have just been processing are important enough to merit storage. He hypothesizes that hippocampus makes the cross-modal associations necessary for classification; amygdala and hippocampus provide an orthogonalized backprojection to those very areas of cerebral cortex that provide their input. Backprojections are posited to facilitate Hebbian learning in neocortex, setting down appropriate representations. (Again, we may need a window of eligibility for this to function appropriately.)

Although hippocampus stores information (for hours or days, as long as it is of continuing relevance), it seems that it *also* installs this processed information elsewhere in cerebral cortex for long-term availability. Buzsáki (1989, and in a modified form Buzsáki 1996) suggested an informal model of memory formation in which cortical information is processed in two stages (see sec. 6.3.1). First, during the theta brain state, cortical activity (through the granule cells) weakly potentiates the CA3 pyramidal cells associated to a labile form of memory trace. This weak potentiation initiates population bursts, implying a transition from theta to an SPW state. Under the SPW state, excitatory synapses between pyramidal cells both within the CA3 region and between CA3 and CA1 regions are enhanced. These enhanced synapses would be the substrate of a long-lasting memory trace. Because SPWs and associated high-frequency oscillation in the CA1 region yield discharge of neurons of deep layers of ENT, it seems likely that hippocampal output may affect other neocortical targets, thus transferring information stored temporarily in the CA3 region to the neocortex for long-term storage.

At least in part, this transfer may occur during sleep. Pavlides and Winson (1989) showed that hippocampal cells active during a waking period exhibit increased firing rates in the following sleep period. To investigate this effect in more detail, Wilson and McNaughton (1994) monitored the simultaneous activity of 50–100 CA1 cells during a running period (RUN) and during both the prebehavioral and postbehavioral sleep periods. During the RUN period, cells with overlapping place fields exhibited highly correlated activity; those with nonoverlapping fields did not. Indeed, cells that were coactive during the RUN period showed a far greater correlation than during the prebehavioral period. Moreover, this correlation was reactivated during the postbehavioral period but declined with a time constant of approximately 12 minutes. Wilson and McNaughton (1994) see this as support for the hypothesis that hippocampal activity during sleep exhibits a reactivation of population activity from the prior waking period. Because CA1 has little direct connectivity between pyramidal cells, these authors suggest that the correlations arise in CA3 (which has many intrinsic connections) or in ENT.

In support of the idea that information is transferred from hippocampus to neocortex especially during the synchronized bursts ("ripples") of SPW activity (Buzsáki 1989), Wilson and McNaughton (1994) found during the postbehavioral period that correlations during ripples were significantly greater than were the correlations in the periods between ripples. Chrobak and Buzsáki (1995; Buzsáki 1996) have shown that SPWs and ripples are initiated in CA3 and that the output layers (but not the input layers) of ENT exhibit neuronal activity correlated with CA1 SPWs. Thus, Wilson and McNaughton (1994) suggest that the induced correlations during SPWs arise from modifications within the hippocampus and are propagated to the output layers of ENT.

6.5.3 Motivation

Rolls (1987) noted that it is only after multiple stages of processing that sensory information is interfaced with motivational systems, with other modalities, or with systems involved in association memory. He described this as necessary so that interference due to lack of orthogonality of the stimuli representations can be minimized, with each level of processing acting like finer and finer grades of filters. Neuronal responses representing the reward value of a stimulus (and thus reflecting an output of association memory) are elaborated along the lateral hypothalamus and substantia innominata but are not fully evident until the ventral forebrain neurons.

Amygdala and Orbitofrontal Cortex

Neurons of the amygdala and orbitofrontal cortex of the primate (see Rolls 1987) are involved in associative memory. Orbitofrontal neurons code that particular visual stimuli are associated currently with reward. The amygdala appears to play a role in rapid learning of associations between complex stimuli. Units in this area have been found to respond to reinforcing stimuli. Emotional conditioning involves the amygdala (LeDoux 1992). The amygdaloid complex is linked directly and reciprocally to both sensory-specific and multimodal cortical association areas. The hippocampal formation also has afferent and efferent pathways linking it with cortical areas (see the next subsection for its links to motivational systems). The amygdala projects directly to association cortex, whereas the ENT acts as a funnel whereby the hippocampus communicates widely with cortical association areas.

The orbitofrontal cortex may be partially responsible for fast and reversible associations in visual tasks. Some units responded to stimuli associated with reward. Changes in the response of these units have been seen during the learning of a reversal. A few units responded both when the appropriate stimulus was received and when a reward was given. The information at this layer could be used to determine when an action no longer elicited a positive response, causing a monkey to begin searching for the appropriate response.

Monkeys without an amygdala fail to make normal associations between such stimuli as the sight of food and reinforcement provided, say, by the taste. The amygdala is implicated strongly in associative memory, because it receives high-level sensory input from visual, gustatory, and somatosensory areas. Lesions of the amygdala impair learning of one-trial associations as well as cross-modal associations. Within the framework of behavioral associative memory, amygdala cells do not show specificity of good-bad or food-nonfood abstractions, though they are implicated in associating sensory information. However, further on in processing in the

lateral hypothalamus, a positive correlation is seen with the stimuli's motivational value. Categorizations made at this level correlate with behavioral responses. Projections are found from the hypothalamus to the autonomical and endocrinal systems, supporting the idea that information flow at this point has reached a response-oriented character. Overall, Rolls (1987) argued that the orbitofrontal cortex encodes the changes between the associations already existing (learned) such that the responses can be altered as needed.

Functional Domains in the Hippocampus

Most of our discussion has focused on the hippocampal pathways to cerebral cortex, including the role of these pathways in cerebral memory systems and in navigation. However, Risold and Swanson (1996) have focused on the rat's unilateral hippocampal projections to the lateral septum, which thence links hippocampus to motivational systems via bidirectional lateral septohypothalamic projections. We emphasize that these authors found variations in these projections along the longitudinal axis of the hippocampus. Via rostral lateral septum, ventral parts of the CA1-subiculum are related to the lateral part of the medial preoptic nucleus (involved in masculine sexual behavior). Progressively more dorsal parts are related preferentially to the ventromediotuberal nuclei (involved in feminine sexual behavior); to the anterior hypothalamic nucleus (involved in agonistic behavior) and to the mamillary body. Ramón y Cajal (1911) observed that a medial part of the striatum of the basal ganglia is innervated by hippocampal cortex. Thus, Risvold and Swanson (1996) stress the importance of exploring the extent to which the motor functions of the circuitry they have charted are similar to those of the adjacent ventral and dorsal striatum, the nucleus accumbens and caudatoputamen, respectively (see chapter 10). Other richly varied data lie beyond the scope of this brief review, but these anatomical results have promising implications for integrated studies in behavior, neurophysiology, and modeling.

6.5.4 Comparisons of Hippocampal Function in Humans, Rats, and Monkeys

A question that has motivated much research is whether episodic-declarative memory in the human is analogous to cognitive map formation in the rat. To focus discussion, we shall pursue the analogy that episode in the human corresponds to situation (i.e., that coded by a single node of the world graph) in a rat. The merging of nodes that is a positive feature of the world graph model for exploring the environment (learning that different cue sets may correspond to the same place) may become a disadvantage in human memory when humans conflate their memory of two distinct episodes. One issue for the rat is identifying the tags needed by a situation. As observed before, one such tag is motivational, but the data show that this already can be quite complex. Contrast "This is where I ate so there's no food left" to "This is where I ate so it's a good candidate to get food again." In the wild, the animal well may learn temporal context for the reappearance of food and thus move somewhat closer to episodic memory in its full sense.

Eichenbaum, Otto, and Cohen (1994) distinguished a hippocampal-dependent capacity for *relational representation* from a hippocampal-independent capacity for *individual representations* in animals that they mapped to the distinction between declarative and procedural memory in humans. They used definitions by Cohen and Eichenbaum (1993):

Relational representations [hippocampal]...maintain the "compositionality" of the items...They support the flexible use of memories by permitting access to items from various sources and by permitting the expression of memories in various, even novel, situations.

Individual representations [nonhippocampal] involve the "tuning" or biasing of items within separate processing modules of the brain operating in isolation....[s]uch processing involves the fusion of stimulus elements into a single representation lacking the property of compositionality....

These definitions raise many problems.

A *skill*, unlike an episode, extracts salient sensorimotor relationships from a wide set of experiences and so seems ill-named as an individual representation.

What is gained by bringing in "separate processing modules of the brain operating in isolation?" Even a humble nonhippocampal-conditioned response may require sensory regions of the brain to work in concert with cerebellum and red nucleus (Thompson 1986). More troubling is that Eichenbaum et al. (1994) offered no way to distinguish "relations" from "fusions" because the same task *will* involve hippocampus when a longer delay is involved, as in trace conditioning (Solomon et al. 1986).

Many skills require the ability to recognize parts in relationship and could not operate without "the property of compositionality." Yet, Cohen (1984) has demonstrated that amnesic patients can learn the Tower of Hanoi problem.

In noting the need for an intact hippocampus for delayed nonmatching to sample, Eichenbaum et al. (1994) stated that "the hippocampal system may also play an important role in the requirement for a non-match response because non-matching requires a 'flexible' response, that is, a choice contrary to that performed during the sample phase." Yet they immediately undermined this by noting that "monkeys with hippocampal system damage are significantly, if not as severely, impaired when the requirement is to 'match' to the sample cue," concluding that on object discrimination learning tasks, "the performance of animals with hippocampal system damage is best predicted by the duration of memory delay and not by appeal to a representational distinction." They argued that the remembered event in timing tasks probably involves a relational rather than an individual representation, but they gave no objective measure of "relational processing" that can predict what will or will not be impaired by hippocampal damage.

Eichenbaum et al. (1994) do seem to be "on to something" with their notion of "relational representation," but they give it an all-or-none role that the data cannot support. Data relating to the basal ganglia and cerebellum subdivide each into subregions, with strong links to brain systems having quite distinctive functions. Correspondingly, future study may show that the longitudinal axis of the hippocampus can take us through territory with different roles. The question of whether the hippocampus is relational then may depend more on what that part of hippocampus is related to than on the intrinsic properties of the hippocampal formation itself.

For example, it is a useful contribution of Eichenbaum et al. (1994) to show that much of the data on spatial learning in rats can make sense in a relational framework, but one still must ask what in hippocampal circuitry mediates the expression of the relations necessary for *spatial* behavior. In figure 6.10, we saw two models that embed hippocampus in a larger system allowing the rat to update its estimate of position (evidenced by place cell firing) even in the absence of visual firing. However, this means that the system must be "wired up" so that corollary discharge and nonvisual cues can be used to update the estimate of place, with a specificity of connections that goes far beyond the generic circuitry for relational representation. It seems that the search for specific mechanisms for specific types of relational processing will prove more fruitful than will attempts at an all-or-none characterization of hippocampal function.

Olton (1979) showed that rats can remember for approximately 4—5 hours the arms of a radial maze that they have entered. He argued that the rat forms a permanent memory of the maze (reference memory) at some extrahippocampal site and then uses the hippocampus to store a transient list of what it has done in the last few hours. Lynch and Baudry (1988) suggested that contextual cues are represented in the hippocampus and that the transient memory is due to interactions (e.g., approach) between these cues. They assume that transient and other memories of events occurring within a given context also are stored outside hippocampus, albeit with facilitation from hippocampus.

Lynch and Baudry (1988) speculated that in small-brained mammals, the map developed by hippocampus is stored there permanently, whereas large-brained mammals use neocortex for further processing of hippocampus functions. (Bolhuis, Stewart, and Forest 1994 showed that rats do lose memory for spatial tasks after hippocampectomy, but this is not quite the same as the animal losing its ability to find its way around a familiar home territory.) Their hypothesis is that the hippocampus outputs signals that a particular context applies. For small-brained mammals and for smell in all mammals, this signal is used also in directing moment-to-moment behavior. For large-brained mammals, the signal might be an impoverished but more rapidly developed and easily triggered version of that found in neocortex. This is reminiscent of our chapter 3 discussion of the visual roles of tectum and superior colliculus in frog and monkey—the region changes from primary visual center to a substrate beneath conscious awareness that is "revealed" in blindsight. Tectal activity has lots of content but signals far less than does pattern vision. Returning to hippocampus, what is lost in amnesiacs is not the ability to form complex cognitive representations but rather the ability to "package" them in such a way as to make them retrievable episodes (e.g., by linking them in a network of temporal relations). Consider what might happen if we had visual cortex but no superior colliculus and had to process a passive sequence of foveal "snapshots." It becomes impossible to form an integrated percept of a scene.

Hippocampus has access to all areas of the neocortex by means of the basal forebrain and to a variety of specific regions through its outputs to the deep layers of ENT. These entorhinal-neocortex pathways are massive, and the medial frontal area is the target of a particularly dense projection (Swanson and Kohler 1986). This area also receives inputs from the subiculum (Swanson and Cowan 1977). If human hippocampus defines the continuing presence of a particular context, its activity might serve to define the onset and offset of particular episodes and might then also serve to facilitate the re-activation of the episodic string. But retrograde amnesia does not extend to established memories, and human amnesiacs also probably lose recently acquired semantic memories. Are older records accurately retained as episodes rather than being converted into a series of associated semantic memories, thus eliminating the necessity of the hippocampus for retrieval? Episodic memory is labile and subject to distortion and in some sense is reconstituted on retrieval (Tulving 1983). On the basis of such considerations, Lynch and Baudry (1988) argued for the following contrast:

In small-brained mammals, the associations are used as primary information, and the context responses are used for navigation through the environment and to direct behavior appropriately. Continued attention directed by continuous hippocampus output is needed for rapid acquisition of new information. In highly encephalized mammals, the associations (except those involving smell) formed in hippocampus are redundant, as in the context map, as far as concerns directing specific behaviors in specific environments. However, hippocampus context signals still are required for rapid encoding of information and possibly are useful in recalling episodes.

Whatever the fate of their hypothesis, we see the necessity for placing the fine details of hippocampal structure, function, and dynamics within the broader context of a cooperative computational analysis of the cortical and motivational systems with which the hippocampus is so intimately linked.

Thalamus

Although the thalamus is treated in section 7.2 for its traditional role as the chief relay for sensory input, this function is only a small fraction of the crucial role of the thalamus in all kinds of pathways: between different parts of the cerebral cortex, between cerebellum and cerebral cortex, between lower brainstem nuclei and cerebral cortex, and additional, more complex neuron circuits involving the striatopallidal nuclear systems (the basal ganglia). We briefly preview the relations of thalamus with cerebellum and basal ganglia in section 7.3. First, in section 7.1, we introduce our view of thalamic structure by describing its nuclei in some detail, although the special objective of this book requires us to be very selective, owing to the huge and diverse range of material available today regarding the nervous system in general and the thalamus in particular.

Section 7.1.1 contains a review of the place of thalamus in the upper brainstem, using an image of an intermediate embryonic stage of the developing brain to provide a basic understanding of the relationship between the diencephalon and the telencephalic vesicles. In section 7.1.2, we introduce the specific nuclei of the thalamus: the lateral nuclear group, the medial nuclear group, and the anterior nuclear group. Then we return to the theme of modular architectonics by noting that frontally oriented successive discs of the cortex from front to aft have a mutual (although more clearly thalamocortical) relationship with close-to-sagittal discs of the thalamus. Finally, we turn to the reticular nucleus of the thalamus, which forms an almost continuous cellular shell around the lateral, inferior, and posterior periphery of the thalamus. The less specific thalamic nuclei are reviewed very briefly in section 7.1.3.

Section 7.2 is a review of the best-known role of the thalamus, namely as a relay in sensory systems; section 7.2.1 is an introduction to synaptic glomeruli, triads, and local circuits; and section 7.2.2 is a review of the major sensory systems, starting with an analysis of the development of the sensory systems. Following that is a review of the commonalities and differences of the somatosensory system (with special attention to the gate control that separates pain-related information from other somesthetic qualities), the auditory system and the visual system.

We devote section 7.3 to thalamocortical loops and cooperative computation. Section 7.3.1 is a review of the descending control of sensory systems in the lateral geniculate nucleus of mammals, and the descending control and thalamocortical oscillations. Then we briefly review the thalamocortical loops involving the striato-pallidal system (sec. 7.3.2) and the cerebellar system (sec. 7.3.3).

7.1 Nuclei of the Thalamus

7.1.1 The Place of Thalamus in the Upper Brainstem

In a wide sense and speaking very loosely, the term *upper brainstem nuclei* can be used on the gross anatomical level for the huge gray nuclear masses engulfed by (and wedged between) the two cortical hemispheres of what is called the *cerebrum*, excluding the lower brainstem (medulla oblongata, pons, mesencephalon) and the cerebellum. Although this is not apparent in the adult brain, the nuclear masses of the upper brainstem belong to two different parts of the developing forebrain (prosencephalic) vesicles: the *diencephalon*, essentially a rostral continuation of the original medullary tube, and the *telencephalic vesicles*, essentially two bulges situated at the rostral end of the original prosencephalic (i.e., most rostral) vesicle and giving rise to the cerebral cortex on their outer surfaces and to two additional large nuclear formations on the inner side of the croissant-shaped vesicles.

Figure 7.1 provides a simplified image of an intermediate embryonic stage of the developing brain, an image from which the nonprofessional reader may gain a basic understanding of the relationship between the diencephalon and the telencephalic vesicles. The two developmentally different structures are welded together by the progressive emergence of fiber tracts (white matter) formed by the axonal processes of neurons—both ascending and descending—that, as seen in the formation of the spinal cord and the lower brainstem, have the tendency to gather in and to occupy the outer surface areas of the original neural tube. In the prosencephalic part of the brain, the fibers of both diencephalic and telencephalic origin or destination become intermixed at the contact surfaces of the three original brain vesicles and give rise to the huge white radiations of intricately intermingled fiber tracts (called the *internal*

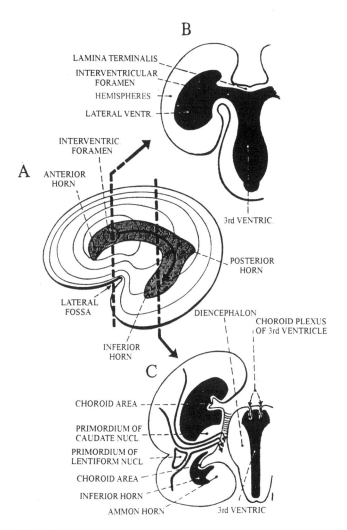

Figure 7.1
An intermediate embryonic stage of the developing brain. (A) The side view shows the lateral ventricle (shaded) in relation to a telencephalic vesicle and the planes of the coronal sections (B and C), in which the cross-sections of the lateral and third ventricles are shown in black. (C) The diencephalon and the telencephalic vesicles are welded together by fiber tracts and the internal capsule covers the primordium of the lentiform nucleus.

capsule, or capsula interna), the internal white cover of the lentiform nucleus, one of the large subcortical telencephalic nuclei.

We shall deal very selectively with parts of the thalamus (and the thalamus is only one part of the diencephalic structures), giving special regard in this Section and the next to sensory and other ascending systems. The thalamus is only the upper part of the diencephalon, other important parts being the hypothalamus, subthalamus, epithalamus (the so-called reticular nuclear formations), and the metathalamus, or geniculate. The geniculate comprises the medial and lateral geniculate nuclear formations that are the major subcortical relay

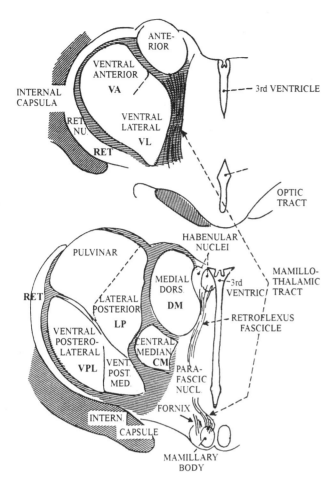

Figure 7.2
Two cross-sections of one-half of the thalamus, surrounded over part of the anterior, lateroventral, and posterior surfaces by the reticular nucleus of the thalamus. The cross-sections show the following thalamic nuclei: ventroanterior (VA); ventrolateral (VL); lateral nuclei; lateralis posterior (LP); pulvinar; ventroposterolateral (VPL); ventroposteromedial; dorsomedial (DM); centromedial (CM). The anterior group receives its chief afferent input from the mamillary bodies (over the mamillothalamic tract), from the hippocampal formation (over the fornix), and from limbic cortical input; its output is mainly toward the limbic parts of the cortex.

systems of the auditory and the visual pathways. Despite their importance, the hypothalamus, subthalamus, and epithalamus will remain outside the scope of our considerations. Chapter 10 deals with the striatopallidal nuclear system of the basal ganglia, closely related to the cerebral cortex treated in chapter 8.

The thalamus proper can be compared vaguely with a hard-boiled egg, with its shell halved, with the two halves separated by the sagittal cleft of the third ventricle, and with the shell removed on the upper side so that it remains continuous over part of the anterior, the lateral ventral, and the posterior surface. Figure 7.2 shows two cross-sections of one "half-egg." The "shell"

is an almost continuous cellular mass (or layer) called the *reticular nucleus of the thalamus.*

7.1.2 The Specific Nuclei of the Thalamus

The specific nuclei of the thalamus can be subdivided into the following major nuclear masses (see figure 7.2):

The lateral nuclear group: the ventroanterior and ventrolateral nuclei subserving mainly the relay of the contralateral cerebellum to the nuclear cortical regions. Backward and directly, this nuclear mass continues into a major system of the lateralis posterior and pulvinar (PUL) complex, subserving mainly intercortical relays. Below this and presenting a rhomboid shape in transversal section (see figure 7.2) is the ventrobasal nucleus subdivided into the ventroposterolateral (VPL) and ventroposteromedial (VPM) nuclei, the main relays of the somatosensory system.

The medial nuclear group: the dorsomedial (DM) nucleus, projecting mainly toward the frontal cortex and receiving probably the ascending systems conveying painful stimuli, and the centromedial (CM) nucleus, an indistinct nuclear mass that appears to be open toward the midline. This mass is continuous over the midline nuclei with the centromedial nucleus of the other side (not really a part of the specific nuclear system).

The anterior nuclear group: the anterodorsal, anteromedial, and anteroventral nuclei. The anterior nuclear mass receives its chief afferent input from the mamillary bodies (over the mamillothalamic tract) and from the hippocampal formations of both sides (over the fornix) and receives cortical input mainly (but not exclusively) from the limbic areas of the cortex (cingulate gyrus). Its output is mainly toward the limbic parts of the cortex.

Irrespective of the nuclear subdivision, the thalamus has a strange overall geometrically organized somatotopic relationship with the cortex, shown for the monkey in figure 7.3 (Kievit and Kuypers 1977). Frontally oriented successive discs of the cortex from front to back have a mutual, thalamocortical relationship with close-to-sagittal discs of the thalamus. These discs depart from the sagittal plane in a double sense. First, the medial thalamic (frontal cortical) discs deviate toward the rear in the lateral direction, partly because the longitudinal axes of the two half-egg-shaped thalamic masses diverge toward the rear and partly to give room (especially in primates) to the increasing masses of the metathalamus. Second (and more importantly) they tend progressively to tilt in fan-shaped fashion laterally toward the horizontal plane. Perhaps the most remarkable feature of this

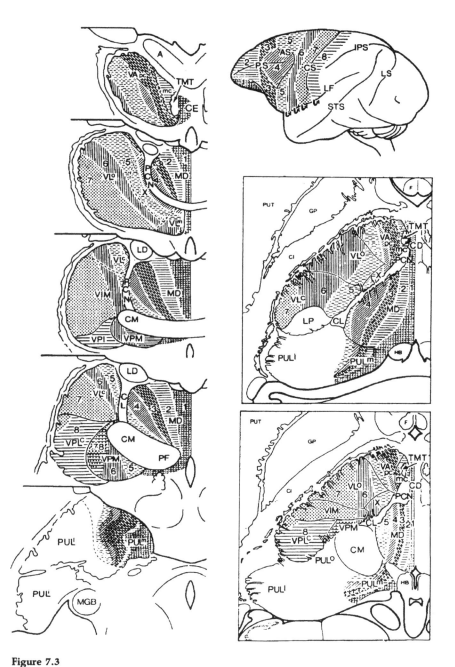

Figure 7.3

Somatotopic relationship with the cortex in monkey. The top right panel shows a succession of frontally oriented discs of the cortex numbered 1–8. The other panels show the close-to-sagittal discs of the thalamus to which they correspond, as indicated by numbering or hatching. These discs depart from the sagittal plane in two ways: (1) The medial thalamic (frontal cortical) discs deviate toward the rear in the lateral direction, and (2) these discs tend to tilt progressively in a fan laterally toward the horizontal plane. The left represents frontal sections, and the framed drawings to the right are horizontal sections

of the thalamus. In the upper right corner, the lateral view of the monkey brain is seen; 1–8 are the frontally oriented cortical discs labeled also with different patterns. (Reprinted with permission from Kievit and Kuypers 1977.) PUL, pulvinar; VPL, ventroposterolateral; VA, ventroanterior; CM, centromedial; VPM, ventroposteromedial; LP, lateralis posterior; VL, ventrolateral; MGB, medial geniculate body; TMT, mamillo thalamic tract; CE, anterior midline nucleus; MD, mediodorsal nucleus; VIM, ventral intermediate nucleus; CM-PF, center median-para fascicular; LD, laterdorsal nucleus.

corticothalamic-cortical projection is that normally it is independent of nuclear borders and crosses quite liberally through the white laminae of the thalamus separating the several specific nuclei of the thalamus. Unfortunately, systematic data on this frontosagittal projection system are available only for the anterior half of the cortex. However, from many bits and pieces of information about thalamocortical (and reverse) relations of the rear part of the brain, one may gather safely that this strange somatotopic projection principle holds true, *mutatis mutandis*, for the whole brain and that the thalamus may receive multiple overlapping cortical projections.

Probably it was unfortunate that Kievit and Kuypers (1977) labeled the system as *columnar*, but this is understandable in view of the fact that until the mid-1970s, brain modules generally were labeled as columns, from the original observations (see sec. 2.3.2) of Mountcastle (1957) of physiological columns in somatosensory cortex to the later observations of Hubel and Wiesel on visual cortex. Because today overuse of the term *column* is the main source of controversial evaluation of the modular architectonics principle of brain structures, it is necessary to speak of columns exclusively in the case of real columns and to define all other types of repetitive modular arrangements with their appropriate labels: *discs, strips, barrels, barreloids,* and the like. In the thalamus, the architectonic subdivisions clearly are discs and can be considered as columns only in a very limited, almost metaphorical sense, as will be discussed later.

The reader well may wonder why we give such disproportionate emphasis to such seemingly trivial matters as overall geometrical principles of gross brain organization; but they are most emphatically not trivial. As discussed at some length in section 2.1, somatotopic relations both on the macroscopical scale and on the minute scale are not minor (or certainly not teleological) chance principles but are an essential result of the embryological underpinnings of neural structure. Wherever it is appropriate and realistic, our main objective is to highlight certain points of contact or agreement between an essentially bottom-up approach to neural structure and dynamics (J.Sz. and P.E.) and the complementary top-down direction of functional analysis (M.A.). Thus, in striving for a coherent view of the brain that integrates multiple perspectives, we try to avoid all-inclusive theories of brain and mind that are in vogue these days, as such attempts are premature.

The brain being a universe of its own and the point of reflection of all the rest of the universe, it is not astonishing that three scientists with backgrounds and philosophies perhaps worlds apart appraise the simple geometrical principles as looming in the background, even in so immensely complex a structure system as the nervous system. Although there are many unexpected, unforseeable, seemingly even completely chaotic aspects of neural organization, very simple basic geometrical principles reveal that there is an elementary geometrical order in the whole neural design. These principles were understood first in euclidean geometry but then progressively enriched by the geometries of Bólyai, Lobachevsky, and Riemann and their further ramifications in pure and applied mathematics.

7.1.3 The Nonspecific Nuclei

Briefly, the less specific thalamic nuclei are the nuclear masses that occupy the medullary lamina system and separate the specific nuclear masses. They also comprise the nuclei close to the midline and those constituting most parts of the ventral thalamus. The CM mentioned previously occupies a position intermediate in many respects between the specific and the nonspecific nuclei, mainly because it is continuous over the midline with the same nucleus of the opposite side (hence its alternative name *nucleus reuniens*).

The reticular nucleus of the thalamus (not to be confused with the reticular formation of the brainstem) forms an almost continuous cellular shell around the lateral, inferior, and posterior periphery of the thalamus. It has a special relationship to the majority of the specific nuclei (as first recognized and described by the Scheibels in 1970) in the perpendicular direction front to aft in the medial part and radially in the lateral part of the thalamus. This simple relationship is obvious only in subprimate mammals, wherein the reticular shell is continuous over the entire lateral aspect of the thalamus. However, the situation becomes blurred in the primates owing to the huge development of the lateral geniculate nuclear system, which has made it impossible thus far to define unequivocally the reticular nucleus associated with the lateral geniculate nuclei. The medial geniculate nuclei cannot be fitted into this simplified thalamic scheme because they already belong to the transition between midbrain and diencephalon.

The so-called epithalamus also belongs to the nonspecific nuclei: It comprises two major nuclei, the medial and the lateral habenular nuclei, and its efferents descend toward the subthalamic region, the fasciculus retroflexus. A major nuclear mass, the parafascicular nucleus surrounds this tract. The afferents of the habenular nuclei come from many sources: lateral hypothalamus, lateral preoptic area, nucleus of the diagonal band, entopeduncular nucleus, septal nuclei, and so on. The efferents can be traced mainly to the interpeduncular and the midbrain raphé nuclei; another group of fibers runs to the ventral tegmental area and also to the substantia nigra. (Because the function of this system is virtually unknown, it will remain largely outside the scope of our considerations.) There are rather vague indications that this whole system may be related somehow to metabolic control mechanisms, possibly temperature regulation and neuroendocrine control of thyroid functions.

The whole subthalamic system is connected so intimately with the striatopallidal nuclei and their pathways that it will be considered specifically in chapter 10. The so-called metathalamic nuclei, the *lateral* and the *medial geniculate* nuclear complexes, will be treated separately in section 7.2.2, wherein the major sensory systems of the nervous system will be discussed in an attempt to give a synthetic view of their comparable organizations.

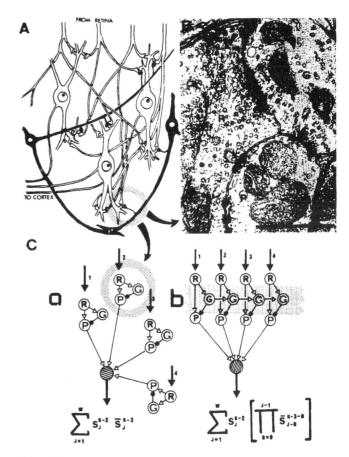

Figure 7.4
The synaptic arrangement in the lateral geniculate nucleus. (A) The circuitry includes several examples of synaptic triads, with input element presynaptic to the dendrite of an interneuron (black), which is presynaptic in turn to the dendritic bulge of a projective neuron (clear). (B) Electron micrograph of a synaptic triad. (C) Models of (a) separately operating and (b) linearly coupled synaptic triads. R, presynaptic input element; G, dendrite of an interneuron; P, dendritic bulge of a projective neuron. Clear arrows indicate excitatory synapses; dark arrows indicate inhibitory synapses.

7.2 Thalamus and Sensory Systems

7.2.1 Synaptic Glomeruli, Triads, and Local Circuits

A special reason for devoting an entire chapter of this book to the thalamus is that virtually all of its nuclei abound in a variety of complex synaptic arrangements, the so-called *synaptic glomeruli*. These arrangements also are known as *encapsulated synaptic zones* if such parts of the neuropil are sufficiently well-separated by glial lamellae from the general intercellular network of axons and dendrites. A standard and characteristic synaptic arrangement is the so-called synaptic triad (Szentágothai, Hámori, and Tömböl 1966), in which the main incoming (input) axon terminals establish a synapse of excitatory nature with a dendritic element (generally a dendritic bulge, or excrescence) of the chief forward-conducting (output, or projective) neuron. Almost invariably, it is the local interposition or juxtaposition of a third element that usually is a presynaptic dendrite of a local inhibitory interneuron. In the standard type of triad (see figure 7.4A for its form in the lateral geniculate nucleus), the input element is presynaptic (by structural standards— that is, by accumulation of synaptic vesicles on the "presynaptic" side and by membrane specializations on the "postsynaptic" side of the contact) to the interneuron dendrite, which is presynaptic, in turn, to the dendritic bulge of the projective neuron. Very often, the presynaptic dendrites of several interneurons participate in

the same glomerulus. Synaptic contacts of opposite polarity often are found in close proximity to one another, both may appear by structural standards to be presynaptic to the other. There are many combinations of such complex synapses with additional contacts of interneuron axon terminals, which then are found to be in presynaptic relation either to the main input or (more often) to the main output element.

Such synaptic complexes by no means are confined to the thalamus. They are found in abundance along the entire sensory neuron chain, from the spinal cord (mainly, of course, in the dorsal horn) to the dorsal column nuclei of the medulla oblongata, all brainstem sensory relay nuclei, and virtually all nonsensory relay nuclei of the thalamus.

This striking structural arrangement led P. Rakic (1975) to develop an entire new concept of so-called local circuit neurons, a general idea picked up and elaborated further by Schmitt, Dev, and Smith (1976) into a general theory reaching far beyond the classic neuron concept (and especially beyond and at variance with one of the major tenets of the neuron theory, the histodynamic polarity of the neuron). This theory assumes that in normal physiological circumstances, conduction of impulses is centripetal in the dendrites (from ending toward perikarya) and is centrifugal in axons. This law seems to hold essentially also for nonspike (e.g., electronic conductance). It is known now that impulse conduction may occur in both centrifugal and centripetal directions in dendrites and in axons and, with the aid of their presynaptic specializations, dendrites are capable of delivering impulses to postsynaptic elements (Rall and Shepherd 1968). Although the structural observations on which the Rakic and the Schmitt et al. concept was based are correct, workers at our laboratory and some other laboratories (notably Pasik et al. 1973a, b; Pasik, Pasik, and Hámori 1976) were looking for less ambitious and more parsimonious explanations. Eventually, the theoretical approach using network logics of Lábos (1977a, b) appeared to become a promising way to explain the ubiquitous occurrence of such triadic arrangements not only in the thalamic nuclei but also in other centers of the main afferent systems and in different combinations.

An explicit formulation of the concept for this type of synaptic organization was given by Szentágothai (1985) for the most frequent type of arrangement in the lateral geniculate nucleus (see figure 7.4C) and by Lábos, Hámori, and Isomura (1980) for an alternative structural combination in the medial cuneate nucleus. Looking through the not strictly sensory thalamic nuclei revealed an even greater variety of such combined synapses (Szentágothai 1965; Hajdu, Somogyi, and Tömböl 1974; Somogyi, Hajdu, and Tömböl 1978). Figure 7.5 is an attempt to summarize the main connections thus far known of the anterior and the PUL nuclei. As can be seen, the basic pattern of synaptic triads is the same.

In the case of the medial cuneate nucleus, a model by Lábos, Hámori, and Isomura (1980) was made of a synaptic triad combining the input from a spinal receptive field (X), a neighboring (Y) spinal receptive field acting via an inhibitory interneuron (IN), and a projective (lemniscal) neuron (R), as shown in figure 7.6. In view of the theory that the spinal afferent X also may have access to the interneuron (IN) participating in the triadic synaptic arrangement (TSA), the situation at the three elements (E_1, E_2, E_3) is as follows: The state module E_3 at

time t is dependent on past events in X and Y, as can be formalized by

$$S_{E_3}(t) = F[X(t - d_1), X(t - d_2), Y(t - d_3), P]$$

where d_1, d_2, d_3 are the delays and P symbolizes other (in this case latent) parameters or sources and is also time-dependent. This model was elaborated further for two alternative explanations for distance-dependent confusion or discrimination of somatosensory stimuli in terms of synaptic triads, as illustrated in figure 7.7. This is just to give an example of the possible functional significance of triadic arrangements considered purely from the viewpoint of network logics.

The network logic approach of Lábos (1977a, b) leads to uniform atomized time axes, (i.e., the time scale is discretized similarly for all units, and the network does not execute asynchronous computation). The dynamics of triadic synaptic arrangements was studied further by network simulations (Lábos et al. 1990). In this study, logical elements were substituted by chaotic elements. Chaotic units have advantages over logical units; because the former are asynchronous, it is possible to simulate temporal summation and also to adjust subthreshold time constants. To allow a clear analysis of signal transmission, only "nonautoactive" elements were used. Technically speaking, piecewise linear interval maps were used. Lábos (1984) showed that this simple mathematical construct can serve as a universal pattern generator, and it was offered as a compromise between biologically detailed compartmental models and the computationally simple McCulloch-Pitts model. It was demonstrated that that ensemble with multiple delay lines most likely was necessary to provide secure ON-gate functions.

From the network logic approach, it appears that there is no need to abandon the classic neuron concept, because there is ample room in its framework for a large variety in interaction between parallel channels and both feedforward and feedback control of transmission. However, it is open to debate whether any fundamental change in our mental strategy is required in regard to the vast new body of knowledge about the many new types of mediators and modulators that are partially coexistent with one another and the new insights about the molecular biology and genetics of mediators and receptors.

7.2.2 The Major Sensory Systems

A broader look here at the major sensory relay systems reflects what we did in an early precursor of this study

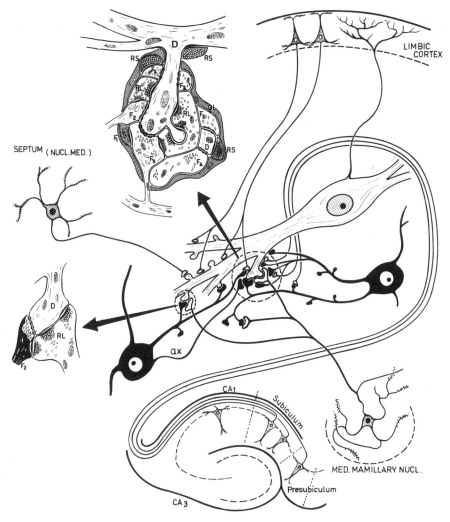

Figure 7.5

The main connections of the anterior and the pulvinar nuclei. (Left inset) based on electron micrograph of a synaptic triad. (Top inset) based on electron micrograph of a glomerulus containing several synaptic triads. RL, synaptic bouton with round and large vesicles; RS, synaptic bouton with round and small vesicles; F2, synaptic bouton with flat vesicles; D, dendrite; ax, axon; CA1 and CA3, hippocampal areas.

(Szentágothai and Arbib 1975). In a somewhat naive way (in retrospect), we made a crude comparison of the overall design of the four major sensory systems—the olfactory, the visual, the auditory, and the somatosensory systems. The olfactory system is distinguished by its lack of a thalamic relay (discussed in chapter 5). The 1975 comparison of sensory systems led us to a crudely oversimplified diagram (reproduced as figure 7.8). Despite obvious inadequacies, this figure at least had the merit of being a first attempt at defining some parallelism for various levels wherein the processing of information occurred and for the various modes of neuron couplings observed at the several major links along the afferent neuron chains. It is here that we find the major flaw of the entire approach: In spite of certain

superficial similarities in neuron couplings, the requirements for the analysis of sensory patterns fed into the central nervous system over hundred of thousands of parallel but separate neuron channels are radically different in the cases of the several senses. The similarities are more apparent than real, although the coupling by means of triadic arrangements (sec. 7.2.1) and the occurrence of local interneurons always are part of the structure.

Development of the Sensory Systems

In addition to the neuroepithelia and the other (supporting) epithelial cells of the inner ear, the sensory nerve cells and additional other epithelia of the head region do not originate from the neural crest cells and their derivatives, as is the case in the main, segmented parts

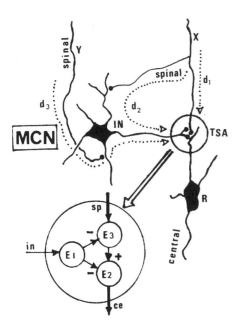

Figure 7.6

Theoretical model of operation of synaptic triads in the medial cuneate nucleus. (Reprinted with permission from Lábos, Hámori, and Isomura 1980.) X, Y, spinal receptive field inputs; IN, inhibitory interneuron; R, projective (lemniscal) neuron; TSA, triadic synaptic arrangement; d_1, d_2, d_3, delays along three pathways. E_1, E_2, and E_3 are three elements of the synaptic triad. MCN, medial cuneafe nucleus.

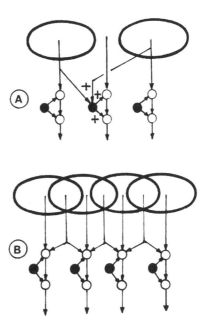

Figure 7.7

Two alternative explanations for distance-dependent confusion or discrimination of somatosensory stimuli in terms of axonal triads. (A) Termination (upper small empty circles) of channels originating in disjoint receptive fields (ellipses) of projective cell modules (lower small empty circles)—that is, outputs of triads. Interneurons (black circles) also receive activation from these respective fields. An AND-gate operates at the medial black circle, and the interneuronal synapses are supposed to be excitatory (+). (B) Symbols are the same as in (A). Overlaps of the four receptive fields explain distance-dependent discrimination of tactile stimuli. Interneuronal influences could be either inhibitory or excitatory. (Reprinted with permission from Lábos, Hámori, and Isomura 1980.)

along the neuraxis. A belt of ectodermal surface surrounds the anterolateral circumference of the medullary plate; it does not become incorporated either into the anterior (encephalic) part of the medullary tube or into the anteriormost parts of the neural crest. This belt is called the *placode*. There is a longitudinal split of the placode into a proximal half (nearer to the closing margins of the medullary plate) and a distal half, giving rise to different neuroepithelia and supporting epithelia. The anteriormost part of the placode becomes invaginated into the original common nose-mouth cavity, gives rise to the epithelia of the anterior and intermediate lobes of the pituitary, and is the unpaired anteriormost derivative of the placode. On both its sides, the nasal placodes also become embedded deeply between the developing frontal maxillary processes so as to give rise to the olfactory neuroepithelia (and supporting cells). Further back along this belt is the lens-placode, giving rise to the later epithelium of the ocular lenses (and hence remaining exclusively epithelial). Epithelial placodal cells positioned behind the lens become incorporated into the sensory ganglia of the Vth and VIIth cranial nerves (geniculate ganglion); it is still unclear whether and how far they are continuous from these nerves with the anteriormost part of the neural crest cells. Some cells in the distal part of this placodal region become incorporated into the ante-

rior part of the tongue as the neuroepithelial cells of the anteriormost tastebuds.

The acousticofacial placode gives rise to the epithelia (both neuroepithelia and supporting and living cells) of the entire membranous inner labyrinth and probably to the majority of the primary sensory neurons and Schwann cells of the VIIIth nerve (and VIIth nerve) ganglia. The postauditory parts of the placodes give rise to both primary sensory nerve cells of the IXth and Xth cranial nerves (probably only partially), because here the neural crest cells increasingly become involved in contributing cell material to the cranial nerves, their sheath cells, and their postganglionic nerve cells. A peculiarity of the VIIIth nerve "primary" sensory ganglion cells is that the process of pseudounipolarization during later development that takes place from amphibia upward to mammals does not occur in the VIIIth nerve ganglia. Many of these cells are surrounded by a myelin sheath and consequently lack all pseudounipolar primary sensory neurons from the point of the T-shaped bifurcation of the unified cell process.

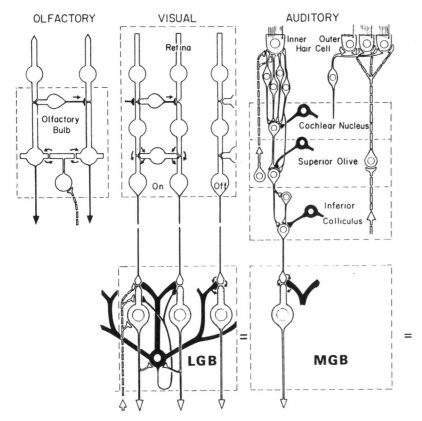

Figure 7.8

Highly simplified comparison of elementary neuron couplings in the four main sensory pathways. Inhibitory interneurons are shown in black; descending control is indicated by dashed axons; convergence and divergence generally is neglected. For the somatosensory pathway, we show two possible interneuron couplings: (A) the older concept of recurrent feedback; (B) dendritic synapses with triads. LGB, lateral geniculate body; MGB, medial geniculate body; VPL, ventroposterolateral nucleus. (Reprinted with permission from Szentágothai and Arbib 1975.)

The visual system differs from all other sense organs in that its neural elements do not arise from cell material of the peripheral nervous system but are derived ontogenetically and directly from the brain's prosencephalic vesicle wall. This process starts as a bulge of the brain wall, the optic vesicle that soon is turned into the optic cup by impression and subsequent impregnation of the outer wall into the posterior half, thus bringing about a double-layered cup (similar to the Dewar vessels for keeping temperature constant). The outer of the two layers eventually is transformed into a pigmented epithelial layer, whereas the posterior part of the inner wall is transformed into the nerve cell layers and glial (Müller) cells of the retina.

The Somatosensory System

The spinal relay in the somatosensory system is complicated by two major routes of forward conduction: the direct dorsal column system and the indirect anterolateral (spinothalamic) system. However, even these two major systems have two side tracts, the dorsal spinocerebellar and the ventral spinocerebellar systems branching off from their original sources. Even this subdivision is valid only for the lower (lumbosacral) spinal segments; there exists a comparable system for the upper (brachial) segments of the spinal cord, with a subdivision of the direct connection over the lateral (cuneate) tract of the dorsal white column and the cuneate nucleus of the medulla oblongata. The indirect (anterolateral) spinothalamic system is organized in the same way as for the lower segments. However, their side tracts over the cerebellum are conveyed at least partially by the reticular nucleus of the cervical cord.

One significant portion of the indirect (anterolateral) spinothalamic system—mainly pathways involved in nociception (i.e., pain mechanisms)—is built at least partially into the so-called substantia gelatinosa (laminae I–II and partially III of Rexed; 1954 see chapter 2 of the spinal dorsal horn). Another more local mechanism, especially the system known as the *flexor reflex afferents*, is

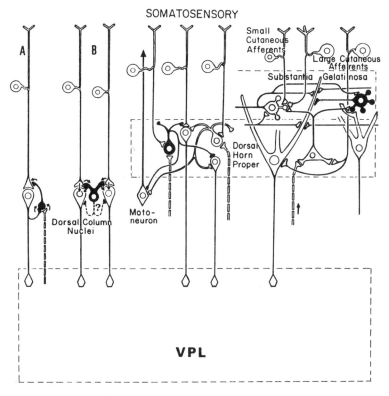

SOMATOSENSORY

Figure 7.8 (continued)

essentially a branch of the somatosensory systems for local reflex functions. Conjecture continues as to how far the primary afferent neurons (having their cells of origin in the spinal ganglia) are individually specific for any of the mentioned systems and as to what portion of the local connections are merely side branches of neurons destined for forward conduction to higher levels. It can be hoped that more specific data on the biochemical or molecular histological properties of the primary afferent neurons will enable us to separate specific groups from one another.

The main thrust of this study—conceptual aspects of neural organization—leads to the mysterious issue of gate control exercised at the very first step of spinal afferent impulse processing: the issue of separating information about physical or chemical forces that cause or threaten tissue damage (effecting their avoidance by causing pain) from other somesthetic qualities that convey information about touch, pressure, tension, temperature, vibration, and the like. Although the concepts concerning the physiology of pain have an ancient history, realistic arguments about the physiological bases of pain started with alternative assumptions. One advocated very forcefully by Marshall (1894) was the assumption that pain would be caused by overstimulation of virtually all types of somatosensory receptors; the

other assumption advocated the existence of specific receptors and nerve fibers and specific pathways for the conduction of painful stimuli.

Emergent knowledge of nerve terminals and of the physiology of nerve fibers increasingly supported the specificity theory. It turned out that two types of nerve fibers; $A_\delta C$ and $A_\delta\beta$ (unmyelinated) fibers were able to conduct mechanonociceptive and thermal (chemical) nociceptive impulses. Melzack and Wall (1965) proposed for neuron coupling (assumed to be in the dorsal horn of the spinal cord) an ingenious model that would remove inconsistencies around the specificity theory by a gate control mechanism. Although elegant, the theory did not satisfy the neurophysiologists engaged in the field. The Hungarian husband and wife team of B. Csillik and E. Knyihár devoted almost a lifetime to the complex study of such a gate control mechanism, summarized in a comprehensive monograph entitled *The Protean Gate* (Csillik and Knyihár 1986) and indicating metaphorically the biological dynamism of the gate control mechanism. Although the theory is subject to serious doubts concerning many of its details and overly ambitious experiments to make clinical use of iontophoretic percutaneous application of drugs that interfere with axoplasmic flow (one of the crucial elements of the entire theory), we deem it worthwhile to give at this point the summarizing diagram

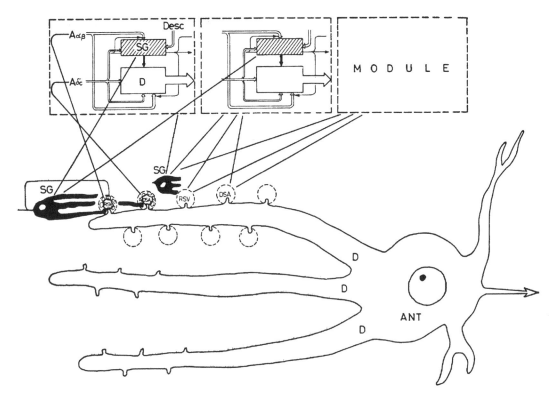

Figure 7.9
The protean gate theory. The row at the top shows the basic inter-actions postulated to occur in units arranged along the dendrites of the antenna cell (ANT). Synaptic triads link impulses arriving from thick $A\alpha\beta$ and thin $A\delta C$ fibers and descending spinal systems (SG), with lateral inhibition between neighboring units. (Reprinted with permission from Csillik and Knyihár 1986.)

of the protean gate theory in figure 7.9. Most of its underlying anatomical facts are clarified convincingly by these authors and are in reasonable agreement with earlier studies by Szentágothai (1964), Réthelyi (1977), and the overview by Kerr and Carey (1978).

"Antenna cells," which showed up in early figures of Ramón y Cajal (1909), were described later by Szentá-gothai (1964) and eventually were analyzed by use of the electron microscope for its triadic arrangements by Réthelyi and Szentágothai (1969) and further by several other authors. Modulelike units are arranged along the dendrites of these antenna cells (much smaller than the modules of many neurons considered elsewhere in this volume). Indeed, these would be suited for (1) equilibrat-ing between impulses arriving from thick $A_\alpha B$ and thin $A_\delta C$ fibers, (2) for imposing an input bias on transmis-sion by descending spinal systems, and (3) for exercising collateral inhibition between neighboring receptive terri-tories. In the Csillik model, the blockage of axoplasmic flow by the so-called vinca alkaloids deranges the minute structure of the modulelike units and prevents the devel-opment of a vicious circle of afferent input that allegedly can cause pain. The reader should realize that in spite of its dynamic properties, the Csillik model essentially is a device for neuronal switching and does not account ex-plicitly for a large variety of mechanisms for selectivity and encoding on the basis of the several biochemical labels (mediator and modulator combinations) of the various primary sensory neurons involved. There is ample proof in the vast territory of vegetative innerva-tion that the combination of such chemical labels is the really crucial factor in determining connectivity by a complex match-mismatch selectivity between neural source and target. One might begin to understand the real complexity in the organization of the afferent systems right at the beginning of the pathways only if the principles operating in the highly autonomous local plexus of the vegetative innervation were extrapolated to the spinal cord and to the afferent systems in general. The short account completely neglects an aspect of crucial importance for nociception and pain mechanisms: the question of opiate receptors and of the entire system of endorphins. By now, it is established that endorphins are present and act on virtually all points of the noci-ceptive pathways (a consideration beyond the scope of this study). Further data on pain pathways and possible directions for future modeling are reviewed by Devor (1995).

The same complexity of switching mechanisms applies along the entire somatosensory path, in the dorsal column nuclei, and eventually in the specific VPL-VPM thalamic nucleus. One illuminating example from the medial cuneate nucleus wherein Lábos, Hámori, and Isomura (1980) have observed an alternative arrangement of the basic triadic situation, is discussed in section 7.2.1 (see figure 7.6).

Eventually, both the dorsal column system and the spinothalamic pathway (the somatosensory pathways) converge on the specific somatosensory subcortical nucleus of the thalamus, the VPL-VPM complex. Information about painful (nociceptive) stimuli virtually is separated from the general somatosensory pathway even before reaching the VPL-VPM complex. The nociceptive fibers are lost progressively from the final part of the spinothalamic tract, partially toward the periaqueductal gray matter of the mesencephalon and the ill-defined regions of the posterior thalamic nuclear mass (the intralaminar thalamic nuclei) and possibly toward the CM and DM nuclei of the thalamus. From the DM, the main cortical projection is directed toward the frontal parts of the cortex.

The Auditory System

The auditory system differs from the somatosensory system in that the auditory system's receptors are not nerve endings (either "free" or "encapsulated" [i.e. organoid]) but rather a system of secondary neuroepithelial cells (in contrast to the olfactory receptors, which are primary). The auditory system is similar to the gustatory afferent system in which the receptors also are secondary neuroepithelial cells located in specific organoid structures, the tastebuds. The auditory-vestibular system is part of a very ancient sense organ system (the lateral-line organ) in the lower vertebrates. This system is widespread in the entire class of the fishes and in aquatic amphibians. This lateral-line organ system consists either of rows of U-shaped canals opening from and returning to the outer body surface walls or of small hills along the side of the animal. They are supplied with neuroepithelial cells, the cilia (or microcilia) of which protrude into the lumina of the canals in order to be stimulated by currents of water in those canals. The predatory larvae of especially the urodeles rely heavily on information received in this way from the immediate neighborhood of the body (especially of the head surface).

Parts of the cerebellum and other centers of the midbrain have a luxuriant overdevelopment in the weakly electric fish (Mormyriforms) representing a specific sense absent in other vertebrates (see chapter 9 in connection

with the phylogenesis of the cerebellum). Part of this lateral-line organ system became separated from the general organ system and differentiated to form a receptor organ sensitive to electrical fields. These receptors develop from the early ampullary vesicle, from which both the vestibular and auditory system of all classes of the vertebrates are derived. Without considering these early phylogenetic origins, neither of the two systems can be understood fully.

The contact between the neuroepithelial cells and the distal branches shows a very great variety, especially in the cochlear part of the VIIIth nerve. From the two main receptor systems, the vestibular part has retained more of the original design of ciliated neuroepithelia of the lateral-line organs. Actually, only one of the cell processes is a real cilium, having the general structure of 11 double tubuli, 9 of them arranged in circular fashion around the periphery and 2 arranged in the center of the cilium. The other apparent cilia lack this inner structure and hence are microcilia in the strict sense.

The single true cilium is positioned systematically on one side of the cell, in the ampullae of the anterior and posterior semicircular ducts at the side of the acoustic crista looking toward the membranous canal. In the lateral semicircular ducts, the true cilium is positioned toward the reticular end of the crista. Because bending of the cilia in the direction of the cilium position triggers the cell to increase impulse frequency, the effective (excitatory) direction of relative endolymph flow in the semicircular ducts is ampullofugal in the anterior and posterior ducts and is ampullopetal in the lateral ducts. Bending of the cilia in the opposite direction reduces the impulse frequencies and hence inhibits the continuous excitatory state of the neuroepithelia.

The neuroepithelial cells are surrounded by calyciform terminals of the distal (dendritic) primary vestibular cells in the centers of the cistae of individual fibers; at the periphery, each vestibular fiber gives rise to several calyciform terminals. The cilia of all vestibular receptors are embedded in a jellylike substance called *cupulae* in the cortical and otolithic membranes in the reticular and saccular maculae. Though the specific weight of the cupulae is equal to that of the surrounding endolymph, that of the otolithic membranes is increased by a layer of diamond-shaped otoliths (calcified grains). Hence, the cupulae act as quasi-valves, moving together with the (relative) flow of the endolymph during angular acceleration of the head and virtually insensitive to the forces of gravitation. Conversely, the maculae are sensitive to gravitation and other accelerations that, for example, lift the head up and down. The positions of the true cilia of the maculae are arranged in complicated patterns (not discussed here).

Many of the calyciform terminals surrounding the vestibular neuroepithelia are supplied on the outer surfaces by terminals of descending fibers that exercise a central inhibitory control of the receptors. The simplest type of contact occurs in the vestibular receptors (both the crista and the macula receptors), when the neuroepithelial cells are surrounded simply by a calyciform ending of the vestibular sensory fibers. The neuroepithelial cells of these vestibular receptors have only one real cilium (i.e., containing the characteristic $9 + 2$ double tubes anchored in the cell surface into the centriolar basal body) positioned systematically at a certain point of the cell surface. The others are stereocilia or micronuclei lacking this mutual structure. As a rule, bending of the cilia in the direction away from the position of the true cilium stimulates the nonadapting neuroepithelial cell to increase its resting frequency of approximately 5–10 per sec to 30 per sec and above, whereas bending the cilium toward the center of the neuroepithelial cell surface decreases the resting frequency toward (and eventually to) zero per second. Knowledge of this general rule and of the position of the true cilia allows deduction of the "effective" direction of the mechanical force (either relative movement of the endolymph, in the case of the cristae, or the deformation of the otolithic membranes by the force of gravity or linear acceleration). Many of the calices surrounding the neuroepithelial cells receive a control from an efferent terminal (on the outside of the calyx) for exercising a central bias on the receptor function.

In the case of the cochlear receptor, the mechanoelectrical transduction is not as well-understood. First, there are no true cilia in the developed state in mammals, rather only a V-shaped row of stereocilia wherein the angle of the V is toward the inner rim of the Corti organ. Also, the sensitivity of the neuroepithelial cells is orders of magnitude higher than could be explained by bending the hairs via any mechanical force caused by displacement of the basilar membrane. The cochlear nerve terminals are arranged at the bases of the hair cells (each of which receives several nerve terminals) or of the outer hair cells, wherein one cochlear fiber is distributed over a large field of outer hair cells, although several cochlear fibers converge on each hair cell also. There is a massive efferent innervation of all hair cells from the olivocochlear bundle. This principle of strong efferent innervation applies not only to the receptors but is implanted at virtually every level of the entire auditory pathway.

The extremely complex connectivity of the lower auditory pathways, and the great wealth of efferent pathways between the cochlear nuclei, superior olive, lateral lemniscus nuclei, and the inferior colliculus, are illustrated in figure 7.10 from the studies of Kiss and Majorossy (many of them still unpublished). The inferior colliculus is an obligatory intermediate subcortical station of the auditory pathway, in contrast to the superior colliculus in the visual system, which (although of the greatest importance, especially in visuomotor coordination in higher mammals) is an alternative to the path through lateral geniculate to primary visual cortex. Also, we may note the colliculoparietal path via PUL (sec. 8.4.3).

In part, the complexity of the auditory pathways has its behavioral correspondence in the sophisticated, probably largely preattentive, ability of mammals to localize the sources of sounds in their close (even in their more remote) environment. Although not exclusively, this performance rests largely on assessing the time difference within which sounds from the same source reach our two ears as dramatically experienced with so called artificial head stereophony. Stereophony is a procedure in which the two microphones for recording sound on a compact disc are positioned in the place of the two tympanic membranes in a dummy-head of roughly human size and shape. The playback of the two sound tracks into the two ears gives us a most vivid demonstration of our unconscious ability to locate the sounds reaching us from a moving source. Albeck (1995) reviewed relevant data and models of sound localization in barn owls and humans.

The medial geniculate is the ultimate subcortical station of the auditory pathway. This nuclear complex consists of three major divisions: the ventral (or principal), the medial (or magnocellular), and the dorsal (or posterior) nucleus. They are localized practically at the rostral end of the brachium of the inferior colliculus, which appears to traverse the ventral nucleus (i.e., the entire medial geniculate complex belongs more to the mesencephalon than to the diencephalon). The dorsal nucleus is particularly large and well-developed in animals using echolocation [bats (Kanwal and Suga 1995), porpoises, and seals], although especially in the bats, such enlargement occurs also for the inferior colliculus. The ventral nucleus has a laminated structure (Morest 1965) in which the collicular fibers terminate tonotopically, with a distribution of high frequencies in medial and lower frequencies in the lateral lamellae. Most of the afferents from the inferior colliculus come from its central nucleus. The tonotopic arrangement also is essential for the last geniculocortical projection.

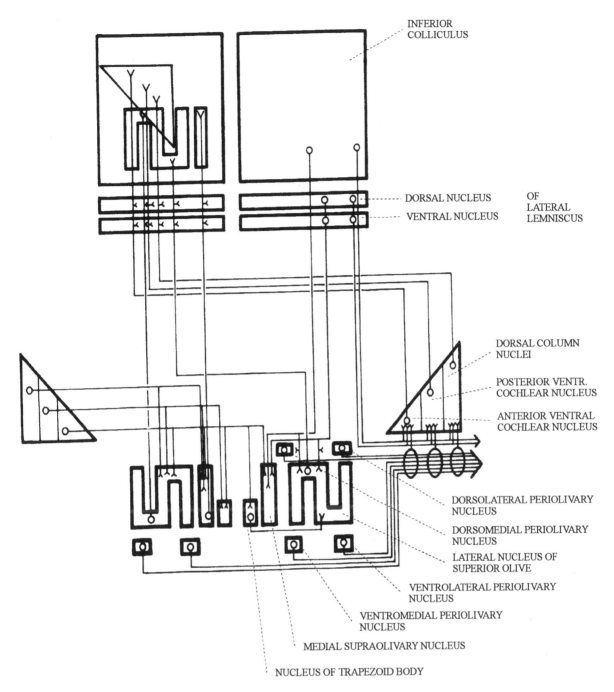

INFERIOR
COLLICULUS

DORSAL NUCLEUS
VENTRAL NUCLEUS

OF
LATERAL
LEMNISCUS

DORSAL COLUMN
NUCLEI

POSTERIOR VENTR.
COCHLEAR NUCLEUS

ANTERIOR VENTRAL
COCHLEAR NUCLEUS

DORSOLATERAL PERIOLIVARY
NUCLEUS

DORSOMEDIAL PERIOLIVARY
NUCLEUS

LATERAL NUCLEUS OF
SUPERIOR OLIVE

VENTROLATERAL PERIOLIVARY
NUCLEUS

VENTROMEDIAL PERIOLIVARY
NUCLEUS

MEDIAL SUPRAOLIVARY NUCLEUS

NUCLEUS OF TRAPEZOID BODY

Figure 7.10
Connectivity of the lower auditory pathways. Shown are the great numbers of efferent pathways among the cochlear nuclei, superior olive, lateral lemniscus nuclei, and the inferior colliculus. (Modified after Kiss and Majorossy.)

The Visual System

Figure 7.11 conveys a simplified idea of the 10 layers of the mature retina.

I. The outer pigment epithelial layer

II. The layer of the rods and cones

III. The external occluding (limitans) layer. This layer is established by the Müller glial cells that surround the bars of both the rods and the cones with a honeycomb of zonula occludens cell membrane contact. The similar zonula occludens honeycomb system that joins neighboring outer pigment epithelium cells encloses a "hermetically" closed receptor space, which communicates with the common tissue space of the body only through living cells. This arrangement is important for the complex biochemical processes needed for the photomultiplier role of the visual receptors.

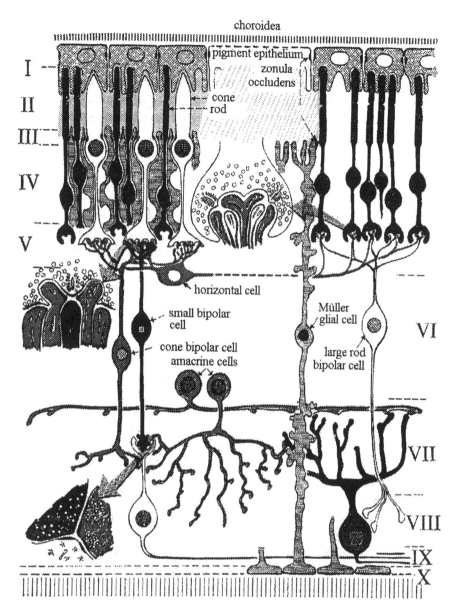

choroidea

pigment epithelium
zonula
occludens
cone
rod

I

II

III

IV

V

horizontal cell

small bipolar
cell

cone bipolar cell
amacrine cells

Müller
glial cell

large rod
bipolar cell

VI

VII

VIII

IX

X

Figure 7.11
The ten layers of the retina. Layer II contains the rods and cones; the external plexiform layer (V) contains the horizontal cells; the internal granular layer (VI) contains the nuclei of bipolar cells, Müller glia cells, and amacrine cells; and the ganglionic layer (VIII) contains the optic ganglion cells, the cells of origin of the optic fibers.

IV. The external granular layer containing the cell nuclei both of the cones in an outer row and those of the rods in a series of inner rows

V. The external plexiform layer containing the first synapses between the receptor cells and the bipolar cells and a complex synaptic system established by the horizontal cells

VI. The internal granular layer containing the nuclei of bipolar cells, Müller glia cells, and (in the inner strata) the so-called amacrine cells

VII. The internal plexiform layer containing the synapses of bipolar and amacrine cells with the optic ganglion cells

VIII. The ganglionic layer containing the optic ganglion cells, the cells of origin of the optic fibers

IX. The layer of the optic fibers, unmyelinated until their exit from the eyeball through the optic disc

X. The internal limitans membrane established by the bases of the Müller glia cells, not connected here by any occluding zonula system

The geniculostriate visual pathway, from the retina via the lateral geniculate nucleus (LGN) to visual cortex is diagrammed in figure 7.12, with an indication of how the visual field is mapped along the pathways. The main subcortical relay center of the visual pathway is the dor-

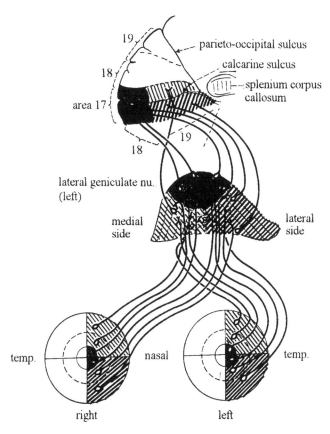

19
parieto-occipital sulcus
18
calcarine sulcus
splenium corpus
callosum
area 17
19
18
lateral geniculate nu.
(left)
medial
side
lateral
side
temp.
nasal
temp.
right
left

Figure 7.12
The geniculostriate visual pathway. Shown is the route from the retina via the lateral geniculate body to visual cortex, with an indication of how the visual field is mapped along the pathways (see text).

sal nucleus of the lateral geniculate body. This nucleus is a layered structure in virtually all mammals. In the primates, the six cell layers are arranged in horseshoe fashion, with the hilus directed ventromedially. The six layers are numbered 1 to 6, starting with two magnocellular layers 1, 2, that have no direct connection with the visual cortex. The crossed optic fibers from the contralateral retina terminate in layers 1, 4, and 6, whereas the uncrossed fibers from the ipsilateral side terminate in layers 2, 3, and 5. The terminal fields of corresponding points in the two eyes are positioned strictly in register over the alternating layers corresponding to "projection lines" of vision. The central retinal fibers corresponding to the territory surrounding the fovea centralis are halved exactly according to a vertical meridian of the retina and are crossed or uncrossed in the same manner as the fibers arising from the peripheral parts of the retina. The termination fields in the LGN occupy the central wedge of the lateral geniculate, the superior retinal quadrant occupying the nasal half and the fibers from the inferior quadrant occupying the temporal half of the wedge.

Ganglion cells have two broad classes: cells with plain receptive fields or those with elaborate receptive fields. X cells respond to stationary spots or gratings in a predictable manner. Y cells respond briskly to changes in illumination or to moving stimuli without clear spatial summation. The axons of the X cells conduct more slowly than do those of the Y cells. Wells, having more complex (elaborate) receptive fields, have the slowest conduction velocities. The synaptic arrangement in the LGN is studied most effectively in the cat, wherein the termination modes of X and Y type fibers are well-demonstrated (see discussion connected to figure 7.4).

7.3 Thalamocortical Loops and Cooperative Computation

The study of the major sensory systems in the previous section emphasizes the classical role of thalamus as a sensory relay, with cortex seen as somehow being at the top of the pyramid. By contrast, here we stress ways in which thalamic nuclei integrate cortex into a cooperative computational system in which many regions are linked in a form of circular causality. This discussion echoes the important theme of the roles of feedback loops and cooperative computation at many levels of organization (chap. 3).

7.3.1 Descending Control of Sensory Systems

Although we have stressed the path from retina through the LGN to visual (striate) cortex, the return pathway is even larger. Descending cortical input from lamina VI of the striate cortex penetrates vertically through successive cell layers of the LGN and contributes to the majority of synaptic contacts in this entire formation. The termination of fibers from the reticular thalamic nucleus (pregeniculate nucleus) are ascertained in the cat, but the analogous system for primates still is unknown. Mumford (1995) discussed models responding to the intimate relation between the reticular thalamic nucleus and the massive descending pathways from cortex to thalamus; a brief discussion of these models follows.

The principal cell type in the specific nuclei of the thalamus is that of medium to large excitatory cells known as *relay cells*; they make up approximately 65%–80% of all cells. Their axons go directly to the cortex, giving off no local collaterals except on cells in the reticular nucleus as they pass through this structure. The remaining cells are inhibitory GABAergic interneurons, which synapse on the relay cells and on each other (for cell counts, see Jones 1985, pp. 166–167). In drowsiness and non–rapid eye movement sleep, thalamic relay cells go into an oscillatory mode (see sec. 8.2).

Every nucleus of dorsal thalamus receives fibers back from all cortical areas to which it projects. Sherman and Koch (1986) estimate that in the cat there are roughly 10^6 fibers from the LGN to visual cortex but 10^7 fibers in the reverse direction. What is the functional significance of this? A widespread belief about the role of feedback is that cortical feedback gates thalamic transmission of subcortical data, allowing the cortex to attend selectively to part of this data (e.g., Crick 1984; Sherman and Koch 1986; Desimone et al. 1990). It is suggested that the synaptic weights from sensory fibers to thalamic relay cells can be adjusted to enhance or suppress selectively parts of the signal. This action occurs either through excitation of the LGN relay cells on the distal parts of their dendrites by direct corticothalamic feedback or by inhibition via an intermediate inhibitory cell in the reticular nucleus (RE) or the LGN. As we have seen, RE forms a thin layer of cells covering the anterior, dorsal, and lateral surfaces of the thalamus (correspondingly, the perigeniculate nucleus covers the LGN). All thalamocortical and corticothalamic fibers must pass through RE, which itself sends inhibitory projections back to the thalamus. Taking this into account, Crick (1984) postulated that the "windows of attention" that seem to be involved in some types of visual processing are created by the RE's suppression of the relay cells outside the current window. Thus, he speaks of the *searchlight* hypothesis (see Sherman and Koch 1986 for possible neural mechanisms).

Why would simply suppressing or enhancing different parts of the subcortical signal require such a massive feedback pathway? One answer was offered by the ALOPEX theory (Harth, Unnikrishnan, and Pandya 1987), which proposed that the feedback pathways enhance and complete sensory input patterns, suppress irrelevant features, and generate quasi-sensory patterns when afferent stimulation is weak or absent. Processing is iterative: Many signals traverse the thalamocortical loop to optimize an objective function that seeks to enhance remembered patterns partially or noisily present in the input.

Mumford (1991–1992) distinguished two distinct ideas in Harth's model: (1) generating completed sensory patterns from memory, when the actual stimulus is noisy and incomplete (see the adaptive resonance theory of Carpenter and Grossberg 1987), and (2) using LGN as an active blackboard on which various patterns can be written, misleading patterns can be suppressed, and a best reconstruction then can be generated. On this basis, Mumford assigned feedback-pattern synthesis to corti-

cocortical feedback loops and active blackboard image processing to thalamocortical feedback loops. He assumed the activity of each specific nucleus in the thalamus to represent the current view of the world for those areas of cortex to which it is connected. He argued further that thalamic regions connected to primary and secondary sensory areas and to associational and multimodal areas contain progressively more abstract representations of some aspect of the world. On this view, top-down data may be used for enhancement of the bottom-up signals, for the purpose of reconstruction of missing data, or to externalize for further processing views created by mental imagery.

Descending Control and Thalamocortical Oscillations

Another consequence of the fact that thalamus and cortex are highly interconnected by reciprocal projections is the generation of characteristic dynamic patterns, a variety of thalamocortical oscillations. High-frequency rhythms are associated with the waking state, whereas low-frequency rhythms are associated with sleeping. The main issue in section 8.3 is to balance the role of oscillations intrinsic to single neurons and network properties in the generation of thalamocortical oscillations.

7.3.2 The Striatopallidal System

The telencephalic part of the upper brainstem (in the sense outlined at the beginning of this Chapter), the striatopallidal complex of the basal ganglia, is so intimately connected with the thalamic system that it warrants a brief anatomical explanation. The term *striatopallidal* results from the fact that the two parts of the complex, the caudate nucleus and the putamen, are connected anatomically by being fused at their rostroventral end by a wider bridge of nuclear tissue and by successively thinner bridges of gray matter piercing the internal (white) capsule to the rear. This configuration gives the horizontal section of the hemispheres a striated gray-white pattern, labeled in classical anatomy *corpus striatum* (striped body). The inner (medial) part of the lentiform nucleus is separated from the putamen by a continuous lamella of white matter and is not as gray, due to a greater dispersal of white substance between the masses of nerve cells; hence its ancient name, *globus pallidus*. (In fact, a third nuclear mass, a thin gray lamella outside the lentiform nucleus, the claustrum, also belongs to this formation, but its inclusion here is unnecessary.)

The basal ganglia is connected thoroughly with the neocortex, the thalamus, and the lower brainstem nuclei.

In great part, but not exclusively, it subserves movement (to be understood in the widest sense) from relatively independent movements of separate body parts (e.g., the limbs) to virtually all stance and locomotion actions in which all parts of the body become invariably involved. Chapter 10 presents the structure of the basal ganglia in more detail and develops a functional account of its role in motor learning, a role strongly linked to modern studies in neurophysiology. Alexander, DeLong, and Strick (1986) found that there are multiple loops of the form

A, B, C in cortex → striatum → SNr → thalamus
    → (pre)frontal A

which embed the basal ganglia in reciprocal interactions with cortex. Each of these loops has a topographical structure that allows each component (with the corresponding parts in the four structures connected) to form relatively separate cortico-basal ganglia-cortical circuits: oculomotor, motor, prefrontal, and 'limbic' (discussed further in sec. 10.1.2).

The Oculomotor Circuit

In addition to influencing movements of the body and limbs, the basal ganglia also influence eye movements by means of an additional projection from the substantia nigra pars reticulata (SNr) to the superior colliculus. The frontal eye fields and several other cortical areas project to the body of the caudate, which projects to the SNr, an output nucleus of the basal ganglia. Then the SNr projects to both the superior colliculus and the frontal eye fields via the thalamus (figure 7.13a).

The Motor Circuit

Those portions of the cerebral cortex most closely related to the control of movement—supplementary motor area, premotor cortex, motor cortex, somatosensory cortex, and the superior parietal lobule—make dense, topographically organized projections to what thus may be called the *motor portion* of the putamen. Somatotopy in putamen is preserved through pallidum and onward. The output of this pathway is directed primarily back to the supplementary motor area and to premotor cortex via thalamus (see figure 7.13b). These cortical areas are interconnected reciprocally with each other and with the motor cortex, and all have direct descending projections to brainstem motor centers and to the spinal cord. Through the projection of the portions of the thalamus that receive input from the basal ganglia to the prefrontal cortex—the premotor cortex, the supplementary

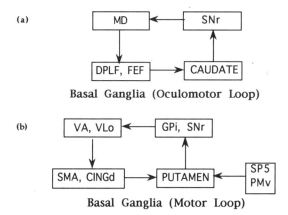

Figure 7.13
The oculomotor (a) and motor (b) loops of the basal ganglia. MD, mediodoral thalamus; SNr, substantia nigra pars reticulata; DLPC, dorsolateral prefrontal cortex; FEF, frontal eye fields; GPi, interior portion of the globus pallidus; VA, ventral anterior nucleus of thalamus; SMA, supplementary motor area; CING, cingulate; PMv, ventral premotor cortex; 5, parietal area 5.

motor area, and the motor cortex—the basal ganglia influences other descending systems, such as the corticospinal and the corticobulbar systems. Thus, the motor functions of the basal ganglia are mediated indirectly by means of these cortical motor areas and their descending projections.

The "Cognitive" (Dorsolateral Prefrontal) Circuit

The dorsolateral prefrontal cortex and several other areas of association cortex project to the dorsolateral head of the caudate nucleus, which in turn projects back to the dorsolateral prefrontal cortex via the thalamus. This circuit probably is involved in aspects of memory concerned with orientation in space and other cognitive functions.

The Limbic (Lateral Orbitofrontal) Circuit

This circuit links the lateral orbitofrontal cortex with the ventromedial caudate. It is thought to be involved in the ability to change behavioral set.

7.3.3 The Cerebellar System

The cerebellum is studied in some detail in chapter 9. The cerebellar cortex can be divided into three zones: the vermis most medially; the intermediate hemispheres on either side of the vermis; and most laterally, the lateral hemispheres. Each zone projects to its own deep cerebellar nucleus: the fastigial nucleus, the interposed nucleus, and the dentate nucleus, respectively. The relations are well-visualized in figures 41-11A,B and 41-12 from Ghez (1991).

The *vermis* receives input from the eyes (see its role in oculomotor control in sec. 9.4.4) neck, trunk, and the vestibular system. It influences both the brainstem and (via thalamus) medial motor cortex.

The *intermediate hemispheres* receive information from the limbs and project via interpositus both to the red nucleus and (via thalamus) to the cortical sources, the corticospinal tracts.

The *lateral hemispheres* both receive cortical input via the pontine nuclei and project to both motor cortex and premotor cortex via dentate nucleus and thalamus. In this last case, we see the cerebellum both instructing and being instructed by cortical activity in a scheme of cooperative computation that cuts across any simple view of hierarchical structure (see section 9.4.4).

Thalamic nuclei integrate cortex into a cooperative computation system in which many regions are linked in a form of circular causality. This theme recurs many times in the next three chapters.

Cerebral Cortex

The structural overview of cerebral cortex begins with its development (sec. 8.1.1), its layered structure (sec. 8.1.2), and its cell types (sec. 8.1.3). In section 8.1.4, we analyze the synaptic connectivity of cortical neurons, noting the interplay of excitation and inhibition, and we analyze the role of neuron chains in cortical function. Finally, in section 8.1.5, we return to the modular-architectonics principle of chapter 2, wherein Szentágothai offers a strong defense of his view of the modular structural organization of the cortex but questions the functional role of such units.

Section 8.2 opens with a very brief look at psychophysical and neurophysiological data on spatial visual perception, discussing the many different aspects of visual information processed by different brain regions (though saying little more about low-level visual processing, in section 3.1.5, we analyzed visual scene interpretation in schema-theoretical terms; in section 8.4, we discuss cortical mechanisms for using vision in the control of movement). After a general discussion of the cortical representation of sensory surfaces (sec. 8.2.1), we offer two striking examples of modular architectonics that have been revealed in primary visual cortex: ocular dominance columns (sec. 8.2.2), and orientation columns (sec. 8.2.3). In each case, the discussion of data establishing the reality of these structures is accompanied by the presentation of models of their development and an analysis of the superposition of these two columnar systems (sec. 8.2.4). Section 8.2.6 contains a brief study of the role of long-range horizontal connections in the integration of information.

Thalamus and cortex are interconnected highly by reciprocal projections, giving rise to characteristic dynamic patterns. High-frequency rhythms are associated with the waking state, whereas low-frequency rhythms are associated with sleeping. The main issue in section 8.3 is to balance the role of oscillations intrinsic to single neurons and network properties in the generation of thalamocortical oscillations. Thus, after a general discussion of rhythms, generating mechanisms, and modulations (sec. 8.3.1), we analyze the intrinsic electrophysiological properties of thalamic neurons, thalamocortical neurons, and reticular thalamic neurons (sec. 8.3.2). A study of data and models for the dynamics of spindle oscillations is found in section 8.3.3, and delta and slow-sleep oscillations are covered in section 8.3.4. In section 8.3.5, we analyze the role of brainstem control and cellular mechanisms in thalamocortical activation and in section 8.3.6 return to the main issue of section 8.3, in which we use a number of models to explore the role of single-cell dynamics and emergent network properties in thalamocortical activation.

Section 8.4 is a return to the functional themes of looking, reaching, and grasping established at the schema-theoretic level in chapter 3. In that section, we focus on frontoparietal interactions in cortex but demonstrate that many other brain regions are involved in the integration of vision with action. In section 8.4.1, we provide a formalism for large-scale models of the nervous system (see also Appendixes). Section 8.4.2 contains a detailed model of corticothalamic systems for saccade control, with particular attention paid to the roles of posterior parietal cortex, frontal eye fields, and thalamus in providing mechanisms for dynamic remapping and target memory. Section 8.4.3 is an analysis of cortical systems for reaching and grasping. First we review data suggesting that visual input to parietal cortex is processed for "where and how" information and visual input to inferotemporal cortex is processed for "what" information. Then we analyze data for "neural codes" in parietal lobe and premotor cortex in relation to schema-based analysis of hand movements (see chapter 3). We conclude by relating a computational model of the neural mechanisms of grasp generation in monkey to the human functional anatomy involved in grasping; we use the technique of synthetic positron emission tomography (PET) imaging.

In section 8.5, we address the theme of learning of coordinated behaviors, providing first a schema-level analysis of motor set and of the neuralization of coordinated control programs, then a specific neural network model of visual-motor conditional learning. Foreshadowed in the study of rat spatial learning (chapter 6), this theme is developed further in our study of cerebellum (chapter 9) and basal ganglia (chapter 10).

Sections 8.4 and 8.5 are focused on action-oriented perception, with special attention paid to the visual control of looking, reaching, and grasping and to visual-motor conditional learning. In section 8.6, we chart a path toward the study of cognition, though from a high-level, schema-theoretical viewpoint that shows relatively little about the relevant neurophysiological data. We argue there that human cognition rests on the integration of schema assemblages "evolutionarily hardwired" into patterns of competition and cooperation between

specific brain regions and those that can yield totally novel forms to develop new skills and represent novel situations.

8.1 Structural Overview

8.1.1 Development of the Cerebral Cortex

The cerebral cortex of mammals is a laminated sheet of gray matter covering the entire outer surface of the telencephalic brain vesicles. It is subdivided into three major parts: the phylogenetically more ancient paleocortex and archicortex and the more recent, six-layered neocortex. As the paleocortex (piriform cortex) has been discussed in chapter 5 and the archicortex (hippocampal formation) has been addressed in chapter 6, here we concentrate on neocortex. The telencephalic brain vesicles develop essentially as two lateral bulges of the original prosencephalic forebrain vesicle, and the main direction of growth (similar to a rubber sac being inflated) is tangential. It is the marginal parts of the outgrowing new vesicles that remain relatively stable and the middle parts of the original wall that are distended maximally. Hence, it is unsurprising that the marginal parts of the telencephalic vesicles are those that stay closer to the archetype of the cortical formation whereas the tissue of the middle parts of the newly formed vesicles has to be quasi-added to the more ancient marginal parts of the vesicles. This grossly oversimplified growth mechanism justified separating the marginal parts as forming "limbic" (marginal) cortex, although the subdivision into archicortex and neocortex does not fit closely with the regions considered as limbic. We remind the reader that these definitions and mechanisms of growth are crude simplifications of an infinitely more complex reality.

In chapter 2, we described the proliferation of the medullary tube epithelium in the inner germinative zone of the original pseudo-stratified epithelium, the progressive differentiation of different cell lines, and the migration of the cells produced by the final division toward outer zones of the tube or the brain vesicle wall. In fact, the migration mechanisms in the segmented part of the neuraxis and even in the cerebellum are less clear than is the relatively straightforward developmental process of the cerebral cortex. Thus, much of our insight and understanding of spinal cord and cerebellar development results from analogies with the mechanisms seen in the neocortex.

What makes the formation of the cerebral cortex a paradigm of neural center formation is the fact that the

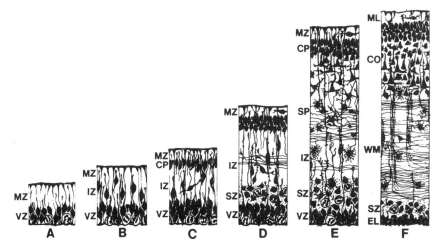

Figure 8.1
A quasi-two-dimensional pattern of the germinative layer. It becomes transformed into a three-dimensional pattern of prismatic columns. (Reprinted with permission from Rakic 1982.) MZ, marginal zone; VZ, ventricular zone; IZ, intermediate zone; CP, cortical plate; SZ, subventricular zone; SP, subplate zone; EL, ependymal layer; WM, white matter; ML, molecular layer.

migrating cells settle progressively into surface-parallel layers in a relatively outer part of the mantle zone of the original brain vesicle. These layered cells give rise to the cell primordium of the cortex, a so-called cortical plate. More strictly, as is seen also in the development of the cerebellar cortex (sec. 9.1.2), the pattern of migration adheres to the rule that the cells formed earliest settle in the deeper layers of the cortical plate, whereas the cells formed later have to transgress the earlier (deeper) cell layers and settle progressively at the outer side of the deeper (earlier-formed) cell layers. The elegance and beauty of this mechanism is shown in a most impressive diagram by P. Rakic (1982), reproduced in figure 8.1. A quasi-two-dimensional pattern of the germinative layer ("quasi" because a cell layer cannot be considered as really two-dimensional) becomes transformed into a three-dimensional pattern of prismatic columns in which the original neighborhood relations of the germinative cell layer are upheld, but the temporal sequence of events is unfolded and transformed into depth relations. We know now that the decision of whether one final cell becomes a neuron or a glial cell and the decision as to cell type and the nature of its mediators (e.g., modulators) are determined at the latest at the time of the final cell divisions of its cell lineage.

Even with the occurrence of horizontal migration taken into account, the elegant developmental mechanisms forcefully suggest a columnar organization principle of cortical tissue, supporting the concept of the modular (columnar) architecture of this central organ. The assembly of major organs by repetitive application of similar structural units is such a general phenomenon (both in living and nonliving matter) that failure to occur would be a priori unlikely in this most complex formation of the central nervous system (CNS). Our study of ocular dominance columns (sec. 8.2.2) and orientation columns (sec. 8.2.3) provides models of self-organization of these modular structures.

8.1.2 The Six Principal Layers of Neocortex

The discovery of the structure of cerebral cortex took its origin from the 1782 observation by an Italian student of medicine, Francesco Gennari, of a delicate pale line (*lineola albidior*) running in a surface-parallel (tangential) direction in the middle of the gray cortex in the medial surface of the occipital lobe of the brain. Soon, this line was observed and illustrated by other authors of the period (Vicq d'Azyr 1786; Soemmering 1788). The characteristic white band in the fourth layer of the primary visual cortex indeed is observable with the naked eye and still is referred to as the *band of Gennari*; it was this band from which the primary visual cortex later received its distinctive name *area striata*.

Radically new insights into the structure of the cortex were obtained by the introduction of cell-staining methods, first by the natural dye, carmine (Berlin 1858), when the general arrangement of the cortical cells in six (at least five–seven) more or less distinct tangential layers was recognized. The early observation of distinct cell types—pyramidal, stellate, fusiform, granular (small polyhedral)—goes back to these early studies, although it was not before the introduction of Golgi's 1873 *reazione nera* (silver chromate precipitation) that the real

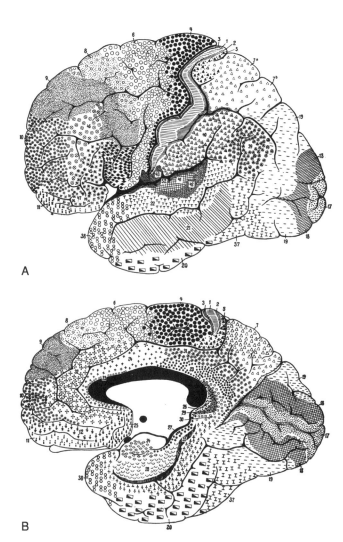

Figure 8.2
Cytoarchitectonic map elaborated by Brodmann in the last period of his studies. More than 50 cytoarchitectonic areas have been distinguished. Various areas are distinguished by different symbols and Arabic numbers. (A) Lateral view of human cerebral hemisphere. (B) Medial view of human cerebral hemisphere.

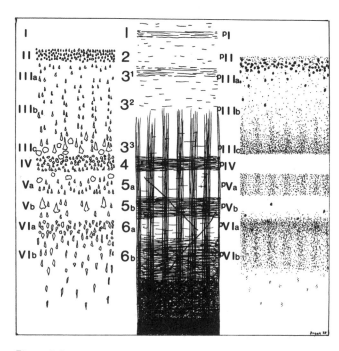

Figure 8.3
A comparison of the lamination nomenclature. Numbers proceed from outside (pial surface) to inside for cyroarchitectonics (left column), given in Roman numerals; myeloarchitectonics (middle column), given in Arabic numerals; and lipofuscin, pigment architectonics (right column) given in Roman numerals with the prefix *p* for pigment. Sublayering is indicated by letters of the Roman alphabet (*a, b, c*); further sublayering is designated by Greek letters (*α, β*) (e.g., IVcα). See text for description of the layers. (Reprinted with permission from Braak 1984.)

shape of the cortical nerve cells was appreciated fully (Golgi 1883).

The most generally accepted human brain map that also could be adapted to that of other primate and nonprimate mammals was published by Brodmann (1908), with a greatly improved version in 1912 and 1914. This map distinguished somewhat more than 50 cortical areas (figure 8.2). However, when the microelectrode exploration of cortical functions began to be used widely in parallel with more recent developments of anatomical tracing methods, the earlier subdivision into architectonic areas was substantiated and the subdivision could be extended on the basis of finer functional and connectivity criteria to territorial subdivisions smaller by one (or often two) orders of magnitude.

The basic six-layered structure of the neocortex gradually was accepted after the architectonics studies of Brodmann (1908, 1912). A unified nomenclature was provided by Vogt and Vogt (1919) on the basis of a careful and systematic comparison (both for different brain regions and for different species) of *cytoarchitectonics* and *myeloarchitectonics*. However, one new aspect can be added fruitfully into our present picture of architectonics. The introduction of aldehyde-fuchsin staining of lipofuscin (Braak 1971) brought a new dimension into architectonics by adding a well-recognizable element of chemoarchitectonics to the two purely morphological sets of criteria: (1) cell size, shape, and density in cytoarchitectonics, and (2) course, density, and fiber thickness in myeloarchitectonics.

The general structure of the neocortex is demonstrated most elegantly and clearly in a synthetic 1984 diagram by Braak (figure 8.3) with a comparison of the lamination nomenclature in the now-traditional sequence from outside (pial surface) to inside.

Lamina I, the *molecular layer*, is almost entirely devoid of nerve cells (apart from a few exclusively inhibitory neurons) and contains varying numbers of tangentially oriented axons.

Lamina II, the *corpuscular layer* (external granular layer), contains small cell bodies rather densely packed, among which it is difficult to distinguish pyramidal from non-pyramidal cells (for reasons to be described later).

Lamina III, the *pyramidal layer*, generally is the thickest layer of the cortex in primates and contains mainly pyramid-shaped cell bodies, which appear to be arranged in vertical columns. The size of the cell bodies gradually increases toward the depth of the layer.

Lamina IV, the (internal) *granular layer*, contains relatively small polyhedral cell bodies. This layer is relatively thin in most cortical regions but becomes widened and subdivided into various sub- or sub-sublayers in the primary sensory cortices.

Lamina V, the *ganglionic layer*, is made up mainly of pyramidal cell bodies, with the exception of the stratum immediately bordering lamina IV, wherein single large polyhedral cell bodies (e.g., Betz and Meynert cells) are relatively frequent.

Lamina VI, the *multiform layer*, contains vertically oriented spindle-shaped and less regular pyramid-shaped cell bodies.

8.1.3 Cell Types of the Neocortex

Pyramidal Neurons

The most characteristic cell type of the neocortex (and of some parts of the archicortex) and, indeed, of the entire mammalian nervous system, is the pyramidal neuron. Pyramidal cells receive their name from their triangular shape (already well recognizable in simple cell stains), an isosceles triangle with the acute angle pointing toward the surface of the cortex. More characteristically, the upper acute angle continues into an ascending apical dendrite or dendritic shaft, which in most cases reaches the border of the two superficial cortical layers, I and II, wherein it breaks up into a terminal dendritic tuft. The apical dendrite gives rise to several side branches of either horizontal or slightly ascending course. The cell body has the shape of an elongated cone. The main part of the dendritic tree takes its origin from the cell body; the so-called basal dendrites form a spherical radiate arborization.

The axon of the pyramidal neuron originates at the base of the cell body and pursues a vertically descending course. Probably the vast majority of pyramidal cell axons leave the cortex toward the white matter. It had been assumed earlier that the axons of the small pyra-

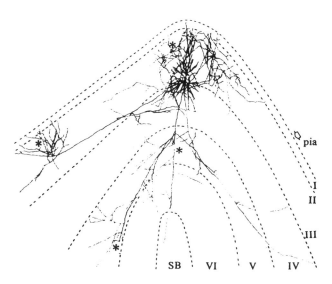

Figure 8.4
A pyramidal cell filled intracellularly by the enzyme horseradish peroixidase (top-center). Asterisks mark the arborizations of the cell's axon collaterals, which are specific and arborize profusely in well-defined patches of the neighboring cortical tissue. SB, "sostanga bianca," white matter. (Reprinted with permission from Kisvárday et al. 1986.)

midal cells of lamina II terminate locally. Before becoming myelinated, the pyramidal cell axons issue a number of collaterals that arborize in a rather large space surrounding the cell of origin. General observation of Golgi-stained pyramidal cells produced the false impression that the branching of the axon collaterals is nonspecific but may reach large distances of up to 1.5 mm and possibly more. Thus, the total span of the collateral arborization of a pyramidal axon was assumed to reach total distances of 3 mm and possibly beyond. However, after cells filled intracellularly by the enzyme horseradish-peroxidase could be observed routinely (figure 8.4), it was revealed that the arborizations of the pyramidal axon collaterals were much more specific and arborized profusely in well-defined patches of the neighboring cortical tissue. On this basis, entirely different classes of pyramidal cells soon would have to be distinguished.

Dendritic Spines Most dendrites of the pyramidal neuron are studded liberally with delicate drumstick-shaped appendages known as *dendritic spines*. These spines already were described by the first investigators by using the Golgi procedure, notably Golgi (1883) and Ramón y Cajal (1899). However, it was only after the advent of electron microscopy that the spines were recognized as the receptive sites of synapses given by the terminal arborizations of terminal axon branches. This fact immediately led students of cerebral cortex to realize the importance of the dendritic spines: their number and presence or absence in certain parts of the dendritic tree under various experimental and pathological circumstances. The density (number per unit length of dendrite) of the spines varies considerably according to species, cortical region, and type of dendrite. However, no clear relations to the phylogenetic position of the species could be detected. It is difficult to find reliable data on spine numbers; the total number of spines in smaller pyramidal cells could be somewhere between 6000 (as an extreme and unlikely minimum) and 30,000. (This would tally with the average of 80,000 spines of Purkinje cells in the cerebellar cortex.) The number of synapses received by any pyramidal cell is higher than that of spines. This is due partially to the fact that some spines receive several (two or three) terminals from presynaptic axons but mainly to the fact that interspine dendritic (shaft) surfaces also receive many synaptic terminals (particularly the spineless initial parts of the dendrites) as does the cell body and the initial segment of the axon. As far as can be judged on the basis of horseradish-peroxidase-labeled terminal axon branches, the number of individual terminal boutons given by any axon to any given cell varies between 1 and 10. Of course, dendritic spines are prevalent in many other cell types and many other regions of the CNS. Holmes and Rall (1995) provide a review of models of their function in neural activity.

Laminar Distribution Pyramidal neurons are found in virtually all laminae, with the exception of lamina I of the cortex. There is a sudden rise of pyramidal cell body size at the border between lamina II and III, then a gradual rise of cell body size over the entire lamina III. In lamina IV, the number of pyramidal neurons varies strongly with cortical areas; fewer pyramidal cells are found in primary sensory fields and very many (a virtual absence of a distinct lamina IV) in motor and premotor regions. Alternatively, it may be that motor areas lack a layer IV because of the dispersion of granular cells such that a clearly coalesced layer IV does not exist. Lamina V contains relatively large pyramidal cells (neurons of excessive size are the giant pyramidal Betz cells in the motor cortex). In lamina VI, the scatter in pyramidal cell size, shape, and orientation becomes so large that it is difficult to decide whether or not a particular cell is a true pyramidal neuron.

Clustering Pyramidal cells are not distributed at random but are arranged quite systematically into clusters. The "core" of each cluster is formed by a small group (three

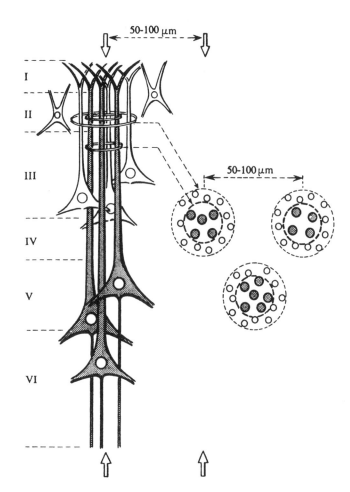

Figure 8.5
The arrangement of pyramidal cells into clusters. A small group (3–5 cells) of large lamina V and VI pyramidal cells forms the core of the cluster, with their apical dendrites forming an ascending dendritic bundle. Smaller lamina III pyramidal neurons in the same cluster have somewhat thinner apical dendrites that also join this ascending dendritic bundle. (Reprinted with permission from Szentágothai 1989.)

to five) of large pyramidal cells of lamina V and VI, the bodies of which are distributed in staggered fashion over a considerable stretch in depth but occurring sufficiently close to a radial (vertical) line of the cortex as to have their apical dendrites form an ascending dendritic bundle. The somewhat thinner apical dendrites of the smaller lamina III pyramidal neurons join the periphery of the apical dendrite bundles (figure 8.5). Although many, if not most, of the lamina II cells are pyramidal neurons, they do not have an apical dendrite, as the dendrite directed toward the surface immediately arborizes, making these cells appear bicuspate in vertical sections. The average distance between "cluster axes" varies between 50 and 100 μm. In spite of such "bundling," there is no electron-microscopic evidence of any synaptic (or any other direct structural) interrelation between apical den-

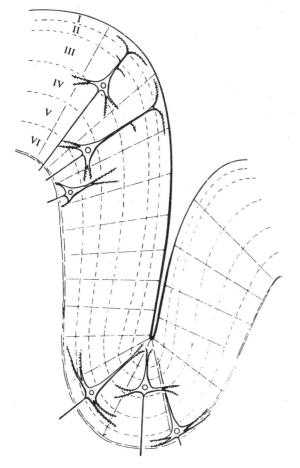

Figure 8.6
Variation of geometry of arborizations of dendrites and axons with folding of the cortex. The superficial lamina I is thickened at the depth of the sulci (center) and thinned down at convexities of the gyri (top left); in lamina VI, the situation is reversed. As a result, the course of the terminal branches of the apical dendrite tufts becomes closer to surface-perpendicular at the depth of the sulci and near surface-parallel at the top of the gyri. Conversely, the main course of the basal dendrites becomes less surface-parallel at the top of gyri and almost completely surface-parallel in the depth of the sulci. (Reprinted with permission from Szentágothai 1989.)

drites belonging to the same bundle. The most parsimonious explanation of this clustering (bundling) of the pyramidal neurons would be the assumption of common origin from a given cell line of the early neuroepithelium of the ventricular germinal zone and of movement along radiate glial bundles as demonstrated in figure 8.1.

As shown much earlier for the cerebellar cortex (Eccles, Ho, and Szentágothai 1967), the folding of the cortical tissue (*folia* in the cerebellar cortex and *gyri* and *sulci* in the cerebral cortex) is reflected in the geometry of arborizations both of the dendrites and (to lesser extent) of the axons. The simplest and probably only realistic explanation of these radical changes in cell and arborization is to consider them as a smooth transformation of

forms, used quite often by scientists trying to elucidate changes of shapes occurring in phylogenesis (e.g., Thompson 1917/1961). Adapted to the circumstances of the cerebral cortex, this basic principle could be illustrated most clearly by such a diagram as figure 8.6, in which it is seen that the superficial lamina I is thickened at the depth of the sulci and thinned down at convexities of the gyri, whereas in lamina VI, the situation is reversed: the lamina thins down in the depth of the sulci and thickens in the convex parts of the cortex. In consequence, the terminal branches of the apical dendrite tufts run close to surface-perpendicular at the depth of the sulci and near surface-parallel at the top of the gyri. Conversely, the main course of the basal dendrites becomes less surface-parallel at the top of gyri and almost completely surface-parallel in the depth of the sulci.

Nonpyramidal Neurons

For reasons of expediency, modern taxonomy labels all other cells of the cerebral cortex as *nonpyramidal*. Apart from the first step in the logical dichotomy of classification, the term has little meaning, because cells that fall into this category have practically nothing in common. Unfortunately, there is little agreement about the next step in the tree of taxonomy; thus, the nomenclature to be used here is arbitrary and reflects the individual views of the authors.

The nonpyramidal neurons can be divided into three major categories: long-axon projective neurons, short-axon projective neurons, and short-axon (true) interneurons. The distinction between the second and third categories is based on an admittedly somewhat shaky criterion. If a neuron is an integral part of a neuron chain for routing impulses through any particular part of the cortex, it can be justly labeled *projective* (the second type). If, conversely, it is a "side-line" (generally inhibitory) for either feedforward or feedback inhibition (or disinhibition), it is a true interneuron. The main neuronal chain for through-conduction also may become inhibitory in the end, as in the cerebellar cortex, but so far there is no evidence for this in the neocortex. Categorization according to the terms *Golgi type 1* (Deiters type) and *type 2* is not used here, because the pyramidal neurons themselves are the best (although by no means the only) examples of Golgi type 1 cells and the classic definition of the Golgi neurons (although an excellent descriptive term) is of little use for distinguishing the preceding second and third categories. The term *local circuit neurons* is not used here because it is suited to obscure matters rather than to clarify them and might lead to unnecessary misunderstandings.

Long-Axon Projective Neurons There are very few (not really reliable) data on nonpyramidal long-axon projective neurons. The visual cortex is the only cortical region of the cortex in which clearly nonpyramidal stellate-shaped neurons with spiny dendrites give rise to cortical efferents. These cells were described by Ramón y Cajal (1899), and this observation has been substantiated by numerous other authors and recently by modern retrograde tracing techniques. No reliable data pertaining to other primary sensory cortices are available.

A special source of ambiguity is the cells of lamina VI, many of which are efferent and in the majority directed toward the thalamus, wherein (due to the irregularity in shape and orientation of the cell bodies and the major dendrites) it is difficult to decide whether any cell could or could not be considered as a pyramidal neuron. Rather, most fusiform or irregular cells of this layer, having spines on their dendrites and an axon that enters the white matter, ought to be considered as genuine but distorted pyramidal neurons.

Short-Axon Projective Neurons *Spiny stellate cells* are among the main target neurons of specific sensory afferents. They are located in lamina IV, especially in the primary sensory cortical areas. Their cell bodies are small and generally stellate-shaped and their relatively short dendrites (usually <150 μm) are studded with spines and occupy spaces of spherical shape. The axon usually originates on the side looking toward the white matter and breaks up immediately into numerous branches. Only a few of the axon branches can be traced for longer distances in the horizontal direction, although many side branches terminate at small distances from the cell body. The main axon branches either ascend or descend (or both) vertically toward the superficial or deeper layers of the cortex. Besides the shorter horizontal axon branches, the main targets for terminal arborization of the spiny stellate neurons are the cells of lamina III, lamina Va, and lamina VI. Figure 8.7 is a general impression of a typical spiny stellate cell in the visual cortex of the monkey. The spiny stellates of other sensory regions (somatosensory, acoustic) are very similar in many different species.

The axonal arborization of the vast majority of the spiny stellate neurons stays within a narrow vertical column of the cortical tissue, so that whatever their input, they can distribute impulses only vertically either in a narrow space around the location of their somas or in the cortical tissue vertically above or below.

Spiny stellate cells do not show any immunocytochemical reactions to either glutamic acid decarboxylase (GAD) or γ-aminobutyricacid (GABA) antibodies. This indication of excitatory synapses corresponds to the

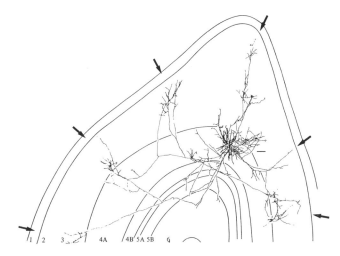

Figure 8.7
A spiny stellate cell of layer IVA in the visual cortex of the cat. (Reprinted with permission from Martin and Whitteridge 1984.)

asymmetric membrane contacts and to the spherical vesicles of all identified terminal knobs of spiny stellate neurons. Hence, the spiny stellate neurons are undoubtedly projective cells that belong to the chain of neurons in continuation of the incoming specific sensory afferents.

Bipolar neurons of strictly vertical orientation have been observed both in lamina II and III of sensory cortices and in laminae IV and V. Having only sparse further arborizations, the two main dendrites ascend or descend vertically and may extend well into neighboring and even more distant layers of the cortex. The dendrites have few, if any, spines. The axons usually originate from the descending main dendrite and have a vertical trajectory. Only their terminal branches run in a horizontal direction, but they terminate at relatively short distances.

Because virtually all cells that give strong reactions with antibodies against vasoactive intestinal polypeptide (VIP) are bipolar and look entirely similar to the Golgi-stained bipolar cells, it generally is thought that this polypeptide is the chief transmitter of the bipolar cells. When applied by microcanullas, VIP acts as an excitatory substance; thus, these cells generally are thought to have excitatory functions. Also, the position of many bipolars in lamina IV—and, if not, many of their dendrites entering and or traversing lamina IV—could be interpreted in favor of the assumption that, like the spiny stellates, they might function as recipients of specific afferent input and transmit it in a vertical direction toward more superficial or deeper layers of the cortex. The bipolars are non GABAergic, but many of these cells contain the enzyme choline-acetyl-transferase, which would be indicative of their cholinergic nature.

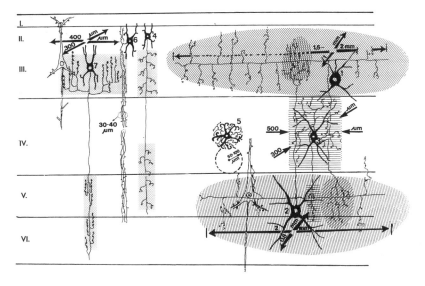

Figure 8.8

Diagrammatic illustration of the seven types of well-characterized (GABAergic) inhibitory interneurons. To facilitate recognition of dendrites and axons, the dendritic trees are simplified and drawn with exaggerated thickness. Fields of axonal arborization are indicated by hatching and stippling where necessary. Horizontal arrows indicate maximal observed extension of the axonal arborizations in the sagittal zone, and oblique arrows are used in the coronal directions. The extension of the axons in depth can be derived from the cortical layering indicated at left margin. *1*, large basket cells of the upper (supergranular) group (Somogyi et al. 1983); *2*, large basket cell of the infragranular group (Kisvárday et al. 1986); *3*, "clutch cell" terminating mainly in lamina IV (Kisvárday et al. 1985); *4*, columnar basket cell (Szentágothai 1983); *5*, microglioform cell (both dendritic and axonal arborization most generally spherical; *6*, *cellule a double bouquet* of Ramón y Cajal; *7*, axoaxonic inhibitory interneuron, the chandelier cells of Szentágothai and Arbib 1975. (Reprinted with permission from Szentágothai 1978b.)

Short-Axon Interneurons For the time being, all known true interneurons of the neocortex (as distinct from the short-axon projective neurons) are of an inhibitory nature. Several types of these inhibitory interneurons were recognized and described on the basis of their characteristic arborization patterns (mainly of the axons) by the classical authors, mainly Ramón y Cajal (1899). Some of these interneurons have been studied and defined unequivocally recently by new more advanced techniques, notably by intracellular labeling with horseradish-peroxidase or, more recently, with *Phaseolus* lectin. These are the *basket cells*, from which at least three subtypes (a1–a3) can be distinguished, the *double bouquet cells*, and the *axoaxonic* (or *chandelier*) *cells*. Other cell types are less well-defined, partly because such cells have not been labeled successfully intracellularly thus far and partly because, although characteristic, their morphological features (particularly the arborization pattern of their axons) do not lend themselves easily to a clear separation of the different types. These types are the following: *neuroglia-form* (dwarf or "spider-web") *cells*; *smooth* or *sparsely spiny* Golgi type 2 *cells* lacking in distinctive patterns of arborization of their axons (by far the most general and probably most frequent and most ubiquitous interneuron type); *axonal tuft cells*; and *dendroaxonal cells*.

A composite diagram of the several inhibitory interneuron types so far identified in the neocortex is reproduced in figure 8.8. The basic message conveyed by figure 8.8 is that there is a kind of mirror reflection of inhibition between the supra- and the infragranular layers (layer IV is the granular layer) in the sense that many of the main inhibitory cell types have a small zone of additional axonal arborization on the opposite side of lamina IV. The large basket cells with their main axonal arborization in lamina III (see *1* in figure 8.8) send a descending axonal branch into lamina V–VI, and the large basket cells of lamina V (*2*) with their main axon arborization in layers V–VI, send an ascending branch arborizing in lamina III (and partially in II). Strangely, these smaller tufts of arborization are positioned very exactly vertically below or above the positions of the parent cell body. The same holds true for two other inhibitory cell types, the layer IV "clutch cells" (*3*) and the axoaxonic cells (*7*). However, we do not have any evidence for a true mirror relation between the supra- and the infragranular layers, but because axoaxonic cell bodies have been observed also in layers V and VI (Tömböl 1978), we may imagine that such an ascending connection does exist for the deeper axoaxonic cells and also for the clutch cells; it is only that such connections have not been observed so far. Also, there is some admittedly tenuous evidence (Somogyi et al. 1983) for vertically ascending columnar connections from inhibitory interneurons positioned in the depth of the cortex, possibly the cells first observed by and named after Martinotti. Their structural information being very indirect, these cells have not been included in figure 8.8. Other probably inhibitory interneurons, such as the cells enumerated earlier (the smooth Golgi type 2, axonal tuft, and dendroaxonal cells) have not been identified by modern methods; thus, they also have been omitted from figure 8.8. However, being found quite regularly in Golgi specimens (especially in the primate cortex), they have been included in a later figure (see figure 8.16) dealing with the illustration of various cell types separated on the basis of the distances that they bridge locally.

8.1.4 Synaptic Connectivity of Cortical Neurons

Although various types of synaptic contacts were known in the late 1880s and early 1890s, the synaptic connectivity of the cerebral cortex was ill understood before the advent of electron microscopy. Synaptic contacts are established with most parts of the cortical cells, notably with dendritic spines, dendrite surfaces, the cell body surface, and (in the case of pyramidal cells) initial segments of the axons. Dendritic spines may receive multiple synapses (up to three), with the restriction that synapses of excitatory axons always are in contact with spine heads, whereas GABAergic terminals of inhibitory cell axons usually have their contacts on the "necks" of the spines, almost invariably "downstream" from the excitatory contact. Single contacts can be traced back exclusively to cells or axons of excitatory nature. Synaptic contacts on the interspine surfaces of spiny dendrites or on nonspiny dendrites may be either excitatory or inhibitory in nature. Synaptic contacts with cell body surface are predominantly inhibitory (i.e., GABAergic), especially in pyramidal neurons; in nonpyramidal cells, either type may occur.

The initial segment proximal to the first collateral branch of the axon of virtually all pyramidal cells is studded with a special kind of synapse, the terminals of the axoaxonic cells [type (7) in figure 8.8; these structures are the *chandelier cells* of Szentágothai and Arbib (1975), so called because of the pattern of their axonal branching]. Invariably, they are GABAergic and hence assumed to be inhibitory in nature. The total number of such axoaxonic contacts per initial segment can be counted easily, and knowledge of the number of contacts given by the individual vertical synaptic stretches (the "candlesticks" of the "chandelier") allows the calculation

of the convergence of different axoaxonic cells on a pyramid neuron (in the order of the tens). Virtually all pyramidal cells in the entire cortex (including the hippocampus, the granule cells of the dentate gyrus, and some cells of the amygdala) have this type of axoaxonic inhibitory synapses.

Although there are no reliable data on the relative (not to speak of absolute) numbers of excitatory and inhibitory synapses, the number of GABA-positive neurons is close to 20% in most layers of the cortex, with the exception of lamina I, which contains very few cells anyway. Thus, we may calculate safely that the number of inhibitory contacts may be less than 20% of the total. This estimate perhaps is reversed in the allocortex, wherein a large number of hitherto unknown inhibitory interneurons have been found and defined recently (chapter 6). In the neocortex, we have to calculate with the several afferent systems either from cortical or from subcortical (thalamic and other specific afferent) sources that are predominantly (if not exclusively) excitatory. The vast majority of corticocortical fibers arise from pyramidal cells that are known to be of excitatory function. The specific sensory and other thalamic afferents also are excitatory in function. However, all of these afferents terminate both on excitatory and on inhibitory interneurons, so that the neuron chain is directed already

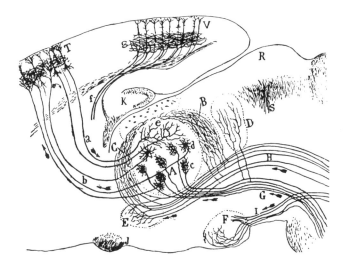

Figure 8.9
A reproduction of Ramón y Cajal's 1911 diagram illustrating the basic "reflex loop" principle of the neocortex, both for the sensorimotor (T) and visual (V) cortex. The monosynaptic connection between specific afferents and some of the (efferent) pyramidal cells is not illustrated explicitly. This is a most impressive example of Cajal's ingenious depth of insight in realizing that connections between incoming and outgoing channels may be monosynaptic in the primary sensory regions but that rarely, if ever, is there an immediate routing of "sensory" input into "motor" cortical output.

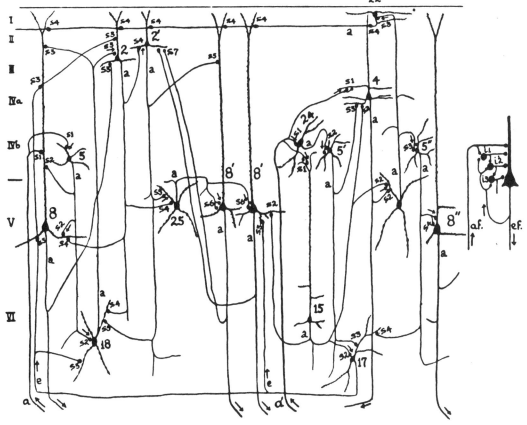

Figure 8.10

Reproduction the by now classic diagram of neocortical structure by Lorente de Nó (1938a). This was the first realistic attempt to understand the neocortex in terms of "neuron chains". Although it is also an ingenious simplification, one limitation of the diagram is the abstraction of the cortical synapse into a single bouton. The reader should remember that although inhibition as a neural phenomenon was known much earlier, the concept of specific inhibitory neurons was not available before the fundamental discovery of J. C. Eccles in the mid 1950s (for a celebrated review, see Eccles 1964). Lorente de Nó recognized the essentially vertical (up-and-down) orientation of the neuron chains. The other fundamental principle of coupling (shown at the extreme right of the figure) was called *reciprocity and multiplicity of synaptic connections.*

at the first synaptic step into an excitatory route and an inhibitory sideline for so-called feedforward inhibition. This effect leads immediately to our next question: the neuron chains of the cortex.

Our principal consideration here is the main neuron chain for routing afferent impulse patterns through the particular piece (or region) of cortex under study. Even without exact knowledge of the details of synaptic connectivity, the early diagrams of Ramón y Cajal (1909, 1911; see particularly figure 8.9) did convey the essence of the main neuron chains involved. The next crucial step was that of Lorente de Nó (1938a) in his magnificent abstraction on cortex written for the 1938 edition of J. F. Fulton's *Physiology of the Central Nervous System* (figure 8.10). Although the abstraction went a bit too far in substituting a single bouton for the entire interneuronal connection, two very basic facts were recognized (though only one of them was interpreted correctly. One fact recognized by Lorente de Nó was

the essentially vertical (up-and-down) orientation of the neuron chains. The neuronal chains of the cortex indeed are oriented preferentially vertically (see sec. 8.1.4). Even if some connections for intermediate (1- to 10-mm) distances are tangential, the final synaptically active parts of the axons are oriented vertically. The other fundamental principle of coupling (extreme right in figure 8.10) was called *reciprocity* and *multiplicity* of synaptic connections. Although the observation was essentially correct (even if perhaps a bit exaggerated), both Ramón y Cajal and Lorente de Nó had a curious blind spot in their field of scientific vision. This limitation is all the more astonishing because nervous inhibition was postulated already by René Descartes and was first observed experimentally by the Russian physiologist Sechenov (1863) and was expanded thoroughly in the works of C. S. Sherrington (1906). However, to our knowledge, the word *inhibition* does not occur in any of the works of Ramón y Cajal and was explained by Lorente de Nó (1938b) as effected by some kind of Wedensky effect (an outdated concept—ingenious but basically wrong).

Especially in the United States, for such scientists as M. A. and A. E. Scheibel, C. Fox, the Lunds, and many others and the Russian neurohistologists (Poljakov, Skolnik-Jaross, Leontovitch) who had kept Golgi studies continuously on very high standards, the revival of Golgi studies was a prelude to efforts aimed at trying to understand neuron chains by a combination of Golgi stains, experimental axon and synapse degeneration, and chronically isolated but vascularized neural tissue block techniques introduced by J. Szentágothai. However, this was only a transitory stage toward the more sophisticated approach introduced in the late 1970s and early 1980s (Somogyi 1977; Somogyi, Hodgson, and Smith 1979; Somogyi and Cowey 1981; Somogyi et al. 1982).

This development (summarized rather cursorily earlier) led Freund et al. (1985a) to the highly simplified diagram still considered valid some years later by Martin (1988a; see figure 8.11). The cell types are drawn in a more natural form and distinguish putative excitatory and inhibitory cells by showing excitatory cells, taxons, and synapses in outline and inhibitory ones in full black. An additional aspect neglected in the original diagram of Freund et al. (1985) was any indication of the forward conduction of excitation over the spiny stellate neurons. Because this activity had been shown clearly in the first studies by P. Somogyi (1977, 1978; Somogyi, Hodgson, and Smith 1979), an incorporation of this type of connection into figure 8.11 seems warranted.

There are infinitely varied possibilities for how such neuron chains arranged in parallel might serve as possible explanations of physiological phenomena observed at the first cortical stages of the major specific sensory pathways. However, the great variety in possible parallel neuronal chains shows immediately that no single such neuron chain would give any satisfactory answer to our quest for a typical reflex arc type of neuron sequence that would explain the routing of any pattern of excitation through any particular piece of cerebral cortex. Only the complete ensemble of parallel neuron chains and their interactions over both excitatory and inhibitory connections would give us a realistic structural image of the path of through-conduction. However, it is also obvious that a composite diagram of only two or three parallel neuron chains and their mutual interconnectivity would render such a diagram too chaotic to be intelligible even to the expert. A way to circumvent this difficulty is to break cortex structure down into manageable architectonic units (see sec. 8.1.5). In section 8.2, we place the development of such units (the ocular domi-

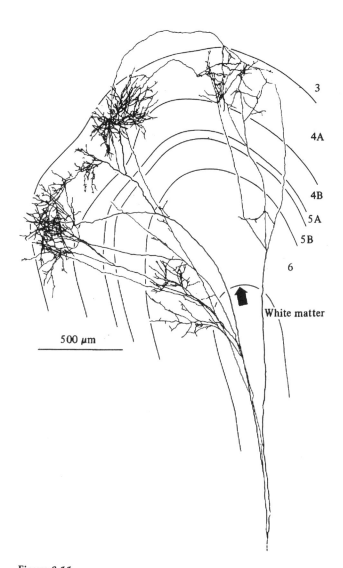

Figure 8.11
Y-type afferent of the lateral geniculate nucleus arborizing in the postnatal gyrus. Its boutons had a patchy distribution and were confined mainly to layers 4A and 6. The arrows indicate the borders of area 17 (to left) and 18. (Reprinted with permission from Freund et al. 1985.)

nance and orientation columns) in the dynamic perspective of self-organization.

8.1.5 The Modular Architectonics Principle

This background on the cellular composition of cerebral cortex serves as a bridge to the theme of *modular architectonics* (see chapter 2, sec. 2.2). The concept of a modular architectonics principle arose from two entirely independent sources: (1) the observation by the Scheibels (1958) of certain spatial regularities in the arborization both of dendrites and of axonal ramification in the lower brainstem and (2) some kind of "columnar" organizations of the somatosensory cortex (Mountcastle 1957) and the even more convincing observation by

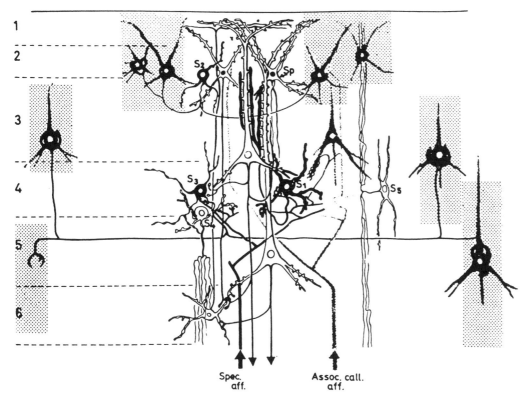

Figure 8.12

An early diagram of cortical circuitry by Szentágothai (1969; reprinted with permission). Putative inhibitory interneurons are shown in full black and excitatory elements are shown in outline. The stippled terri-tories are assumed places where inhibition might prevail if the inhibi-tory interneurons were active. In 1968, the basket cells were the only cells that could be assumed realistically to be inhibitory in function.

Hubel and Wiesel (1959) of so-called orientation columns in the visual cortex. Though the observations of the Scheibels had their main follow-up in our studies in the spinal cord (reported at some length in chapter 2), the observations of Mountcastle and of Hubel and Wiesel prompted efforts to adapt new findings in cortical histology to the new insight gained from emergent cortical physiology. Actually, a very first attempt by Szentágothai (1967) anticipated the concept of the modular architectonics principle under a different name: *elementary integrative unit.* This expression was abandoned later by Szentágothai, because it was misleading and, in fact, led to certain misinterpretations (very unfortunately in some otherwise fundamental writings of Sir John Eccles). The first explicit modular neuron connectivity model of the cortex was proposed for the somatosensory cortex in a diagram reproduced in figure 8.12 (Szentágothai 1969). This model (and the earlier 1967 integrative unit model) still was under the influence of (and mimicking) the earlier cerebellar cortex model of the same author (Szentágothai 1963, 1965). It took an additional 10 years before the more realistic model could be devised, still

using the earlier "pre-Somogyi" guesswork strategy (Szentágothai 1975, 1978b, 1983), and reproduced with slight modifications in figure 8.13. This model was reproduced many times in various modifications, although the labeling and reconstruction of single cells by microinjection, with or without previous physiological testing (Martin and Whitteridge 1984), revealed many hitherto unknown features of the cat visual cortex, and the definition of many inhibitory interneuron types (see figure 8.8) made considerable progress.

Under the influence of G. M. Edelman's concepts of "group confinement" (figure 8.14; Edelman and Finkel 1984) a certain change occurred in our understanding of cortical architectonics in the direction of compressing the piecemeal, but spatially coexisting, arborization spaces into some simpler synthetic view of the whole ensemble. Although the diameter of the size of neuron groups assumed by the Edelman hypothesis was a bit small (a 50-μm diameter against an anatomically realistic 200- to 300-μm diameter), the conjecture was anatomically sound. This prompted us to simplify our overcomplicated original model of the corticocortical (determined

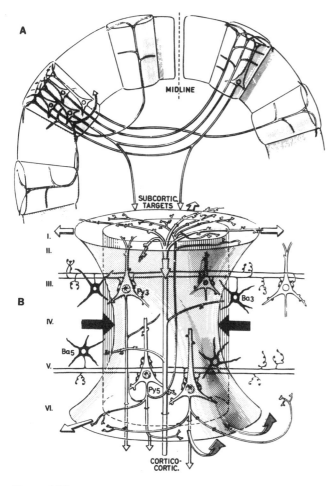

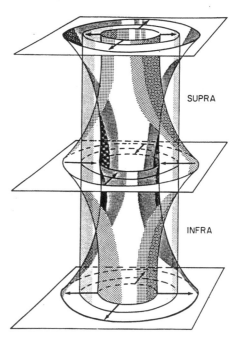

Figure 8.14

Schematic conceptualization of the hypothesized process of group confinement. Three different group configurations are shown as demarcated by the three surfaces. A group will tend to expand in the supragranular layers, owing to excitatory horizontal connections. This expansion leads to increased inhibition in layer IV, in turn leading to constriction of the group. However, constriction of the group in supragranular layers lead to expansion in layer IV. The intermediate cylinder represents an equilibrium configuration for the group. The infragranular portion is depicted as symmetrical with the supragranular but, in reality, probably differs, owing to the existence of direct supragranular input. (Modified after Edelman and Finkel 1984.)

Figure 8.13

A more realistic diagram of cortical circuitry than that shown in figure 8.12. It illustrates the principle of corticocortical modular architecture of the neocortex. (A) Corticocortical connectivity on the large scale. *Supragranular pyramidal cells* (in laminae II and III; two cells of the outer row in left middle column) connect preferentially with columnar tissue spaces in the ipsilateral or in the contralateral cortex. *Infragranular pyramidal cells* (lower row of cells in middle column at left and one cell in one column at right) send their axons to subcortical targets, but some of them are addressed to (or give major collaterals to) contralateral cortical columns. Local (intracortical) connectivity extending over approximately 10 neighbouring columns is neglected in this diagram. (B) The architecture of a single corticocortical column (vertically hatched inner cylinder) of 200–300 μm width and extending through the entire depth of the cortex, radically stripped down to a few essentials. Elements (and direction) of excitatory nature are indicated in outline, inhibitory cells (and directions of connections) are shown in black. A single corticocortical afferent arborization is placed into the center of the drawing (representative for a few of the 10 corticocortical afferents coming probably from the same source). Representative pyramidal cells of the supragranular (Py₃) and the infragranular layers (Py₅) are indicated. Relatively long-range inhibitory cells are represented by two large basket cells (Ba₃ and Ba₅). Terminal branches of corticocortical afferents and pyramidal cell collaterals extend over the limits of the basic cylinder in lamina I and lamina VI (emphasized by outline arrows pointing in outward direction in the two layers). Conversely, dark arrows indicate that horizontally oriented basket (and other inhibitory) cells would tend to narrow down activity in the columnar unit. The original cylinder (vertical hatching) hence would become distorted dynamically into the shape of an hourglass (rotation hyperboloid (stippled). (Adapted from Szentágothai 1987a.)

primarily by the arborization of corticocortical connections) into a hyperboloid-toroid (hourglass) shape (Szentágothai 1985, 1987).

The modular architectonics principle recently has come under criticism either explicitly by Swindale (1990) and Purves, Riddle, and La Mantia (1992) or indirectly by other authors. However, on close inspection, these objections appear to be irrelevant—or, more accurately, missing the point—by giving undue emphasis to: (1) areal and animal species differences in the size and pattern of the observed discontinuities and repetitiveness in cortical architectonic patterns; (2) to differences in the description and definition of columns given by different authors on the basis of different and inconsistent criteria; and (3) to loose speculations on the possible functional significance of such discontinuities. The chief argument of the explicit criticism is that although these discontinuities undoubtedly do exist, such a variety of patterns cannot be the explanation of some so-called fundamental principle.

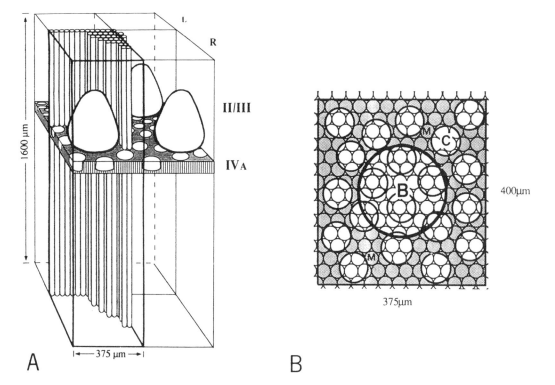

A   B

Figure 8.15

Diagrammatic representations of the relationships between CO "blobs," layer IV cones, and pyramidal cell modules of the primary visual cortex of primates. Shown are "quasi-crystalline" structures of regular patterns formed by structural units coexistent with and superimposed on one another. (A) Three-dimemsional representation. The "blobs" in layer II/III are aligned in single rows along the 400-μm-wide ocular dominance columns (R and L), and they have a center-to-center spacing of 375 μm. Each blob (the focus of a blob-centered module) lies above the cones of neurons in layer IVA, and throughout the entire cortex is a matrix of long, thin pyramidal cell modules. (B) A diagram of the contents of a blob-centered module as though looking down from the pial surface. The blob (marked B) is approximately 200 μm on the side. An average of 20 layer IVA cones (C) would occupy such an area, which also would contain some 190 pyramidal cells modules (M). (After Peters and Sethares 1991.)

The most recent studies of cortical structure (e.g., Peters and Sethares 1991), do indicate that cortices, especially the primary visual cortex of primates, far from being less modular than was imagined some 20 years ago, are in fact "quasi-crystalline" structures of regular patterns formed by structural units coexistent with and superimposed on one another (figure 8.15). Although this quasi-crystalline structure does not give us much more understanding of the several superimposed maps, it is fully in accord with the histogenetic mechanism suggested by Rakic (1982).

Returning, briefly, to the anatomical reality of cortical structure, we ought to realize that local connectivity has to be viewed in the context of the most recent direct anatomical information. As mentioned earlier, the spread of axonal arborizations (with that of dendritic arbors added) does not allow for finer-grain overlap (shared spaces) of more than approximately 20 μm. Anything smaller than that has to be the outcome of narrowing down any kind of effect by some complex mechanism of inhibition. On the other end of the scale, there are dis-

tances measured in a few millimeters. This is illustrated tentatively in figure 8.16, wherein relatively large range connections are shown at the left side of the diagram and shorter range connections are shown at right. Some less well-defined inhibitory cells omitted from figure 8.8 are included in this figure. There is no doubt about their existence, but their axonal arborizations are not sufficiently well-known.

However, the main afferent systems, both specific and secondary, and corticocortical connections have arbors confined to narrow tissue spaces ±300 μm wide. Although this structure is true for individual neurons, the vertical borders of the arborizations are most conspicuous under circumstances in which the arborizations of groups of similar neurons are labeled simultaneously. It is this finding that is so striking in the observations of corticocortical connections by Jones, Burton, and Porter (1975), Goldman and Nauta (1977), and Goldman-Rakic and Schwartz (1982). In the last study, convergence on the same general cortical area of cortical afferents from two widely different sources shows a strikingly system-

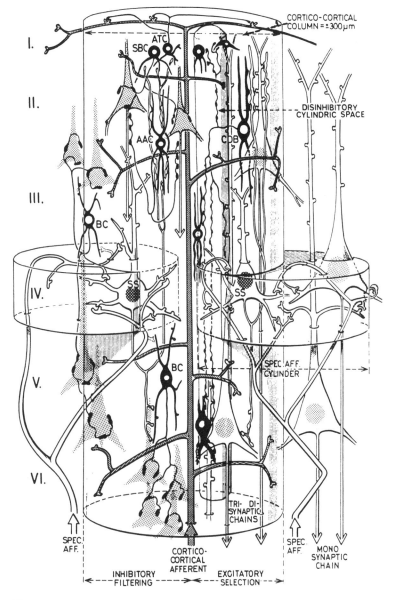

Figure 8.16

The spread of axonal arborizations (with that of dendritic arbors added). Relatively large range connections are shown at the left side of the diagram, while shorter range connections are shown at right. Some less well-defined inhibitory cells omitted from figure 8.8 are included here.

atic interdigitation, with very little overlap of the two afferent systems (figure 8.17). Although relevant information is scanty, there can be little doubt that if other cortical regions and various animal species were studied, the convergence of other systems would be found everywhere, either to the "empty" spaces left free between the elements of such repetitive arborization patterns or probably superimposed on other repetitive patterns. Certainly it would be irrational to assume that such regularities were meaningless.

One of the strongest manifestations of a modular architectonic principle is the well-known cortical barrels of the primary sensory cortex in rodents that are clearly isomorphic with the mobile whiskers of the upper lip. This isomorphy is kept up from the periphery, over the sensory nucleus of the thalamus, and straight into the cortex. The complex neuronal network corresponding to the barrels was described much earlier by Lorente de Nó (1922), although then he did not realize that it was the somatosensory cortex that he was studying. Short of appropriate microelectrode studies, we do not have any idea what this isomorphy means for the analysis of the impulse patterns transmitted by the whiskers, but it indicates that the existence of some isomorphy between

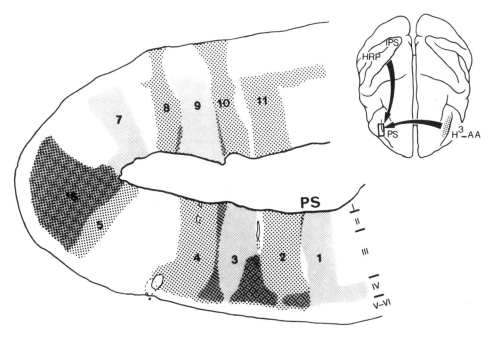

Figure 8.17
Composite diagram of two adjacent coronal sections through the principal sulcus (PS) in the right hemisphere following injections of tritiated amino acids (H³-AA) into the PS of the right hemisphere. Autoradiographically labeled callosal fiber columns (1, 3, 6, 7, and 9) are indicated by coarse stippling; associational fiber columns (2, 4, 5, 8, 10, and 11) originating in the parietal cortex, labeled by anterograde transport of HRP, are shown in fine stippling. Blood vessels in the section reacted with HRP are shown by dashed lines; those from autoradiograph are outlined by continuous lines. (From Goldman-Rakic and Schwartz 1982.)

sensory periphery and the cortex cannot be rejected flatly, although certainly this is not one of the major principles governing sensory pathways. Conversely, the barrels certainly are no useful argument against the general concept of the modular architectonic principle.

The present trend of observations runs counter to the view of architectural modules (columns) as functional units. Considerations of the large number of synaptic sites per neuron and the large number of synaptic sites (boutons or synaptic swellings) per axon arborization always suggested both a large convergence and divergence in cortical connectivity. Although this would not be a logical necessity, this situation always suggested some stochastic mass action of neurons.[1]

When cortical physiology studied in parallel with synaptic connectivity gradually became more sophisticated, authors' guesses about how many simultaneously active synapses would be needed to discharge a cell came down radically. Unfortunately, the neocortex is ill-suited for conducting such experiments with simultaneous observation of two interconnected neurons both in their

actions and in the identified histological loci of their contacts. Such studies are possible in the dentate-hippocampus formation. In that area, there is clear and direct evidence for the fact that a single synapse given by a pyramidal neuron to an inhibitory interneuron can elicit an excitatory postsynaptic potential and cause the cell to fire (Gulyás et al. 1993b). Considering the large number of boutons in the total axonal arbor of a pyramidal cell, the divergence to certain groups of inhibitory cells may run as high as 1,000. This same principle was observed by Buhl, Halasy, and Somogyi (1994), although for the inhibition of hippocampal pyramidal cells by a few (5–10) synaptic boutons. If it could be extrapolated to the neocortex, it ought to be possible to estimate the number of individual combinations of chains consisting of very few neurons within a module. It is relevant to recall here at least the spirit of a celebrated theorem on random graphs. Erdős and Rényi's 1960 theorem implies that the average distance between two arbitrarily chosen nodes of even a rather interconnected graph is relatively short. It is realistic to assume that any

---

1. An alternative view consistent with the models in sec. 8.4 would ascribe more functional importance to the columns but would still be "somewhat" statistical in that the functional role of cortex would rest on widely distributed patterns of cortical activity, rather than on ever "handing responsibility" to a single column. Földiák and Young (1995) discuss a number of related issues for face coding in visual cortex.

neuron of the neocortex is connected with any other over chains of not more than five neurons on the average.

Although attention was originally called to it in the cortex by physiological observations on primary sensory cortices, the modular principle is an architectonic (i.e., structural) principle. In chapter 2, we tried to show that in the segmented part of the neuraxis, the modular nature is clear and almost exclusively architectural and that its relevance for functions is only rather remote and not even secondary, even if ultimately of crucial importance.[2] Following the mechanism of cortical development as elucidated in the studies of Rakic (see figure 8.1), the columnar architectonics of the cortex are a logical consequence of its histogenesis, and if there are exceptions to the general pattern by sidewise movements of individual cells, certainly these are not major aspects of the entire mechanism. In chapter 9, we show that the early development of the cerebellar cortex and the inferior olive involves mass movements of quickly proliferating cell masses in early neuroblast stage (in a manner comparable to lava flows in geology), masses that are an essential mechanism of neural center development coexistent with and superimposed on the fundamental radiate movement mechanism of the main cell types. This type of cell movement also exists in certain parts of cerebral cortex formation. However, the discussion of these in any detail would be beyond the scope of this book.

Like the apical dendrite bundling of the pyramidal cells described earlier, many of the most apparent discontinuities of the cortex cannot have any immediate functional significance, because nothing in the synaptic connections of the cortex gives even the remotest suggestion of a significance in impulse-processing functions of this bundling, which is explained most parsimoniously by the histogenetic movements in the cortex. However, there is the rather remote possibility of a major role of volume diffusion—primarily of nitrous oxide—as a mechanism for information-processing without connection in the nervous system. Everything and the opposite are possible, but we choose to neglect such possibilities as mere speculations until more substantial evidence becomes available. On the same basis, the concept of minicolumns always was left out of the considerations of Szentágothai. Although functional periodicities of 10–20 μm have been observed (and undoubtedly exist) in the visual cortex of primates, we always have stressed that they have to come about not by any existent pattern of afferent convergence but as the result of some refined mechanism of inhibitory processing. The coexistence of up to five or six different maps in the same piece of cortical tissue does show in itself that any single functional principle of cortical function is absurd from the very beginning.[3]

What follows is the study of primary visual cortex as the paradigm for modular architectonics and a look at dynamic models of the process of self-organization of ocular dominance and orientation columns therein. In section 8.2.6, we look briefly at long-range horizontal connections and their role in the integration of information. This discussion leads to the study of thalamocortical oscillators (sec. 8.3) and of fronto-parietal interactions (sec. 8.4). Regardless of which "module of structural analysis" we interpose between single neurons and the brain regions that contain them, it is the connections both between the modules of a given region and linking different regions that yield the cooperative computation that integrates sensory data, internal state, and proprioception into dynamic patterns of perception, thought, and action.

8.2 Primary Visual Cortex: The Paradigm of Modular Architectonics

The following overview of the structure of the primary visual cortex (V1) sets the stage for our discussion of dynamic models of the development of visual cortex. In section 8.2, we link two quite different themes of the book: modular architectonics and the dynamics of development.

Psychophysical evidence suggests that visual information is processed in parallel by separate channels tuned to different spatial frequencies. [See Spillman and Werner (1990) for many aspects of the psychophysical and neurophysiological approach to visual perception.] A seminal paper by Campbell and Robson (1968) describes the visual cortex as a kind of Fourier analyzer, whereas neurophysiological studies suggest that the visual cortex might be interpreted as a population of feature detectors (e.g., Hubel and Wiesel 1962; Barlow 1969). Many efforts have been made to unify the results obtained by

2. Arbib and Érdi would phrase this somewhat differently: that columns come first as the result of patterns of network self-organization and that adaptive exploitation of them for functional specialization then follows.
3. On a more positive note, later sections provide illustrative models of the many functional roles that cortex can play. However, it must be confessed that such models have made little use of modular architectonics. On the other hand, dynamic models (sec. 8.2) do relate modular architectonics to the process of self-organization of cortical networks. Much remains to be done.

the two approaches. Some physiological and anatomical evidence supported the multiple spatial channel view (DeValois and DeValois 1988). There are some substructures of the visual cortex that respond selectively to limited ranges of spatial frequency (Hubel and Wiesel 1968; Maffei and Fiorentini 1977), and a 2-deoxyglucose study has suggested a columnar organization of spatial frequency specificity in primary visual cortex (Tootell, Silverman, and DeValois 1981).

In fact, there are many cortical visual areas, and neurons of the different areas encode the visual information differently. Though neurons in the V1 respond well to edges or bars of light, those of later stages of the visual cortex can be very selective (i.e., they may respond to specific, complex patterns). Summarizing the converging results of many studies, Maunsell (1995) suggested that "while the early stages of processing in the visual pathway provide a faithful representation of the retinal image, later stages of processing in the visual cortex hold representations that emphasize the viewer's current interest." These many visual areas are defined by retinotopography, cytoarchitecture, and function, and there are reciprocal connections between many of these areas. Forward connections "up the hierarchy" go out from cortical layers II and III and into layer IV, whereas the the corresponding feedback connections proceed out from layers V and VI to layer IV. Ungerleider and Mishkin (1982) assign "what" and "where" functions to temporal and parietal visual cortex, respectively (sec. 8.4). Among the cues for "what" are those of three-dimensional form—shape, size, and rigidity—and of intrinsic surface properties: color, shininess, texture, and transparency. Cues for "where" include both static spatial relations—location and orientation relative to the observer and other objects—and the way in which the object is moving. Clearly, these different properties can cooperate. In relation to our design of schema-based vision system (sec. 3.1.5), these "pure" visual areas correspond to the low-level vision processes that create the intermediate database. These include segmentation processes, depth analysis, and optic flow.

We reiterate our theme of cooperative computation: These processes can work together to provide a more reliable intermediate representation of the visual scene. Marr's (1982) emphasis on the $2\frac{1}{2}$ D (two-and-a-half-dimensional) sketch involved two claims: That a "bas-relief" provided *the* intermediate database and that this database did not need updating by hypothesis-driven requests. We reject both claims. For the first claim, we replace the $2\frac{1}{2}$ D sketch by the dynamic sketchbook (Arbib 1989), in which many processes cooperate to provide di-

verse sources of information on which higher-level processes may operate. The success of the VISIONS system (sec. 3.1.5) shows that high-level vision can proceed on the basis of monocular cues alone. This in no way denies that schemas may converge on an interpretation more quickly if the "sketchbook" contains other "pages" with information about depth and motion and other properties of the visual input. For the latter claim, we recall the way in which schemas in VISIONS could invoke low-level processes to find missing edges, merge regions, and so on. The intermediate database is highly imperfect in our current machine model, and the system continually must use the top-down invocation of low-level processes to refine it. Cooperation between different partial representations also can be crucial, depending on the visual task at hand. For example, depth and texture can cooperate to separate figure from ground, yet a camouflaged object may become apparent only when it moves against its background. Again, both disparity and contour orientation cues can contribute to processes inferring shape and distance, and shape also can be inferred from shading.

We will not offer a functional analysis of V1 in any detail but address the function of the visual system in section 8.4, wherein we develop the observations that V1 projects to many other visual areas of the primate brain and that these areas can be seen as forming the what and where-how visual systems. Then we study the role of visual areas of parietal cortex in looking, reaching, and grasping.

8.2.1 Cortical Representation of Sensory Surfaces

Sensory information is represented in primary sensory areas of the cortex according to "topical" principles (i.e., in a topographically ordered way). Skin surface and retina are mapped onto the cortex somatotopically and retinotopically, respectively. Topographical principles preserve spatial relationships (i.e., the neighborhood relations at large), but local variations may occur at the level of individual cells, and there is fan-in and fan-out rather than point-to-point connectivity. Though one may describe a topographical mapping by a mathematical function, assigning a location y in $\Re^2$ in the target area to every point x in $\Re^2$ in the source area, y should be considered as the center of the patch rather than as the sole point, to which x projects.

Schwartz (1977) suggests that visual topographical mappings should be conformal (angle-preserving), using the complex logarithm for the retinogeniculocortical projection. This hypothesis is based on empirical facts

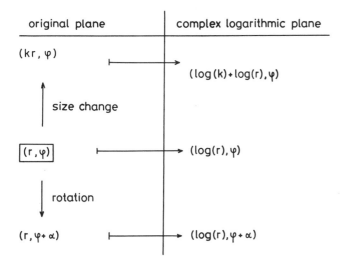

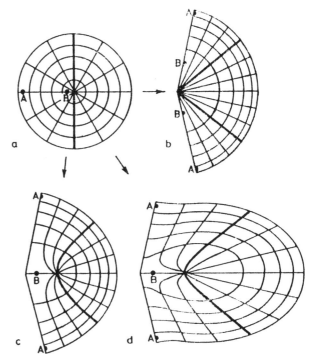

Figure 8.18
The complex logarithm postulated to describe the mapping from retina to visual cortex (see the transformation from (a) to (b) in figure 8.19). Here (r, ϕ) provide polar (radial, angular) coordinates. Size change and rotation in the image plane each imply shift in the complex logarithmic plane.

Figure 8.19
Three transformations of a polar grid (a) compatible with anatomical data on the mapping from retina to visual cortex: (b) transformation of a polar grid by a complex power function (see figure 8.18); c) by an eccentric power function; and (d) by a two-step modification. The images of the two points (A, B) on the negative real axis are indicated.

referring to the geometrical structure of the retina and cortex: The retina shows evidence of radial symmetry, and cortical structures exhibit translational symmetries. The complex logarithm fulfills the criteria of mapping radial symmetries into translational symmetries; it has invariance properties under the size and rotation transformations (figure 8.18). The determination of the functional form of the topographical mappings in the visual system exemplifies the interplay between experimental neurobiology (i.e., neuroanatomy) and mathematical analysis (i.e., the theory of two-dimensional mappings and complex analysis) and led to the emergence of computational anatomy (Schwartz 1980).

The appeal of the properties of the complex logarithm mapping should not render them unique. In fact, complex power functions have been suggested for describing the overall behavior of the cat's visual cortex (figure 8.19: Mallot 1985; von Seelen, Mallot, and Giannako-poulos 1987).

8.2.2 Ocular Dominance Columns

The V1 is considered as the best paradigm of modular organization of the neural centers. Ocular dominance columns are characteristic examples of such units of organization. In fact, they are not columns but stripes akin to those of the zebra. Recording from layer IVc reveals alternating stripes in which physiological recordings are dominated first by one eye, then by the other. (Of course, the input from the two eyes is combined

rapidly in the other layers of V1.) In normal cats and monkeys, each lamina of the lateral geniculate nucleus (LGN) receives its inputs from a single eye. When the afferents from the laminae innervate common target structures (e.g., layer IV of the visual cortex), they form partially overlapping bands dominated by one eye or the other. Showing approximately a 300- to 400-μm periodicity, this alternating termination of LGN afferents is thought to be the anatomical substrate for the physiologically defined ocular dominance columns (Hubel and Wiesel 1972; LeVay, Hubel, and Wiesel 1975; Shatz, Lindstrom, and Wiesel 1977; Ferster and LeVay 1978; Hubel 1982; Wiesel 1982). Ocularity domains likely are formed incompletely in monkeys and are absent in kittens immediately after birth. Though normal development leads to nearly periodic spatial patterns, visual deprivation during the critical period results in severe breakdown of the alternation of ocularity domains (figure 8.20).

Activity patterns heavily influence the formation of ocularity domains. Treatment with tetrodotoxin of one eye of a 2- to 6-week-old kitten prevents the normal development of ocular dominance columns. Tetrodotoxin

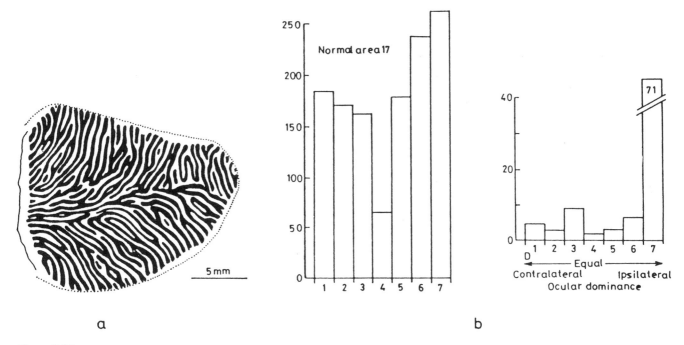

a   b

Figure 8.20

(a) Reconstruction of ocular dominance columns in layer IVc of the visual cortex of a normally developed macaque monkey. (b) Ocular dominance histograms in normal (left) and monocularly deprived (right) macaque monkeys. Cells in bar 1 are dominated by the contralateral eye, those in bar 4 are dominated equally, whereas those in bar 7 are dominated by the ipsilateral eye. Monocular deprivation caused a significant symmetry breaking in the ocular dominance. (Reprinted with permission from Hubel and Wiesel 1977.)

blocks discharge of retinal ganglion cells. Because binocular impulse blockade of even spontaneous discharge activity prevents the normal segregation of geniculocortical afferents, it was concluded that activity plays a role in the columnar segregation and that *spontaneous* activity (having random character) must be sufficient (Stryker and Harris 1986).

Recently, new mathematical models have been given for the development of cortical structure on the basis of cellular activity patterns. (An early model based on chemical markers, not on activity patterns, was given by von der Malsburg 1979.) Miller, Keller, and Stryker (1989) dealt specifically with the development of ocular dominance columns and derived differential equations for synaptic modification without taking into consideration (at least implicitly) the single neuron activity. Tanaka (1990, 1991) introduced a model, as did Thomson et al. (1990) and Cowan and Friedman (1991) based on the analogy of statistical mechanics of spin systems. This model does not generate simultaneous retinotopy and ocular dominance columns but assumes that retinotopy already has been completed (see our modeling of the development of retinotectal connections in section 4.4.2). Chernjavsky and Moody (1990) studied the general features of spontaneous development of cortical modularity, emphasizing the collective excitations sup-

porting modularization even in the absence of spatially correlated afferent stimulations. However, the variants of this model family do not deal specifically with the problem of the alternating termination of the LGN afferents: two presynaptic sheets projecting to one postsynaptic sheet. There are models (Obermayer, Ritter, and Schulten 1990; Obermayer, Blasdel, and Schulten 1991; Obermayer, Ritter, and Schulten 1991) that generate simultaneous topography, ocular dominance, and orientation selectivity on the basis of an artificial neural network algorithm—the Kohonen feature map algorithm (Kohonen 1982, 1988). The Kohonen algorithm implements a general map formation technique and sacrifices biological plausibility for computational efficacy, as was also remarked in a recent comparative study of models of ontogenetic formation of ocular dominance (Goodhill 1992). Originally elaborated as an approximate method of a combinatorial optimization problem (the "elastic net" of Durbin and Willshaw 1987), the application of the elastic net algorithm to the formation of ocular dominance columns (Goodhill and Willshaw 1990) suffers in part from the same lack of biological plausibility. Still, it is based on neurobiological arguments, such as the principle of the minimal cortical wiring (Mitchison and Durbin 1986; Durbin and Mitchison 1990; Mitchison 1991).

The model discussed here in more detail is slightly different from other models, because it implements a two-level realistic neurodynamic model and it uses the beneficial (even indispensable) role of environmental noise during the development of ordered neural structures (Érdi and Barna 1984, 1985, 1987, 1991a,b; Barna and Érdi 1986). Recalling the treatment in section 4.1.2 (equation 8), a two-level neurodynamic model describes the activity change of single neurons and the modifiability of the synaptic efficacy:

$$\frac{da_i(t)}{dt} = f(a(t), \Theta(t), \mathbf{W}(t), I_i(t))$$

$$\frac{dw_{ij}(t)}{dt} = g_{ij}(a(t), \mathbf{W}(t), u, R_{ij}(t))$$

Here a is the activity vector, Θ is the threshold, $\mathbf{W}$ is the matrix of synaptic efficacies, I is the sensory input, $R(t)$ is an additive noise term to simulate environmental noise, u scales the time, and f determines the rate of presynaptic information transfer and the spontaneous activity decay. The function g may contain the modification due to the local cooperation among neighboring synapses and global competition of ingrowing axons for receptor molecules, as will immediately be shown in a special case.

The specification of this model follows: The formation of mapping between 2 two-dimensional presynaptic sheets (m^L, m^R) and one postsynaptic sheet of cells (a) is investigated. The connections between them are denoted by 2 four-dimensional synaptic matrices ($\mathbf{s}^L, \mathbf{s}^R$). Simulation may start with zero postsynaptic activity and uniform connectivity strength:

$$a_j = 0; j = 1, \ldots, 1;$$

$$s_{ij} = \text{const.}$$

(The indices i and j each denote elements of two-dimensional arrays. For the sake of simplicity, they are shown as if they were indices of one-dimensional arrays.) The activity of the presynaptic cells is determined by unstructured stimuli: only one randomly selected element in each presynaptic sheet has nonzero activity value at a given time instant:

$$m_n^N = c_1; N \in \{L, R\}; n \in \{1, \ldots, k\};$$

$$m_i^j = 0; i = 1, \ldots, k^J; J = L, R; i\_n \text{ or } J\_N.$$

Spatially correlated stimulation of afferents supports modularization (e.g., Chernjavsky and Moody 1990), but the present model can work even without this assumption. However, in accordance with the assumption of

spatial correlation, it can be assumed also that if a cell becomes active, its neighbors also get some (reduced-size) activity.

Postsynaptic activity is determined by two factors: the presynaptic information transfer and a spontaneous decay process. The evolution equation is:

$$a_j = a_j + c_2 \sum_{j=LR}^{kJ} s_{ij}^j m_i^J - c_3 a_j$$

Synaptic strengths are modified by three different factors. First, synapses are changed due to correlation of activity patterns. A Hebbian association rule was extended by a selective decreasing term:

$$s_{ij}^J = s_{ij}^J + c_4 m_i a_j - c_5 (a_j - s_{ij}^j m_i); J = L, R$$

Second, there is a tendency to take into account the effect of immediate neighbors (see Kohonen 1982):

$$s_{ij}^j = s_{ij}^j + c_a((s_{i,j-1}^J + s_{i,j+1}^J)/2 - s_{ij}^J),$$

$$s_{ij}^j = s_{ij}^j + c_b((s_{i,j-1}^J + s_{i,j+1}^J)/2 - s_{ij}^J); J = L, R$$

Third, a normalization procedure (not repeated here; see Érdi and Barna 1991) is adopted. (Normalization procedures, which violate locality, seem to be indispensable in the modeling of spatial segregation (sec. 4.2.2). The learning procedure can have some random character; therefore, a superimposed noise term is taken into consideration:

$$s_{ij}^J = \max\{0, s_{ij}^J + c\xi_{ij}^J\}; J = L, R$$

where $\xi_{ij}^J \in \mathcal{N}(0, 1)$ is a gaussian probability variable.

Simulation experiments with one-dimensional pre- and postsynaptic sheets demonstrated that the model is capable of describing the simultaneous formation of retinotopy and of the alternating segregation of the thalamic afferents. Local and global order was generated for ocular dominance (figure 8.21). In the first case (see the upper two of the four parts of the figure), the strengths that characterize the synapses coming from the left and right presynaptic afferents do not show spatial periodicity, whereas in the second case (lower two parts), the incoming fibers show spatial segregation. Simulation experiments with two-dimensional pre- and postsynaptic sheets consume much more time. However, the formation of alternating segregation of afferents was demonstrated even in this case (figure 8.22; this figure is the two-dimensional analog of the lower part of figure 8.21). To reduce computational time, these experiments were started from connectivity patterns corresponding to topographical order.

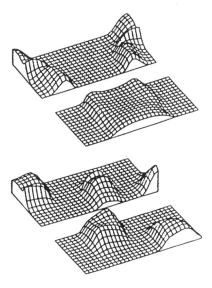

Figure 8.21
(a) Locally ordered structure formed by a deterministic learning rule. (b) Globally ordered structure formed by a stochastic learning rule. The alternating innervation of the postsynaptic sheet can only be seen in (b).

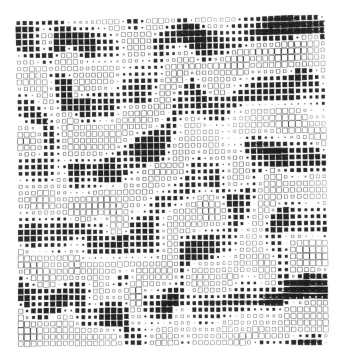

Figure 8.22
Simulation experiment with two-dimensional pre- and postsynaptic sheets. Shown is the formation of alternating segregation of afferents. Compare the reconstruction of ocular dominance columns in layer IVc of the visual cortex shown in figure 8.21a. To reduce computational time, these experiments started from connectivity patterns corresponding to topographical order. (Reprinted with permission from Érdi and Barna 1991.)

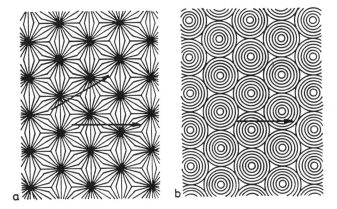

Figure 8.23
Alternative ways of interpreting centric arrays of orientations. (a) Radial. (b) Concentric. Arrows indicate movement of an electrode through the cortex, producing regular changes of orientation. (Reprinted with permission from Braitenberg and Braitenberg 1979.)

8.2.3 Orientation Columns

It is a well-known neurophysiological fact that neurons in the primary visual cortex give selective response for the orientation of the stimulus (Hubel and Wiesel 1974). More precisely, (1) the change of orientation specificity with the movement of the recording electrode across the cortex is "regular;" (2) the change of orientation with the movement of the electrode is clockwise for part of the trajectory and counterclockwise for another part, and (3) a sudden jump might occur in an otherwise smooth progression of the orientation along a straight line in the cortex.

The anatomical substrate of the orientation columns is not understood as well as that of the ocular dominance columns. The application of modern anatomical techniques—2-deoxyglucose, a metabolic marker for labeling active neurons (Hubel, Wiesel, and Stryker 1978); voltage-sensitive dyes (Blasdel and Salama 1986); studies of the distribution of the mitochondrial enzyme cytochrome oxidase (Wong-Riley 1979; Horton and Hubel 1981; for a short review, see Wong-Riley 1989); and activity-dependent intrinsic optical changes (Frostig et al. 1990)—gradually offered new ideas regarding the functional structure of the orientation columns and that of the whole visual cortex.

A concentric arrangement of orientation columns was suggested by Braitenberg and Braitenberg (1979; Braitenberg 1985). They suggested circular symmetry around centers, either radially (figure 8.23a) or along concentric circles (figure 8.23b), as a natural explanation for the observed facts. The Braitenbergs' hypothesis is based on the analysis of electrical recordings of Hubel and Wiesel (1974, 1977). According to this suggestion, the

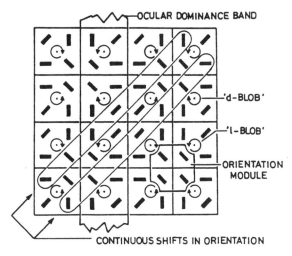

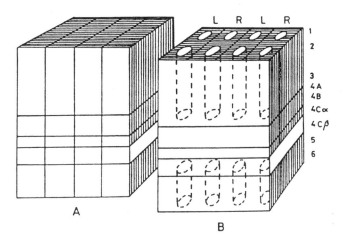

Figure 8.24
Illustration of the two types of hypercolumns having different "handedness" (l-type and d-type). (Reprinted with permission from Goetz 1987.)

Figure 8.25
The functional architecture of the primary visual cortex. (A) The original "ice cube" model illustrating the connections among ocular dominance columns and orientation columns. (B) The modified ice cube model takes into account the existence of the "non-orientation-selective" blobs. (Reprinted with permission from Martin 1988b.)

orientations rotate by 360 degrees around centers. On the basis of the optical recording pictures of Blasdel and Salama (1986), Goetz (1987, 1988) suggested that orientations rotate by only 180 degrees and that there are alternating (dextrorotatory and levorotatory) orientation circles (figure 8.24). An assembly of neighboring columns of the assumed basic modules would be interpreted as hypercolumns, and Goetz believed in the existence of two types. This apparent contradiction was resolved by Braitenberg (1992), who stated that Goetz's 180 degree-columns do not represent the orientation columns proper but rather the whirls at the points where the orientation columns meet. Newer optical recording experiments (Grinvald and Malach 1994) seem to be in accordance with this resolution: Centers around which the orientation turn in optical recording usually do not coincide with the cytochrome oxidase blobs (Livingstone and Hubel 1981) in (see sec. 8.2.4).

The developmental mechanisms by which neurons acquire their orientation selectivity and aggregate in columns and slabs are less well investigated than those regulating the expression of binocular receptive fields. However, there are numerous indications suggesting that the two processes are based on similar mechanisms and differ only because they occur at a different level of cortical processing (von der Malsburg and Singer 1988).

There are some mathematical models for the formation of orientation columns (von der Malsburg 1973; Bienenstock, Cooper, and Munro 1982; Swindale 1982; Linsker 1986, 1990; Barrow 1987; Obermayer, Ritter, and Schulten 1990; Costa 1994). Swindale (1982) does

not use learning rules but gives a phenomenological explanation for the form of the patterns. The main conceptual difference between the von der Malsburg and Bienenstock models is that the former implements spatial competition and the latter implements temporal competition. Linsker separated the problem of orientation specificity into two parts and asked how selectivity emerges and specifically how orientation selectivity emerges. The Linsker model (based on a linear summation response, a simple hebb-type learning rule, and feedforward connections) demonstrates that the properties of sensory neurons could arise spontaneously during ontogeny, whereas the former models required structured input patterns. Linsker used saturation; once synaptic weights reach the limits, they are not allowed to change further. One criticism of the Linsker-type treatment is that it does not pay particular attention to the possibility of full spatial congruence between the orientation maps in the cortical layers and the visual field (Costa 1994).

8.2.4 The Superposition of the Two Columnar Systems

Although the term *hypercolumns* is used as an organizing concept for the orientation columns, it was introduced by Hubel and Wiesel (1974) as a conceptual device for visualizing the idealized relationship between ocular dominance columns (slabs) and orientation columns (slabs). According to this approach, a hypercolumn consists of a pair of ocular dominance columns and a complete set of orientation columns (figure 8.25A). Of course, this illustration is not in accordance with the Braitenbergs' view of circular symmetry of orientation.

The most important finding, which has modified this "ice-cube" model of the primary visual cortex, was the demonstration of cytochrome oxidase-rich "blobs" (Livingstone and Hubel 1981). Surprisingly, cells in these blobs show high spontaneous activity and selectivity for, say, color and brightness but do not exhibit orientation selectivity (for a review on the role of cytochrome oxidase, see Martin 1988b). The modified ice-cube model is visualized in figure 8.25B (based on Martin 1988b). This picture agrees with the previously introduced view that the visual system is a functionally organized, parallel, and distributed system wherein form, color, and spatial information are processed along independent channels (Livingstone and Hubel 1988; Zeki and Shipp 1988). The functional organization of the human visual cortex has been studied extensively (Gulyás, Ottoson, and Roland 1992).

8.2.5 Long-Range Horizontal Connections and Their Role in the Integration of Information

In a vertical column, cells have overlapping receptive fields with similar eye preference and orientation specificity. Furthermore, the axon collaterals of cortical pyramidal cells traveling parallel to cortical surfaces form horizontal connections (Gilbert and Wiesel 1979, 1989; Rockland and Lund 1983; Martin and Whitteridge 1984; Gilbert 1993). These connections promote the integration of information from a wide area of cortex and contribute to context-dependent changes in receptive fields. Because of the topographical character of the visual mapping, information is integrated from a large part of the visual field. The horizontal connections show remarkable target specificity: The axon collaterals do not contact all the cells within a certain radius; rather they form discrete clusters (see figure 8.4). It seems likely that horizontal connections mediate communication between cortical columns, as follows both from physiological measurements (cross-correlation analysis; Ts'o, Gilbert, and Wiesel 1986) and from anatomical demonstrations (Gilbert and Wiesel 1989). Approximately 20% of target cells of horizontal connections have an inhibitory character, and their contribution to the horizontally evoked synaptic potentials may be even larger than is proportional because of the relative excitability and density of local collaterals. Similar clustered connections have been demonstrated both in the primary visual cortex and in other visual and nonvisual cortical areas (Gilbert 1993).

Size and orientation specificity can be changed by context, and horizontal connections now are thought to

contribute to the context-dependent changes in the receptive fields. Furthermore, the strengths of horizontal connections may be the subject of synaptic modification. Both short-term and long-term changes may occur in response to partial retinal or CNS lesions.

8.3 Thalamocortical Oscillators

Having now looked at dynamics on a developmental time scale (the formation of the modular structure of visual cortex) and early stages of visual processing, we now turn to a dynamical analysis of thalamocortical oscillations, a study related to the analysis of oscillation and chaos in the olfactory bulb (sec. 5.2.2) and of hippocampal mechanisms for the theta rhythm and sharp waves (sec. 6.2.2) and epileptic seizures (sec. 6.2.3). This analysis is reminiscent of the reciprocal interaction of thalamus and cortex, a particular example of the many loops within which regions of cerebral cortex are embedded (see sec. 7.3).

8.3.1 Rhythms, Generating Mechanisms, and Modulations

Both the aroused and the sleeping brain exhibit particular dynamic activity patterns. The aroused brain is characterized by high-frequency rhythms, whereas during sleeping, the dominant spatiotemporal pattern is synchronized, low-frequency activity. These patterns are generated in the thalamus and the cortex, which are interconnected intimately by reciprocal projections (sec. 7.3.1). The detailed analysis helps to classify the different rhythms and to understand the mechanisms and functional consequences of rhythm generation. Thalamocortical oscillations can be demonstrated both at the single-cell and the network levels, and the interplay between them should be more clearly understood. We know already that the interaction among simple single-cell oscillators through synaptic coupling may lead to more complex temporal patterns. Awakening (i.e., the transition from the sleeping to the aroused state) is associated with change from high-amplitude electroencephalographic (EEG) oscillation to low-amplitude fast rhythms. The process of awakening associated with desynchronization is activated by the neuromodulators of various ascending systems.

In the early stage of quiescent sleep, the high-frequency of the aroused state (20–80 Hz) is reduced to the "spindle waves" that occur at a frequency of 7–14 Hz. Deepening of sleep implies the appearance of slower frequencies (0.1–4 Hz) in the EEG. The sleep state associated with rapid eye movements (REMs) is characterized by abolition of the low-frequency oscillations and an increase in cellular excitability. Transition from quiescent sleep to REM sleep also is activated by the ascending modulatory system, specifically by cholinergic activation.

In addition to the oscillatory mode characterized by the alteration of silence and bursts, thalamic cells are capable of functioning in a tonically active relay mode exhibiting sustained repetitive activity. In this latter mode, which correlates with desynchronized brain states, cells serve as relay elements. Of course (as noted in sec. 7.3.1, Descending Control of Sensory Systems), the idea of a relay per se is too simplistic because the descending signals from cortex well may gate or otherwise modify the sensory signals as they pass through thalamus en route from the sensors to primary sensory cortex.

The physiological bases of the thalamocortical oscillations, the related state-dependent activities of thalamic and cortical neurons, and the effect of the ascending modulatory systems have been reviewed several times in the past decade (Steriade and Deschenes 1984; Steriade and Llinás 1988; Steriade and Llinás 1988; Steriade, Jones, and Llinás 1990; Steriade, McCormick, and Sejnowski 1993; Llinás et al. 1994). These works form a basis for a discussion of the different rhythmic phenomena. Illustrative model studies help provide a coherent view of the effects of the intrinsic properties of neurons and of synchronizing synaptic coupling mechanisms on the emerging spatiotemporal activity patterns.

8.3.2 Intrinsic Electrophysiological Properties of Thalamic Neurons

Intracellular recordings performed both in vitro and in vivo have revealed the intrinsic electrophysiological properties of the neurons in the thalamocortical circuit. The properties of thalamic neurons are reviewed in the following section.

Thalamocortical Neurons

Cortically projecting thalamocortical cells exhibit almost uniform behavior electrophysiologically. Their firing patterns are implemented by a few other conductance changes in addition to the conventional sodium and potassium conductances necessary for the electrogenesis of fast action potentials.

A calcium conductance leading to a high-threshold dendritic calcium spike controls the duration of the normal spike after-hyperpolarization; the blockade of this channel reduces this duration drastically because the calcium-dependent potassium conductance is not activated. A low-threshold somatic calcium conductance generates the so-called low-threshold calcium-dependent spike. These channels allowing inward calcium flow are inactive at rest and are deactivated with membrane hyperpolarization. A nonactivating sodium conductance associated with inward current generates long plateau potentials. Voltage-dependent potassium conductances also are present.

Thalamocortical cells exhibit multirhythmicity. Oscillation of 6 Hz occurs if the cell is hyperpolarized, whereas slightly depolarized cells may oscillate at 10 Hz (Llinás 1988). Oscillations with lower frequency also were reported (Leresche et al. 1991; Soltesz et al. 1991).

As noted previously, thalamocortical cells also function as "relay" elements. Though the oscillatory mode occurs when the membrane potential is negative to −70 mV, the relay mode appears when the cell depolarizes from −60 mV. This operational mode corresponds to the brain state of wakefulness.

Reticular Thalamic Neurons

Neurons in the reticular thalamic nucleus use GABA as transmitter. Compared with cortically projecting thalamocortical neurons, these neurons contain additional conductances. These cells demonstrate sodium-dependent dendritic spikes and a second rebound excitation produced by a calcium entry. These neurons are more susceptible to showing oscillation than are thalamocortical cells.

8.3.3 Spindle Oscillations

From a behavioral physiological point of view, spindle oscillation is considered as the physiological correlate of drowsiness and the early stage of sleeping. In the EEG records, it appears as a high-amplitude waxing-and-waning field-potential wave with a 7- to 14-Hz frequency. These oscillations are grouped in sequences that last 1–3 sec and recur every 3–10 sec.

It was first suggested by Bremer (1938) that spindles are generated in the thalamus; a few years later, Adrian (1941) demonstrated the survival of spindles after cortical ablation. Further demonstration of the thalamic origin of spindle rhythmicity was given by Morrison and Bassett (1945). The intrathalamic spread of rhythmic activity was suggested by Jasper (1949).

Intracellular studies allow us to study the synaptic events underlying synchronizing and desynchronizing processes in the thalamus. Purpura (1970) considered the synchronization as "complex organizations of excitatory and inhibitory neurons." More precisely, he demonstrated that similar postsynaptic potentials (PSPs) are produced in very heterogeneous thalamic neuronal populations during synchronization, and the key event was identified as a long-lasting inhibitory PSP (IPSP). Furthermore, Andersen and Andersson (1968) formulated the facultative pacemaker hypothesis, assuming that no particular thalamic area serves as a general pacemaker. In their model, spindle rhythms are generated by cyclical excitation and recurrent inhibition via local interneurons.

The synaptic organization of the thalamus now is moderately well-understood (see figure 7.4) and, in the light of this knowledge, spindle oscillation may be considered as an emergent property of the network consisting of excitatory neurons (e.g., thalamocortical cells and cortical pyramidal cells) and (GABA-containing) inhibitory neurons of the reticular thalamic nucleus. As stressed in section 7.3.1, connections are reciprocal between different dorsal thalamic nuclei and the cerebral cortex, whereas the reticular cells do not project back to cerebral cortex but are connected reciprocally to dorsal thalamus. The inhibitory connections among reticular cells play an important role in the rhythm generation.

The facultative pacemaker hypothesis has been falsified on the basis of some findings: Spindles disappear in the remaining part of the thalamus and the cerebral cortex if the reticular nucleus is removed, and survive in deafferented reticular thalamic nucleus. Consequently, the latter now is considered to be the pacemaker of spindle rhythmicity. Axonal as well as dendrodendritic mutual inhibitory interconnections between reticular cells may promote the formation of synchronized spindle rhythmic activity in the reticular thalamic nucleus (Destexhe et al. 1994).

Thalamocortical and reticular cells show mirror-image activity during spindle rhythms. Bursts with 7–14 Hz generated by low-threshold Ca^{2+} spikes in the reticular cells imply the inhibition of thalamocortical cells, which inhibition finally leads to the appearance of an IPSP in these neurons. This IPSP produce rebound excitation followed by bursts of action potentials. These periodic bursts in the thalamocortical cells transfer to both the reticular and the cortical neurons. In the latter, excitatory PSPs are generated and form the EEG spindle waves.

The mechanism for waxing and waning is not well understood. It was speculated (Steriade, McCormick, and Sejnowski 1993) that the waxing stage "could be generated by a recruitment of neurons through divergence of axonal connections between reticular and thalamo-

cortical neurons as well as through the effects of cortical pyramidal cells that are entrained in the oscillation and impinge back onto reticular thalamic neurons." The waning is explained by a shift in the properties of the ionic conductances or by the failure in operation of the pacemaking reticular thalamic nucleus.

The impairment of the mechanism leading to spindle oscillation may lead to spike-and-wave discharges at 3 Hz in patients with petit mal (absence) epileptic seizures. In accordance with knowledge regarding the mechanism of epilepsy generation in the hippocampus (chapter 6), the general idea is that the decrease of the efficacy of the inhibitory effects can result in epileptic seizures (Buzsáki 1991; Steriade, McCormick, and Sejnowski 1993).

8.3.4 Delta and Slow-Sleep Oscillations

The frequency of thalamocortical oscillation is reduced in the last stages of sleep. According to recent intracellular analysis, there are at least two different classes of oscillators as characterized by their characteristic frequency: The delta oscillation corresponds to 1–4 Hz, whereas the frequency of the so-called slow oscillation is less than 1 Hz. Though delta waves were shown to have cortical origin, the thalamus also contributes to their generation. Even more is true: As opposed to spindle oscillators, wherein synaptic coupling plays a crucial role in rhythm generation, the interaction between two intrinsic currents within a single thalamocortical cell can generate the delta oscillation. Specifically, these so-called pacemaker oscillations are generated by an inactivating low-threshold calcium current (I_T) and a hyperpolarization-activated, noninactivating, mixed sodium-potassium inward current (I_h). The latter current seems to be a control parameter according to numerical studies: Modification of its value drives the system from the hyperpolarized resting state through delta and spindle frequencies to the depolarized resting state (Babloyantz 1992; see sec. 8.3.6).

Although delta oscillations most likely are generated by intracellular mechanisms, they are also visible in the EEG because of the existence of some efficient synchronization mechanisms (locally, by axonal collaterals of thalamocortical neurons or by connection from the reticular nucleus or from the cortex). However, it should be remarked that there is a significant difference between the delta rhythms of single thalamic cells and the EEG delta waves, because the former are regular, whereas the latter show polymorphic irregularities.

Lesion studies suggested that slow oscillations (<1-Hz frequency) have mostly cortical origin (Steriade, Nunez, and Amzica 1993a,b; Steriade et al. 1993). Both cortical pyramidal and local inhibitory cells show this slow oscillatory activity on which action potentials are riding. Slow cortical rhythms are reflected in thalamic neurons.

The major step in the cellular mechanism of sleep oscillations seems to be clear. During waking and REM sleep, the I_t current is mostly inactive. With increasing hyperpolarization, spindle, delta, and slow oscillation consequently occur.

8.3.5 Thalamocortical Activation: Brainstem Control and Cellular Mechanisms

Moruzzi and Magoun (1949) found that brainstem stimulation results in EEG desynchronization (i.e., slow high-amplitude rhythms are replaced by fast low-amplitude waves. It was concluded that the activity of the brainstem reticular system contributes to the waking state and that its absence leads to sleep. In particular, it was demonstrated (Steriade, McCormick, and Sejnowski 1993) that the spindle, delta, and slow waves can be suppressed by specific brainstem stimulations. The operation of these ascending modulatory systems is based on the release of a few transmitters, such as acetylcholine (ACh), norepinephrine (NE), serotonin, histamine, and glutamate. Cholinergic projections originate from certain brainstem nuclei, NE fibers originate from the locus coeruleus, serotonergic projections form the dorsal and median raphe, and the histaminergic projections start from the hypothalamus. Though each transmitter system is involved in its control, thalamocortical processing is modulated dominantly by the cholinergic and the noradrenergic systems (McCormick 1989; Steriade, Jones, and Llinás 1990).

The investigation of the ascending modulatory system (and specifically the effect of cholinergic and noradrenergic innervation on both thalamic and cortical cells) led to a better understanding of the cellular mechanisms of transition from sleep to arousal.

Electrical stimulation of brainstem cholinergic and noradrenergic neurons, or direct application of ACh or NE, yields depolarization of thalamocortical cells, which is associated with the disappearance of the sleep rhythms. Such depolarization results from the reduction of a specific potassium conductance associated with muscarinic ACh receptors and α_1-adrenergic receptors by means of G proteins.

The cerebral cortex is innervated densely by cholinergic and noradrenergic fibers. ACh reduces three different potassium currents and establishes a remarkable inhibition, owing to the excitation of intrinsic inhibitory neurons. NE results in both excitatory and inhibitory effects on spontaneous cortical activity, depending on the type of the adrenoceptors.

Cortical EEG recording shows that low-frequency oscillations transit to higher frequencies (20–80 Hz, mostly near 40 Hz) at arousal. Such synchronized rhythms were found in sensory systems (Eckhorn et al. 1988; Gray and Singer 1989; Gray et al. 1989; Ahissar and Vaadia 1990). It was found that neurons within cortical columns separated by even a rather large distance (7 mm) may work synchronously if activated by a single stimulus.

By and large, cortical oscillations may be explained by the interplay of oscillatory thalamic inputs and of internal rhythm generation due to the interaction between excitatory and inhibitory cells. Inhibition also is involved in synchronizing a large population of pyramidal cells.

Rhythmic brain activity occurs at different frequencies and with a distinct degree of spatial coherence. Higher frequencies were found in specific localized cell assemblies, whereas lower frequencies may involve the entire neocortex during sleep and petit mal epilepsy. Inhibitory neurons are considered to have a major role in synchronization and in the determination of the spatial extent of spatial coherence. Neuromodulatory systems take part in shifting the brain through different functional states, as from EEG-synchronized states to arousal.

8.3.6 Models: Single-Cell Dynamics and Emergent Network Properties

Rhythmic thalamic activities have been studied by mathematical models at both single-cell and network levels. An ambitious goal would be to build large network models composed of biophysically detailed models of single cells. Because of the discovery of more and more intrinsic membrane conductances (e.g., in the thalamocortical cells), the Hodgkin-Huxley-type equation for such cases contains many more terms than does the original. In a recent model (Wallenstein 1994), eleven currents were taken into account. A relatively good compromise has been shown (Babloyantz 1992) by including three currents in the single-cell model to describe the most important bifurcations and changing the value of only one current (the noninactivating mixed sodium-potassium inward current I_h) and simulating the global oscillatory properties of the network of 400 cells with 24 connections per neuron.

In the last 10 years, the enormous increase of knowledge about single-cell properties has been reflected in the complexity of models of thalamocortical oscillation.

A simple phenomenological model was introduced by Rose and Hindmarsh (1985). In the two-variable version of the model, the interaction between the membrane potential and an adaptation variable is taken into consideration. The time-independent input served as the control parameter because its change led to transition from resting to oscillatory states.

A single-compartment model based on quantitative data from current and voltage clamp experiments for the generation of delta oscillations in thalamocortical cells (Tóth and Crunelli 1992a,b) takes only the soma into account and neglects dendritic effects. The use of a single-compartment model is approximately justified by the findings that the two channels (I_T and I_h) mostly responsible for delta rhythms are concentrated on the soma. In the spirit of the original Hodgkin-Huxley model (Hodgkin and Huxley 1952), the change of the membrane potential is supplemented with the voltage-dependent channel kinetics, so that the equation for the membrane potential change reads:

$$C\frac{dV}{dt} = I_L + I_{Na} + I_K + I_T + I_h + I_{in} \tag{1}$$

where V is the displacement of the membrane potential from its resting level, I_L is the leakage current, I_{Na} and I_K are terms responsible for the fast spikes in the classic Hodgkin-Huxley model, I_T denotes the low-threshold, voltage-dependent calcium currents, and I_h represent the hyperpolarized induced mixed sodium-potassium current. The passive leakage current can be written as

$$I_L = g_L(V - V_L) \tag{2}$$

where g_L is the leakage conductance, and V_L is the relative leakage reversal potential. The sodium and potassium currents are described by the form used in the Hodgkin-Huxley model. Inactivating currents are characterized by the p and q activation and inactivation variables, and I_T is given as

$$I_T = g_{Ca}p^3q(V - V_{Ca}) \tag{3}$$

where g_{Ca} is the maximal conductance, and V_{Ca} is the relative reversal potential. The (actually slow) noninactivating current is described by

$$I_h = g_h s^3(V - V_h) \tag{4}$$

Here the activation variable is denoted by s, and g_h and V_h are the maximal conductance and reversal potential, respectively.

The activation and inactivation kinetics are given formally with the same type of equation:

$$\frac{dx}{dt} = a_x - x/\tau_x \tag{5}$$

where x represents the activation or inactivation (the so-called gating) variables, τ_x is the time constant, and $a_x\tau_x$ is the steady-state value of x. Through the voltage-dependence of a_x and τ_x, the kinetic equations for the channel activation-inactivation are coupled to equation 1.

Simulation studies are necessary if many currents are to be included (e.g., see Abbott 1994). Single-compartment models can be integrated relatively easily because of the specific structure of the interactions. First, the gating variables interact with each other indirectly through the membrane potential alone. Second, though the equation for the membrane potential contains nonlinear functions of the gating variables, it is linear in the membrane potential itself. Formally, it can be described as

$$C\frac{dV}{dt} = D - BV. \tag{6}$$

Where all the dependence on the gating variables has been absorbed into B and D. However, in the case of calcium-dependent conductances, the intracellular calcium concentration has to be calculated simultaneously with the membrane potential.

Simulation results (Tóth and Crunelli 1992a,b) showed that the model is capable of describing the generation of delta rhythms within the voltage range between -55 mV and -75 mV (figure 8.26). The effects of GABA-

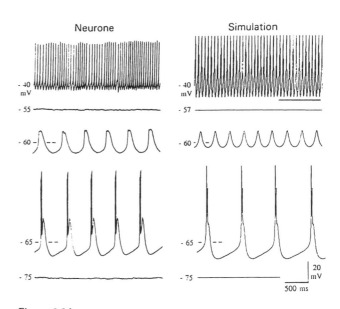

Figure 8.26

Comparison of experimental and simulation results. Shown is the generation of delta rhythms within the voltage range between -55 mV and -75 mV. (Reprinted with permission from Tóth and Crunelli 1992a.)

mediated synaptic currents particularly have to be taken into account. Specifically, IPSPs are generated through GABA_B-activated potassium channels, and a single IPSP is sufficient to activate the low-threshold calcium response. In a study of the relationship between the frequency of the presynaptic repetitive stimulation and that of the thalamocortical cells (Wallenstein 1994), it was hinted cautiously that oscillations in the thalamocortical cells may occur not (only) in consequence of their intrinsic biophysical properties but also owing to (GABA-mediated) synaptic effects. Destexhe et al. (1994) have studied the mechanism of spindle generation.

An early model of thalamocortical activities was given by Wilson and Cowan (1973) and was based on a simplified anatomical structure, taking into account excitatory-excitatory, excitatory-inhibitory, inhibitory-excitatory, and inhibitory-inhibitory interconnections. The model treats populations of neurons by statistical methods and gives a (phenomenological) explanation for the occurrence of thalamocortical oscillations. A kinetic theory (in the sense of statistical physics) for describing global cortical activity was given by Ventriglia (1988, 1990, 1994), and coherence in cortical networks induced by a thalamic pacemaker was modeled by Destexhe and Babloyantz (1991). Even if only a small percentage of cortical cells get periodic thalamic input, the entire cortical network shows both spatially and temporally coherent behavior.

We expect that models in the near future will try to make a compromise between using very detailed single-cell models at the expense of describing relatively small populations of neurons and large networks of oversimplified elements. Cellular mechanisms and global dynamic behavior should be understood simultaneously by using models that balance the intracellular details with the emergent properties of large networks.

8.4 Frontoparietal Interactions

We now return to the study of looking, reaching, and grasping initiated in sections 3.3 and 3.4. In chapter 3, we offered schema-based models of each of these three functions. Our understanding of these functions is enriched by a wealth of neurological and neurophysiological data on the primate brain. In the present section, we will emphasize the contributions of parietal and prefrontal cortex, studying saccade control (sec. 8.4.2) and reaching and grasping (sec. 8.4.3). The next chapter addresses the role of cerebellum in the adaptation and

coordination of a number of these functions, and chapter 10 completes our "neuralization" of looking, reaching, and grasping with an analysis of the role of basal ganglia.

The first subsection of our discussion of cortico-thalamic systems for saccade control bears the title "Matching Brain Regions to Schemas." Before proceeding further, it is important to establish what this title means. It does *not* imply that the matching is one-to-one. In chapter 3, we stressed that a given schema defined functionally may be distributed across more than one brain region; conversely, a given brain region may be involved in many schemas. Also, we saw how brain function can be analyzed in a process of "evolutionary" refinement in which basic systems serve as the substrate for the evolution of more refined systems. We noted that the evolutionary path may not be the actual path of evolution by natural selection but rather helps us understand a complex behavior by the evolutionary design of successively more complex models to approximate increasingly the neural realization of that function. This evolving schema methodology is used in defining and refining neural models for looking, reaching, and grasping by the successive addition of more brain regions to those that can offer a first approximation to the given function. What needs to be added here is that the definition of the overall function that we are seeking to understand is a "moving target." At first, we may define the function only crudely and in a limited set of experiments. The continued cycle of theory and experiment leads both to more detailed description of familiar behaviors and to the description of related behaviors that extend our understanding of the given function. For example, experiments on delay saccades and double saccades not only extend the body of data that constrain our schema and neural modeling but also extend our description of the functionality of saccades; similarly, perturbation experiments extend our description of the functionality of reaching and grasping. Thus, as we study data and build neural models for looking, reaching, and grasping in this chapter and the two that follow, we involve more and more brain regions in the neuralization of our schemas and also update the specification of the schemas that underlie these three key functions of visually guided behavior.

8.4.1 A Formalism for Large-Scale Models of the Nervous System

Connections between two-dimensional arrays of neurons are defined in terms of interconnections masks that describe the synaptic weights. The following equation, where m, B, and C are arrays of neurons and $M1$ is a 3×3 connection mask

$$S_m = C + B * M1$$

says that, for each cell (i, j) in array m, the input $S_m(i,j)$ is the sum of the output of the i, j^{TH} cell in C, plus the sum of the outputs of the nine cells in B centered at i, j times their corresponding weights in $M1$:

$$S_m(i,j) = C(i,j) + \sum_{k;l=-1}^{1} M1(k,l)B(i+k, j+l)$$

That is, the $*$ operator in "$B * M1$" indicates that mask $M1$ is *convolved spatially* with B.

To complete the specification of the dynamics of the array, we simply specify τ_m, the membrane time constant for cells that we describe as leaky integrator neurons. Thus, the membrane potential m_{ij} of the (i, j) cell of array m is given by

$$\tau_m \frac{dm_{ij}}{dt} = -m_{ij}(t) + S_m(i,j)(t).$$

However, in the spirit of our Neural Simulation Language (NSL) (see appendix A), we do not write out the equation for every element but simply consider it as a matrix differential equation

$$\tau_m \frac{dm}{dt} = -m(t) + S_m(t).$$

In what follows, then, we represent the dynamics of each array simply by listing τ_m and S_m.

The way in which we represent the cells in the arrays and the interactions between them in NSL is described more fully in Appendix A. Appendix B describes Brain Models on the Web, which provides full access to the Dominey and Arbib (1992) (D&A) model, including a tutorial, complete NSL code, and interfaces designed to make it easy to run a number of basic experiments.

8.4.2 Corticothalamic Systems for Saccade Control

Matching Brain Regions to Schemas

Figure 3.9 (sec. 3.3) established a basic set of schemas involved in the control of simple saccades, memory saccades, and delay saccades: the retinotopic mapper, hypothesized to be implemented by the superior colliculus (SC); the saccade burst generator (SG), hypothesized to be implemented in the brainstem; and the target memory schema and the remapping schema. The present section introduces the cortical and thalamic networks

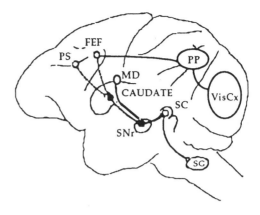

Figure 8.27
Anatomical localization of brain regions involved in sequential saccade generation. *VisCx*, visual cortex; *PP*, posterior parietal cortex; *FEF*, frontal eye fields; *CD*, caudate nucleus; *SNr*, substantia nigra pars reticulata of the basal ganglia; *MD*, mediodorsal thalamus; *SC*, superior colliculus; *SG*, brainstem saccade generator. (Modified from Hikosaka 1989.)

that the D&A model posits to be involved in implementing the target memory schema and the remapping schema: the posterior parietal cortex (PP) and the frontal eye fields (FEF) and the mediodorsal nucleus of the thalamus (MD). However, in chapter 10, we show that the schemas for saccade control also involve the basal ganglia, with the caudate nucleus (CD) and substantia nigra pars reticulata (SNr) working with cortex, thalamus, and SC to control the oculomotor regions of the brainstem. Moreover, in chapter 9, we show how the cerebellum serves to adjust the parameters of saccadic eye movements, modulating the contributions of the various motor pattern generators.

In the following subsections, we marshal neurophysiological evidence that, based on the anatomy of figure 8.27, leads to the model depicted in figure 8.28. The use of target memory and remapping schemas to provide a functional explanation of simple, delay, and double saccades does not imply that these two schemas are implemented in a single brain region or that they are implemented in disjoint brain regions. In particular, we must not insist that the role of SC be limited to implementation of the retinotopic mapper. The major neural elements of the model are two-dimensional neural surfaces to which we refer as *arrays*. The labeled arrays represent two-dimensional surfaces of neurons that form an interdigitated mosaic of task-related response types. In the original implementation of the model, the resolution is rather coarse; each array is only 9×9. Connections between arrays preserve topography of saccade dimensions. The model specifies each array in terms of leaky integrator dynamics (sec. 8.4.1).

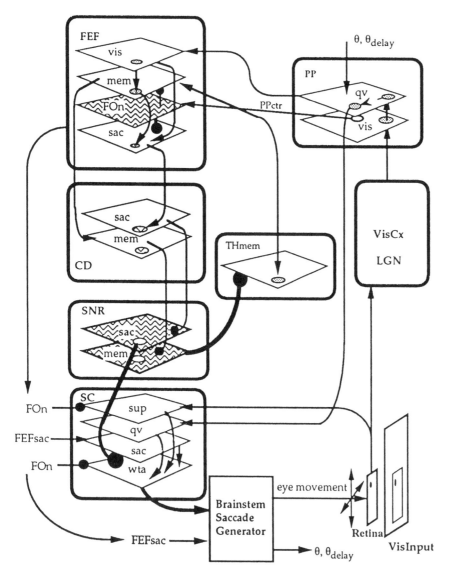

Figure 8.28

An expansion of the schema and model of figure 3.9b. Shown is the posited role of the brain regions of figure 8.27. Connections between arrays preserve topography of saccade dimensions. The labeled arrays represent two dimensional surfaces of neurons that form an inter-digitated mosaic of task-related response types within the topography of saccade dimensions. The FEF-to-SC path includes both an excitatory topographical projection of saccade dimension and a distributed inhibitory fovea-on (FOn) projection that inhibits SC and prevents saccades while a target is fixated. FOn is activated by the central element of PP. Output from FEF and SC drives the brainstem saccade burst generator, which in turn drives a linear oculomotor plant, moving the retina with respect to the visual input projection screen (VisInput), thus updating the visual image as the result of a saccade. VisCx, visual cortex; PP, posterior parietal cortex; FEF, frontal eye fields; CD, caudate nucleus; SNR, substantia nigra pars reticulata; SC, superior colliculus; LGN, lateral geniculate nucleus; TH, thalamus. Specific arrays are related to visual input (vis), memory during a delay period (mem), and the motor command for a saccade (sac). wta, winner-take-all circuit; sup, superficial layer of SC; qv, quasi-visual cells.

Topographical Organization of the Retinal Input

Output from SC drives the brainstem SG, which, in turn, drives a linear oculomotor plant, moving the retina with respect to the visual input (VisInput) projection screen, thus updating the visual image as the result of a saccade. Before detailing the rest of the model and the data that support it, we must explain how the VisInput is "read" by the retina and passed both to SC and [via LGN and visual cortex (VisCx)] to PP.

The sampling of the VisInput by the retina is given (using the conventions of sec. 8.4.1) by

$$\tau_{\text{RETINA}} = 8 \text{ msec}$$

$$S_{\text{RETINA}} = \text{Eyemove}(\text{VisInput}, \theta_H, \theta_V * SACCADEMASK.$$

(7)

Here, (θ_H, θ_V) give the coordinates of the direction of gaze relative to the visual field, Eyemove(VisInput, a, b) $(i, j) = $ VisInput$(a + i, b + j)$ for $-4 \leqslant i, j \leqslant 4$, thus passing the current "field of view" to the retina. SACCADE-MASK is a 9×9 mask wherein elements are 1 when the eye velocity is less than 200 degrees per second, and 0 otherwise. Thus, the retina just registers the visual input "where the eye is looking."

Because the concern of the model is with saccades to point targets, we model the pathways from retina to SC and PP without including any model of "feature extraction." The visual pathway from retina to PP simply is reduced to:

$\tau_{\text{VisPath}} = 8$ msec

$$S_{\text{VisPath}} = \text{RETINA}. \qquad (8)$$

$\tau_{\text{PP}} = 8$ msec

$$S_{\text{PP}} = \text{VisPath}. \qquad (9)$$

Basically, SC will respond to retinal input unless inhibited from doing so by "higher centers." The FEF to SC path includes both an excitatory topographical projection of saccade dimension (described later) and a distributed inhibitory fovea-on (FOn) projection that inhibits SC and prevents saccades while a target is fixated. FOn is activated by the central element of PP. Leaving aside the topographical projection (and the basal ganglia activity described in chap. 10), the retinal input to SC is modulated by the target fixation signal FOn:

$\tau_{\text{SCsup}} = 8$ msec

$$S_{\text{SCsup}} = \text{RETINA} - 2 * \text{FOn}. \qquad (10)$$

(In the living brain, the anatomical implementation of this simple inhibition is more subtle. The FOn cells of FEF project to the rostral pole of SC, in which activity serves to maintain fixation, having inhibitory connections to the rest of SC, activity in cells of which can induce saccadic eye movements.)

To monitor whether a target is on the fovea (which, in the present crude model, involves nothing more than retinal activity at the center of the retina), the FOn cells monitor the retinal input as stored in the PP layer of posterior parietal cortex to signal whether the fovea (corresponding to coordinates $[X_{\text{Center}}, Y_{\text{Center}}]$ of the PP array) currently is being stimulated:

$\tau_{\text{FOn}} = 6$ msec

$$S_{\text{FOn}} = (\text{PP}[X_{\text{Center}}, Y_{\text{Center}}]). \qquad (11)$$

To complete the initial description of SC, we note that the model of FEF will include a layer of cells called *FEFsac*, whose activity signal FEF's decision as to appropriate targets for saccades. SC saccade cells are excited by FEFsac but also receive inhibition from SNr (basal ganglia output described in chap. 10) and from the fixation-related cells in FEF:

$\tau_{\text{SCsac}} = 10$ msec

$$S_{\text{SCsac}} = \text{FEFsac} - 1.1 * \text{SNRsac} - 2 * \text{FOn}. \qquad (12)$$

The motor output of SC then is obtained by using a winner-take-all circuit to locate the peak of activity summed over the other three SC "layers" as long as this surpasses fixation-related inhibition:

$\tau_{\text{SC}} = 6$ msec

$S_{\text{SC}} = $ winner-take-all

$$(2 * \text{SCsup} + 1.5 * \text{SCqv} + \text{SCsac} - 2 * \text{FOn}) \qquad (13)$$

where the population SCqv will be described later.

Does Superior Colliculus Provide the Only Input to the Saccade Generator (SG)?

Previously, we stated that output from SC drives the brainstem SG. Evidence shows that output from FEF also drives the generator. Bruce and Goldberg (1984) found that, as in SC, stimulation at a particular location of the FEF yields saccades of a particular direction and amplitude, largely independent of stimulation parameters and the position of the eyes in their orbit when the stimulation is applied. Although FEF does project to the intermediate and deep layers of the SC, Keating and Gooley (1988) used reversible cold lesions of both FEF and SC to show that saccades can be triggered from FEF even when SC is inactivated. Cooling the FEF increased saccade latency by an average of 68 msec and shortened the amplitude of the initial saccade. Saccades following the initial one successfully acquired the target. Cooling SC increased the saccade latency by an average of 98 milliseconds and also shortened the first saccade's amplitude. Unlike FEF cooling, a subsequent corrective saccade brought the eyes closer to the target but ultimately fell short by some three degrees. These observations led to a change in the model of figure 3.9B, namely, to provide a direct path from target memory to SG and a path via SC. Following, we review evidence that led Dominey and Arbib (1992) to make FEF a part of the working memory.

Remapping

In the double-saccade task, Mays and Sparks (1980) detected a class of cells in intermediate layers of SC that discharge with the topographical metrics of the second saccade, even though a visual stimulus with this retinal error did not appear in the receptive field of these cells. They call these cells *quasi-visual* (QV) cells. The QV cells predict the updated motor error for the extinguished second target as if it were still visible after the initial saccade. More recently, in the SC of the cat free to move its head, a caudal to rostral shifting of activation across SC tectoreticular cells was recorded by Munoz, Pelisson, and Duhamel (1991) during gaze shifts.

Gnadt and Andersen (1988) found cells in PP that appear to code for future eye movements and show behavior similar to that reported for the QV cells of SC. In a double-saccade task, they found cells in the lateral intra-parietal sulcus (LIP) that code for the second eye movement even though a visual stimulus never falls in the cells' receptive field. They propose that PP may receive corollary feedback activity of saccades, suggesting that PP has access to eye position information that could be used in generating the QV shifting activity. Goldberg, Colby, and Duhamel (1990) reported on similar cells in PP that perform a retinal-to-oculomotor transformation. In the simple saccade, this is just an identity transformation, whereas in the double saccade, the transformation is the shifting of the second target to compensate for the initial saccade. In addition, there are neurons in FEF that have response properties similar to those of QV cells. Coding for the second saccade in the double saccade, these cells demonstrate the *right movement field* and the *wrong receptive field* responses characteristic of QV cells and are referred to as *right-MF* and *wrong-RF* cells (Goldberg and Bruce 1990). This raises the question of whether remapping occurs in one of these areas or occurs cooperatively in several. Dominey and Arbib (1992) postulate that PP is the locus of the remapping schema and that projections from PP to SC and FEF yield the QV activity in these latter areas.

Droulez and Berthoz (1991) proposed a computational model for this shifting. An eye velocity signal, applied to the array coding the location of a future target, continuously shifts the representation of that location. If position information were used to update the map, it would allow for a single shift to update the map but would require long connections between neurons in the map. The use of a velocity signal requires only local connectivity in the map. The temporal variations of the activity of a target representation due to eye velocity are the scalar product of the velocity with the spatial gradient of the original target activity. This results in a displacement of target activity loci in the direction opposite to the ongoing eye movement, thereby compensating for the movement. The shifting thus predicts where the target would be if it were still visible.

This notion of remapping goes back to Pitts and McCulloch (1947), who offered two approaches: moving the eye to bring a pattern into a standard position or shifting the pattern among layers of a neural network wherein there is one layer for each element of a group of transformations. In the current model, the transformations are simple translations corresponding to eye movements. Activity is shifted on a single layer within a neural network to compensate for eye movements in updating the internal representation of a pattern that no longer is visible. These various models are related to studies of selective attention, both those based on eye movements (Didday and Arbib 1975) and those based on internal "shifts" (Koch and Ullman 1985). Anderson, Olshausen, and Van Essen (1995) addressed "routing" of visual input to cortex to compensate for eye movements. Pouget and Sejnowski (1995) offered a general review of models of dynamic remapping.

Dominey and Arbib (1992) implemented remapping by a mechanism that shares the notion of continuous shifting with Berthoz and Droulez (1991) but used an alternative mechanism for achieving the remapping. Whereas Berthoz and Droulez used learning to find the appropriate connectivity in the network, Dominey and Arbib explicitly defined the shifting via a spatial convolution mask generated as a function of the temporal codes for horizontal and vertical eye velocity. The convolution mask causes the activity of a neuron to be influenced by its neighbors whose spatial relation to the neuron is opposite to the direction of the saccade. For example, if the saccade is horizontal and to the right, the update will shift activities to the left. This is implemented in a convolution mask that specifies a cell's activity to be determined from the activity of its neighbor to the right. The biological claim is that connections between neurons can be modulated by velocity signals. This kind of modulation has been seen in retinotopical maps in parietal cortex area 7a (Gnadt and Andersen 1988).

More specifically, the model of PP (see figure 8.29) is expanded to contain not only the cells, PP, that receive visual input but also an array of cells, PPqv, corresponding to the cells studied by Gnadt and Andersen (1988). The convolution mask, QVMASK, is created dynamically on the basis of corollary discharge signals, HTN and VTN, respectively, copying the horizontal and vertical eye movement commands from tonic neurons of the SG in comparison with damped delayed copies of those commands (see Dominey and Arbib 1992 for details). QVMASK then is employed in

$$\tau_{PPqv} = 6 \text{ msec}$$

$$S_{PPqv} = PP + QVMASK * PPqv \tag{14}$$

to yield a shift in topographical PPqv activity opposite but approximately equal to the current eye movement. The PP input allows retinal input (see equation 3) to update PPqv when this input is available.

The FEFvis layer (the QV-like cell layer of FEF) and the SCqv layer of SC are both driven solely by PPqv:

$$\tau_{FEFvis} = 6 \text{ msec}$$

$$S_{FEFvis} = PPqv \tag{15}$$

$$\tau_{SCqv} = 10 \text{ msec}$$

$$S_{SCqv} = SACCADEMASK * PPqv \tag{16}$$

Thus, in this model, neither FEF nor SC has its own intrinsic mechanisms for dynamic remapping. However, recent neurophysiology does suggest the existence of such mechanisms in SC. An interesting topic for future research is the analysis of the cooperative computation whereby this function is distributed across many brain regions.

The Structure of Working Memory

Alexander and Fuster (1973) found that MD, which projects to FEF in a topographical and reciprocal fashion, is implicated in spatial memory, with MD neurons showing sustained activity during the delay period of a delay response task. This led Dominey and Arbib to model target memory as resulting from reciprocal interactions between FEF and MD. FEF is innervated by, and closely related to, the cortical tissue surrounding the principal sulcus, which has parallel but distinct connections with areas including MD and PP (Selemon and Goldman-Rakic 1985). In the delay-memory saccade, a sustained tonic activity is seen in FEF neurons that code for the location of the remembered target (Bruce and Goldberg 1984), and a similar sustained activity has been found in PP of macaque monkeys (Gnadt and Andersen 1988). Like the FEF neurons, these PP neurons have receptive fields tuned for saccades of a particular amplitude and direction and show a sustained activity in the delayed-saccade task. Both areas show sustained activity in tasks that require memory of a spatial location (Goldman-Rakic 1987).

Once again, Dominey and Arbib (1992) choose to localize a function in one region, leaving to later research the exploration of how multiple brain regions cooperate in its implementation. Rather than consider PP as part of target memory, they consider it the recipient of such a memory signal from FEF. They propose that reciprocal connection between FEF and MD implements the spatial memory

$$\tau_{FEFmem} = 8 \text{ msec}$$

$$S_{FEFmem} = 8 * THmem + FEFvis - 0.25 * FOn \tag{17}$$

where FEFvis initiates storage, the interaction with THmem sustains it, and the FOn term yields an increase in activity at removal of the fixation point.

In addition to its reciprocal interaction with FEFmem, THmem receives input SNrmem from the substantia nigra (part of the basal ganglia; sec. 10.4). Once a saccade has been made to a remembered target, the memory trace must be erased to prevent generation of further saccades of equal magnitude and direction. The SC projects to the dorsal thalamus (Ilinsky, Jouandet, and Goldman-Rakic 1985), possibly erasing the remembered target location. This erasure is modeled by the "−8 * SC_Delay" term in equation 18, where SC_Delay provides a delayed copy of the SCsac command signal:

$$\tau_{THmem} = 100 \text{ msec}$$

$$S_{THmem} = 2.0 * FEFmem - 2.0 * SNRmem - 8 * SC\_Delay \tag{18}$$

The FEF saccade cells, FEFsac, are driven by both FEFvis and FEFmem:

$$\tau_{FEFsac} = 8 \text{ msec}$$

$$S_{FEFsac} = FEFvis + FEFmem - 2.2 * FOn \tag{19}$$

An Illustrative Simulation

The spatial memory for targets maintained between FEF, thalamus, and PP is updated following the saccade to accommodate the change in eye position. How these components cooperate to produce a double saccade (see section 3.3.1 for a description of the experiment) is illustrated in certain features of the D&A simulation of the double-saccade task (figure 8.29). The task begins with the "animal" fixating the central spot. When the fixation point is removed, the two targets are presented successively for 40 msec each. This is not long enough for the signal to propagate from retina to brainstem via FEF and SC before both targets are removed. Shortly after the second target is removed, the first stimulus has

a)

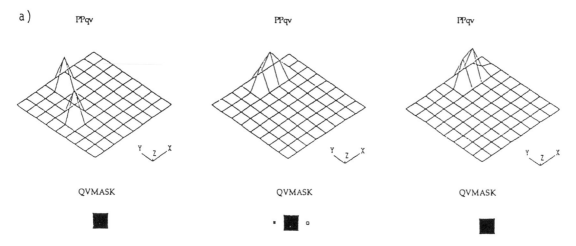

b)

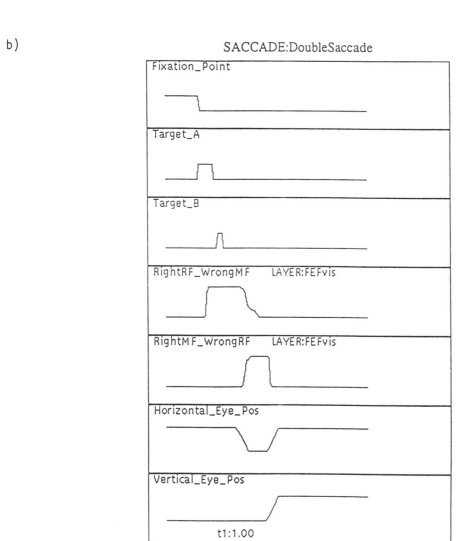

Figure 8.29

Dynamic spatial remapping simulation: double saccade. Illustrated is the convolution mask (*QVMASK*) and resultant shifting activity that is seen in posterior parietal cortex (PPqv) during the course of the double-saccade task. QVMASK is generated from temporally offset horizontal and vertical eye position components. When convolved with PPqv,

QVMASK represents local cellular interactions posited to implement the QV shifting in parietal cortex. The result is that the new locus of activity that codes for a saccade has been updated by shifting in the opposite direction and magnitude of the initial saccade. (A) The first frame (left) shows the configuration just following the presentation of propagated through the system and initiates the first saccade. By this time, the second signal has reached the PP and FEF.

Recall that the convolution mask, QVMASK, varies with eye movement to yield a shift in topographical PPqv activity opposite (but approximately equal in magnitude to) the current eye movement. As the eye velocity becomes nonzero, QVMASK makes a transition from the identity mapping to the mapping that implements the shift, as discussed earlier. This shifting originates in the PPQV array and then is distributed to FEF and SC. During the course of the saccade, the mask continues to generate this shifting, effectively simulating the change in position of the second target were it still visible. The activity for the first target also is shifted, but as it is shifted to the foveal region, it is erased. Following completion of the first saccade, this shift leaves the second target properly adjusted to compensate for the first saccade. This recorded position serves as the primary activity in the colliculus, wherein a winner-take-all network selects the maximum signal and projects it on to the brainstem to command the next saccade.

Figure 8.29 illustrates QVMASK and resultant shifting activity that is seen in PP and in SC during the course of the double-saccade task. The simulation accurately generates activation of the QV cells that code for the second saccade. QVMASK is generated from the horizontal and vertical eye velocity components. For each time step of the simulation, a linear relation between velocity and eye displacement holds (i.e., in a given time step, a particular velocity will generate a particular displacement). This relation is exploited in generating QVMASK that (when convolved with an array representing topographical motor error) will shift the center of mass of an activity pattern a distance opposite to that of the eye displacement. When convolved with PPQV, QVMASK represents local cellular interactions thought to implement the QV shifting in PP. The result is that the new locus of activity that codes for a saccade has been updated so that it represents the new movement-map locus for a saccade that will take the eye to the target location in space. Updating a retinotopical map by shifting activity profiles in the direction opposite to the eye movement yields the functional equivalent of a spatiotopic map embodied in retinotopic coordinates. A side effect of the shifting is that the activity patterns are dispersed. Because the areas involved (i.e., SC, FEF, PP) code in populations, the shifting is not necessarily a problem.

Role of the Basal Ganglia

Figure 8.28 contains two regions that we have not discussed: the CD and the SNr of the basal ganglia. This is surprising, because we seem to have captured already the full functionality called for by the schema level analysis. However, their addition is necessary because data on the monkey (Hikosaka and Wurtz 1983a,b) and the rat (Chevalier et al. 1985) have shown that these systems can provide an important inhibitory role, blocking the release of saccades by the SC. The detailed analysis of the neurophysiology leads to a further refinement of the schema model which we present in section 10.2. Because the studies that reported this important role of the basal ganglia led Dominey and Arbib (1992) to analyze the memory saccade, the involvement of the basal ganglia in their model was always an important consideration. Nonetheless, we have attempted here to provide a conceptual path rather than a historically accurate chronology of the research in which we first establish the cortical systems in the model before "evolving" their refinement by the action of the basal ganglia. The point is that the analysis of the brain is neither purely top-down

the two stimuli, prior to the first saccade. In the second frame, during the initial 20-degree leftward saccade, QVMASK indicates that PPqv cells are excited by their neighbors on the left and inhibited by those on their right, generating a rightward shift. The third frame shows that following the completion of the first saccade, the updated locus of activity for the second target (now shifted 20 degrees to the right) becomes the next saccade target. (B) The time course of presentation of the central fixation point and two targets is shown. FEFvis (the array of frontal eye field visually driven cells) receives its input from PPqv. The two traces labeled *FEFvis* indicate the activity of two FEF cells: one with a visual and movement field corresponding to the retinal location of the second target when it is presented (right-RF/wrong-MF) and a second cell with the visual and movement fields corresponding to the dynamically remapped retinal error of the second target (wrong-RF/right-MF). Note: The (x, y) coordinates in these 9×9 layers are num-

bered with the lower left corner as 0, 0 and the foveal element at (4, 4), so FEFvis (4, 7) is at (0, 30 degrees), and FEFvis (6, 7) is at (20, 30 degrees). Thus, by using PPqv as input to FEFsac (the array of FEF cells that can drive saccades) we see the same responses as recorded in FEF by Goldberg and Bruce (1990) during the double saccade. The horizontal and vertical eye positions (EyeH, EyeV) are provided by the horizontal are vertical tonic firing rates HTN and VTN, respectively, in our model. In this instance, the first target is 20 degrees left, indicated by the downward deflection of EyeH. The second target is 30 degrees up, but it must compensate for the 20-degree rightward saccade, so the compensatory movement from A to B is an oblique saccade 20 degrees right and 30 degrees up, shown in the EyeH and EyeV traces. Both the first and second saccades brought the eye to its respective targets with less than 1 degree of error.

(from function to neural network) nor purely bottom-up (from neural or synaptic components up to function) but rather that it requires a continual middle-out dialog.

8.4.3 Cortical Systems for Reaching and Grasping

The discussion of reaching and grasping in humans (sec. 3.4) provided a functional analysis of interacting schemas that further exemplified the principle (based on our study of approach and avoidance in frog and toad; sec. 3.2): A multiplicity of different representations must be linked into an integrated whole in action-oriented perception. In this section, we look at the way in which these representations are played out over the human brain and extend our understanding of coordinated control programs (e.g., figure 3.4) and how they may be created and modified by learning.

Animal perception has evolved so as to estimate the parameters needed for control of movement. Nothing guarantees that the estimate is correct, but survival depends on schemas that are correct enough often enough—as when we estimate the "time until collision" parameter of oncoming traffic to decide whether to cross the road. The parameters required by each schema then must be specified to tune the movement, "filling in the details." The notion of parameterized motor schemas is related closely to the view of motor control in terms of selecting and coordinating from a relatively short list of synergies of groups of muscles (Bernstein 1967; see sec. 3.1.4). These motor schemas are akin to control systems but are distinguished in that they can be combined to form coordinated control programs that control the phasing in and out of patterns of coactivation, with the passing of control parameters from perceptual to motor schemas.

From "What and Where" to "What and How"

Before turning to an exposition of neurophysiological studies of cortical correlates of grasping, we briefly review data that establish a useful overview of cortical function. Ungerleider and Mishkin (1982; Mishkin, Ungerleider, and Macko 1983) noted that monkeys with lesions of inferotemporal (IT) cortex were impaired profoundly in visual pattern discrimination and recognition but less impaired in solving "landmark" tasks, wherein the location of a visual cue determines which of two alternative locations is rewarded. Quite the opposite pattern of results was observed in monkeys with lesions to PP. Thus, they distinguished two visual systems in extrastriate visual processing, both originating in V1 (figure 8.30):

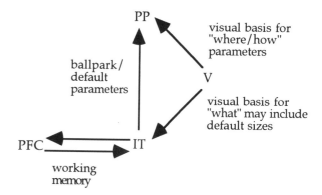

Figure 8.30
The "where," "what," and "how" of vision. Recognizing what an object is (V → IT) may also yield "default parameters" concerning, say, its size, which can be used (IT → PP) to provide ballpark estimates to aid in the control of movement. The areas of cortex shown are early visual (V), inferotemporal (IT), posterior parietal (PP), and prefrontal (PFC) cortex.

What: The ventral system, V1 → V2 → V4 → IT, was characterized as the cortical "what" (pattern recognition) system.

Where: The dorsal system, extending from V1 to PP, was characterized as the cortical "where" (object location) system and was seen as mediating spatial memory.

This is at first sight confusing, because we saw in chapter 3 that SC and its homolog, the tectum, functions as a where system. However, note the crucial choice of *a* rather than *the*: Our study of frogs has taught us that a function that might appear unitary to introspection may involve diverse schemas distributed across multiple brain regions. The where of approach and the where of avoidance in the frog brain involve different (though overlapping) sets of brain regions. Similarly, though the where of making an eye movement in response to a flash of light involves SC, subtle patterns of reaching that involve analysis of object patterns require cortical structures. For example, Lawrence and Kuypers (1968) performed a bilateral pyramidotomy (removing cortical pathways for controlling arm and hand movements but not brainstem pathways) on macaques, resulting in the loss of fractionated finger movements in both hands. Within the 5-month follow-up period, use of the precision grip never was recovered. The monkeys could run and climb normally, but there remained difficulty in relaxing voluntarily their grasp from food (though not in relaxing the grasp for climbing or clinging). Brinkman and Kuypers (1972) concluded that finely coordinated, visually guided behaviors involve the cooperative computation of cortex via the corticospinal tract (controlling the distal muscles and relatively independent finger movements) and the brainstem (controlling undifferentiated hand movements).

Observations of human patients allow us to refine the what-where distinction considerably. Patients with visual agnosia following brain damage involving the occipito-temporal region often are unable to recognize or describe common objects, faces, pictures, and abstract designs, even though they can navigate through the world (at a local level, at least) with considerable skill (Farah 1990). Conversely, patients suffering from optic ataxia following damage to the PP region are unable to reach accurately toward visual targets that they easily recognize. Patients with optic ataxia have difficulty in reaching in the right direction and in positioning their fingers or adjusting the orientation of their hand when reaching toward an oriented object (Perenin and Vighetto 1988). Such patients also may have trouble adjusting their grasp to reflect the size of the object they are asked to pick up.

Goodale et al. (1991) studied a patient (DF), who (following carbon monoxide poisoning) developed a profound visual-form agnosia in which most of the damage to cortical visual areas was apparent in areas 18 and 19 but not in area 17 (V1), which allowed signals to flow from V1 toward PP but not from V1 to IT. When asked to indicate the width of a single block by means of her index finger and thumb, she exhibited finger separation bearing no relationship to the dimensions of the object and showed considerable trial-to-trial variability. Yet, when she was asked simply to reach out and pick up the block, the aperture between her index finger and thumb changed systematically with the width of the object, as in normal controls. A similar dissociation was seen in her responses to the orientation of stimuli. In other words, DF could preshape accurately, even though she appeared to have no conscious appreciation (either verbal or pantomime) of the visual parameters that guided the preshape.

On the basis of such data, Goodale and Milner (1992) refined the Mishkin-Ungerleider description of the visual system. They noted that a patient with a ventral lesion was able to carry out a variety of object manipulations even though unable to report verbally on the object parameters used to guide these actions. Thus, though still accepting that the ventral system plays a major role in the perceptual identification of objects, they suggest that the dorsal system mediates the required sensorimotor transformations for visually guided actions directed at such objects, They replace the where system with the how system (top right-hand arrow in figure 8.30):

How: The dorsal system more properly may be called the *how* system because location (where) is only one of many properties needed to determine how to interact with an object.

A grasping arm movement can be elicited without the instruction of refined distal control. Cortical signaling fractionates the undifferentiated hand movements controlled by lower centers. Paillard (1991) notes the way in which visual systems frame action, with SC more involved in the peripheral cues for "approach" and cortical systems more involved in the object-centered "frame." We should note also the distinction between the viewer-centered and the allocentric frames, involved in reaching for objects and navigating through terrain, respectively. Both the reach with generalized grasp and precise adjustment of the fingers to conform to the object are how systems but involve different visual systems (Kuypers 1987). The role of central and peripheral retina in the guidance of arm movement makes it necessary to consider two independent visual subchannels that convey position information for the arm in a body-centered representation and shape information for the hand in an object-centered representation (see Paillard 1991). Indeed, Goodale (1993) emphasized that some patients with damage to PP "have difficulty with hand postures, some with controlling the direction of their grasp, and some with foveating the target. Indeed, depending on the size and locus of the lesion, a patient can demonstrate any combination of these visuomotor deficits. Different sub-regions of the posterior parietal cortex, it appears, support different visuomotor components of a skilled act" (Goodale 1993).

Having accepted that *what and how* is a better description of the visual system than is *what and where*, we must seek a more extensive view of the interaction of what and how. Jeannerod (1994) has advanced the terms *semantic* and *pragmatic* for the ventral (IT: what) and dorsal (parietal: how and where) streams, respectively. There are multiple how systems for, say, looking, reaching, and grasping. Moreover, it is only in the simplest circumstances that we can expect the how of interacting with an object to be divorced from the what of the object's structure and function. Quite to the contrary, we would say that it is the utility of object analysis to modulate courses of action that provided the prime evolutionary pressure for the evolution of the ventral (i.e., the what) system. For example, the perception of whether a piece of fruit is ripe (a what question) plays a crucial role in deciding whether to pick it, whereas the perception of a screwdriver as a screwdriver to be used rather than as an object to be moved from one place to another determines which of the possible "affordances" for grasping it one will act on.

Jakobson et al. (1991) studied visually guided grasping in a patient who had recovered from Balint's syndrome, a disorder in which bilateral parietal damage causes profound disorders of spatial attention, gaze, and visually guided reaching. Though this patient had no difficulty in recognizing line drawings of common objects, when she reached out for a small wooden block that varied in size from trial to trial, there was little relationship between the magnitude of the aperture between her index finger and thumb and the size of the block as the movement unfolded. Also, she made very many adjustments in her grasp as she closed in on the object, adjustments rarely observed in normal subjects. Such studies suggest that damage to the parietal lobe can impair the ability of patients to use information about the size, shape, and orientation of an object to control the hand and fingers during a grasping movement, even though this same information still can be used to identify and describe the objects. Additionally, we may recall the data (sec. 6.4.5) showing that damage to other areas of the parietal lobe differentially may impair topographical learning, orientation with respect to objects, localization of stimuli in peripheral vision, visually guided maze learning, locomotor map following, and the ability to perceive two objects simultaneously.

In summary, the visual projection system to the human parietal cortex provides action-relevant information about the structural characteristics and orientation of objects and not just about their position, whereas projections to the temporal lobe may furnish visual perceptual experience of the kind that appears to be damaged severely in the patient DF studied by Goodale et al. (1991). Even though we relate both the reaching and grasping systems to the ventral how system, even here we see the further decomposition of specialized subsystems, with a corticosubcortical arm-guidance system integrated with a parietal-premotor grasp-guidance system. As we explore further the relation between the what and the how systems, it is not enough to dissect more carefully a variety of specialized subsystems. In general, the various aspects of our visual recognition of, and motor interaction with, an object are joined seamlessly. Thus, we must solve the *binding problem*: linking representations of a single object, task, or action widely distributed over many brain regions. Some current approaches to this problem were presented in the study of invariant pattern recognition and dynamic links (sec. 4.5.2), but the role of oscillations here still is highly controversial.

Castiello, Paulignan, and Jeannerod (1991) report a study of impairment of grasping in a patient (AT) with a lesion of the visual pathway that left PP, IT, and the pathway V → IT relatively intact but grossly impaired the pathway V → PP. This patient is the "opposite" of DF; she can use her hand to pantomime the size of a cylinder but cannot preshape appropriately when asked to grasp it. Instead of forming an adaptive preshape, she will open her hand to its fullest and begin to close her hand only when the cylinder hits the web between index finger and thumb. However, there was a surprise: When the stimulus used for the grasp was not a cylinder (for which the semantics contains no information about expected size) but rather a familiar object—such as a spool of thread or a lipstick—for which the "usual" size is part of the subject's knowledge, AT showed a relatively adaptive preshape. This leads to the labeling of the IT → PP pathway (see figure 8.30) with *default parameters*, providing a representation of the approximate (default) size of a known object to help the pragmatic system.

We assume, then, that the ventral and dorsal systems often will be activated simultaneously (with somewhat different visual information), thereby providing visual experience during skilled action. We assume also that the two systems engage in direct cross talk. Indeed, PP and IT themselves interconnect (Cavada and Goldman-Rakic 1989) and both in turn project to areas in the superior temporal sulcus (Boussaoud, Ungerleider, and Desimone 1990; Baizer, Ungerleider, and Desimone 1991). There, cells that are highly form-selective lie close to others that have motion specificity (Perrett, Mistlin, and Chitty 1987), providing scope for cooperation between the two systems. In addition, there are many polysensory neurons in these areas, so that both visual and cross-modal interaction may be enabled by these networks.

We can grab an object whose movement is sensed in the peripheral visual field if only a "generalized" grasp is required (recall our discussions of Kuypers earlier in this section), but if we wish to preshape the hand to grasp the object appropriately, we first must foveate the object. We see here the continuity in discontinuity in the evolution of cognitive architecture. In section 2.3.2, we showed that the role of tectum in directing the whole body movements of frog and toad is akin to the role of SC both in directing eye movements and in setting the frame for arm and hands movements in monkey and human. This is the *continuity*. The *discontinuity* is that the SC need not commit the monkey or human to an overt course of behavior, as in approach or avoidance, but instead can gather information that can be used in "planning" before the organism is committed to action. To this must be added that shifts of attention are not only overt (i.e., involving eye movements). For example, neural circuitry can enable us to attend to different letters of a word even while we maintain the same fixation point. Many cells (e.g., in area 7a) are modulated by such covert switches of attention to different parts of the visual field (Bushnell, Goldberg, and Robinson 1981). However, attentional modulation can be found in neurons in many parts of the cortex, including area V4 and IT within the ventral stream (Moran and Desimone 1985).

In general terms, attention needs to be switched to particular locations and objects whenever they are the targets either for intended action (Rizzolatti, Gentilucci, and Matelli 1985) or for identification (Moran and Desimone 1985). In either case, this selection typically seems to be spatially based. Thus, human subjects performing manual aiming movements have a predilection to attend to visual stimuli within the action space of the hand. In this instance, the attentional facilitation might be mediated by mechanisms within the dorsal projection system; in other instances, probably it is mediated by the ventral system. Indeed, the focus of lesions causing the human attentional disorder of "unilateral neglect" is parietotemporal, unlike the superior parietal focus for optic ataxia (Perenin and Vighetto 1988), as is the focus for object constancy impairments. We conclude that spatial attention is physiologically nonunitary (Rizzolatti, Gentilucci, and Matelli 1985) and may be associated as much with the ventral system as with the dorsal. For further discussion of many of the issues raised in this section, see *The Visual Brain in Action* (Milner and Goodale 1995).

"Neural Codes" in Parietal Lobe and Premotor Cortex

Section 8.4.2 demonstrated the important relationship between the PP and the FEFs in the visual guidance of saccades. In this section, we summarize data on the parietofrontal relations underlying grasping movements of the hand (a similar story can be told for the reaching movements that bring the hand to its target) (Mountcastle et al., 1975). The inferior parietal lobule of PP receives visual inputs from occipitotemporal areas and from the visual field periphery of V3 and V2 (Andersen et al. 1990; Baizer, Ungerleider, and Desimone 1991). Inferior parietal lobule is subdivided functionally into three areas buried in the intraparietal sulcus: the *lateral intraparietal* area (LIP), the *ventral intraparietal* area (VIP), and the *anterior intraparietal* area (AIP)—and into areas 7a

and 7b and the *secondary somatosensory* area (SII). These areas have specific sensoimotor functions, including those for saccadic eye movements (LIP), ocular fixation (7a), reaching (mostly 7b), and grasping (AIP). A similar modular organization is seen in the motor sector (agranular cortex) of the frontal lobe related to body movements (except for the supplementary eye fields).

In monkeys trained to grasp objects requiring different types of grip, approximately half the task-related neurons related to hand movements located in AIP fired almost exclusively during one type of grip, with precision grip being the most represented grip type (Taira et al. 1990; Sakata et al. 1992). Approximately 40% of the AIP neurons discharged equally well if the appropriate grasping movement was made in the light, with the monkey looking at the object, or in the dark. They have been called *motor-dominant neurons*. The remaining neurons discharged more strongly (visual and motor neurons) or exclusively (visual-dominant neurons) in the light. Half of the visual-dominant neurons and a part of the visual and motor neurons became active when the animal fixated the object in the absence of any movement. For these last neurons, the visually effective object and the type of grip coded (assessed in the dark) coincide. Therefore, they appear to match the visual representation of the objects with the way in which the objects can be grasped.

The area of agranular frontal cortex involved in grasping in the monkey is called *F5* (Rizzolatti and Gentilucci 1988) and forms the rostral part of inferior area 6. Its main anatomical connections are with AIP and the hand field of the precentral motor area (Matsumura and Kubota 1979; Muakkassa and Strick 1979; Matelli et al. 1986). Rizzolatti et al. (1988) described various classes of F5 neurons, each of which discharge during specific hand movements (e.g., grasping, holding, tearing, manipulating). The largest class is related to grasping. The temporal relations between neuron discharge and grasping movements vary among neurons. Some of them fire only during the last part of grasping (i.e., during finger flexion). Others start to fire with finger extension and continue to fire during finger flexion. Finally, others are activated in advance of the movement initiation and often cease discharging only when the object is grasped. Of these grasping neurons, 85% were found to be selective for one of precision grip, finger prehension, or whole-hand prehension, with precision grip again the most frequent (Rizzolatti et al. 1988). This finding is reminiscent of the motor schemas discussed in (sec. 3.4), with the specification of a movement in response to a visual object reduced to the task of passing its size and orientation to the appropriate schema. "Visual" responses are observed in approximately 20%–30% of F5 neurons, with two separate classes being distinguished. One set of neurons responds to the presentation of graspable objects (Rizzolatti et al., 1988); another class of cells ("mirror" neurons) responds when the monkey sees movements executed by the experimenters or by another monkey, which movements are similar to those coded by the neurons (di Pellegrino et al. 1992).

We may compare the AIP data with those for F5. In F5, the discharge of a given neuron usually is limited to one motor act (e.g., grasping or holding) or even to a segment of the act (e.g., hand closure), but parietal neurons most often start to discharge during hand shaping and continue also during object holding, suggesting that AIP neurons code actions in a more global way than do F5 neurons. Visual responses to three-dimensional objects are more frequent in AIP than those in F5. Both areas respond to complex biological stimuli (e.g., the vision of the hand). However, mirror neurons have not been reported yet in AIP. Thus, it is likely that the hand neurons described by Sakata et al. (1992) could have a role in hand control during manipulation rather than in recognition of biologically or socially relevant movements.

The motor responses in AIP may be explained as corollary discharges sent by F5 back to PP. If the F5 motor command matches the visual signals, the parietal cells are fully activated and send a positive feedback signal to the premotor cortex to carry on the correct movement until the object is grasped and held successfully. Otherwise, the parietal activity is suppressed, and the movement is interrupted or modified (Sakata et al. 1992). It is unclear at present whether there is a set of neurons, genetically preformed or determined by learning, for each type of grip or whether different types of grips result from a joint action of a limited series of fundamental grip neuron types. However, what is clear is that grip movements are not organized on the basis of a direct link between visual neurons and motor neurons controlling individual muscles or simple finger movements. Moreover, general commands (e.g., grasp with the mouth or hands) often are not distinct from a precise specification of how the action has to be performed (e.g., precision grip). What to do and how to do it seem to be processed together.

The FARS Model and Synthetic PET

Based in great part on the data of Rizzolatti and Sakata, a detailed model of the neural mechanisms of grasping has been developed by Fagg and Arbib (to appear; Fagg 1996) and thus is called the *FARS model*. This model makes numerous predictions. One simulation study showed how the model performs when a delayed instruction stimulus is used to inform a subject how to grasp an object. The model is presented with a single object (a small cylinder) and is asked to perform one of three different tasks: to grasp the cylinder by using a precision pinch, to grasp the cylinder by using a side opposition; and to grasp the cylinder by using either a precision pinch or a side opposition, as a function of an instruction stimulus (e.g., the color of a light).

(We speak rather loosely here. The model is not a robot; it transforms visual codes for objects to neural codes for movements via neural network models of diverse brain regions.) In the model, area F2 (dorsal premotor cortex) has a high level of activity in the conditional task, as this region is involved only when the model must map an arbitrary stimulus to a motor program (in this case, a grasp), and the region does not receive instructional stimulus (IS) inputs in the nonconditional task. F5 receives inputs from F2, causing an increase in the region's activity level that is passed on through excitatory connections to AIP.

Rizzolatti et al. (1988) found that the number of neurons in F5 involved in the execution of the precision pinch was greater than those involved in either the side opposition or the power grasp (the fewest neurons were observed in the latter case). In the construction of the model, this information was used to select the distribution of neurons for each type of grasp. For the precision pinch versus other grasps (in the nonconditional case), there was an increase in the number of active units only in F5 and AIP.

This background permits a review of the methodology of synthetic PET imaging and a comparison of the results of modeling the monkey with brain imaging studies on humans. $H_2{}^{15}O$ PET is an imaging technique that allows the measurement of regional cerebral blood flow (rCBF). Because rCBF appears to be related to the local synaptic activity within a region (Brownell et al. 1982), it is possible to observe differences in the measured rCBF as a function of the task that a subject performs (e.g., Decety et al. 1994; Grafton et al. 1995; Grafton et al. 1996a). Current resolution of the technique is on the order of 1.5 mm in each spatial dimension and temporally is approximately 80 seconds.

In humans, then, PET and functional magnetic resonance imaging (fMRI) techniques allow us to achieve a global view of the systems involved in performing a task, but at the expense of a very coarse spatial and temporal resolution. On the other hand, in monkey we are able to examine individual cells and resolve single spikes, but we have tremendous difficulty in examining entire circuits. Thus, it is important to develop techniques that allow experimental results at both levels to be brought together as we attempt to understand the different systems. Arbib et al. (1995) proposed *Synthetic PET* imaging as a way to draw conclusions in one domain from experimental results in the other. This method starts with a computational model of the neural networks involved in some task, with subsets of the neurons in the networks assignable as modeling the activity in specific regions of the primate brain. The synaptic activity of a region A under condition 1 is computed from the model as follows:

$$\text{PET}_A(1) = \int_{t_0}^{t_1} \sum_B w_{B \to A}(t) \, dt \qquad (20)$$

where $w_{B \to A}(t)$ is the absolute value of the activity of the synapses (firing rate × |synaptic strength|) connecting region B to region A at time t, B runs over the set of regions (which may or may not include A) that have synapses in A, and $[t_0, t_1]$ is the time interval for (simulated) execution of task 1. The measure of instantaneous synaptic activity in region A then is integrated over the time required to perform a task (which might involve multiple trials).

The simulated synaptic activity of a region then can be compared over several conditions. To create a synthetic PET comparison, we compute the raw PET activity during task 1 and during task 2, then compute the comparative activity $\text{PET}_A(1/2)$ for task 1 over task 2 for each region A. This measure is given by

$$\text{PET}_A(1/2) = \frac{\text{rPET}_A(1) - \text{rPET}_A(2)}{\text{rPET}_A(2)} \times 100 \qquad (21)$$

to compare the change in PET_A from task 2 to task 1.

Note that the positive and negative projections into a region are treated equally in their contribution to the synthetic PET measure (owing to the absolute value operator applied to the connection weight in equation 20). Thus, from the PET measure alone, it is impossible to distinguish the case in which a positive input is given from the situation where an equally negative input is given.

With this background, we can summarize the predictions made by applying Synthetic PET to the FARS model. The conditional task is to grasp a cylinder using either a precision pinch or a side opposition, the choice being determined by an instruction stimulus (the color of a light). Fagg, Arbib, and Grafton (to appear) tabulated in the model regions that demonstrate a change in synaptic activity in the conditional task above and beyond those involved when the subject knows a priori which of the two grasps to perform. The most significant change predicted by the model is the level of activity exhibited by area F2 (dorsal premotor cortex). Its high level of activity in the conditional task is due to the fact that this region is involved only when the model must map an arbitrary stimulus to a motor program (in this case, a grasp). In the nonconditional task, the region does not receive IS inputs, and thus its synaptic activity is dominated by the general background activity in the region. The additional IS inputs in the conditional task have a second-order effect on the network, as reflected in small changes in activity in F5, basal ganglia, and AIP. The increased synaptic activity in F5 is due to the additional inputs from F2 (into the supporting inputs of some columns in F5). These inputs also cause an increase in the region's activity level, which is passed on through excitatory connections to AIP.

As noted previously, the model reflects the fact that the number of F5 neurons involved in the execution of the precision pinch was greater than that of those involved in either the side opposition or the power grasp. To show how this distribution is reflected in the Synthetic PET measures, we compare these measures for the precision pinch and side opposition. Among other effects, there is an increase in the number of active units only in F5 and AIP.

The previous Synthetic PET experiments raised some important questions about how instruction stimuli are mapped to arbitrary motor programs and about the relative representation of different grasps. These predictions were tested in a human PET experiment (Fagg, Grafton, and Arbib, to appear).

The model predicted that the conditional task should yield much higher activation in F2 (dorsal premotor cortex), some activation of F5, and a slight activation of AIP. The human experiment confirmed the F2 result but failed to confirm the predictions for F5 and AIP. In fact, in humans there is an activation of the inferior parietal cortex (AIP) but no significant activation of ventral premotor cortex. The model involved reciprocal connections between regions F5 and AIP and a projection from F2 to F5, but the strength of the projection from F2 to F5 essentially is a free parameter of the model: There is a wide range of values over which the model will perform the conditional and nonconditional tasks correctly. The implication is that by tuning this parameter, we can control this projection's contribution to the synaptic activity measure in F5. However, the original FARS model was such that difference in AIP synaptic activity from the nonconditional to the conditional task will always be less than the difference observed in F5. One possibility for repairing this problem in the model was to reroute the F2 information so that it enters the grasp decision circuitry through AIP rather than through F5.

In the other case, studied both by Synthetic PET and by PET study of human subjects, the model predicted an increase of synaptic activity in both F5 and AIP in the precision pinch case as compared to side opposition. Although we saw an increase in activity in the inferior parietal area in the human experiment, we failed to see any such change in the ventral premotor cortex (specifically F5). One possibility is that F5 is involved in the grasp but that the effect is masked by force-related activity in the region. In the human experiment, performance of the power grasp required application of a reasonable level of force to the block that the subject is required to grasp. In monkey, force-related activity has been observed in F5 (Hepp-Reymond et al. 1994). The implication is that even though there are fewer neurons involved in encoding the power grasp, they are achieving a higher level of activity because of the force requirements of the task. Thus, the rCBF measures still could be relatively similar in both conditions.

The low-level details of the FARS model were derived primarily from neurophysiological results obtained in monkey. The Synthetic PET approach extracts measures of regional synaptic activity as the model performs a variety of tasks. These measures are compared to rCBF observed during human PET experiments as the subjects perform tasks similar to those simulated in the model. In some cases, the human results provide confirmation of the model behavior. In other cases, where there is a mismatch between model prediction and human results, it is possible (as we have shown) to use these negative results further to refine and constrain the model and, on this basis, design new experiments for both primate neurophysiology and human brain imaging. Our point here is not to highlight (or hide) the flaws in the present FARS model but rather to suggest that it provides a useful platform for further modeling and that Synthetic PET provides a technique (itself open to fruitful modification) to ensure that future modeling is responsive (and contributory) to future developments in both monkey neurophysiology and human neurology.

8.5 Learning of Coordinated Behaviors

8.5.1 Motor Set and the Neuralization of Coordinated Control Programs

Can the general notion of coordinated control programs (see figures 3.4 and 3.14 in chapter 3 for such programs for reaching and grasping) be related to—or constrained by—data regarding the brain? Iberall and Arbib (1990) postulated how the various functions of figure 3.6 may be distributed in the primate brain after their refinement in terms of our subsequent theory of preshaping on the basis of opposition space (see figure 3.10).

Here, we view prehension as controlled by the coordinated activity of four schemas.

1. *Target location and grasp selection:* These elements emanate from occipital cortex, involve dorsal and ventral pathways, and enter into the motor system in different places.

2. *Eye movement and spatial memory:* Closely coupled, these functions have been modeled previously (sec. 8.4.2; the role of basal ganglia is explained in chapter 10). Their contribution to prehension becomes particularly relevant when targets must be grasped from memory.

3. *The arm movement schema:* This schema is based on well-defined cortical and subcortical anatomical circuitry (DeLong, Georgopoulos, and Crutcher 1983; Kalaska and Crammond 1992).

4. *The grasp-shaping schema:* It includes the insula, SII, and ventral premotor cortex. The involvement of SII, presumably mediating tactile expectations and feedback, is a major innovation of the model and is based on the finding of Grafton et al. (1995). Their PET study of humans showed that the SII was significantly more active in reaching to grasp than in reaching to point. Thus, for example, the role played by the "early" somatosensory areas 1, 2, 3a, and 3b in the Iberall and Arbib figure (not shown here) now is played by the more "perceptual" SII.

Together, these schemas integrate visual and tactile input into an appropriate motor plan for successful reaching and grasping. Here, the connections in the coordinated control program map well to those given by the anatomy, though even here we must face the question, "How are the regions involved in the grasp-shaping schema deployed first in the preshape and later in the enclose schema?" More generally, when we learn a new skill, there is nothing anatomical about the relationship between the constituent motor schemas. If one learns the sequence, "Pull your left ear, touch your nose, pull your left ear, touch your chin," it seems reasonable to postulate that a separate neural assemblage code is required to specify how the activity of the various pull and touch schemas is to be coordinated in the coordinated control program for this new skill. Without denying that they might overlap, we must distinguish the circuitry that implements the schemas from the circuitry that implements the assemblage code specifying how these are coordinated. In some cases, much of this "code" is implicit: The simple linkage of the output of one brain region to the input of another provides fixed connections between the schemas that *in this case* do not require explicit circuitry to implement (though we take a less simplistic view in chapter 10). However, when we learn a skill, we learn to deploy schemas that are already available so as to provide a coordinated control program that then may be tuned by experience. A verbal description may tell us how to assemble a network for a task, but synaptic plasticity then may reshape the neural net to achieve (on the basis of experience) properties that were not explicit in the original high-level specification. Thus, we now suggest one way in which patterns in one region of cerebral cortex (implementing the assemblage code) may coordinate schemas implemented in the neural circuitry of other regions. (In chapter 10, we suggest what the basal ganglia may add to this description.)

In describing learned behavior, the coordinated control program is to express the way in which a number of already available skills (expressed as perceptual or motor schemas) may be combined, on the basis of instruction or experience, in diverse ways to constitute a variety of novel skills. Here, the *effective connectivity* between the neural networks implementing the schemas is to be changed, depending on which skill is being exercised. Moreover, that pattern is to change dynamically during a single episode of skilled behavior. Thus, going beyond the case of fixed connections, the issue is how the connections between a set of neural circuits can be under the dynamic control of neural activity (probably elsewhere in the brain) encoding a coordinated control program. Arbib (1990) presented a preliminary account of one way in which this might be done. The starting point is the notion that the coordinated interweaving of motor schema activations might be enforced through the neural mechanism of *motor set*.

In work that provides background for our later study of visuomotor conditional learning, Evarts and Tanji (1976; see also Evarts, Shinoda, and Wise 1984) monitored premovement neural activity in the primary motor

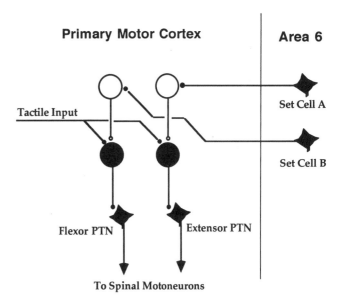

Figure 8.31
Neural gating in motor cortex. (Reprinted with permission from Arbib 1990.) PTN, pyrimidal tract neuron.

cortex of monkeys. They found evidence that sensory information is selectively gated to pyramidal tract neurons (PTNs), depending on the premovement signals from *set cells* that relay the current intention of the animal to primary motor cortex. The set cells, located perhaps in area 6, are able to facilitate or block sensory input to primary motor cortex regions concerned with specific movements, depending on the desired movement. Such a neural gating mechanism is illustrated in figure 8.31, which uses single cells to represent cell populations in the monkey brain. Here SI is somatosensory area one, the primary area of cortex for receipt of tactile and kinesthetic information; correspondingly, MI is primary motor cortex. When set cell A is highly active, it stimulates an inhibitory neuron that blocks the flow of tactile information (from somatosensory cortex SI) to the arm flexor pool of PTNs in MI. Because sensory input to the arm extensor PTN remains unchecked, a tactile stimulus then will produce an arm extension. On the other hand, if set cell A is dormant and set cell B is active, the arm extensor PTN's access to the sensory input will be blocked, leaving the arm flexor PTN's input open, and a tactile signal will trigger an arm flexion. Thus, we see how set cells can change the effective connectivity of the underlying circuitry for tactile control of arm movement.

In what follows, we view each basic motor schema as having its own neural representation, and we explore the hypothesis that higher motor centers implement a coordinated control program by controlling the activity of motor schemas through the regulation of sensory information to each motor schema's neural representation. (We focus on motor control here. The build up of a complex perceptual representation appears to involve coordination of multiple instances of a given schema that must be coordinated, as when we see a scene with several houses. Because the example of a skill given earlier involves multiple instances of a motor schema, the differences in mechanism may not be so great.) Through the same neural gating mechanism, the higher motor centers also might regulate excitatory or inhibitory flow among the schemas.

It is the pattern established in the neural circuitry of the "higher center" that encodes the schema assemblage; it is the interaction of these patterns with the circuitry encoding the schemas that enables the brain as a whole to execute the assemblage. A possibly dynamic connection to circuitry implementing a schema controls the activation transitions of the coordinated control program. To illustrate various aspects of such "administrative control" of MI, consider four uses of neural gating in enforcing an orderly sequence of submovement executions.

1. The selective denial of topographically relevant PTNs' access to different sources of sensory input (see figure 8.32) could enable the higher motor centers to establish loops between sensory trigger stimuli and arbitrary functional synergies, as in the long-latency reflex and the intention-related grasping reflex. Hence, the higher motor centers can program reflexes as needed. The crucial point here is that rich excitatory pathways exist to link a large variety of circuits; much of higher level control is provided by *inhibitory sculpting*.

2. The mutual exclusion of a given pair of motor schema activations could be implemented by setting up symmetrical inhibition between the schemas' networks via neural gating. Conversely, schemas can be made to "cooperate" by establishing lines of excitatory communication or by blocking lines of inhibitory communication. In this case, the blending of the two prototypical movements could take place in MI or further downstream.

3. If asymmetrical inhibitory communication is set up between two motor schemas' patterns of activity, the recipient schema will be inhibited whenever the other is activated. Thus, the higher motor centers could enforce the sequential ordering of any pair of submovements by priming their schemas for activity and by establishing an asymmetrical channel of inhibitory communication between them.

4. By priming a chosen set of motor schemas, either through direct neural excitation of PTNs or by the gat-

ing of sensory stimuli to PTNs, coupled with the establishment of inhibitory lines of communication among those motor schemas (to ensure that only one schema activates as in (2) above), the higher motor centers may initiate competition between a set of favored motor schemas, leaving the final decision to the intermediate motor level. This possibility distributes the processing of sensorimotor information through the motor hierarchy, allowing efficient use of resources through parallelism.

It should be apparent now that the interweaving of motor schema activations can be accomplished through various neural gating tactics involving the temporary establishment of excitatory or inhibitory interactions among the patterns of neural activity corresponding to different motor schemas. It is possible to envision the motor hierarchy as a directed graph structure, with coordinated control programs for complex skills parenting low-level coordinated control programs and motor schemas. Each coordinated control program has a characteristic pattern of neural activity that involves the imposition of motor set on the neural structures subordinate to the coordinated control program, effectively interweaving the activations of "child" coordinated control programs and ultimately the basic motor schemas. What remains to be discovered is how the various assemblages that exercise such restructuring are themselves acquired and updated through experience. Also, we need simulation studies to probe what patterns of activity in the competing networks do and do not trigger action and how the "decision time" for an act increases with the complexity of competitive interactions.

Of course, an important distinction between the hierarchical organization of motor activity and the perceptual organization of complex object categories is the temporal-sequential nature of a skilled action. A skill's motor hierarchy unfolds in the course of its submovements instead of "all at once" during the preparatory phase. Indeed, during the execution of movement sequences, the motor hierarchy is in a constant state of flux. Motor schemas in the hierarchy do not activate until necessary, and each motor schema remains active only as long as necessary.

Tanji and Kurata (1985) trained monkeys to perform key presses in response to different stimuli. In the tactile mode, an instruction stimulus (the tactile instruction) warned the animal to perform a key press in response to a tactile trigger stimulus (tactile stimulus) and to ignore an audio signal. In the audio mode, a different instruction warned the animal to respond instead to an audio stimulus and to ignore a tactile signal. The experimenters recorded the activity of neurons in MI and area 6 during

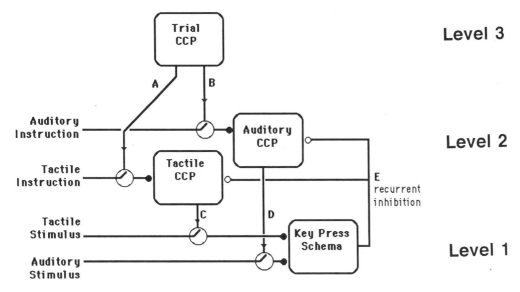

Figure 8.32
Schema hierarchy for the Tanji-Kurata experiment. (Reprinted with permission from Arbib 1990.) CCP, coordinated control program.

the trials. A total of 128 neurons in area 6 responded to the instruction and, of these, 44 responded with greater magnitude to one instruction than to the other (i.e., some neurons responded to the tactile instruction but not the auditory instruction, and vice versa). All area 6 neurons responding to an instruction resumed normal activity on arrival of the stimulus that triggered the key press. Thus, the activity of neuronal populations associated with the high-level establishment of MI's motor set dissipated at the start of the movement's execution, their influence no longer being required. Neurons in primary motor cortex responded to the instruction without preference to one instruction or the other.

Figure 8.32 illustrates the schema hierarchy for a schema-theoretical interpretation of these results. At level 1, we have the key press schema. At level 2, we have the tactile coordinated control program (shown as tactile CCP), which links tactile stimulation to the key press schema, and the auditory coordinated control program, linking auditory stimulation to the key press schema. At level 3, we have the trial coordinated control program, which can be activated (in ways not shown here) in response to the organism's goals or to the environmental situation.

Though the definition (learning) of these assemblages flows up the hierarchy, the activation flows down. (In the present example, we shall assume that instantiation of a schema or assemblage is identical with the attainment of some threshold level of distributed activity in the neural circuitry that embodies it.) Activation of the trial coordinated control program opens channels of communication

from the source of the anticipated tactile instruction to the tactile coordinated control program, and from the source of anticipated auditory instruction to the auditory coordinated control program. In figure 8.32, arcs A and B represent the axons of set cells whose activity establishes the sensory communication pathways to the tactile and auditory coordinated control programs, respectively, via neural gating. Note that at this point, the active motor hierarchy for the task we are considering consists of only the trial coordinated control program, the other components not yet having been activated. If a tactile instruction now occurs, the tactile input to the tactile coordinated control program raises that coordinated control program's activation level above its activation threshold, allowing the tactile coordinated control program to open a pathway of communication via arc C from the source of the tactile stimulus to the key press motor schema. On receipt of the tactile stimulus, the latter schema finally activates, producing the key press movement. In this case, an auditory stimulus would not evoke any movement because a pathway has not been opened to the motor schema.

Alternatively, the event of an auditory instruction activates the Auditory coordinated control program, which establishes a pathway of communication via arc D from the auditory stimulus source to the key press motor schemas. Now, the event of an auditory stimulus (but not a tactile stimulus) will lead to the activation of the key press motor schemas, eliciting a key press response.

The preferential responses of the area 6 neurons to one instruction or the other are interpreted here as hav-

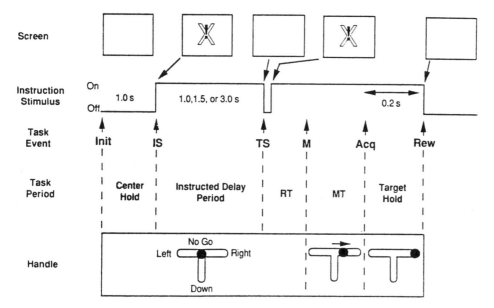

Figure 8.33
The protocol for visual-motor conditionary. Top row, visual stimulus as seen on the video screen; second row, temporal trace of the visual stimulus; third and fourth rows, primary events and periods of the experimental trial; fifth row, expected motor response. (Reprinted with permission from Mitz, Godshalk, and Wise 1991, fig. 1.) IS, instruction stimulus; TS, trigger stimulus; M, movement initiation; Acq, acquisition of motor target; Rew, reward; RT, reaction time; MT, movement time.

ing been due to the separate coordinated control programs (tactile and auditory) that activated in response to the respective stimuli. The nonpreferential nature of the primary motor cortex neurons to the different stimuli follows from the fact that whichever coordinated control program activated (tactile or auditory), the anticipated stimulus was channeled to the same motor schemas.

Finally, we consider the evidence that coordinated control programs deactivate in the course of movement execution. Recall that 128 area 6 neurons resumed normal activity on the arrival of the stimulus. In figure 8.32, this may be interpreted as follows: Once the stimulus arrives and the motor schemas activate, the motor schemas suppress the parent coordinated control program through inhibition (arc E), deactivating the coordinated control program, which has fulfilled its role. Though the descending arcs A, B, C, and D are shaped by learning, it may be that the arcs E represent an innate feedback path for broadcasting a "reset" to area 6 whenever execution of the next step of a plan is initiated. The reader may compare this to the way in which the activation of a saccade is accompanied by an SC signal that "clears" the working memory (sec. 8.3.2; see equation 18).

8.5.2 Visuomotor Conditional Learning

Mitz, Godshalk, and Wise (1991) examined learning-dependent activity in the premotor cortex of two rhesus monkeys required to move a lever in a particular direc-

tion in response to a specific visual stimulus. Figure 8.33 shows the protocol and expected response for one such trial. Initially, the monkey was given a ready signal, which was followed by a visual stimulus (instruction stimulus, IS). Then the monkey was expected to wait for a flash in the visual stimulus, the trigger stimulus (TS), and to produce the appropriate motor response. The four possible motor responses were to move the handle left, right or down or not to move. When a correct response was produced, the monkey was rewarded and a stimulus was picked randomly for the next trial. On the other hand, when an incorrect response was produced, no reward was given, and the same stimulus was kept for the next trial.

Phase I, Shaping: During the initial training phase, two monkeys were trained to perform the task with a fixed set of visual stimuli. Albeit incredibly time-consuming, this phase taught the monkeys the four appropriate motor responses and the fact that they would be rewarded for learning to associate one of these responses with each new visual pattern.

Phase II: Once shaping was complete and the monkeys had learned the "rules of the game", they required remarkably few trials to learn the rewarded response to a novel stimulus (table 8.1). The left-hand column shows the correct response, and each row of the right-hand column shows a monkey's response in one trial over time. In a number of cases, the monkey exhibited an incorrect

Table 8.1
Samples of responses to novel stimuli, given example-specific expected motor responses

Correct response	Trial number														
	1	2	3	4	5	6	7	8	9	10	11	12	13	14	15
Down (D)	L	+	+	+	+	+	+								
	R	L	L	+	R	+	+	+	+	+	+	+	+	+	
	R	+	R	L	+	+	+	+	+	+	+	+	+	+	+
	+	+	+	+	+	+	+	+							
	N	R	+	+	R	+	+	+							
	N	L	N	R	+	+	+	+	+	+	+	+	+	+	+
Right (R)	N	L	N	D	L	+	+	+							
	N	+	+	+	+										
	N	N	N	L	+	N	N	N	+	+	+				
	N	N	N	N	N	+	+	+	+						
	N	N	L	+	+	N	+	+	+						
Left (L)	R	D	+	N	+	+	+	+	+	+	+	+	+	+	+
	+	+	+	+	+	+	+	+	+	+	+	+	+	+	
	N	D	+	+	+	+	+	+	+	+	+	+	+	+	+
	N	D	+	+	+	+	+	+	+	+	+	+	+	+	+
	N	N	D	R	+	+	+	+	+	+	+	+			
	N	R	D	+	R	D	+	R	+	R	+	+	+		
No-go (N)	R	+	+	+	+	+	+	+	+	+	+	+	+	+	+
	+	+	+	+	+	+	+	+	+	+	+	+	+	+	+
	+	+	+	+	+	+	+	+	+	+	+	+	+	+	+
	L	L	R	D	L	+	L	+	+	+	+	+	+	+	+
	+	+	+	+	+	+	+	+	+	+	+	+	+	+	+
	D	R	D	+	D	L	R	+	L	D	R	D	+	+	+

Correct responses are indicated with a plus sign (+). Each row shows responses to a different novel stimulus, and only the first 15 responses are shown.

Note: Each row represents only those trials from an experiment that correspond to a specific desired motor response.

response, and even though it did not receive a reward, it may continue to output the same response for several additional trials. In most of these cases, the no-go response appeared to be the "default" response. In almost half of these response traces, the monkey may give one or more improper responses after first exhibiting the correct response, before producing the correct response consistently.

Mitz et al. (1991) recorded from a variety of cell types in the premotor cortex. *Anticipatory* cells tend to fire between the ready signal and the IS. *Signal* cells respond to the presentation of a movement-related stimulus, whereas *set-related* cells fire after the IS in preparation for a particular motor response, corresponding to FEF cells that fire during the delay period in delayed saccades. *Movement-related* cells respond to the presentation of the TS, and in some cases stay on for the duration of the movement. Most cells exhibit multiple response properties (e.g., combined set- and movement-related responses).

Signal-, set-, and movement-related cells typically fired in correlation with a particular motor response. Thus, for any particular visual stimulus, only a small subset of cells fired significantly during the execution of the corresponding motor program. As learning progressed, some cells were seen to increase in their response activity toward a stimulus, whereas others decreased in their response. Figure 8.34 shows normalized activity and performance curves for one experiment plotted against the trial number. The normalized activity is computed for a particular stimulus by observation of the activity of the ensemble of units that show an increase in activity over the course of learning. The performance curve is computed as a sliding window over a set range of trials. Mitz et al. (1991) identified a number of key features of learning-dependent activity in these experiments:

• *The increase in cell activity.* For those cells that increased their activity over the learning period, it was correlated closely with but was preceded (though only

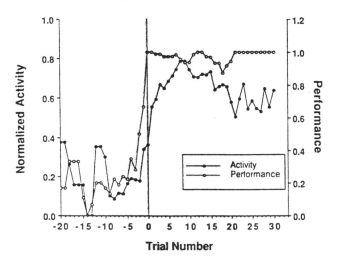

Figure 8.34
Normalized activity and performance curve plotted as a function of trial for the presentation of a novel stimulus. The rise in overall performance precedes that of cellular activity by approximately three trials. (Reprinted with permission from Mitz, Godshalk, and Wise 1991, fig. 3.)

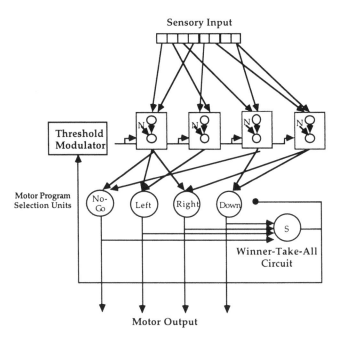

Figure 8.35
The motor program selection model. Each motor selection column comprises a feature detector that detects specific events from the sensory input and a voting unit that produces a vote for an appropriate set of motor programs. Along with the noise and the threshold modulator, each unit implements a search mechanism. The votes of the motor selection columns are collected by units representing the activity of the schemas for each legal motor response. The winner-take-all circuit ensures that only one motor program is selected. (Reprinted with permission from Fagg and Arbib 1992.) N, noise; S, summed activity of motor columns.

slightly) by the improvement in performance. Similar relations were seen in signal-, set-, and movement-related units.

- *Activity of a particular unit for correct responses.* In most cases, it was higher than that during incorrect responses in the same movement direction.

- *Activity for correct responses.* During times of good performance, it exceeded that at times of poor performance.

- *Similar learning-dependent responses of the signal-, set-, and movement-related cells.* When multiple sets of novel stimuli were presented to the monkey, were observed for stimuli that yielded the same motor response.

The researchers also noted that the activity pattern resulting from a familiar stimulus closely correlated with the activity due to novel stimuli (after learning), although this correlation was not a perfect one. This pattern and the fourth feature demonstrate that a similar set of premotor neurons are involved in responding to all stimuli mapping to the same motor output. Thus, we can conclude that the pattern discrimination probably is not happening within the premotor cortex. If this were the case, one would expect separate groups of cells to respond to different stimuli, even if these stimuli mapped to the same motor output.

In modeling these data, Fagg and Arbib (1992) sought *distributed representations* in which a single pattern (or task) is coded by a small subset of the units in the network. Although different subsets of units are allowed to overlap to a certain degree, interference between two patterns is minimized by the nonoverlapping compo-

nents. A unit that has not learned to participate in a motor program is able to respond to a wide range of different inputs. As learning progresses within this unit, its response increases significantly for some stimuli and decreases for the remainder. The primary computational unit in the proposed model is the *motor selection column*, each consisting of two neurons: the *feature detector unit* and the *voting* unit. The overall network (figure 8.35) is composed of a large number of these columns, each performing a small portion of the stimulus-to-motor program mapping. (*Column* is being used here as the name of a small neural circuit that acts as a functional unit in the model. No claim is made as to whether it maps onto a column in the structural sense of section 8.1.5, or, indeed, whether all its circuitry is localized within cerebral cortex.)

Each column (see the row to the right of the threshold modulator in figure 8.35) receives input via a feature detector, the feature detector drives the voting unit, and the voting unit sends "vote signals" to the motor program selection units. The *feature detector* recognizes small portions (microfeatures) of the input stimulus. Due to the distributed construction of the circuit, a particular signal unit is not restricted to recognizing patterns from a single stimulus but may be excited by multiple patterns, even if these patterns code for different responses. A particular signal unit is connected physically to only a small subset of the input units. This connection enforces the constraint that only a small subset of the columns will participate in the recognition of a particular pattern. As will be discussed later, this reduces the interference between patterns during learning. The *voting unit* receives input from its corresponding feature detector and from a noise process and the threshold modulator. Based on the resulting activity, the voting unit instantiates its "votes" for one or more motor programs. The strength of this vote depends on the firing rate of this neuron and on the strength of the connection between the voting unit and the motor program selector units. As shown in figure 8.35, the votes from each column are collected by the *motor program selection* units, labeled *left, right, down,* and *no-go.* The final activity of these units determines whether a particular motor program is activated, and thus executed. The winner-take-all circuit (Didday 1976; Amari and Arbib 1977) ensures that when more than one motor program selection unit becomes active, this unit sends an inhibitory signal to the array of motor program selection units. The result is that all the units will begin turning off until only the unit receiving the largest total of votes from the motor columns is left. At this point, the one active unit will cue the execution of its motor program.

The reception of the TS causes the execution of the selected motor program (this occurs outside the scope of figure 8.35). Although only a single motor program selection unit typically will be active when the TS is received, two other cases are possible: none active, and more than one active. In both cases, the no-go response is executed, irrespective of the state of the no-go motor program selection unit. Thus, the no-go response may be issued for one of two reasons: explicit selection of the response or the system's uncertainly as to an appropriate response by the time the TS is received.

The global threshold modulator and the local noise processes play an important role in the search for the appropriate motor program to activate. When a new visual stimulus is presented to the system, the feature detector units often will not respond significantly enough to bring the voting units above threshold. As a result, no voting information is passed on to the motor program selection units. The threshold modulator responds to this

situation by lowering the threshold of all of the voting units slowly. Given time (before the TS), at least a few voting units are activated to contribute some votes to the motor program units. In this case, a response is forced, even though the system is very unsure as to what that response should be.

Learning in this model is reinforcement-based and is implemented by modifying two sets of synapses: the sensory input–to–feature detector mapping and the voting unit–to–motor program selection unit mapping (i.e., the weight matrices $\mathbf{W}_{\text{in, feature}}$ and $\mathbf{W}_{\text{vote, motor}}$ corresponding, respectively, to the fan-in and fan-out of the columns in figure 8.35). Only those columns that participated in the current computation adjusted their weights. In the experimental setup, positive reinforcement was given when the monkey exhibited a correct response, but not otherwise. Similarly, in the model, a scalar quantity called *reinforcement* was set by the teacher to +1 if the selected motor program was correct and to −1 otherwise. However, a special case occurred when the system was unable to make a decision within the allotted time (causing the no-go response to be selected).

First, if more than one motor program selection unit became active at one time, the reinforcement term was set by the system to −1. This decreased the response of all columns involved, adjusting the input to the two (or more) motor program selection units until one was able to achieve threshold significantly before the other(s). It was at this point that the symmetry between the two was broken.

Additionally, if no motor program selection units were active, the reinforcement term was set to +1 by the system itself, regardless of the teacher feedback. Therefore, the currently active columns were rewarded, ensuring that the next time the pattern was presented, these columns would yield a greater response. Thus, they would have a greater chance of activating one of the motor program selection units. Without this additional term, negative reinforcement from the teacher was disastrous. The negative reinforcement further decreased the response of the already poorly responding columns, further decreasing their response. The result would be a self-reinforcing situation that can never discover the correct response.

When positive reinforcement was given, the weights leading into the feature detector units were adjusted such that the feature detector better recognized the current sensory input. In the case of negative reinforcement, the weights were adjusted in the opposite direction such that the current input was recognized by the feature detector unit to an even lesser degree. Note that this reinforcement depends on whether or not the overall system response was correct, not on the output of any individual motor selection column.

$$l_{gain} = \begin{cases} negative\_factor\_f & \text{if reinforcement} < 0 \\ 1 & \text{if } 0 \leq \text{reinforcement} \end{cases}$$

$$\Delta \mathbf{W}_{in,feature} = \text{reinforcement} \cdot l_{gain} \cdot l_{rate_f} \cdot (\text{Input} \cdot \text{Voting}^T)$$
(22)

where l_{rate_f} is the learning rate coefficient for the stimulus-to-feature and $(\text{Input} \cdot \text{Voting}^T)$ is the outer product of the input and movement vectors. The l_{gain} factor is used simply to scale the effect of negative reinforcement relative to positive reinforcement. In this case, the effect of negative reinforcement on the weights is intended to be less than that of positive reinforcement. This is done because negative reinforcement can be devastating to columns that are just beginning to learn the appropriate mapping.

To weaken simultaneously those weights that are not strengthened by reinforcement, we then set

$$\mathbf{W}_{in,vote} = \text{Normalize}(\mathbf{W}_{in,feature} + \Delta \mathbf{W}_{in,feature}$$
$$\wedge \mathbf{W}\_in\_feature\_mask)$$
(23)

where $\text{Normalize}(\mathbf{x}) = \mathbf{x}_i / \left(\sum_j |x_j| \right)$.

$\mathbf{W}\_in\_feature\_mask$ is a matrix of ones and zeros that determines the existence of a weight between the corresponding voting and motor program selection units. The elements of this matrix are point-wise multiplied with those of $\Delta \mathbf{W}_{in,feature}$ to mask out weight deltas for weights that do not exist (see Appendix A of Fagg and Arbib 1992 for further details).

Equation 23 produces a competition between the weights associated with a particular unit. Thus, the weights are self-regulating, forcing unneeded or undesirable weights to a value near zero. If a column continues to receive negative reinforcement (as a result of being involved in an incorrect response), it becomes insensitive to the current stimulus and is reallocated to recognize other stimuli.

The voting unit–to–motor selection mapping is adjusted similarly. Positive reinforcement increases the weight of the synapse to the correct motor program. When negative reinforcement is given, the synapse is weakened, allowing the other synapses from the voting unit to strengthen slightly through normalization. Thus, more voting power is allocated to the other alternatives:

$$\Delta \mathbf{W}_{vote,motor} = \text{reinforcement} \cdot l_{gain} \cdot l_{rate_v}$$
$$\cdot (\text{Voting} \cdot \text{Motor}^T)$$
(24)

$$\mathbf{W}_{vote,motor} = \text{Normalize}(\mathbf{W}_{vote,motor} + \Delta \mathbf{W}_{vote,motor})$$
(25)

where l_{rate_v} is the learning rate coefficient for the voting–to–motor response mapping. A similar type of reinforcement learning is used in Barto et al. (1983). $\mathbf{W}_{in,feature}$ and $\mathbf{W}_{vote,motor}$ initially are selected at random (again, see Appendix A of Fagg and Arbib 1992 for more details). When a response is generated, learning is applied to each of the columns that currently are participating in the computation.

The learning objective of an individual column is to recognize particular patterns (or subpatterns) and to identify which of the possible motor programs deserves its votes. As these feature detectors begin more adequately to recognize the correct patterns, the activity of the signal units will grow with respect to the pattern, thus giving the column a larger voting power (see the competitive learning of von der Malsburg 1973; Grossberg 1976; and Rumelhart and Zipser 1986). Individual columns learn to become feature detectors for specific subpatterns of the visual stimulus. However, a column does not recognize a pattern to the exclusion of other patterns. Instead, several columns participate in the recognition at once. In addition, a column is responsible for generating an appropriate motor output directly. Therefore, the update of the feature detector weights depends not only on recognition of the pattern (as in competitive learning) but also on whether the network generates the correct motor output. In the case of a correct response, the feature detector weights become tuned better toward the incoming stimulus. For an incorrect response, the weights are adjusted in the opposite direction such that recognition is lessened for the current input.

Note that in this scheme, all the columns that participate in the voting are punished or rewarded as a whole, depending on the strength of their activity. Thus, a column that votes for an incorrect choice still may be rewarded as long as the entire set of votes chose the correct motor program. In general, this method works because this "incorrect column" always will be active in conjunction with several other columns that do vote appropriately and always are able to overrule its vote. As a result, the model satisfactorily reproduces the data shown in Table 8.1 and figure 8.34, predicting both the number and pattern of trials required to learn the correct response to a new visual stimulus and the way in which overall behavior leads the response of newly trained neurons.

Completing our introduction to the cerebral cortex, this model of reinforcement learning explains satisfactorily how the monkey can learn variations rapidly once it has been trained on the overall task (in this case, matching lever pulls to visual patterns) and shows variations in cellular responses that match those seen by Mitz et al. (1991) in premotor cortex. However, the Fagg and Arbib (1992) model does not rest on any claim that all the circuitry of the model represents premotor cortex. In fact, there is increasing evidence that conditional and sequential behaviors rest on the cooperation of cerebral cortex with basal ganglia (see Role of the Basal Ganglia, in sec. 8.4.2, Corticothalamic Systems for Saccade Control). Between them, the next two chapters will make clear that the cerebral cortex does not act in isolation as executive controller, so to speak, but relies heavily on the cerebellum to tune its activity and on the basal ganglia for scheduling of behaviors.

8.6 From Action-Oriented Perception to Cognition

Our trajectory in this chapter has been from structure through dynamics (both developmental, and as exhibited in thalamocortical oscillations) to function, and our discussion of function has focused on action-oriented perception, with special attention to the visual control of looking, reaching, and grasping, to visuomotor conditional learning, and to the relationship of motor set to the neuralization of coordinated control programs. We also offered a number of promissory notes, for we suggested that much activity of cerebral cortex (including its roles in visual-motor conditional learning and sequential behavior) can be fully understood only when we view the activity of cerebral cortex in its interaction with the basal ganglia, which we will do in chapter 10. Meanwhile, we have already discussed empirical data or models that shed light on a number of crucial issues such as the action-perception cycle, attention, working memory, remapping, and sequential behavior, while demonstrating the utility of both schema theory and various levels of neural analysis.

However, we have not attempted to review data on the role of the diverse regions of cerebral cortex in functions that might be described as being cognitive rather than sensoimotor. We restrict ourselves to an essay on such cognitive functions from a high-level schema-theoretical viewpoint and refer the reader to Fuster (1995) for a wealth of relevant neurophysiological data.

8.6.1 From Visual Perception to Distributed Planning

In section 3.1.5, we gave an abstract account of schemas for visual scene interpretation: the VISIONS computer vision system. It is possible to view the computations underlying visual perception as constituting a distributed form of planning. This allows a brief mention of ways in which a single schema may support multiple instances and also shows how schema theory extends to realms more cognitive than the basic patterns of sensorimotor coordination. In the VISIONS system, it is the user who starts the interpretation process by invoking general goals. However, it is the current goals of the autonomous organism, not the demands of some user, that guide the process of action-oriented perception. The crucial transition is as follows:

(P1) In VISIONS, an image is supplied, goals are set, and the process of scene interpretation proceeds to conclusion. The result is a network of parameterized schema instances linked to portions of the image. (Miikkulainen and Leow 1995 offer a preliminary account of how these schema instances may be implemented in nonbiological neural networks.)

(P2) In a human or animal, the sensory input is changing constantly, in part because of the organism's control of its sensors. The process of interpretation in action-oriented perception involves a network that links instances of perceptual schemas to motor schemas, providing parameters and changing confidence levels. As their activity levels reach threshold, certain sets of these motor schemas create patterns of overt behavior. Thus the action-perception cycle continues.

To see the way in which perceptual demands change as action proceeds, consider a driver instructed to turn right at the red barn. At first, the person drives along looking for some crude perceptual event (something large and red), after which the perceptual schema for barns is brought to bear. Once a barn is identified, the emphasis shifts from identification of the barn per se to recognition of spatial relations appropriate to executing a right turn "at" the barn but determined rather by the placement of the roadway, the position of cars, and the like.

In "classic" artificial intelligence, explicit planning precedes execution, taking the form of a centralized sequential deliberation based on goals and a world model to yield a sequence of actions. Such an approach may impose unrealistic requirements for modeling and perception, because all relevant information must be available before planning begins. This necessity makes it hard to adapt the plan to events not predicted by the model. In reaction to this, some critics have advocated *reactive planning*, in which selection and execution of actions are intertwined inextricably. Such reactive systems (e.g., the subsumption architecture of Brooks 1986) are parallel and distributed, with a hard-wired priority scheme fixed at "compile-time." There is no deliberation and no model. Inhibition-suppression rules determine which modules will control action, on the basis of current input. Similarly, *Rana computatrix* (chapter 3) is controlled by the interaction of hard-wired schemas to react in situations in which multiple targets, predator and prey, and obstacles, and moving targets must be taken into account.

All this process is a form of "planning," as the result of activity emerging in a flexible network, but the analysis of the VISIONS system makes it clear that schema theory embraces not only reactive schemas but also a more general form of planning, generatively forming patterns of schema activation that may involve creation of novel networks. The transition from (P1) to (P2) suggests how to extend the VISIONS computational strategy to provide a computational analysis of action-oriented perception in which planning is intertwined with execution. As we know from chapter 3, schema instances can combine their effects by distributed processes of *competition* and *cooperation* (i.e., interactions that, respectively, decrease and increase the activity levels of these instances) rather than by the operation of an inference engine on a passive store of knowledge. Cooperation yields a pattern of strengthened alliances between mutually consistent schema instances. This cooperation allows them to achieve high activity levels so as to constitute the overall solution of a problem (as perceptual schemas become part of the current short-term model of the environment or motor schemas contribute to the current course of action).

Here, planning is a process emerging from the cooperative computation of multiple agents rather than that being imposed by a separate executive planning system. Planning is intertwined with execution, and the plan may be updated as action proceeds. As such, this approach to planning provides a valuable complement to the direct consideration of neural networks for specific subsystems that has been the focus of so much of neuroscience. It also points the way to the extension of schema theory into the cognitive realm.

In light of this background, there are some ways in which the VISIONS system falls short of being a model of the brain mechanisms of visual perception. In doing so, we make explicit the outlines for a fresh appreciation of how different regions interact in visual perception, and they extend our understanding of cognitive architecture in general.

VISIONS takes a single photograph and produces a generic interpretation. In action-oriented perception, current sensory stimulation is assimilated to an already formed schema assemblage: the structure of working memory, and the structure of that representation is conditioned strongly by the current goals, tasks, and motivational and emotional state of the organism. Encouragingly, however, schema instantiation in VISIONS can be both hypothesis-driven and data-driven; thus, its general architecture is well-suited for use in the action-perception cycle. In section 3.1.5, we stated, for example, that the "sky-schema runs on the segmented image and finds a region reasonably high in the image and with a high value for m_{sky}." However, creating an instance of every schema for every region of an image to determine for which pairs (s, r) of schemas and regions there is a high value of $m_s(r)$ is prohibitively expensive, whether in time on a serial computer or in space in a fully parallel implementation. The mechanism in the brain is likely to be something more like this: Low-level mechanisms can isolate regions with sufficient "salience" to become the focus of attention (see our review of certain neural correlates of attention in sec. 8.4.3). These regions provide input to a variety of networks—some specialized, as for face recognition, others tuned more by experience than evolution—that proceed through a hierarchy of interacting descriptors to provide vigorous firing of those neural patterns that code for certain generic schemas. These then provide the inputs to working memory (coding both the schema and the locus where it has gained a high confidence level), which allow the process of scene recognition to proceed, by both data-driven and hypothesis-driven mechanisms.

8.6.2 Attention and Planning

The original VISIONS architecture has no focus of attention mechanism. It allows unlimited spawning of schema instances that then all compete and cooperate before a final consensus is formed. In a serial computer implementation of the system, a rigid schedule must be enforced, with one process active at a time. In the brain, the matter is more subtle. We have seen that a multiplicity of different brain regions are dedicated to a variety of processes of the kind referred to as *low-level vision* or to specialized schemas for tasks from face recognition to reaching and grasping to navigation. They also provide vital control structures, such as the ability to perceive more than one object at a time. On the other hand, we do have a conscious experience of shifting our attention to one or another aspect of a scene, and we have reviewed some of the brain mechanisms related to shifts of attention. What remains to be understood is how these shifts are nonetheless integrated with the unfolding structure of STM as perception proceeds. Didday and Arbib (1975) provided an early account of how the driving of eye movements by the SC might be "co-opted" (another example of evolutionary modulation) by cortical mechanisms generating the schema assemblage. The idea may be understood in terms of the goal-setting of the VISIONS system. We saw that activation of a schema instance for a roof in one region might create a hypothesis for a house and that this would seek confirmation by creating an instance of the wall schema to check the region beneath the roof. In general, there may be many such instances activated. Didday and Arbib modeled the attentional shift needed to obtain the necessary data on which to act. We postulated that the cortical system can generate a signal for each region of the visual field, indicating the likely utility of further analysis of that region. This signal is mapped retinotopically to a winner-take-all process in SC that determines which eye movement will occur and thus which schema instance will get the necessary data to change its confidence level effectively. The SC model was a simple modification of our earlier model of tectal mechanisms for prey selection in the frog (Didday 1970, 1976). A related model of cortical mechanisms for shifts of *covert* attention has been offered by Koch and Ullman (1985).

This discussion leads to a hypothesis that may reverse the view of activity-passivity of schemas and instances adopted in the VISIONS system. There, the schema in long-term memory is the passive code for processes, whereas the schema instance is an active copy of that process. By contrast, it may be that in the brain the active circuitry *is* the schema, that therefore only one instance can apply data-driven updating at a time, but that the structure of STM maintains a graphical representation of the world, which can create schema instances not as active processes but as patterns that link a schema to a region of the world not necessarily visible or within reach, and encode the current schema parameters, both confidence levels and perceptual or motor descriptors. Then, this working memory can mediate processes of competition and cooperation between schema instances, but the data-driven updating of a particular instance must await the shift of attention that can provide appropriate input to the active circuitry of its schema, which

will then update the STM for that schema instance accordingly.

In our proposed cognitive architecture, the short term memory is a working memory that holds a representation of data relevant to action, a memory that must be updated as action proceeds or as unexpected contingencies arise. This ability underlies the capability of the system to combine explicit planning based on look-ahead evaluation of multiple alternatives with reactive "planning" that enables an autonomous system to act promptly should an unexpected emergency arise. However, our earlier analysis of neurological data makes it clear that STM is not a unitary structure embodied in one brain region but is distributed across many brain regions maintaining diverse partial representations of the organism, its world, and the state of their interactions.

Our hypothesis is that even if object recognition is mediated by the ventral system in the manner proposed by Mishkin, Ungerleider, and Macko (1983), the question of which objects to recognize is mediated through dynamic interaction of the ventral system with a variety of prefrontal areas that elaborate, store, and update a plan of action during the course of behavior (Fuster 1989). At each stage of action, we hypothesize that through its extensive system of reciprocal interconnections with parietal cortex (Goldman-Rakic 1987), prefrontal cortex "focuses the attention" of the dorsal system so that it may elaborate visually based parameters for action. Again, through these reciprocal connections, parietal cortex can apprise the prefrontal system of the progress of motor execution as controlled by premotor cortex and can report any obstacles to execution of the current plan. This arrangement allows the prefrontal system to update the plan through a mixture of off-line and reactive planning as the task unfolds by using mechanisms akin to (but more powerful than) those used in prefrontal-parietal interactions subserving STM in the much simpler domain of eye movements to point targets (Dominey and Arbib 1992; sec. 8.4.2).

8.6.3 The Evolution of Intelligence

Newell (1990) speaks of the *Great Move* in the evolution of intelligence. Here, we review this concept and relate it the foregoing material to update our view of cognitive architecture. Newell notes that ethologists study specialized circuits for specific behavioral adaptations (such as those studied for the frog in sec. 3.2) but that

[F]inding feasible representations gets increasingly difficult with a richer and richer variety of things to be represented

and richer and richer kinds of operational transformations that they undergo. [He thus suggests that] ... instead of moving toward more and more specialized materials with specialized dynamics to support an increasingly great variety and intricacy of representational demands, an entirely different turn is possible. This is [the Great Move] to using a neutral, stable medium that is capable of registering variety and then composing whatever transformations are needed.... [T]his path opens up the whole world of indefinitely rich representations (Newell 1990, p. 61).

More subtly, we propose to combine ethological mechanisms with more flexible cortical mechanisms that can accommodate the efflorescence of human cognitive and intellectual abilities, including the capability for culture. We would explain a complex cognitive function through the interaction of instinctive schemas implemented in specifically evolved circuitry and of abstract schemas that are developed through learning and experience in general purpose (highly adaptive, post–Great Move) circuitry. An intelligent system must combine the ability to react rapidly (jumping out of the way of an unexpected vehicle when crossing the street) with the ability to weigh alternatives abstractly (deciding on the best route to get to the next appointment).

In summary, a satisfactory account of Newell's Great Move should not seek a complete break from using specialized materials to support different schemas (i.e., making exclusive use of a medium in which it is possible to compose copies of whatever schemas are needed to form novel representations). Rather, we should analyze how instinctive behavior provides a basis for and is intertwined with rational behavior. The contrast between frog visuomotor coordination and the flexibility of human visual perception makes explicit the contrast between those schema assemblages that are hard-wired evolutionarily into patterns of competition and cooperation between specific brain regions and those that through multiple data- and hypothesis-driven instantiations can yield totally novel forms for developing new skills and representing novel situations. The integration of this viewpoint—cooperative computation between special purpose and general purpose neural mechanisms—with the increasing accumulation of data from both animal neurophysiology and human brain imaging regarding cerebral mechanisms of cognition provides one of the most exciting challenges for twenty-first century neuroscience.

Cerebellum

The cerebellum is a mystery and a miracle within a mysteriously miraculous organization, the brain. This description is valid for all its possible aspects: overall function, phylogeny, ontogeny, structure, and physiological functions. Understanding of cerebellar machinery has advanced remarkably at many levels: as an assembly of specific molecules and cells, as a complex system with unique structures, as a set of adaptive control systems, and even as a partner in certain mental activity. In this chapter, we begin to integrate diverse knowledge to draw out the computational principles implemented in the actual cerebellar circuitry.

The human cerebellum is shown in figure 9.1. The cerebellar cortex is folded and projects to the rest of the central nervous system (CNS) via three pairs of deep cerebellar nuclei, corresponding to three paired regions of cerebellar cortex. The vermis (V) is oldest in evolutionary terms and has connections to the spinal cord via the flocculus; the pars intermedia (PI) communicates via the interpositus with both the spinal cord and neocortex; and the hemispheres (H), the most recent part of the cerebellum to evolve, communicate only with the neocortex, via the dentate nucleus. We may think of V and PI as refining spinal algorithms for movement, whereas PI and the cerebellar hemispheres both refine the cerebral planning of movement.

As seen in chapter 2 and in figure 9.2, cerebellar cortex contains five major neuron types—Purkinje, basket, stellate, Golgi, and granule cells—and four types of afferents (the mossy and climbing fibers that we discuss in this chapter and noradrenaline- and serotonin-containing fibers). The only output of the cerebellar cortex is provided by the Purkinje cells, which provide inhibitory input to the cerebellar nuclei. The neurotransmitter for this inhibition is γ-aminobutyric acid (GABA) but in some Purkinje cells, motilin also may be a neurotransmitter. The function of this inhibition is understood best by seeing how activity of a Purkinje cell modulates the activity of the cerebellar nucleus to which it projects (see the discussion of microcomplexes in sec. 9.3.2).

Our structural view of the cerebellum is contained in section 9.1 (the phylogeny and ontogeny of the cerebellum) and section 9.2 (the structural organization of

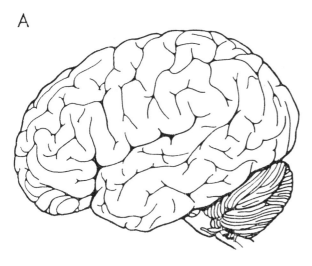

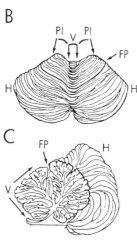

Figure 9.1
The human cerebellum. (Reprinted with permission from Eccles, 1973, fig. 4-9). V, vermis; PI, pars intermedia; H, hemispheres.

the cerebellar cortex and nuclei). We also trace the delicate mechanisms (cell growth, migration, and interaction) that yield the quasi-crystalline structure of the mature cerebellar cortex. In section 9.2.1, we look at this structure and the "space economy" of the cerebellar cortex in some quantitative detail. Sections 9.2.2 and 9.2.3 contain reviews of the circuitry of both cerebellar cortex and cerebellar nuclei. In section 9.3.2, we return to this circuitry to stress its integration in a "microcomplex" that unites a microzone of cortex with the region of nucleus to which it projects and with which it shares afferents. However, in section 9.2.4, we study the simulation of a single Purkinje cell as a very detailed compartmental model with realistic ion conductances and synaptic currents in each compartment. Because it takes massive computing resources to simulate a single cell, the models of cerebellar function in sections 9.3 and 9.4 use simpler, single-compartment models; the "aside" in section 9.2.4

points the way to future multilevel modeling that will relate system behavior to the fine details of neuronal function.

Section 9.3 contains clinical data on the role of the cerebellum in skilled movements, then focuses on the issue of how these skills are acquired, viewing the cerebellum as a learning machine. Section 9.3.1 is an introduction to the most influential model of cerebellar cortex: the Marr-Albus model, which views the Purkinje cell as a perceptron. We note that data on long-term depression (LTD) support the Albus version of the model, namely that "coincidence" of climbing fiber and parallel fiber activity on a Purkinje cell *depresses* the efficacy of the synapses of parallel fibers active during the conjunction. In section 9.3.2, we stress that cerebellar models should integrate cerebellar cortex into a cerebellar system, we introduce the microcomplexes mentioned earlier, and we stress the idea that cerebellar nuclei modulate motor pattern generators (MPGs), whereas the cerebellar cortex learns how best to modulate the cerebellar nuclei (i.e., modulating the modulator). The role of the cerebellum in motor-reflex learning has been most widely studied in two behavioral paradigms. The first is the adaptive modification of the vestibulo-ocular reflex (VOR) (section 9.3.3). The second is the classical conditioning of the rabbit eye-blink response (section 9.3.4).

In section 9.4, we present models of the function of the cerebellum in adapting the metrics of movement to changing circumstances. The Boylls model (sec. 9.4.1) shows that detailed circuitry of the cerebellar cortex and of various nuclei with which it interacts could modulate activity in MPG-related loops on a short-term basis. Section 9.4.2 discusses debate about the primary role of climbing fibers as being "teacher" or "on-line". Then we note approaches that argue the primacy of cerebellum as a timing organ and those that emphasize its sensory role. Notwithstanding, we devote sections 9.4.3 and 9.4.4 to models that emphasize adaptation of motor control based on climbing fiber control of LTD of parallel fiber → Purkinje cell synapses.

Section 9.4.3 is a presentation of various models of cerebellar activity and, in section 9.4.4, we present our own current models. Section 9.4.3 presents Kawato's model of feedback-error learning, Houk and Barto's model of the role of cerebellar plasticity in adaptive pattern generators, and Miall et al.'s view of the cerebellum as a "Smith Predictor." In section 9.4.4, we present our own current models, in which the cerebellar microcomplex is the unit of cerebellar adaptation, with its role being to modify the parameters of MPGs existing elsewhere in the brain. We model the cerebellar role in sac-

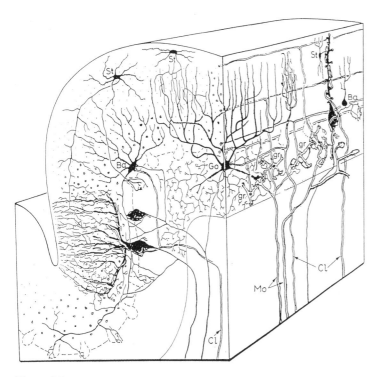

Figure 9.2
Stereodiagrammatic illustration of a fragment of the cerebellar cortex, redrawn from the color diagram in Eccles, Ito, and Szentágothai 1967; reprinted with permission). The cut surface at left is perpendicular to the folium axis; the right runs parallel to the folium. A Golgi cell (Go) is positioned at the anterior edge of the tissue block. Inhibitory cells are shown in full black; excitatory elements are shown in outlines. The full expansion of the dendritic tree of a Purkinje cell is shown at left, and another Purkinje cell at right is cut at right angles to the dendritic tree. The row of Purkinje cell bodies is indicated by their dashed outlines.

The cell body of an additional Purkinje cell at left is shown in full black to indicate the expansion of the Purkinje axon collaterals. The dendritic and axonal expansions of basket cells (Ba) and stellate (St) cells are indicated. The course of incoming climbing fibers (Cl) and some of their collaterals (to basket and Golgi cells) are visible. The mossy afferents (Mo) synapse with the short dendrites of the granule cells (Gr) wherein axons divide in T-shaped fashion into parallel fibers. The axon of the Golgi cell participates in the mossy afferent, granule cell synapses.

cade adaptation and in adaptation of dart throwing to wearing prisms, and we extend our view of LTD, introducing the notion of a window of eligibility to constrain the timing relation between the parallel fiber context and the climbing fiber "training signal." Section 9.4.5 is a discussion of how these ideas regarding adaptation may be extended to the coordination of MPGs, and section 9.5 is a look at some provocative ideas about the role of the cerebellum in mental activity.

9.1 Phylogeny and Ontogeny of the Cerebellum

In the present section, we provide perspectives on the structure of the cerebellum on the basis of both phylogeny and ontogeny.

In *phylogeny*, the cerebellum reaches a peak of development—a veritable luxuriant overgrowth—in the lowest class of the vertebrates, the fish. This view does not apply to all fish, because already it is reduced to general vertebrate size in the teleosts; the luxuriant overgrowth

is found in the weakly electric fish, the *mormyriforms*. The great size of the cerebellar hemispheres in humans is understandable from the many cultural skills in the human, such as speech, the making and use of tools, technologies for survival under vastly different environmental conditions, and symbolic speech-equivalent expressions (e.g., dance, music, pantomime, and the like). At best, all these expressions are rudimentary in humankind's closest relatives, the apes but are developed fully and are highly sophisticated in every human society. Different parts of the cerebellum may vary in importance among species. As demonstrated by figure 9.3, it is not the same part of the cerebellar hemispheres that makes the bulk of the volume in human and whale. Though the frontal parts of the cerebellar hemispheres are preponderant in the human, it is the rear parts of the hemispheres (modestly sized in the human) that are so oversized in the whale. What kind of neural function might require in the whales such a large "inferior" hemisphere of the cerebellar cortex? The skills in swimming

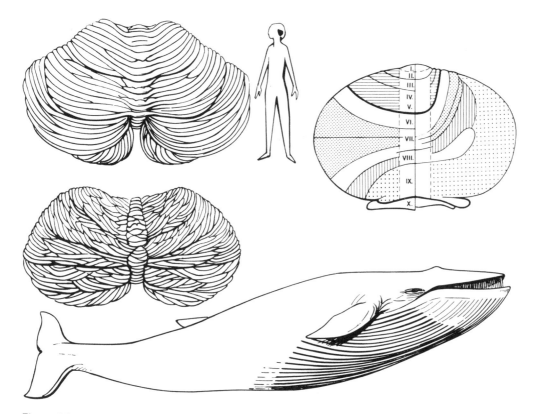

Figure 9.3

A comparison between the cerebellum in the human (upper left, as viewed from above) and in the cetaceans (left below). Of course, the cerebella, of *roughly equal* size and shape in human and whale, are out of proportion to body size; here the human is shown in comparison with a smaller whale. At right above, the main lobes of the cerebellum are shown slightly unfolded: on the left side for the human and on the right for the whale. It is apparent that most of the whale hemisphere belongs to Larsell's vermal lobes VIII and mainly IX of the inferior cerebellum. (After Jansen 1969.)

are at least equal in conventional fish, which have relatively small cerebella. Two possible special behavioral skills may come to mind: sonar and other acoustical communication in the whale and the technique for concentrating the chief source for food (krill) by their ability to emit air bubbles in a highly sophisticated geometrical pattern. The sonar function in other vertebrate classes (birds) or mammalian genera (bats) does not seem to require major cerebella, but this may show simply the diversity of evolutionary pathways for neural structures in view of, for example, the development of a specialized auditory cortex for echolocation in bats (Suga and Kanwal 1995).

The *ontogenesis* of the cerebellar cortex proceeds, at least partially, according to the typical pattern of morphogenesis of all "laminated" brain structures. The intracranial part of the medullary tube originally has only one flexure, resembling the handle of a walking stick or an umbrella, with its convexity toward the head end of the embryo. In the human embryo stage of approximately 9 mm, this single flexure gradually becomes more pro-

nounced in the neck region (the cervical flexure) and with a much sharper flexure in the region of the later mesencephalon (the mesencephalic flexure). Due to restrictions in space, an additional flexure develops in the opposite sense, with a convexity in the ventral direction at the border between what later are called the *metencephalon* and the *myelencephalon*, into which the original rhombencephalic vesicle becomes subdivided. (The restricted space of the cranium ought not to be understood only as an operative mechanical function during ontogenesis but as a geometrical restriction for the entire phylogenetic evolution program of the brain.) The major part of the roof of the fourth (rhombencephalic) ventricle becomes extended and reduced to a thin epithelial lamella. However, there remains a thicker part of the fourth ventricle roof, separated from the mesencephalon by a deep furrow called the *isthmus of the rhombencephalon* (also known as the *dorsal rhombic lip*), which will become the cerebellar primordium. The neuroepithelial cells in this rhombic lip begin to multiply, first producing (in the rat from the thirteenth embryonic day onward)

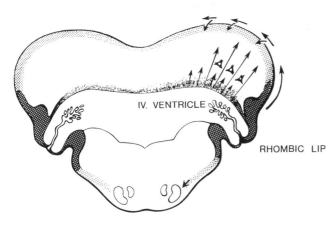

IV. VENTRICLE

RHOMBIC LIP

Figure 9.4
Development of the cerebellum, shown diagrammatically in a transverse cut of the rhombencephalon at the level of the cerebellar velum. Arrows originating from the roof of ventricle IV indicate the successive origin and emigration of the three successive generations of cells: first, the cells of the cerebellar nuclei; second, the Purkinje cells traversing between the earlier nuclear cells (longer arrows); and third, the Golgi cells (not indicated) that eventually settle below the Purkinje cell layer. Darkly stippled areas at the lateral rhombic lips show the rapid proliferation of cells that overflow the cerebellar primordium as the external granular layer (light stippling at upper surface) the cells of which will migrate inward to settle both within and beneath the Purkinje cell layer (see figure 9.5). Also shown is another proliferating cell mass in the ventral part of the rhombic lip, giving rise eventually to the inferior olive (this level) and to the pontine nuclei in more rostral levels (not seen in this transverse section).

the cells that eventually will become the cerebellar nuclei, then (on the fifteenth embryonic day) producing the Purkinje cells. They penetrate through the layer of the earlier nuclear cells and gradually are ordered into a single surface-parallel layer of cells across the entire cerebellar cortex. The last generation of nerve cells— the Golgi cells of the cerebellar granular layer—departs from the basic morphogenetic pattern of laminated brain structures in not penetrating through the Purkinje cell layer but settling below the Purkinje cell layer (figure 9.4).

On day 17 in the rat, a radical change in the morphogenesis of the cerebellar cortex occurs with the development of a great multitude of neuroblasts in the lateral part of the dorsal rhombic lip. By dividing very rapidly, this cell mass moves in the dorsomedial direction and soon overflows the entire external surface of the cerebellum, very much like the icing on a cake. In this way, an external granular layer (EGL) develops and covers the entire early primordium of the cerebellar cortex. By rapid cell divisions in the outer surface, the EGL will give rise to an exceedingly large number of cerebellar cortical nerve cells, of both excitatory and inhibitory nature, moving in reverse direction (i.e., inward toward the

depth of the cerebellar cortex) and yielding the vast majority of the nerve cells in the later EGL (described in some detail later and illustrated in figure 9.5).

One of the greatest mysteries of the cerebellum is the very curious fact that the cerebellum contains at least half the nerve cell population of the entire body in higher mammals and at least five times as much as other parts of the nervous system in humans. (We do not have any reliable data on this curious ratio in whales, but it may be even more "absurd" than in humans.) This is all the more curious because, as we see in the later description of the numerical and geometrical analysis of cerebellar circuitry, the granule cells of the cerebellar cortex (i.e., the cells that contribute to this immense number) are embedded into the neuron network of the cerebellar cortex with a huge degree of redundancy (i.e., approximately 2,000 granule cells and Purkinje cells in the cat and probably four times as many in humans). Our later analysis of cerebellar function (secs. 9.3 and 9.4) offer the hypothesis that the granule cells provide a combinatorial richness of context crucial for subtleties of motor coordination and adaptation.

In regard to phylogeny, another, more ventral contingent of alar lamina cells, those lying ventral to the rhombic lip of the unfolded medullary tube, begin to proliferate and move ventrocaudally outside the cell mass of the abasal lamina but inside the original marginal zone of the original tube. These cells contribute to two large masses of cells in the rhombencephalon: a caudal group forming the inferior olive (IO) and a cranial group forming the pontine nuclei. Hence, it should be realized that both large cell formations of the rhombencephalon that are the main origins of immediate input into the cerebellum are themselves derivative of the alar lamina of the medullary tube and not, as it might appear, of the basal lamina.

The migration of the cells rapidly proliferating in the EGL of the cerebellar primordium is illustrated in four steps in figure 9.5. As seen in part A of the figure, the outgrowth of axons begins in the deepest layer of EGL by the transformation of some cells into spindle shape by sending out two axons in opposite directions that begin to make synaptic "contacts of passage" with the first (lowest) dendritic spines of the Purkinje cell dendrite arborization. These are the prospective granule neurons that are of excitatory nature, their transmitter being glutamate. At approximately the same time, the later basket neurons begin to issue axons that soon are attached to the "necks" of the Purkinje cell dendritic tree. We do not know when the separation of the prospective granule cells and the inhibitory (GABAergic) basket cells (BCs) is

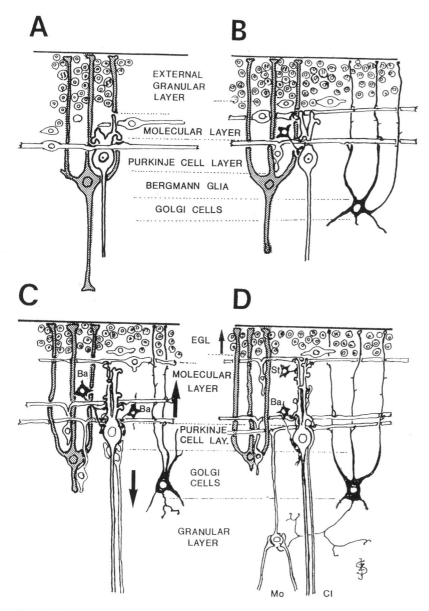

Figure 9.5

Schematic drawing of the transformation of the external granular layer into the molecular layer, giving rise to most cells of the granular layer. Radiate Bergmann glia cells are shown stippled; inhibitory interneurons are indicated in full black. Ba, basket cells, St, stellate cells. Purkinje cells, although inhibitory, are illustrated in outlines. Cell layers are indicated by dashed horizontal lines. Coarse arrows indicate the direction of growth (or reduction) of the several layers. (A) The earliest stage when the first (deepest) cells of the granule cells are transformed into spindle shape and grow out their horizontal processes, which will become the parallel fibers. The first synapses are established with the first (lowest) dendritic spines of Purkinje cells. (B) A somewhat later stage in which the lowest (deepest) granule cell has taken up its characteristic T-shape and is beginning to climb downward along the upper processes of the Bergmann glia cell. Meanwhile, the first Ba has formed and makes its primary synapses with the upper part of the Purkinje cell bodies. The next upper generation of granule cells and parallel fibers are formed and synapse with the next synapses of the growing Purkinje

cell dendrites. A Golgi cell at extreme right penetrates the external granular layer (EGL) as far as the pial surface and establishes synapses with the early parallel fibers. (C) A subsequent stage of tissue development with two granule cells climbing downward along the lower process of the Bergman glia cell. Two Bas already have been formed, and the Purkinje cell dendrites have grown upward to establish synapses with successively higher primary granule neurons (parallel fibers). A climbing fiber arriving from below synapses with the lower part of the Purkinje cell body. (D) Gradually, the EGL is exhausted, and the first stellate cells (St) are formed. Meanwhile, the translocation of the Ba axons toward the lower part of the Purkinje cell bodies and toward the initial axon segment has occurred, and the climbing fiber (Cl) has begun its ascent along the dendritic tree of the Purkinje cells. In the granular layer, the first generation of granule cells already has met two ingrowing mossy fibers (Mo), and the first synapses with the Golgi cell axons are established. (Diagram developed after the studies of P. Rakic 1971.)

determined. However, from recent observations in the developing cerebral cortex (Rakic 1988), we know that this separation may occur simultaneously with (or slightly before) the last division of the EGL cells. We may assume that the "single-layer" character of the germinative zone is not strictly kept up in the EGL for two reasons: because the entire EGL may be considered as a translocated germinative zone of the original medullary tube epithelium and because mitoses do occur in most vertebrates (especially in humans) well after birth (or hatching) and mitoses are found not exclusively in the outermost cell strata.

As seen in figure 9.5B, the next step is a gradual transformation of the early granule cells into a T by downward movement of the perikarya. This type of morphogenetic movement is not unique to the cerebellar cortex, because exactly the same process occurs in the transformation of primary sensory (spinal and cerebral nerve sensory) ganglia, wherein the process of pseudo-unipolarization of the cell bodies is a similar process. The cell bodies of the granule cells attach themselves to the ascending branches of the Bergmann glia cells (as clarified by Rakic 1971).

At this stage, one of the most mysterious histogenetic processes begins, a unique feature in the brain: The granule cell axons are oriented strictly in parallel with the axes of the later cerebellar folia. Though the consequences of this rigid, almost crystalline, order in orientation are treated at some length in later sections, we still are in absolute darkness about its possible causes. One might speculate about some specific spatial (geometrical) constraint forcing two elements to grow exclusively at right angles, but it is difficult to imagine that such a constraint could act at larger distances. However, because growing Purkinje cell dendritic trees are found all over the emerging molecular layer, the rectangular growth constraint has to be present equally in every piece of the molecular layer. Though there is a large class of dynamic models for explaining the ontogenetic formation (and even plasticity) of ordered structure of the cerebral cortex (sec. 8.2), now we do not have models of a self-organizing mechanism of the formation of the cerebellar lattice. However, the primary factor has to be the orientation of the primordial granule cell axons that subsequently become the parallel fibers, with the transverse orientation of the Purkinje cell dendritic arborizations being secondary. This is obvious simply from the fact that Purkinje cell dendrites never penetrate the EGL before the parallel fibers are formed. There is good experimental evidence for this fact from agranular cerebella, caused either by X-irradiation of newborn rats

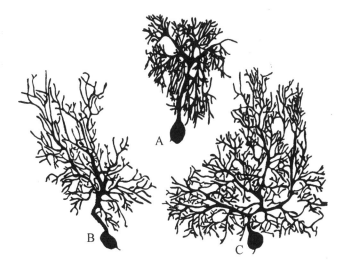

Figure 9.6
Weeping-willow type of Purkinje cell after x-irradiation of the newborn cerebellum has wiped out all but the earliest granule cells wherein parallel fibers already had established their synapses with the lowest dendrites of Purkinje cells. The further upward growth of the Purkinje dendritic tree was arrested. (Reprinted with permission from Bradley and Berry 1976.)

and kittens (Bradley and Berry 1976; Shofer, Pappas, and Purpura 1964), of intrauterine viral infection of fetuses in various stages of their development, and of strains with genetic defects. In all these cases, the deepest stratum of parallel fibers establishes synapses with the lowest dendritic branches of the Purkinje cells. However, if the EGL then is wiped out by experimental interference (or by some genetic disorder), the upper part of the Purkinje cell dendritic tree is blocked from further development. Eventually, the Purkinje cells look like weeping willows (figure 9.6; Bradley and Berry 1976), "as if they were searching for synaptic input from the earliest parallel fibers." We use this provocative phrasing deliberately to show how our logic may run into the *post hoc ergo propter hoc* fallacy.

A related issue is the spatial discreteness of the Purkinje cells (i.e., their noninterpenetration to each other's arborization spaces). In principle, there would be two different ways to achieve this goal, and we have good examples for the two mechanisms in several parts of the CNS. One extreme solution would be to restrict the growth of dendrites in the preferred direction, as occurs in the cerebellum, wherein the outgrowth of dendritic branches proceeds as the parent cells of the later granule cells are transformed into the parallel fibers (see figure 9.5). The other (opposite) mechanism would be to let the dendrites grow out freely in all directions and cut them back by a pruning process, thus establishing individual arborization spaces for each cell.

Interestingly, the Golgi cell dendrites do not care about the EGL, their bodies being situated less regularly but still completely filling the entire space available while confined to discrete space compartments. Their dendrites grow out to the external pial cover (see Eccles, Ito, and Szentágothai 1967; figure 15D). Their dendritic trees are not restricted to the transversal plane of the later folia. Emerging relatively late, both BCs and stellate cells are oriented, both with their axons and dendrites, with preference in the transversal plane of the folia (see figure 9.5D). However, one has the feeling that the spatial constraints are caused by the Purkinje cell dendritic trees and are (as it were) "forced" on the BC and stellate cell arborizations.

The spatial arrangement of neurons is one of the most fascinating aspects of neurogenesis. Spatial interpenetration versus discrete arborization spaces are the two extremes of a continuum. This problem has been discussed at some length in the forerunner of the present volume (Szentágothai and Arbib 1974) mainly on the basis of a subdivision of neuronal arborization types by Ramón-Molinar and Nauta (1966) into isodendritic (radiate), allodendritic (tufted), and idiodendritic (recurving) dendrite patterns. Bodian (1952) and Szentágothai (1953) have proposed related observations as a basis for various categorizations of the several neuron types. However, this is a major problem of neural organization of its own, to which we can only allude in this book.

The further histogenesis of the cerebellar cortex is illustrated in parts C and D of figure 9.5. As in parts A and B, the progressive outward differentiation of the EGL cells continues well into the postnatal life of most mammals (and probably also in other vertebrates). However, in talking of postnatal life, a relation between "fetal maturity" and competence for movement ought to be confronted systematically with the developmental states of the cerebellar cortex in those mammals born as miniature quasi-adults (e.g., the guinea pig) versus those born as helpless semimature fetuses (e.g., in most rodents). As one logically might expect, human proliferation in the EGL and differentiation into neurons continues well into the second year of life. Figure 9.5D shows the translocation of the BC synapses toward the axonal pole of the Purkinje cells and the climbing of the climbing fibers along the major dendrites of the Purkinje cells. Figure 9.7 (from Szentágothai 1983) shows the later transformation and maturation of the granule cells in the complex glomerular synapses by mutual spatial adjustment of the participating constituents. This figure might serve also as an illustration of neural tissue growth that is interstitial and not appositional, as in the initial stages of laminated

structure development (i.e., by some kind of "free-market type" space economy under conditions of both supply and demand).

9.2 Structural Organization of the Cerebellar Cortex and Nuclei

9.2.1 Structure and Space Economy of the Cerebellar Cortex

Having learned something of its ontogeny, we now look in some quantitative detail at the amazing quasi-crystalline structure of the cerebellar cortex. The admirable economy in the use of available tissue space became especially evident when the arrangement of Purkinje cells was analyzed by suitable methods of stereology (Palkovits, Magyar, and Szentágothai 1971a). One single possible mode of arrangement satisfied the rigid geometrical requirements and rules that could be deduced from the quantitative histological studies. It is seen in plan view, as if looked at from the surface (figure 9.8)—that is, as if it were assumed that the Purkinje cell bodies were arranged in parallel rows, deviating from the transverse axis of the folium by 11 degrees (of course, in an ideal case and for a flat piece of the folium). Evidently this picture is idealized highly and is distorted according to the curvature of the folium, whether it is a convexity at the top of the folium or a concavity in the depth of the furrows between neighboring folia. The transformation going hand in hand with surface curvature has been described and illustrated (see Eccles, Ito, and Szentágothai 1967, figure 2). Occurring in all laminated nervous tissue formations, these transformations are not irrelevant for theoretical considerations, especially (as with Purkinje cells) if conductions of spikes along the dendrites come into the picture, so that the dendritic arborization pattern and the distances between the branching points become important elements with which to calculate (see sec. 9.2.4). Both the Purkinje cells and the Golgi cells are confined to quasi-discrete spaces of cerebellar cortex tissue, both in the molecular and in the granular layer and both for axons and for dendrites. This has been discussed at some length in the quantitative histological studies of Palkovits, Magyar, and Szentágothai (1971b). In an idealized case, the space and numerical arrangement of the Golgi cells (Go : P = 1 : 3), with their dendritic and axonal arborizations, would occupy hexagonal tissue compartments resembling the pattern of beeswax honeycombs (figures 8, 9 in Palkovits et al. 1971b). However, certain irregularities do exist in reality, includ-

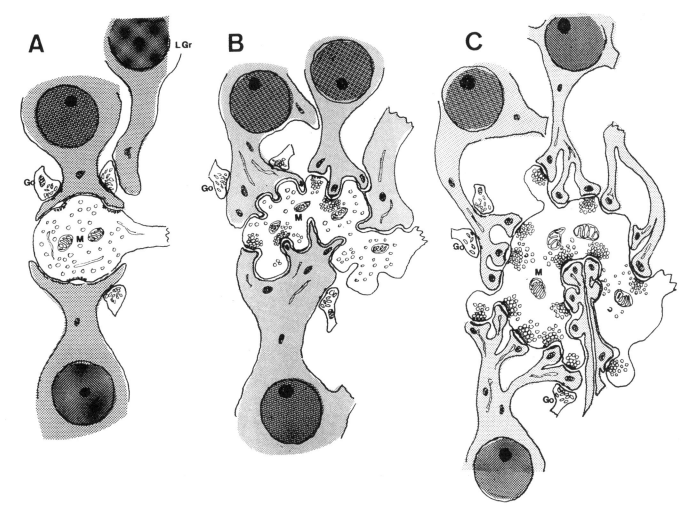

Figure 9.7
Three successive stages of cerebellar glomerulus development. (A) The mossy fiber terminal has been engulfed by two calyciform processes of two early granule cells (stippled), but the first synapses of Golgi cell axons (Go) already are present. A later granule cell (L Gr) "gropes" its way toward the glomerulus. (B) A somewhat later stage of development with four granule cells shown in surface contact with the mossy fiber terminal that now assumes a sinusoid shape. (C) The granule cell dendrites have developed their dendrites and the synaptic digits. The Go terminals were continuously present but were translocated to "downstream" parts of the granule cell dendrites. (Modified after Szentágothai 1983.)

ing Golgi cells that do not have dendrites reaching the molecular layer.

The quantitative parameters of cells and axons in the molecular layer have been studied at considerable length by Palkovits, Magyar, and Szentágothai (1971c), the main results being that the BC–Purkinje cell ratio would be 6:1, and that the stellate cell–Purkinje cell ratio would be 16:1 (in the cat), much larger than hitherto had been assumed. Conversely, the number of Purkinje baskets in which the average basket axon would participate was found to be much lower than expected (8–7), but the two results would compensate for each other; thus, earlier assumptions on the territorial expansions of BC inhibition (Eccles, Ito, and Szentágothai 1967) do not

need to be reconsidered radically. The parallel fibers traversing the dendritic arbors of many Purkinje cells appear to give one synapse to every fifth Purkinje cell (Palkovits, Magyar, and Szentágothai 1971c). However, it appears from studies in progress that the synapses given by any parallel fiber are distributed very unevenly along the course of the axon; there are more synapses given close to the T-shaped bifurcation of the parallel axons and far fewer in their distal courses. However, the conclusion reached in the quantitative studies—that the average length of the parallel fibers is 2 mm in the cat (Palkovits, Magyar, and Szentágothai 1971c)—was subject to question later on the basis of results of degeneration experiments in the vermis (Brand, Dahl, and

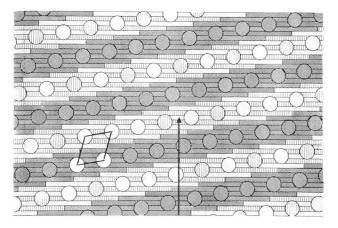

Figure 9.8
An idealized arrangement of Purkinje cells according to Palkovits et al. (1971a) in a flat piece of the cerebellar cortex surface in plane view (as if seen from above). Purkinje cells are represented by circles and their dendritic trees are designated by horizontal bars (hatching tries to show which belongs to which). The rhombic shape at left indicates the statistical average of cell body–to–cell body distance as established empirically. The long arrow indicates the axis of the folium. Purkinje cell rows ideally would deviate by 11 degrees from the transverse folium axis.

Mugnaini 1976; Mugnaini, 1983). According to the degeneration studies, many parallel fibers had a length of 5–6 mm. This disagreement could be explained partially by the fact that the total length of many folia in the cat is less than 2 mm. In fact, this revised view—that parallel fibers are much longer than were previously thought—will play an important role in our later theorizing about the role of cerebellum in motor coordination.

9.2.2 Cerebellar Circuitry

One "goal" achieved by the curious arrangement of the Purkinje dendritic trees is to secure maximum divergence and convergence in a very highly redundant system: the mossy fiber → granule cell → parallel fiber → Purkinje cell chain. Characterized by an enormous divergence, the mossy fiber input exerts both excitatory actions and (via interneurons) inhibitory actions on Purkinje cells. The mossy fibers activate granule cells wherein axons rise up into the layer of Purkinje cell dendrites (which are flat, with the planes of all their dendritic trees parallel to one another) to form Ts. Their cross-bars run parallel to one another at right angles to the planes of the Purkinje dendritic trees. Some 200,000 parallel fibers run through a single Purkinje tree in humans, with perhaps 1 in 5 synapsing as they pass through. The mossy fibers also synapse on Golgi cells, and the parallel fibers (granule T-bars) also synapse on BCs and stellate cells. BCs project a dense array of inhibitory synapses on the bodies of the Purkinje cells. Golgi cells control mossy fiber to granule cell synapses. There would be little point in this arrangement if it were not for the other input system, the climbing fibers, in which locally a strict one-to-one ratio between the input and the output lines is guaranteed. However, an axon leaving the IO will branch to provide a number of Purkinje cells, each with their own private climbing fiber. Physiologically, each arriving climbing fiber impulse generally elicits a short series of discharges in its target Purkinje cell (Eccles, Ito, and Szentágothai 1967): the *climbing fiber response*. The number of discharges can be reduced but not completely blocked by the state of readiness of the Purkinje cells, depending on the integrated excitatory-inhibitory influences exercised on it by the parallel fiber excitatory and interneuron inhibitory input. Hence, the climbing fiber input could be considered as the "readout of the changing readiness of each Purkinje cell." In keeping with the approximate firing periodicities of the olivary cell ensemble (Bell and Kawasaki 1972), climbing fiber input occurs approximately two to four times per second "at rest" and perhaps twice as much when "signaling." Controversy continues as to whether the complex climbing fiber spike is the "secret" of the climbing fiber or whether the silent period lasts as much as 100 msec after the complex spike (Murphy and Sabah 1970). In any case, this real-time view of the role of the climbing fiber signal is to be contrasted with the role suggested by modeling and confirmed by experimentation in providing a "training signal" for adjusting the efficacy of parallel fiber → Purkinje cell synapses. Thach (1968) recorded Purkinje cell activity in monkey during alternating wrist movements. Mossy fiber–induced spikes are in phase with alternations, but climbing fiber responses had no correlation with the movement. Though the models in sections 9.3 and 9.4 emphasize the training signal role of the climbing fibers, future models must integrate this role with the real-time effects of climbing fiber activity.

9.2.3 Cerebellar Nuclei

Because of the beautiful quasi-crystalline structure of the cerebellar cortex, relatively little attention has been paid to the cerebellar nuclei, although it has been known since classical times that virtually the entire output of the cerebellar cortex is conveyed to the rest of the CNS via the cerebellar nuclei, the one exception being that the axons of the Purkinje cells belonging to the so-called "vestibulocerebellum" (mainly, but not exclusively, the flocullomodular lobe) terminate in one of the vestibular nuclei, the Deiters nucleus. The gross topographical organization of the efferent cerebellar systems and the organization's basically sagittally oriented nature were discussed first by Jansen and Brodal (1940, 1942; see also 1954). The preliminary data on synaptology given in Eccles, Ito, and Szentágothai (1967) clearly were inadequate for a real understanding of the position of the cerebellar nuclei within the whole ensemble of the cerebellar system. A major change in attitude resulted from three different sources:

In his studies of VOR. Ito (1970; 1972a, b; 1974; 1982) assumed that the cerebellum, mainly the flocculus, would provide the necessary feedforward correction in a side-path, adding a corrective term to the noncerebellar pathway (see sec. 9.3.3).

Eccles (1973a) developed elegant ideas on how the cerebellar hemispheres, deprived of direct input about things happening in the spinal mechanisms, achieve access to information about the evolving movement from cortical motor centers via the pontine, olivary, and lateral reticular nuclei. By some kind of learning process this ability would contribute to the high sophistication of limb and body movements in general.

Ablation experiments (especially observations about restoration of movement) show that there was a radical difference between whether the lesion was restricted to the cerebellar cortex or whether the nuclei also were affected. This finding also was known earlier from human pathology.

The studies of Victoria Chan-Palay (1977) on the lateral (dentate) cerebellar nucleus showed that whatever was known in the classical period (mainly Ramón y Cajal's studies) and in the postclassical period (prior to the 1967 monograph of Eccles et al.) was barely more than the raw skeleton of the real connectivity of the cerebellar system. Although in showing cerebellar corticonuclear (and reverse) neuronal connections figure 9.9 uses some of the information given by the Chan-Palay study, the figure still remains a highly selective diagram of the basic neuron circuit. A detailed inquiry by Palkovits et al. (1977) into the synaptology of the cerebellar nuclei in the cat yielded data on an average divergence of Purkinje axons on 35 nuclear cells; convergence is much higher, with more than 800 Purkinje cell axons giving synapses to the average nuclear cell. Four different kinds of synapses could be identified: Purkinje axon terminals, mossy or climbing afferent terminals, nuclear recurrent axon terminals (partially excitatory), and local GABAergic interneuron terminals (Hamori and Mezey 1977).

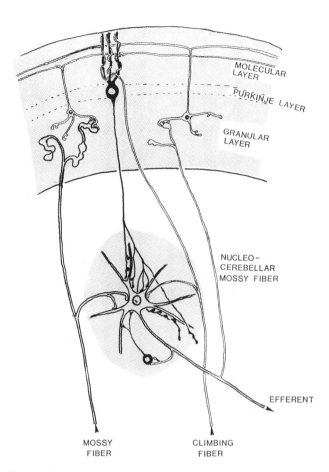

Figure 9.9

The principal connection between cerebellar cortex (above) and cerebellar nuclei (middle) stripped down to the bare minimum. Inhibitory neurons and their processes are shown in full black, and excitatory elements are shown in outline. Arrowheads indicate the direction of conducted impulses (where this is not obvious). Note the inhibitory intrinsic interneuron that in reality is not self-inhibitory, as indicated here for the sake of simplicity. Both mossy fibers and climbing fibers send collaterals to the nuclei en route to the cerebellar cortex, and nuclear cells themselves send collaterals to cortex.

9.2.4 Modeling the Cerebellar Purkinje Cell

Our look at the detailed modeling of the Purkinje cell uses detailed compartmental modeling of the kind presented in sections 5.2 and 6.2. The availability of new data regarding the types, kinetics, and distribution of voltage-dependent channels, the increase of computer power, and software tool kits made it possible to formulate and test a detailed multicompartmental Hodgkin-Huxley–type model of the Purkinje cell (De Schutter and Bower 1994a, b). The main intention of this modeling effort was to simulate under realistic assumptions the cell response to current injection (i.e., the fundamental spiking modes and plateau potentials) and the effects of excitatory and inhibitory synapses. Because of the lack of sufficient available data, the numerical values of some parameters (e.g., channel densities expressed as maximum conductance) had to be estimated. Those values were chosen for which the simulations gave the best fit to physiological measurements. The models of cerebellar function in sections 9.3 and 9.4 use simpler, single-compartmental models, but we include the present detailed modeling of the Purkinje cell to point the way to future multilevel modeling that relates system behavior to the fine details of neuronal function.

On the basis of earlier measurements, 10 different ion channels have been incorporated into the model: a fast and a persistent sodium current, a low-threshold and high-threshold calcium current, an anomalous and a delayed rectifier, an A-type and a noninactivating potassium current, and a low-threshold and a high-threshold calcium activated potassium current. The channel densities are considered as free parameters of the model and the distribution of channels and the decay constant of the calcium concentration also were tuned to simulate biologically realistic behavior. The main source of the experimental data concerning the intracellular response properties to current injections came from in vitro studies (Llinás and Sugimori 1980a, b). Basically, the ionic channels were distributed over three zones: sodium channels in the soma, fast potassium channels in the soma and the main dendrite, and calcium channels and calcium-activated potassium channels in the entire dendrite.

Simulation studies contributed to an understanding of the mechanism of the generation of the two types of spike generation (somatic and dendritic). Fast somatic spikes, which are responses to small current injections, are generated by sodium channels and is repolarized by the delayed rectifier. Increasing the amplitude of current injections increases the frequency of sodium spikes until large dendritic calcium spikes are generated. The generation of this spike is caused by the high-threshold calcium channel and is repolarized by one of the calcium-dependent potassium channels. In addition to spiking behavior, a plateau potential also occurs in both the dendrite and soma. By and large, the somatic plateau potential was caused by sodium currents, whereas the dendritic plateau potential was generated by calcium channels.

The robustness of the model has been tested by (1) varying morphological data, (2) adding channel blockers, and (3) varying channel densities. The model showed high sensitivity mostly for the changes of those conductances that are involved in spike generation and repolarization. They are the high-threshold calcium cur-

rents and the two types of calcium-activated potassium current. The model was shown to be rather robust to changes in channel densities. Consequently, initial assumptions on channel distributions were "approved" by the simulations whenever they were within a reasonable range.

The effect of different excitatory and inhibitory synapses on a cerebellar Purkinje cell were studied by extending the Hodgkin-Huxley-type model of the membrane to include proper synaptic currents. In particular, excitatory inputs from climbing fibers and granule cells and inhibitory inputs from intrinsic neurons (the stellate cells and BCs) were taken into account. Currents mediated by these synaptic channels have to be added to the model. Describing the synaptic effects required the specification of the locations, the pharmacology and kinetics, the conductance, and the specializations and the activation of synapses. In particular, the excitatory inputs are mediated by α-methyl proprionic acid (AMPA) receptors, with glutamate released by granule cell synapses also activating metabotropic receptors on Purkinje cell dendrites, whereas inhibition is assumed to be mediated by GABA receptors. The maximum synaptic conductances provided the free parameters to tune the model to reproduce physiologically recorded responses. In the presence of inhibition due to stellate cells, dendritic calcium spikes are suppressed, and only somatic action potentials are generated. Simulation results led the authors to suggest cautiously that stellate cells may have a special role in controlling the firing patterns of the Purkinje cell.

Though the bottom-up model is sufficiently detailed to reproduce the nature of the complex dendritic calcium spike and the dual reversal potential (both as responses for climbing fiber inputs), other important features (e.g., the LTD of the parallel fiber synapses; see sec. 6.3.5) admittedly are outside the scope of the present version of the model. Even with this simplification, the simulation of a single Purkinje cell as a very detailed compartmental model with realistic ion conductances and synaptic currents in each compartment takes massive computing resources. Our strategy in developing system models of the cerebellum (secs. 9.3 and 9.4) thus is drastically different, using rather simple models of individual neurons but then modeling very large numbers of neurons. In our view, even the most optimistic advances in computing resources will not make simulation of realistically large networks practicable if each cell is modeled in immense detail. Rather, we see the detailed modeling of single neurons and small networks as necessary to validate the selection of key properties to be included in the models of

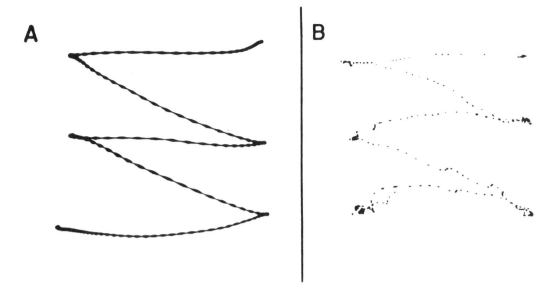

Figure 9.10
(A) Normal and (B) dysmetric movements of a hand in which ipsilateral cerebellum is normal (A) and destroyed by gunshot wounds (B). (Modified after Holmes 1939.)

individual neurons when the contribution of these neurons to large-scale neural systems is under investigation.

9.3 The Cerebellum as a Learning Machine

With this background, we address the mystery of the cerebellum: What is the real concept (or purpose, if one might say so) of such a structure? Our ideas regarding the role of the cerebellum have been shaped by clinical data about movement abnormality in patients with cerebellar lesions (Plaitakis 1992). A classic example is that of Holmes (1939): A subject can form smooth alternating movements with the hand on the side of the body with a normal cerebellum, whereas on the side with cerebellar lesions, the hand movements are dysmetric (i.e., inaccurate and jerky; figure 9.10). This suggests that in concert with the basal ganglia, the neocortex is capable of strategic planning of movement (see chaps. 8 and 10), that the spinal cord has "algorithms" for reflex control of posture and for locomotion, and that the cerebellum plays a role in refining and extending the basic motor repertoire. Though the usual caveats about lesion experiments must be borne in mind, it does seem reasonable to suggest that the cerebellum helps the predictive computation required to start decelerating in time for the smooth reversal of motion at the endpoints of the trajectory (figure 9.10). The Holmes experiment shows the loss of smooth transition from one phase of a sequence of voluntary movement to another (decomposition of movement) that results from cerebellar impairment.[1] Thus, the hypothesis is that in, say, playing the piano, the learning of the sequence of notes involves neocortex and basal ganglia but that the smooth skillful running off of the notes, including coordination of the two hands and of the fingers on each hand, requires cerebellar learning to "tune" the other systems (as in the Holmes experiment). Sections 9.3 and 9.4 explore a number of variations on this theme of the cerebellum as a learning machine.

9.3.1 The Marr-Albus Model: Purkinje Cell as Perceptron

The first explicit model of the function of cerebellar circuitry, and a very attractive one from the viewpoint of its aesthetic appeal, was formulated by Braitenberg and Onesto (1961) by considering the cerebellar cortex network as a timing device for the starting and stopping of rapid ballistic-type movements. The basic mechanism involved the slow propagation of a signal down the length of a parallel fiber from an initial position to a target Purkinje cell "labeled" by the activating influence of a

---

1. Note that this is *not* to claim that cerebellar damage is the direct cause of this decomposition. Rather, we claim that in finding that loss of cerebellum impairs the ability to coordinate diverse movements, a cerebellar patient learns that one movement at a time is a good strategy to reduce gross errors in behavior.

climbing fiber. The time required could be read out to time a movement. Unfortunately, the model required far slower propagation of signals on parallel fibers than was later measured, and ascribed an excitatory role to Purkinje cells.

The old timing hypothesis in its original form ... had to be abandoned. What is left is the idea that the cerebellar cortex reacts specifically to sequences of input signals when they are presented along a folium or "beam" in the right tempo (Braitenberg and Preissl 1992).

In fact, the most influential model of the cerebellar cortex viewed it as a learning machine. This is the model we describe.

Using the anatomical and physiological information provided by the 1967 monograph of Eccles, Ito, and Szentágothai, Marr (1969) proposed a model of learning and associative memory in which each of the five neuron types found in the cerebellar cortex played a role. In this model, each Purkinje cell acts as a perceptron (i.e., a simple learning device) whose output encodes an "elemental movement." The climbing fiber input to a Purkinje cell both triggers the elemental movement of the cell and (the key idea of Marr's theory) acts as a teacher to enable it to learn which sensorimotor patterns conveyed by mossy and parallel fibers are appropriate to trigger its elemental movement. Marr suggested that the climbing fiber input serves to increase the strength of simultaneously active parallel fiber → Purkinje cell synapses. Independently, Albus (1971) developed a similar theory but hypothesized that parallel fiber synapses should be *decreased* rather than increased because this would increase the activity of cells in the cerebellar nucleus inhibited by the Purkinje cell. Due to the fact that a given parallel fiber does not contact all the Purkinje cells through which it passes, and because synapses may vary in efficacy, neighboring Purkinje cells in the longitudinal direction of the folium are not stimulated necessarily in similar situations.

As noted in section 6.3.5, when signals reach a Purkinje cell through climbing fibers and parallel fibers in approximate synchrony, LTD results (Ito 1989). Synaptic transmission from parallel fibers is depressed, and this depression lasts a long time. This supports the Albus version of the Marr-Albus hypothesis regarding synaptic plasticity (see also Gilbert and Thach 1977; Ito and Kano 1982; Ito 1984). With LTD incorporated, the cerebellar cortical network can be conceived as a distributed, adaptive parallel processing computer (Marr 1969; Albus 1971) or as an adaptive filter (Fujita 1982a, b). The notion of eligibility (sec. 6.3.5) is discussed in section 9.4.4 as a solution to the following problem: If parallel fibers are continually active and a climbing fiber "error signal" depends on the result of earlier parallel fiber activity, how does LTD affect only the "relevant" synapses?

To repeat the essential points, a signal on the climbing fiber input to a Purkinje cell causes an update to active parallel fiber synapses on that Purkinje cell. The parallel fiber inputs to the Purkinje cell act as a context for the particular movement. The term *codon* denotes the subset of mossy fibers that encode an event. Having learned the context via synaptic weakening on temporal correlations between climbing fiber and parallel fiber (which translates into increased activity in the nuclear cells that now receive less Purkinje inhibition), the Purkinje cell is "turned on" by the "context" from the parallel fibers—mossy fibers. According to this model, the lack of climbing fiber input in an adult animal should not create any performance deficits *after learning has occurred* (i.e., after patterns of parallel fiber input have been trained to disinhibit elemental movements whenever appropriate). This does not appear to be the case. Lesion of the olive (the source of the climbing fibers) can result in the abolition of the cerebellar coordination function (Murphy and O'Leary 1971).

Marr (1969) further argued that the granule cells decorrelate input patterns arriving along the mossy fibers, consequently increasing the efficiency of the associative memory linking mossy fiber patterns to elemental movements. In this codon model, the activities of granule and Purkinje cells are controlled by Golgi cells and by BCs and stellate cells, respectively (see the use of such ideas in modeling the hippocampus, sec. 6.4.6). Cowan (1995) points out that in a frame of nonlocal representation for enhanced reliability, the Marr codon is related to fundamental issues in coding theory. Reliability of computation in this system comes from redundancy in function encoding, from computing functions by computing approximations (or portions) of the function over a subset of the actual inputs, and from using random subsets of inputs.

9.3.2 From Cerebellar Cortex to Cerebellar System: Microcomplexes

The Marr-Albus theory focuses on the cerebellar cortex and associates each Purkinje cell with an elemental movement. However, the cerebellar cortex is part of a cerebellar system, and the cerebellar system interacts with MPGs elsewhere. We are thus interested in studies that take account of Marr-Albus learning mechanisms in a broader motor system context.

The spinal input to the cerebellar cortex is carried by approximately 20 different paths. However, only two paths—the dorsal spinocerebellar tract and the cuneocerebellar tract—provide mossy fiber inputs that carry signals from the body about peripheral events. These projections are arranged topographically in relation to adjacent body parts. Other mossy fiber and climbing fiber inputs carry signals from auditory and visual systems to the cerebellum. Interestingly, exteroreceptive inputs favor the top of the folia, with the proprioceptive mossy fiber inputs favoring the deeper part of the sulci. It would appear that foliation is not just a way of fitting a large cortical sheet into the skull. The sagittal climbing fiber zones and the transverse mossy fiber bands subdivide the cerebellar cortex into an orthogonal lattice. Oscarsson (1973) showed that mossy fibers carry primarily information about the state of lower motor centers (efferents) but also carry some information from the sensors. Voogd (1969) reported that the cerebellum shows a sagittal compartmentalization (see Murphy, MacKay, and Johnson 1973a; Armstrong, Harvey, and Schild 1973a,b). Each compartment projects to restricted regions in the cerebellar nuclei. The compartments are sagittal strips (parallel to midline), so the compartments are bridged by parallel fibers. Voogd's delimitation of the sagittal cerebellar corticonuclear projection describes the cortex in its flexor-extensor influence (as the muscular effects from the cerebellar nuclei are known). Oscarsson's 1969 maps of climbing fiber zones divide the same cortex into hindlimb and forelimb regions. The projection of climbing fibers to cerebellar cortex also is organized in sagittal strips. It is not known whether the strips and compartments are the same, but the Boylls model described later *assumes* identity.

A small area of the cerebellar cortex called a *microzone* receives climbing fibers from a small group of IO neurons and, in turn, sends Purkinje cell axons to a small group of vestibular or cerebellar nuclear neurons. Other signals from precerebellar nuclei in the brainstem and spinal cord flow through vestibular or cerebellar nuclei but also reach the microzone via mossy fibers. Thus, the major signal flow through nuclear neurons is modulated by inhibitory output signals of the cerebellar microzone. We stress that the cerebellar cortex and nuclei form an integrated system, and we view this system as divided into small structural and functional units inserted into various extracerebellar systems. Figure 9.11 reproduces one of these units named a *cerebellar corticonuclear microcomplex* (Ito 1984). A microcomplex is composed of a cerebellar microzone and a small number of nuclear cells

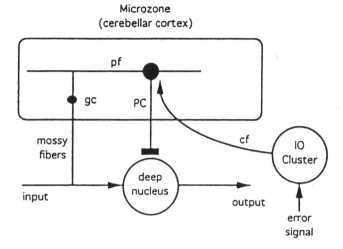

Microzone
(cerebellar cortex)

Figure 9.11
A corticonuclear microcomplex, the structural-functional unit of the cerebellum, involving a patch of cerebellar cortex and the patch of cerebellar nucleus to which its Purkinje cells project. cf, climbing fiber; PC, Purkinje cell; gc, granule cell; IO, inferior olive.

and (to simplify) receives two kinds of input, mossy fibers and climbing fibers, the output being carried by the deep nuclear cells. Both mossy fibers and climbing fibers supply collaterals to the nuclear cell group and pass to the corresponding microzone of cerebellar cortex. The set of mossy fiber inputs is transformed by the granule cells whose axons form the parallel fibers. Later, we study various hypotheses on how synaptic plasticity can turn such a microcomplex into a component of a learning machine.

The parallel fibers are long enough to provide synapses across many microzones (Mugnaini 1983). In the models to be developed later, we hypothesize that the set of parallel fibers crossing a given microzone constitutes a general context for the present sensorimotor actions in the form of a large set of signals providing information about the state of activity of various structures, from the higher to the sensory level. The granule cells ensure that the parallel fibers each carry some combination of activity on several mossy fibers rather than simply relaying their activity. On the strength of this discussion, we note several crucial facts and hypotheses.

First, the only output cells of a microzone are Purkinje cells. As Purkinje cells have inhibitory action on nuclear cells (while collaterals of mossy fibers excite the nuclear cells), the signal flow from the nuclear cells is modulated by the microzone action.

Second, most of the modeling and experimentation studies described later considered the climbing fibers to encode control errors in the operation of the system in which a given corticonuclear microcomplex is involved (see Ito 1990 for a review). In this view, climbing fibers convey signals encoding errors in the performance of the system in which a given microcomplex is installed. However, the Boylls model shows the possible importance of real-time effects of climbing fibers, posing a dichotomy that currently is contentious and awaits its proper resolution in further research. (See Bloedel and Bracha 1995 for a review of much pertinent information.)

Third, climbing fiber signals induce LTD of synaptic strength in those parallel fiber → Purkinje cell synapses that were coactivated with the climbing fiber (within a certain time window). Signal transfer characteristics of the microzone and (accordingly) dynamic characteristics of the corticonuclear microcomplex will be modified toward minimization of control errors.

In section 9.4.4, we see how this general mode of cerebellar learning can be applied to model conditioning of simple reflexes and in adaptation both of the saccadic system and of throwing to wearing prisms. Our later discussion provides a new perspective on the phrase "the system in which a given corticonuclear microcomplex is involved," for we shall see that many microcomplexes may be involved in assisting a "focal" microcomplex to achieve its goal; consider the coactivation of arm and posture required to bring the hand to grasp a target successfully.

9.3.3 Adaptation of the Vestibulo-Ocular Reflex

By generating compensatory eye movement, the VOR stabilizes the retinal image during movement of the head. The VOR is able to adapt to both natural changes (cell loss, disease, and aging) and artificial changes (e.g., induced by prisms) of the visual field (Robinson 1972, 1975, 1981). Ito based his notion of the microcomplex on a study of the adaptation of the VOR. Experimental support for this model was given by experimental results from the rabbit, some lesion experiments performed on the cat, and some inconclusive data regarding the monkey. Correlated stimulation of vestibular nerve and IO depresses the early excitation of Purkinje cells by the vestibular nerve. This is not the case if the vestibular nerve is not involved in the correlated stimulation.

The gain of the VOR can change when vestibulovisual interactions are modified by, say, prisms or magnifying lenses, but this accommodation can be abolished by ablation of the flocculus or of the dorsal cap of the inferior olive. In rabbit flocculus, responsiveness of Purkinje cells to vestibular mossy inputs changes in parallel with the VOR adaptation. Debate continues over the

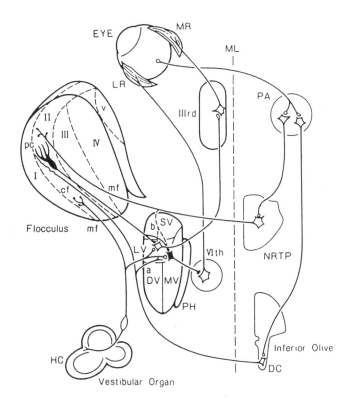

Figure 9.12
The vestibulo-ocular reflex pathway is connected to a part of the cerebellum called the *flocculus*, exactly in the manner of a corticonuclear microcomplex. LR, lateral rectus; MR, medial rectus; ML mid-line; NRTP, nucleus reticularis tagmenti pontis; DC dorsal cap; HC, horizontal canal; DV, LV, MV, SV, dorsal, lateral, medial, and superior parts of vermis; mf, mossy fiber; pc, Purkinje cell. (From Ito 1982. Reproduced with permission from the Annual Review of Neuroscience, Vol. 5, © 1982, by Annual Reviews Inc.)

precise location of the plasticity. Ito (1982) argues that it is the cerebellar cortex, more precisely the parallel fiber → Purkinje cell synapses, whereas, on the basis of monkey data, Du Lac et al. (1995) argue that plasticity must occur in both cerebellar cortex and the relevant (here the vestibular) nucleus. The Fujita (1982a,b) adaptive filter model of the cerebellar role in the adaptive VOR is in accordance with Ito's approach.

The VOR is controlled by the flocculus. Vestibular inputs come via mossy fibers and visual inputs via climbing fibers. These visual inputs reflect the instruction nature of the climbing fiber input of the Marr-Albus model. The VOR pathway is connected to the flocculus (vestibulocerebellum), exactly in the manner of a corticonuclear microcomplex (figure 9.12; sec. 9.3.2). Ito argues that the normal feedforward path from the vestibular organs to the motoneurons is modulated by the inhibitory influence of the Purkinje cells using the flocculus as a gain control mechanism. If VOR compensation for head movement is inadequate, an indication of the retinal error will be forwarded to the flocculus through climbing fiber afferents and will there modify signal transfer characteristics across the flocculus through induction of LTD; thus, dynamics of the VOR will be improved toward minimizing retinal errors (Ito 1982). VOR adaptation can be induced by introducing artificial retinal errors. Floccular Purkinje cells are involved in monitoring eye movements rather than in recognizing patterns. Floccular stimulation represses oculomotor response to vestibular stimulation. Each eye muscle receives both excitatory and inhibitory vestibular input, but only one of each of these two inputs is under floccular control, so the flocculus is not fighting itself. Caudocranial slippage indicates excessive floccular inhibition; craniocaudal slippage implies the reverse. If climbing fibers adjust the inhibition, to which slippage do they respond? One view is that if caudocranially moving visual stimuli excite floccular climbing fibers, then there is a long-term depressive influence of mossy fiber input on Purkinje cell inhibition. The slow mossy fiber signal appears to be timed to coincide with the output of the Purkinje cells stimulated by the fast mossy fiber signal initiated at the same time.

9.3.4 A Cerebellar Circuit for Conditioning

The involvement of the cerebellum in classical conditioning has been shown by studies of many types of movement, including limb flexion, neck turns, and facial movements as well as rabbit eyelid and (nictitating membrane) conditioning (Gormezano, Kehoe, and Marshall 1983) on which we focus here (see Bartha and Thompson 1995 for a review of basic data and models). For the rabbit eyeblink task, the *conditioning stimulus* (CS) usually is a tone or light, and the *unconditioned stimulus* (US) usually is a corneal air puff or shock. The US evokes a defensive blink reflex or *unconditioned response* (UR) that includes both eyelid closure and nictitating membrane (third eyelid) extension. The CS does not evoke a blink initially but, after repeated pairings of the CS followed by the US, rabbits eventually learn to blink in response to the CS, and this is called the *conditioned response* (CR).

A key variable of the experiments is the interstimulus interval (ISI), defined as the time between the CS onset and the US onset, whereas other parameters are the intensity, duration, number, and type of stimuli. The optimal ISI is approximately 200–400 msec. As in conditioning experiments in general, the efficacy of the CR depends on the number of trials. After 200 trials, the CS

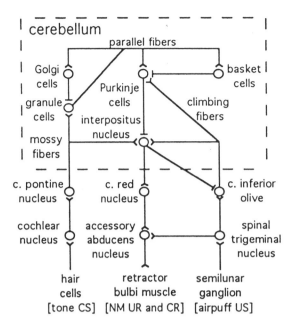

Figure 9.13
Neural network for conditioning of the nictitating membrane (NM) response. The unconditioned stimulus–unconditioned response (US–UR) pathway (i.e., the pathway that mediates the reflex "blink" in response to an air puff) consists of the semilunar ganglion, spinal trigeminal nucleus, and accessory abducens nucleus; the accessory abducens nucleus contains retractor bulbi motoneurons controlling the rectractor bulbi muscle to yield retraction of the eyeball and consequent extrusion of the nictitating membrane. The conditioned stimulus–conditioned response (CS–CR) pathway (i.e., the pathway wherein adaptation comes to yield a "blink" in response to a conditioning auditory tone) consists of auditory hair cells, cochlear nucleus, pontine nucleus, cerebellum, red nucleus, and again the accessory abducens nucleus. The reinforcing pathway begins with US information in the spinal trigeminal nucleus and consists of the inferior olive and its projections to the cerebellum. The interpositus nucleus provides inhibitory feedback to the inferior olive. Angled synapses are excitatory, straight synapses are inhibitory. c, contralateral. (Reprinted with permission from Bartha and Thompson 1995.)

may yield the CR on more than 90% of the subsequent trials.

In Search of the Basic Circuitry

In determining which brain structures are responsible and which mechanisms of plasticity are involved, extensive anatomical, lesion, and physiological studies led Thompson (1986) to propose the brain circuit shown in figure 9.13 as being essential for classical conditioning of the nictitating membrane response. The CS is carried along mossy fibers via the pontine nuclei to the cerebellum. Originating from the IO, the climbing fibers convey the US. This is considered to be the reinforcement pathway but, to unify it with other studies in this chapter, we may consider it instead as an error signal:

"You did not blink in time to avoid the aversive stimulus." The site of the conditioned response resides in the Purkinje cell modulation of the interpositus nucleus. The efferent pathway from the interpositus has two different collaterals: First, there is an inhibitory pathway to modulate US activation by inhibition; second, CR information is projected back into the cerebellar cortex through granule cells (see figure 9.9). Note that this pathway is not included in the basic microcomplex model of figure 9.11, providing another target for refinement of models based on this construct in section 9.4. Note also that the US and CS information must have pathways that bring them together for associative learning of the CR to occur. Further note that the US elicits the UR and provides the error-reinforcement signal by using distinct pathways. An important feature missing in other models discussed in this chapter is that the interpositus provides inhibitory feedback to the IO that increases during the course of learning; this process is consistent with the view that the IO represents an error signal.

For blink and related forms of conditioning, the neural substrates shown in the figure constrain what can be learned. Interestingly, the hippocampus appears to be important for long ISI trace conditioning; when there is a delay of 500 msec or more between CS and US, the hippocampus seems to be required to maintain a "trace" of the CS until the US is available. By contrast, the hippocampus is not required for delay conditioning, i.e., when the delay between CS and US is short. The data also strongly suggest that the cerebellum is the primary site of plasticity, although the respective contributions of the cortex and deep nuclei are not known. Thompson (1990) concluded that "evidence to date demonstrates that the cerebellum is absolutely necessary for both learning and memory in classical conditioning eyeblink" and more emphatically "essential memory traces are in fact formed and stored in the cerebellum." (See Blum et al. 1993 for a related network simulation using compartmental models). However, Bloedel (1992) has argued that conditioning also may occur in the absence of cerebellar cortex.

One of the more interesting features of classical conditioning of the rabbit nictitating membrane is that of the well-timed response. Over the course of training, the timing of the response to the CS (tone) becomes more precise. In the earlier phases of training, the CR occurs at long latencies. Over the course of training, the onset of the CR moves forward in time. Eventually, in the later stages of training, the peak of the CR coincides exactly with that of the US (air puff).

Modeling the Role of Cerebellum in Classical Conditioning

The Albus model (sec. 9.3.1) stated explicitly that climbing fiber spikes are the US and mossy fiber activity patterns are the CS for Purkinje cell conditioning. This view is supported by eyelid-conditioning studies. However, this model does not account for CR phenomena, such as rate of acquisition, optimal ISI, and CR timing. Conditioning behavior has been simulated by applying the Rescorla-Wagner rule (1972; Donegan and Wagner 1987; Moore and Blazis 1989):

$$\Delta w_i = \alpha_i (\lambda - \sum w_i x_i)$$

where any w_i is a CS associative weight, α_i are CS-dependent learning rate parameters, λ indicates the presence of the US, and x_i are CS activities. The Rescorla-Wagner rule is a special case of the least–mean squares error-correction rule (Widrow and Hoff 1960; see Widrow and Lehr 1995 for a recent review of its use in the artificial neural network community). Like the perceptron rule adopted by Marr and Albus, this is a supervised rule as distinct from the unsupervised learning rules emphasized in section 4.5. The underlying biophysical and cellular mechanisms are to be sought in such mechanisms as the LTD reviewed in section 6.3.

Moore, Desmond, and Berthier (1989) derived a neural network model from mapping functional considerations onto the cerebellum. Each CS stimulus trace was represented internally as a spectrum of time delays by using a tapped delay line. Stimulus traces are activated by both CS onsets and offsets and make contact via modifiable connections with so-called V- and E-units (Purkinje cells and Golgi cells, respectively); both units can learn with conjoint parallel and climbing fiber activity. The CS also generates a "CR image," a short-latency increase to a plateau of activity that lasts as long as the US. The Purkinje cell is the output element, and the Golgi cell acts to gate learning in the V-unit near the expected time of the US. The delay-line structures are not specified, but delays occur before the parallel fiber outputs. The Golgi cell gates the association of the CR image with the Purkinje cell. The authors suggest that the CR image is learned in the brainstem in parallel with learning in the cerebellar cortex and that release of interpositus nucleus inhibition by Purkinje cells is responsible for generation of CRs.

Purkinje and Golgi cell plasticity combined with the model's tapped delay lines yields anticipatory CRs for delay and trace conditioning at all ISIs. CRs initially develop near the US onset, begin earlier in trial over the course of training, and peak near the US onset as observed experimentally. The model also reproduces discrete shifts in CR timing and double-peaked CRs with mixed ISI training. The learning rules follow the form of Rescorla-Wagner's model (1972) and thus account for some of the same stimulus context effects (e.g., blocking and conditioned inhibition). As noted earlier, experimental evidence suggests that the hippocampus is required for long ISI trace conditioning but, unfortunately, this model accounts equally well for delay and trace conditioning without including a model of the hippocampus. Finally, the proposed delay lines must be more than 1 second long, and no physiologically plausible mechanism has been suggested for this (see the earlier critique of the classic Braitenberg model in the introduction to sec. 9.3.1).

Gluck et al. (1996) provided a simple "connectionist" model that aggregates the cerebellar cortex and interpositus nucleus into a single node, the inputs to this node being filtered through a system of higher-order combinations corresponding to the mossy fiber → parallel fiber transformation effected by the multitude of granule cells. As for Moore et al.'s (1989) model, the main approach of this model was to take an algorithm of conditioning and map its computations onto the cerebellum. The mapping included negative feedback from cerebellum to IO and a recurrent cerebellar connection. Cerebellar output was identified with the CR. It was assumed that Purkinje cell dendrites transform CS input and CR information from the recurrent connections into a higher-order CS * CR input. Negative feedback to the IO implemented the subtractive term $(\lambda - \sum w_i x_i)$ in Rescorla-Wagner's formula. This allowed plasticity for the lumped cerebellum node to follow a hebbian rule conjoining cerebellar inputs and IO activity. The model qualitatively accounted for cerebellar output after delay conditioning for a short range of ISIs. Peak CRs occur near US onset, but this does not account for output pathway delays. Consistent with behavioral data, CRs are broader for longer ISIs, but the delay in CR onset does not increase at longer ISIs, as it should. The model accounted for extinction and reacquisition that is faster than initial acquisition, but reacquisition was slower than that in rabbits. The model also accounted for blocking and conditioned inhibition but was unable to account for trace conditioning or even long ISI delay conditioning. In accord with lesion data, Gluck et al. assumed that the hippocampus is required for long ISI trace conditioning but that this is not the case for shorter ISIs. Because the CR is driven by the CS, removal of the CS quickly ter-

minates the CR, a result inconsistent with experiment. Early in training, the model appeared to produce CRs that peak too early in the trial and only later peak near the US.

Bartha (1992) developed a realistic network simulation of the cerebellum and associated circuitry responsible for the acquisition of the nictitating membrane response. He stressed the importance of neural input and output representations by using neural recordings to constrain mossy fiber input and by studies of a detailed CR pathway and oculomotor plant model to constrain cerebellar output. The oculomotor plant model showed that the relation between neural firing and movement of the nictitating membrane can be highly nonlinear (Bartha and Thompson 1992). The cerebellar cortex model consisted of a Purkinje cell, Golgi cell, 200 granule cells, 50 mossy fiber inputs, and 10 BC inputs. The divergence and convergence of the connections were scaled in proportion to the level of scaling of the neural populations. Neural activity was modeled as spike trains by using conductance-based, single-compartment neuron models. Two populations of granule cells—one responsive to the tone CS and one unresponsive—existed within this model. The granule cells changed their synapses with the Purkinje cell, which generated the CR by disinhibiting the interpositus.

With the support of early experimental work (Eccles, Ito, and Szentágothai 1967), Bartha's primary hypothesis was that Golgi cells inhibit granule cells for periods of tens to hundreds of milliseconds. Purkinje cell LTD can decrease selectively the synaptic weights from granule cells that are active around the time of the US. In this way, Purkinje cells can learn to reduce their firing near the time of the US and thus release inhibition on interpositus cells that in turn may drive the CR. Tone-responsive mossy fibers synapse with a Golgi cell and a population of tone-responsive granule cells. The Golgi cell inhibits both the tone-responsive and the unresponsive granule cells. Bartha hypothesized that during learning, the tone-unresponsive parallel fiber → Purkinje cell synapses active during the US are decreased, whereas synapses that have been inhibited by the Golgi cell for the proper time period are left alone. (The model itself only simulates the untrained and naive responses and does not include a learning rule.) The Golgi cell's inhibitory influence on the tone-unresponsive granule cells is to produce a variety of firing patterns in which the granule cells display differing periods of depression. The Purkinje cell then selects the granule cells that display the proper time interval of depression to produce a properly timed eyeblink.

9.4 Cerebellar Adaptation of Movement Generation

The Marr-Albus theory emphasizes the turning on or off of elemental movements. The studies of classical conditioning address the pairing of a new stimulus with a response but also bring in the study of the timing of the response. In this section, we study cases in which the cerebellum has been implicated in adaptation of the metrics of movement to changing circumstances (as in the VOR studies of sec. 9.3.3). For a controller, the appropriate choice of control signal that will move the controlled system into ever greater conformity with a given plan depends on having a reasonably accurate model of the controlled system (e.g., the appropriate thrust to apply must depend on an estimate of the mass of the object that is to be moved). Because the controlled system may change over time, it is useful to provide an "identification" algorithm that can update a parametric description of the controlled system; in that way, the observed response of the system to its control signals comes into greater and greater conformity with that projected on the basis of the parametric description (Narendra 1995). When (i) a controller is equipped with an identification algorithm, (ii) the controlled system is of the class whose parameters the algorithm is designed to identify, and (iii) the changes in parameters of the controlled system are not too rapid, then the combination of controller and identification algorithm provides an adaptive control system able to function effectively despite continual changes in the environment.

The Boylls model (sec. 9.4.1) shows how the detailed circuitry of the cerebellar cortex and of various nuclei with which it interacts could serve as an identification algorithm to tune the parameters of various motor control systems on a short-term basis (i.e., one appropriate to the current circumstances). The remaining subsections review three approaches to modeling adaptation of motor control wherein the adaptation takes far longer than, say, adjusting to step height in a flight of stairs and wherein the adaptation persists on a long-term basis. First, we review Kawato's model of feedback-error learning (sec. 9.4.2) as a process whereby the cerebellum takes over motor control from other parts of the brain, but we argue that the cerebellum works by modulating and coordinating multiple MPGs. Though the Boylls model used the control of reverberating loops to set motor parameters in the short term, the later models emphasize the role of synaptic plasticity in acquiring long-term changes in such plasticity. Interestingly, both features

are combined in a model by Houk and Barto of the role of cerebellar plasticity in adaptive pattern generators (sec. 9.4.3). Our current models (sec. 9.4.4) build on Ito's study of the VOR, viewing the cerebellar microcomplex as the unit of cerebellar adaptation; its role is to modify the parameters of MPGs existing elsewhere in the brain. These models also depend on the important notion of a window of eligibility, which suggests basic constraints on the timing relation between the parallel fiber context and the climbing fiber training signal.

9.4.1 The Cerebellum as a Setter of Motor Parameters

Sherrington (1910) viewed locomotion in the spinal cat as a coordinated series of flexion reflexes, but the view of Graham Brown (1911, 1914) that this is a programmed activity is substantiated by the finding that, injected with the dopamine precursor DOPA (to raise the tonus sufficiently), a spinal cat will locomote even if deafferented. Stepping is not as regular and precise as in the deafferented cat, but the overall pattern appears to be the same. Locomotion in a DOPA-injected spinal cat will proceed at some fixed rate even in the absence of a treadmill. However, if the cat is not deafferented, it can adjust its speed to that of a treadmill above which it is placed, with shift from trot to gallop when appropriate (see Lundberg 1969; Forssberg and Grillner 1973; Grillner and Zanger 1974). Without feedback, the spinal cat no longer can adjust the rate to that of the treadmill. In any case, the stepping of the spinal animal is underpowered grossly.

As a working example, we outline cerebellar function in locomotion of the higher decerebrate cat as described by Shik, Severin, and Orlovskii (1966a,b). As we have just seen, the locomotory MPG is available even in the spinal cat (see Székely's 1968 work on the segmental programming of stepping discussed in chapter 2). Shik et al. have described the supplementary role for the cerebellum in tuning the locomotor MPG. Driven principally by the cerebellum in the decerebrate cat, the red and Deiters nuclei are found to have activity modulated in accordance with contraction of flexors and extensors. However, this modulation is impressed on already substantial levels of background activity in both nuclei, which is present whether or not the associated musculature is active currently. It is as though nuclear contributions (and hence cerebellar influences) are directed or switched into the muscles only at appropriate times. The existence of similar switching phenomena (which appears to be a spinal process) were discussed long ago, relative to peripheral inputs to the spinal reflexes (Magnus's classic demonstration of *die Umkehr*) by Sherrington (1910). Deiters nucleus stimulation yields limb *extension* in the passive cat (a reasonable strategy because Deiters nucleus normally is activated by the vestibular system, and rigid extension of all limbs is the appropriate response to a nonspecific "falling over" message). We may tabulate the effects of stimulating various nuclei on the muscles of the static animal as follows:

Deiters $\xrightarrow{++}$ Extensors

Medial bulbar RF; rubrospinal and corticospinal tracts $\xrightarrow[-]{++}$ flexors; $\longrightarrow$ extensors

Ventral bulbar RF $\xrightarrow[-]{}$ flexors; $\xrightarrow[-]{}$ extensors

But how might these "strengthening pathways" be used by the spinal MPGs during locomotion? Orlovskii (1972b) has demonstrated that stimulation of either red or Deiters nucleus is effective in augmenting contraction of the related musculature only when that musculature is being employed actively. Indeed, red and Deiters nuclei do show maintained activity even when their related muscles are silent during locomotion (Orlovskii 1972a,b). In hip movement during walking, muscle activity is enhanced by stimulation of the appropriate nuclei only during its active phase in locomotion, and timing of the stepping is not affected with weak stimulation. Thus, in the high decerebrate cat, stimulation of Deiters nucleus during locomotion would not affect extension during the swing phase but would yield increased extension during the support phase. On this basis, Arbib, Boylls, and Dev (1974) posited that the climbing fibers specify the muscle groups involved and their covariances, whereas the mossy fibers carry metric information (see also Szentágothai and Arbib 1975). This is in contrast to the Marr-Albus family of models in which the climbing fibers play at most a secondary role in generating motor activity but do play the role of training signal as synergies evolve over time.

In summary, we have the following view of locomotion: (1) A spinal mechanism generates the stepping movements; (2) the cerebellum provides adjustment *within* this phasing by descending control; and (3) the spinal cord "pays attention" only during the extensor phase of the locomotion algorithm. This view clearly extends to many other forms of motor control and holds that the cerebellum modulates brainstem nuclei to compute "tuning parameters" "called" by MPGs at appropriate stages of execution.

Boylls (1975, 1978, 1980) provided a model of this style of motor control that also builds on Tsukahara's

1972 demonstration of the possibility of activity reverberating between the reticular and cerebellar nuclei following removal of Purkinje cell inhibition of activity in the nuclei. Brodal and Szikla (1972) and Brodal et al. (1972) demonstrated the anatomical substrate for such loops, suggesting that the cerebellofugal projection may display more topographical precision than does the reverberatory return in the projection between the interpositus and the nucleus reticularis tegmenti pontis. The model is built on spatiotemporally significant inhibition from the cerebellar cortex of "reverberatory" or positive feedback connections between the cerebellar nuclei and particular reticular nuclei that then provide parametric adjustment for the spinal schema.

Boylls developed a synergy controller model of cerebellum that creates synergically meaningful excitation profiles on a cerebellar nucleus via spatiotemporally significant inhibition from the cerebellar cortex. There is a sagittal orientation of cerebellar cortex inputs and outputs. Synergic agonists cocontract, and synergic antagonists corelax. The purpose of the cerebellar "computer" diagrammed in figure 9.14 is to create synergically meaningful excitation profiles on a cerebellar nucleus, which subsequently are transmitted via an output nucleus to spinal levels. The principal instrument of this pattern sculpting is spatiotemporally significant inhibition from the cerebellar cortex, but this, in turn, results from activity on climbing fibers from the IO and on both slow and fast mossy fiber paths. As we see in figure 9.14, loop activity also must reach the cerebellar cortex on slow mossy fibers, thereby creating a negative feedback check on an otherwise unstable situation. In accord with Tsukahara's 1972 data, simulation of this loop region involves the use of two populations of model neurons interconnected in space by reciprocal, quasi-topographical projections.

The model posits that the climbing fiber plays a real-time role rather than a training role. At first, climbing fiber input yields a relatively balanced effect on the cerebellar nucleus, as climbing fiber excitation is counteracted by the inhibitory climbing fiber response of the Purkinje cells. However, the firing of nuclear cells from Purkinje inhibition serves to release the reverberations between the reticular nucleus and the cerebellar nucleus. (Purkinje cells have a very high level of resting activity.) Boylls's simulation showed that once reverberation has started, only intermittent climbing fiber activation is required to block Purkinje inhibition sufficiently for reverberation to be maintained, just as gentle brake pressure will stop a stationary car from rolling but will have little effect once the car has gained momentum.

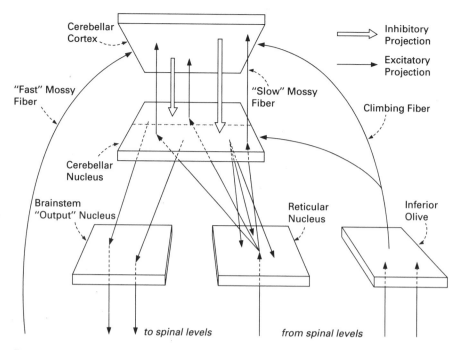

Figure 9.14

Components of cerebellar-related circuitry and their interconnections in the Boylls model of cerebellar function in mesencephalic locomotion. Activity in loops between verebellar and other nuclei encode "motor parameters" that tune the activity of motor pattern generators downstream. The value of these parameters is adjusted by inhibition from Purkinje cells in the cerebellar cortex. In this model, climbing fibers play a real-time role in adjusting Purkinje cell activity, rather than serving as "training signals" for synaptic plasticity. (Reprinted with permission from Arbib, Boylls, and Dev 1974.)

The Boylls model of the cerebellar cortex ignores the inhibitory interneurons, and simply studies granule and Purkinje cells and parallel, mossy, and climbing fibers, along with the related geometry. In figure 9.15, the cerebellopetal fibers of the reticular nucleus are shown continuing to the cerebellar cortex as slow mossy fibers after having made nuclear collateral synapses. Boylls treats the branching of the mossy fibers as if they were lying mostly in a sagittal plane but with a substantial mediolateral excursion. This proved qualitatively sufficient to establish the observations that follow. The crucial point is the spread of the parallel fibers, which provides a mechanism to spread the reverberatory excitation over a range of Purkinje cells. The reverberation is maintained at the center (figure 9.16), but the spread of Purkinje cell activation provides lateral inhibition for nearby regions. Thus, a key postulate of the Boylls model is that adjacent regions code antagonistic parameters. Thompson's (1990) data on activity during eyeblink-conditioned behavior are consistent with this. Purkinje neurons that appear directly involved in the eyeblink response show learning-induced decreases in simple spike activity in the CS period in trained animals. Many other Purkinje neurons show learning-induced in-

creases in activity in the CS period, possibly as a means of suppressing irrelevant responses.

Computer simulation demonstrated the control of a ballistic movement of a limb, with excitation local to the individual Purkinje cell and depression of activity around it. The physical analog of this behavior is that the excitation would relate to the agonist contraction and the depression would relate to the antagonist relaxation. Only a few of the more interesting results of the computer simulation of this cerebellum model can be given here. Climbing fiber inputs produce an initial collateral activation of the cerebellar nuclei followed by a brief, strong burst of Purkinje cell activity prior to the so-called inactivation response of Granit and Phillips (1965). The last is a silencing of the Purkinje cell for a highly variable length of time, depending on the preparation employed (e.g., see Murphy and Sabah, 1970; Murphy, MacKay, and Johnson 1973b). Etiology of the inactivation continues to be in dispute. Boylls's simulation employs a brief, 16-msec inactivation following a very strong Purkinje burst, with sagittal zone distribution of the affected cells (supposedly as would be produced by activation of a small region of the IO; Armstrong, Harvey, and Schild 1973a). When climbing fiber activity is

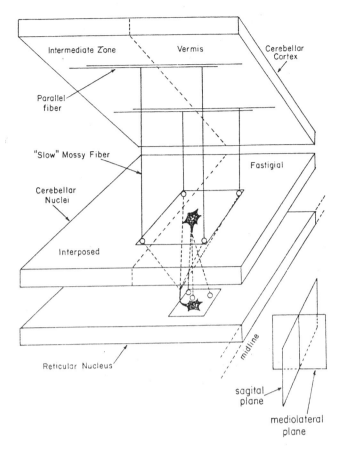

Figure 9.15
Template diagram illustrating the routing of reverberatory loop activity to a simplified cerebellar cortex via a subset of slow mossy fibers. These mossy fibers, collaterals of the "loop return" from reticular nucleus to interpositus, ascend to the cerebellar cortex via granule cells (not shown) to spread their activity via parallel fibers. We show neither the granular and Purkinje layers nor the actual spatial geometry of mossy fibers as they arrive at the cortex. (Reprinted with permission from Arbib, Boylls, and Dev 1974.)

provided at a rate well above its resting level, Purkinje cell activity is inhibited long enough to release loop activity (the cerebellar nuclear aftermath of which is shown in figure 9.16). Above the nucleus, a rolling surface indicates by its height the degree of excitation of nuclear cells. The central, sagittal "hill" is located at the homolog of the activated cortical strip and is flanked by two depressed regions. This hill was created when the Purkinje inactivation response released underlying nuclear cells from cortical inhibition. However, at the same time, the rebounding nuclear activity was amplified greatly through the reticulonuclear reverberation (positive feedback), which serves to maintain the hill and also is transmitted back to the cortex; there, it spreads mediolaterally along parallel fibers, activating more Purkinje cells and thus leading to simple lateral inhibition of the nuclear areas

adjacent to the hill. The persistence of this spatial excitation configuration is regulated partially by the ratio of positive to negative feedback gain in the system. In the simulation, the pattern (which otherwise fades) is "refreshed" by climbing fiber input approximately every 100 msec, though this may be somewhat too frequent, given the firing periodicities of the olivary cell ensemble (Bell and Kawasaki 1972). Spread of loop activity via parallel fibers yields a lateral inhibition effect.

What do such patterns mean? Boylls looked initially at the synergic interpretation (i.e., at the encoding implied by the pattern of figure 9.16). Regardless of specific cerebellar nuclear topography, if this pattern directly modulates the musculature, those muscles represented within the sagittal hill of excitation would tend to cocontract: They would be agonists of a synergy. On the contrary, muscles within the adjacent "valleys" simultaneously would corelax as synergic antagonists. In cerebellar cortical coordinates, one concludes that along any sagittal climbing fiber zone of the cortex, certain synergic agonists can be recruited by climbing fiber action, whereas along the mediolateral dimension, their antagonists are suppressed on either side of the zone. The data of section 9.3.2 lead us to suggest that Voogd (1969) and Oscarsson (1969) have mapped out the cortex in a way that allows some specification of the actual synergic linkages wrought in each region of cerebellar cortex. Voogd's delimiting of the sagittal cerebellar corticonuclear projection describes the cortex in its flexor-extensor influence (because the muscular effects from the cerebellar nuclei are known). Oscarsson's maps of climbing fiber zones divide the same cortex into hindlimb and forelimb regions. Consequently, applying the previous synergic formula to each cortical sector can define the flexor-extensor, hindlimb-forelimb synergic modulation possible there. Divisions of the IO similarly can be assigned synergic significance (specifically, agonist recruitment). More generally, the patterns transmitted to various brainstem motor nuclei are interpreted topographically as motor parameters for the MPGs resident there.

9.4.2 The Controversial Functions of Cerebellum

Do Climbing Fibers Teach?

Most of this chapter focuses on the role of the cerebellum in the acquisition and storage of learned-coordinated motor behaviors. Instead, Bloedel (1992, Bloedel, Bracha, and Larson 1993) argues that the cerebellum is not a plastic storage site but is involved in regulating the coordination of real-time motor activity (as in the Boylls model).

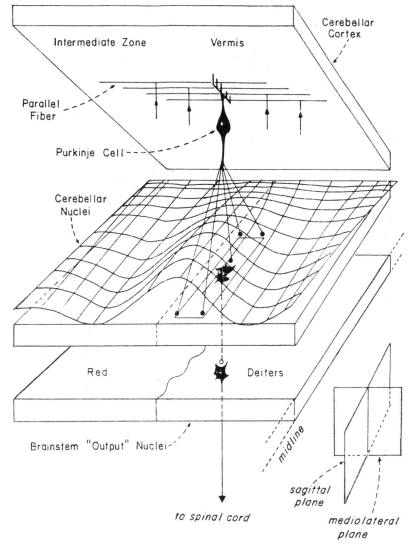

Figure 9.16
Spatial pattern of activity created in cerebellar nuclei by climbing fiber action along one saggital strip in Boylls's computer simulation. Height of the functional surface indicates the magnitude of excitation at each locus. The active climbing fiber strip was located in the cerebellar cortex above the central hill of excitation. This hill and the depressed val- leys flanking it persist for a considerable time beyond the initiating climbing fiber bursts. Such patterns are transmitted to various brainstem motor nuclei, where they are interpreted topographically as "motor parameters" for the motor pattern generators resident there. (Reprinted with permission from Arbib, Boylls, and Dev 1974.)

In one study (Ebner and Bloedel 1984), parallel fibers to some Purkinje cells were excited or inhibited either randomly with respect to the occurrence of the cells' climbing fiber input or at specific time intervals following the occurrence. Simple-spike responsiveness of Purkinje cells was found to be enhanced for a brief period following the activation of their own climbing fiber input, this enhancement occuring for excitatory as well as inhibitory response components. It is not at all clear how to reconcile this finding with the "inactivation response" described as part of the experimental basis for the Boylls model: a silencing of the Purkinje cell for a highly vari- able period following climbing fiber input. Activity of sagittally aligned Purkinje cells also was recorded during unperturbed and perturbed movements in cats. Synchronous activation of climbing fiber inputs (indicated by occurrence of complex spikes) and associated enhancement of simple-spike modulation consistently were observed during perturbed movements.

Ebner and Bloedel (1984) formulated the *gain change hypothesis* as a descriptive framework for characterizing the enhanced activity in the Purkinje cells. According to this hypothesis, when activated within a critical period prior to the arrival of other synaptic inputs to Purkinje cells, the climbing fibers are capable of inducing an enhanced responsiveness or an increased gain in the neuron's response to its other synaptic inputs. Bloedel et al. (1993) argue that the olivocerebellar system is involved in on-line, real-time processing rather than in processes restricted to the establishment of memory traces in the cerebellum, as proposed by the LTD hypothesis. However, there is no reason to adopt an either-or position here, though how these two roles for climbing fiber signals might be combined poses challenges for both modeling and experimentation.

Another study adopted the paradigm used by Thompson (1990) (sec. 9.3.4): standard paired-trial delay conditioning using a tone as the CS and an air puff as US, but this time applied to a decerebrate, decerebellate rabbit. The animal still could be conditioned. The same conditioning task was applied to an intact rabbit with microinjection of lidocaine into specific brainstem nuclei (pars oralis of the spinal trigeminal nucleus) after conditioning. The injection caused substantial reduction of conditioned responses for a short period. Examination of the activity in that brainstem region during acquisition of the conditioned behavior revealed cell activity correlated with CRs or URs. On the basis of these results, Bloedel et al. (1993) concluded that cerebellum is not a storage site for plasticity. Instead, cerebellum ablation disrupted a critical action of cerebellar output projections on brainstem nuclei required for establishing plasticity; it is a performance deficit rather than a memory or learning deficit. However, again the claim seems stronger than necessary. The evidence certainly calls into question a view of the cerebellum as the one and only site for plasticity in this type of conditioning but does not exclude the claim that cerebellum may work cooperatively with other regions to enhance learning.

The Cerebellum as a Timing Organ

As mentioned earlier, Braitenberg and Onesto (1961) considered the cerebellar cortical network as a timing device. Keele and Ivry (1991) argued that timing is a general computation that can be used by a variety of tasks and that cerebellum is the neural structure that implements this clock. They argued that in this way, the cerebellum plays the prominent role in motor control because most coordinated actions require fine timing. More strongly, their argument seems to be that the cerebellum provides a *common* internal clock. In one study, human subjects were asked to produce extensive series of timed taps using a forefinger or a foot. Each trial began with the presentation of a series of computer tones,

separated by isochronous intervals. By pressing a response key, the subject attempted to synchronize his or her responses with the tone. After a series of paced responses, the tones ceased and the subject's task was to continue tapping at the target rate until producing 30 unpaced intertap intervals. Accuracy with the finger correlated with accuracy of the foot with a coefficient of approximately 0.6. Subjects also were asked to perform a timing perception task, comparing the intervals between tone pairs and stating which interval was longer. Temporal acuity on the perception task correlated with a coefficient of approximately 0.5 with the standard deviation of timing on the timed tapping task.

However, do these studies imply a common system computing time across different motor effectors and across diverse tasks? In learning the general skill of tapping, repetitive movements of each motor system will have been learned in conjunction with rhythmical auditory stimuli. Successful learning of the tasks thus should yield correlations in performance irrespective of whether common neural circuitry is involved in their control.

Diener et al. (1993) and Keele and Ivry (1991) used studies on neurological patients to demonstrate that the cerebellum is the candidate neural structure for temporal computation. Timed tapping tasks were given to patients with lesions in premotor cortical areas, patients with Parkinson's disease, and patients with cerebellar lesions. The result showed that patients with cortical and cerebellar lesions were impaired on the task, whereas Parkinson's disease patients performed comparably to the control subjects. The patients also were asked to perform the time perception task. In this case, only the patients with cerebellar lesions were impaired. Taken together, the impaired performance of the cerebellar patients on both tasks was understood to provide evidence that the cerebellum can be considered an internal clock.

Is a timing mechanism separable from the motor system as the source of increased variance in timing in the cerebellar patients, or is motor implementation itself the source? A solution to this problem was proposed by Wing and Kristofferson (1973), who assumed that the clock process is not dependent on receipt of feedback from each response but operates independently of the response outcome. (By contrast, the Boylls model assumed that in repetitive operations, the performance on early repetitions can adjust the parameter settings for later repetitions.) When this method was applied to the data from the cerebellar and cortical patients, the decomposition showed that clock and motor components both were affected in both patient groups. To explain why the cerebellar patients show impairment on both clock and implementation components, Ivry, Keele, and Diener (1988) offered the hypothesis that the lateral cerebellar regions are responsible for the clock component of timing, whereas the medial regions are part of the implementation system. (See the Smith Predictor, another example of invocation of different roles to be implemented in control of the same task, sec. 9.4.3.) On the basis of this hypothesis, widespread cerebellar damage may cause both clock and motor damage because both systems may be involved. Indeed, Ivry et al. (1988) showed data that support this fact. On the other hand, to explain why cortical patients show no deficit in the perceptual timing test but appear to show both a clock and an implementation deficit on the tapping task, Ivry et al. suggested that selection of the appropriate effector and the goal of the action might be expected to involve such cortical structures as portions of parietal cortex and motor cortex. For them, it is not until these various computations are assembled that a response can be released for final implementation, which takes place via descending commands, some of which involve medial regions of the cerebellum. Simultaneously, with release of a response, the next cycle can begin to prepare the next response, including the circuit through the cerebellum to provide the temporal computation.

However, timing does not require a clock in the conventional sense of a device that has a regular beat and can be used to measure off the length of time intervals. Unfortunately, the very method used by Keele and Ivry (1991) applied a data analysis method (Wing and Kristofferson 1973) that assumed, rather than tested, the notion of an internal clock and, moreover, assumed that the clock is unaffected by motor feedback. For example, a dynamic system (such as a tapping effector) may have an intrinsic period of oscillation; the device that controls its rate of oscillation thus may act by adjusting dynamic parameters rather than by making use of explicit clock signals. Consider a leaky integrator with a special threshold function that gives zero output unless the membrane potential reaches the input value, then immediately drops the membrane potential back to zero, and has an adjustable time constant. Certainly the notion of time exists in this simple system, and the temporal behavior of the system can be controlled explicitly by the adjustment, but it is not a clock in the common sense. By extending this thinking to motor systems, we can see that it is possible to control a system's temporal behavior (e.g., response time, settling time) by adjusting its parameters, but we would not call the motor system a timing device.

Additionally, if damage is done to a motor system, the timing behavior obviously is affected.

In summary, Keele and Ivry (1991) have drawn our attention to important timing phenomena that involve the cerebellum. However, they have not proved that the cerebellum is an internal clock. Moreover, because their work rests exclusively on behavior and lesion studies, much remains to be done to establish the role of cerebellar circuitry in the phenomena that they have reported.

The Cerebellum as a Sensory Organ

Paulin (1993) has been one of those who challenged the view of the prime function of cerebellum as motor control and coordination. He marshaled a variety of evidence in different species to argue that the structure is involved directly in certain sensory tasks and that the cerebellum's function is to track and predict states of dynamical systems. He offered two main lines of evidence: (1) the presence of a cerebellarlike structure related to some sensing capability in certain species and (2) the presence of an expanded cerebellar cortex that seems to be associated with species with a certain specialty in sensation and perception. Paulin (1993) also gave some evidence that cerebellar dysfunction can cause perceptual deficits.

Paulin viewed the cerebellum as a sensory processor whose correct operation is essential for motor control. According to Paulin (1989), the cerebellum is necessary for tracking movements, and its function is similar to that of a Kalman filter, a device for tracking and predicting states of dynamical systems (Kalman and Bucy 1961). However, in arguing for this similarity, Paulin was not arguing that cerebellar cortex is an implementation of Kalman and Bucy's mathematics. Rather, his idea was that when dynamics vary rapidly during movements, the cerebellar cortex would alter time constants in the underlying loops by altering loop gains or by shunting loop activity. Indeed, Paulin cited the work by Tsukahara (1972) that underlies the Boylls model (and the Houk-Barto model described later) that showed that when the cerebellar cortex is poisoned with picrotoxin, electric shocks delivered to the red nucleus cause an explosive buildup in the red nucleus, the interpositus nucleus loop, showing that time constants in this loop normally are controlled by cerebellar cortical inhibition of the interpositus.

Thus, for Paulin, it was plausible to assume that the long time constants required for the Kalman filter dynamics actually are being constructed in loops between cerebellar nuclei, reticular nuclei, and the red nucleus and that the function of the cerebellar cortex is to vary filter dynamics during filtering operations so as to optimize the accuracy of filter output. Paulin conjectured that the IO can act as a bias detector, triggering corrections to filtering dynamics when significant errors are detected. The correcting signal also would be a performance signal, telling the cerebellar cortex that it has chosen the wrong dynamics for the current task. Then an adaptive Kalman filter could be constructed by computing a measure of temporal correlation or bias in the innovations and applying a reinforcement learning rule.

In line with the filtering theme, Nelson and Paulin (1995) modeled the dorsal cochlear nucleus. Studies in weakly electric teleosts (Bell et al. 1993) and elasmobranchs (Montgomery and Bodznick 1994) show that the major function of this area is to strip self-movement-related noise and distortions from incoming signals. This finding is in accordance with the findings of Schwartz (1987) that demonstrated that tapping the paw of the cat resulted in IO activity, whereas the stimulation of that same site as a result of normal locomotion did not elicit this response. This suggests also that the cerebellum is a location that contains an internal model of the system and therefore can filter out expected peripheral feedback as not important to learning. Nelson and Paulin (1995) modeled the dorsal cochlear nucleus as a system that nulls reafference in two ways: by common mode (a signal common over all of the sensory afferents is subtracted from the sensory signal) and by adaptive filtering (efference copy of the motor commands is correlated with the sensory input, and any correlated signal is removed). Through these mechanisms, the adaptive filter becomes habituated to periodic sensory signals that persist over time.

A different argument implicating the cerebellum in sensory acquisition and discrimination comes from Gao et al. (1996), supporting the theory proposed in Bower and Kassel (1990). The experimenters had human subjects undergo functional magnetic resonance imaging (fMRI), and measured activity in the cerebellum during each of four tasks:

1. The subjects' hands were restrained and passive while experimenters rubbed one of four different grits of sandpaper across their fingertips for 3 seconds each.

2. The procedure was the same as in item 1, but the subjects were instructed to think about which hand was being stimulated by the rougher sandpaper.

3. The subjects held their hands inside tightly woven socks, each one with four wooden-ball stimuli inside.

The four wooden balls were differentiated by their number of extra flat sides. The subjects were instructed to pick up with a precision pinch a pair of balls, raise them, drop them, and start again.

4. The subjects did the same thing as in item 3, but they were instructed to determine whether the balls were the same and, if they were, to drop both; if they were not, they were to drop one and pick up another.

Gao et al. (1996) focused on activity primarily in the dentate nucleus, the primary output for the cerebellar hemispheres (lateral cerebellum). The magnitudes of stimulation in the dentate nucleus were ordered: 3 < 1 < 2 < 4. They emphasized that activity of the dentate nucleus was correlated with those aforementioned tasks 2 and 4 requiring sensory acquisition. There was almost no activation of the dentate nucleus during task 3. The authors argued that therefore, cerebellar regions primarily are involved in "coordinating the acquisition of tactile sensory information." However, one might argue that task 4 is a task in which a far more complex series of movements is required than there is in task 3 and that this is why the cerebellum is involved so heavily.

In summary, Paulin (1993) and Bower and Kassel (1990) argued that the existence of cerebellar projections to motor regions of the CNS does not imply that cerebellar function is restricted to some aspect of motor control but only that the cerebellum performs some computation useful for motor control. This theory does not seem inconsistent with models developed later in this chapter, in which the cerebellum learns part of the inverse model of the motor system and sends compensatory signals to the appropriate MPGs. Because the compensation depends crucially on sensory signals (as well as on proprioception and corollary discharge), one can expect a huge enlargement of cerebellar structures when the cerebellum has access to large sensory systems. However, this does not preclude the view that the prime role of the sensory processing is to compute sensorimotor transformations in the service of improved, adaptive motor control. Then, the size of the cerebellum would be attributable to the sheer number of contingencies required to be represented to yield satisfactory motor control.

9.4.3 Varieties of Cerebellar Learning

Feedback-Error Learning

The nonplastic model of Boylls emphasizes the real-time role of the cerebellum in adapting motor activity to current circumstances. We now turn to the first of several

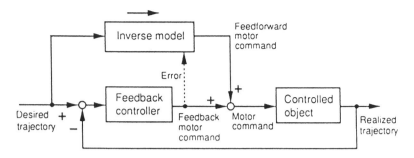

Figure 9.17
Feedback-error learning: parallel combination of a feedback and an adaptive feedforward system operating on one and the same control object. In this model, training adapts the feedforward system so that it becomes an "inverse model" (i.e., one that can compute "the inverse of plant dynamics" to convert the desired trajectory to the complete motor command). (Reprinted with permission from Kawato and Gomi 1992.)

models which emphasize the role of cerebellar plasticity in motor learning (as in the Marr-Albus model). Voluntary movement control is characterized by learning through repetition (but with parametric variations). At the beginning of learning a new skill, its execution will rely on sensory feedback but, after repeated practice with conscious effort, the movement becomes almost automatic and is executed in a feedforward mode. This situation may be represented by a parallel combination of feedback and adaptive feedforward operating on one and the same control object (figure 9.17).

The crucial control theory notions for this scheme are those of forward and inverse models of the dynamics of a controlled system. The *forward* dynamics model mimics the controlled system: It predicts how the system will respond to a given sequence of input commands. Conversely, the *inverse* dynamics model provides crucial control information: Given a desired output trajectory, it computes a sequence of inputs designed to cause the controlled system to behave in this way. In Kawato's view, training adapts the feedforward system of figure 9.17 so that it becomes an inverse model (i.e., one that can compute "the inverse of plant dynamics" to convert the desired trajectory to the complete motor command). The error signal drops to zero, and the feedback controller then issues no further command, effectively dropping "out of the loop" as long as the inverse model is accurate. Models developed later in this chapter view the sidepath as providing a correction to a controller that continues to provide signals that approximate the trajectory, rather than as replacing that controller. In this regard, the discussion of the Hoff-Arbib model (sec. 3.4.2) showed that the distinction between feedback and feedforward is more subtle than most people realize: A movement may appear to be feedforward, yet exhibit its feedback character when perturbations apply or high

accuracy requirements are imposed. When we are confident that the parameters of a skill are accurate, we may move quickly, because we need not be concerned about errors; otherwise, we must move slowly to allow time for feedback to be effective.

Kawato et al. (1988) formulated a hierarchical neural network model (figure 9.18) in which many regions are involved in the learning of distinct motor skills, each computing various nonlinear transformations of input signals and adapting to circumstances, owing to heterosynaptic plasticity (i.e., changes of synaptic weights are assumed proportional to a product of two kinds of synaptic inputs).

The Kawato model is composed of four elements, the first of which is the transcortical loop (visual feedback control). The association cortex provides a desired trajectory in body coordinates (θ_d) to the motor cortex (which provides higher-level premotor commands) wherein the motor command (torque, T) is calculated with the use of long-loop sensory feedback.

In addition, the cerebellum uses error signals from the IO (not shown in the figure) to adapt the way in which it transforms sensory signals into control signals applied to the premotor networks. The spinocerebellum plus the magnocellular part of the red nucleus receive the results of the movement (θ) and an efference copy of the motor command (T) and adapt to acquire a forward model of the musculoskeletal system. Once formed, it can provide an internal feedback loop, updating the motor command by predicting the movement (with prediction $\bar{\theta}$), thus yielding a possible error of movement ($\theta_d - \bar{\theta}$). The cerebrocerebellum plus the parvocellular red nucleus system (prominent in humans and primates) monitor the desired movement (θ_d) and the feedback motor command (T_f) but do not receive information about the actual movement. This system learns the inverse dynamics model for

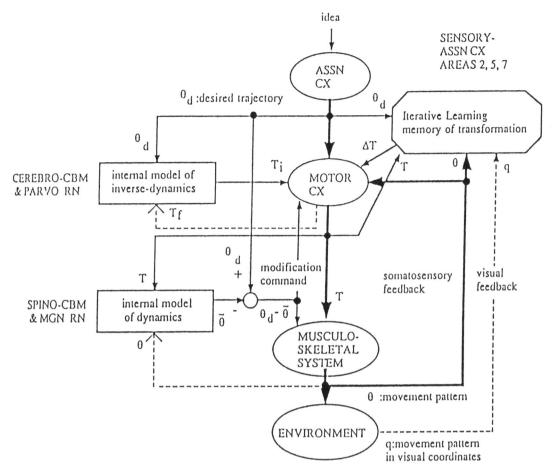

idea

ASSN
CX

SENSORY-
ASSN CX
AREAS 2, 5, 7

θ_d :desired trajectory

θ_d

θ_d

CEREBRO-CBM
& PARVO RN

internal model of
inverse-dynamics

Iterative Learning
memory of transformation

ΔT

MOTOR
CX

T_i

T

θ

q

T_f

θ_d
+

SPINO-CBM
& MGN RN

internal model
of dynamics

modification
command

somatosensory
feedback

visual
feedback

T

$\bar{\theta}$

–

$\theta_d - \bar{\theta}$

T

θ

MUSCULO-
SKELETAL
SYSTEM

θ :movement pattern

ENVIRONMENT

q:movement pattern
in visual coordinates

Figure 9.18

Hierarchical neural network model for the generation of motor commands through the interaction of multiple brain regions. The spinocerebellum (SPINO-CBM) plus the magnocellular part of the red nucleus (MGN RN) adapt to acquire a forward model of the musculoskeletal system, whereas the cerebrocerebellum (CEREBRO-CBM) plus the parvocellular red nucleus (PARVO RN) adapt to acquire an inverse dynamics model for which the trajectory is the input and motor command is the output. This model is hypothesized to substitute for other brain regions in complex computation of the motor command (see figure 9.17). (Reprinted with permission from Kawato, Isobe, and Suzuki 1989.) T, motor command; θ, movement pattern; θ_d, desired movement; $\bar{\theta}$, prediction of movement; T_f, feedback motor command; T_i, inferred motor command.

which the trajectory is the input (θ_d) and inferred motor command (T_i) is the output. This model substitutes for other brain regions in complex computation of the motor command. (This part of the model corresponds to Kawato's generic scheme of figure 9.17.)

The sensory-association cortex serves as an associative memory for iterative learning control. The parietal cortex (areas 2, 5, and 7) receives visual and somatosensory information and solves problems of coordinate transformation and generation of motor command via an iterative learning algorithm. This is trial-and-error learning of a single repetitive motor pattern (e.g., repetitive training to learn a tennis stroke).

Control and learning performance of the model were investigated by computer simulation, in which a robotic manipulator was used as a controlled system. Both the

forward and inverse dynamics models were acquired during control of movements. As motor learning proceeded, the inverse dynamics model gradually took the place of external feedback as the main controller. Concomitantly, overall control performance became much better. However, in the Schweighofer-Arbib model discussed later, we argue that the cerebellum does not take the place of other controllers but rather supplies a "correction term" that permits fast and accurate motor performance.

Once the neural network model learned to control some movement, it could control quite different and faster movements. The neural network model worked well even with only very limited available information about the fundamental dynamical structure of the controlled system. Consequently, the model both accounted for learning and control capability of the CNS and offered a parallel-distributed control scheme for a large-scale complex object the dynamics of which are known only partially. The goal of the movement is transformed via trajectory determination into a desirable trajectory in task-oriented coordinates, this trajectory in turn is transformed via a coordinate transformation into a desirable trajectory in body coordinates, which is transformed into a motor command (muscle torques).

Feedback-error learning of the inverse dynamics is performed by the cerebellar system with a synaptic rule wherein it is assumed that the synaptic weight changes when there is conjunction between the input and the error signal. This architecture is said to have advantages over other learning schemes. First, no external teaching signal is required; the feedback torque (assumed coded by climbing fiber activity) is used as the error signal, which tends to zero as learning proceeds. Second, control and learning are done simultaneously. The problem with the feedback learning network is that it requires a significant amount of learning time (30 minutes on-line for a three-degrees-of-freedom arm). Also, even though the controller generalizes well, there are parts of the space that it does not learn. If these areas are encountered later, the performance will be poor.

The cerebral (iterative learning) network, the transcortical (negative feedback) loop, and the cerebellar (feedback-error learning) network are arranged hierarchically and are used for motor control at the same time. The combination of the different learning loops increases control stability and also dramatically improves accuracy of control and shortens required learning time. The most important idea in the model is that the three neural networks complement each other's shortcomings. The results of the study are taken to indicate the superiority of the design concept of the brain, which hierarchically overlays a phylogenetically new and rather unstable (but precise) network on a phylogenetically older and dull (but robust) network.

This model is not without problems. Though the spinocerebellum and the magnocellular part of the red nucleus receive information from proprioceptors and from the motor command, it does not necessarily mean that they are using this information to develop an internal model of the musculoskeletal system. They could be calculating an error signal instead. The authors give no support to their statement that the cerebrocerebellum plus the parvocellular part of the red nucleus are acquiring an inverse dynamics model of the musculoskeletal system, nor do they discuss the issue of delayed feedback information. This problem could show itself in poor

learning of functions, because the torque and desired trajectory are not correlated entirely.

Figure 9.19 shows how the basic configuration of figure 9.17 can be modified to suggest how four regions of the cerebellum may be involved in the learning of distinct motor skills: (1) the flocculus in the vestibulo-ocular reflex, (2) the vermis in control of posture, (3) the intermediate part of the cerebellar hemisphere in control of locomotion, and (4) the lateral part of the hemisphere in voluntary movement.

Loops and Motor Learning

Houk and Barto (1992) and Houk, Keifer, and Barto (1993) modeled the role of cerebellum and red nucleus in sensorimotor leaning. Control of limb movements is shared by the rubrospinal and corticospinal movements. To study this concept, Houk et al. (1988) trained a monkey to make a variety of hand movements and studied firing in red nucleus cells. They found cells firing prior to a "twistor" movement and, as the animal was tracking a moving target, they found bursts corresponding to rapid velocity changes in compensating for departures from the "ramp." Thus, this red nucleus activity is tied to velocity of movement rather than to sensory data. Houk et al. (1988) recorded from up to 20 muscles and red nucleus cells, computing the cross-correlation of arm activity with electromyography, and found strong correlation of a cell with certain muscle groups. For example, they saw a cell correlated with preshaping of the hand while reaching for a raisin. Another cell was correlated more aptly with intrinsic muscles during actual grasp of the raisin. They looked for population effects and direct linkages for single neurons so as to get both polysynaptic and monosynaptic effects.

Houk and Barto (1992) thus view the red nucleus as driven by a tunable central pattern generator. Just as the Boylls-Arbib model is based on Tsukahara's work on the ventral loops, so do Houk and Barto base their analysis on loops: cerebellum → red nucleus → lateral reticular nucleus → cerebellum (figure 9.20), stressing their importance in generating motor commands. Similarly, the model takes account of the parasaggital zonation of cerebellum. For example, the zones for climbing fiber hindlimb input and Purkinje cells associated with hindlimbs show a nice alignment. This zonation may have evolved to solve the problem of *credit assignment*: routing the reinforcement (and other) signals to the right place.

Learning is viewed as distributed in many sites, not just in cerebellum. The premotor network comprising motor cortex, red nucleus, and spinal circuitry has loops

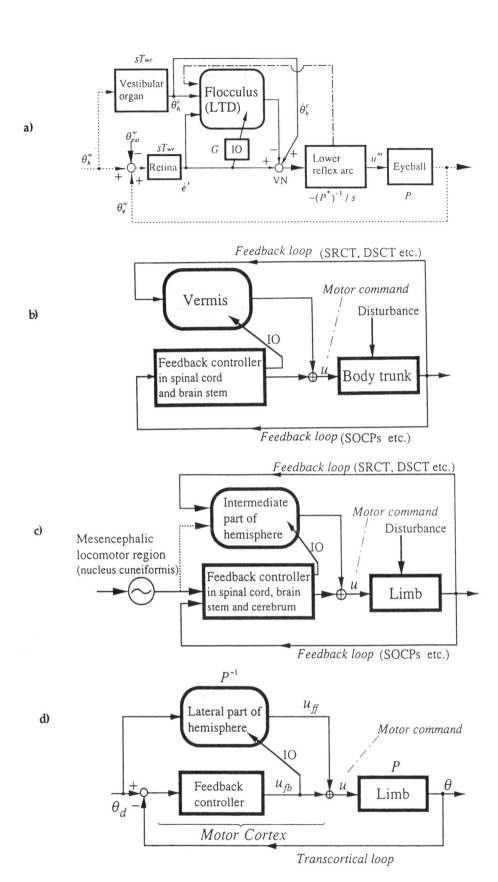

Figure 9.19
Variants of the basic configuration of figure 9.17, designed to suggest how four regions of the cerebellum may be involved in the learning of distinct motor skills. (a) The flocculus in the vestibulo-ocular reflex. (b) The vermis in control of posture. (c) The intermediate part of the cer- ebellar hemisphere in control of locomotion. (d) The lateral part of the hemisphere in voluntary movement. See the cited paper for further de- tails. (Reprinted with permission from Gomi and Kawato 1992.)

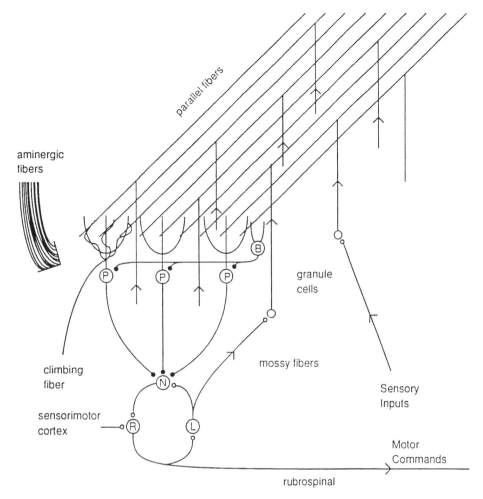

aminergic
fibers

parallel fibers

granule
cells

climbing
fiber

mossy fibers

sensorimotor
cortex

Sensory
Inputs

Motor
Commands

rubrospinal

Figure 9.20
A model of cerebellum's role in motor control based on adaptive modulation of loops: cerebellum → RN → LRN → cerebellum, taking into account the parasaggital zonation of cerebellum. (Reprinted with permission from Houk et al. 1990.) B, basket cell; P, Purkinje cell; N, cerebellar nucleus cell; R, red nucleus cell; L, lateral reticular nucleus cell.

through multiple regions of the cerebellar nuclei, thus suggesting that cerebellar nuclei be viewed as an integral part of the premotor apparatus. Given Tsukahara's demonstration of the excitatory nature of the red nucleus loop, Houk and Barto (1992) viewed each loop as a positive feedback loop. Buildup of positive feedback may correlate with latency of response; Purkinje cells may set movement parameters by adjusting loop activity. Going beyond the Boylls model, Houk and Barto employed synaptic plasticity to effect the learning of motor patterns. The model used the LTD induced by climbing fibers to store a command in Purkinje cells. Moreover, Purkinje cells can be "toggled," according to this model, between states of relatively high and relatively low firing. (Such toggling actually is seen [sec. 10.1.1] for the medium spiny neurons of the striatum.) The learning algorithm learns the *end point* of a movement by en-

abling the cerebellum to recognize when a movement is getting near the target on the basis of visual and kinesthetic input. Aminergic input can speed up or slow down the process.

One study wired 34 of these adjustable pattern generators to control the paired muscles of a two-jointed limb to yield population vectors and fairly accurate trajectories. Sensory triggers activate a few motor cortical cells (as different stimuli may trigger a given cell); positive feedback binds the trigger to a motor program stored in cerebellar cortex; and positive feedback brings the activity back to the level that controls an actual pathway. The buildup of positive feedback may explain the length of reaction times, with different inputs yielding different reaction times. [For a more recent view of this modeling project and a perspective on other models, see Houk, Buckingham, and Barto (in press).]

The Smith Predictor Approach to Long Delays

Many cells of the dorsal accessory olive are responsive to passive movement of the limb or to tapping or squeezing of particular portions of the paw of a cat; yet, when these paw areas are stimulated during the course of volitional movement, as when the paw touches the support surface, these same cells are unresponsive (Schwartz 1987). Gellman, Gibson, and Houk (1985) suggested that in active movement, an efferent copy of the motor command elicits an expectation of particular feedback and that if that feedback occurs, no error signal is generated. However, to be effective, this efferent copy would require explicit timing of the feedback (see the look-ahead in Hoff and Arbib 1992). If the feedback signal came too early or too late, an error signal would occur even if the results of the action were as anticipated. Gellman, Gibson, and Houk (1985) suggested that the cerebellum might be the source of the computation needed to adjust the efferent copy to the time of the expected feedback.

Miall and Wolpert (1995) described the results of an experiment wherein cerebellar patients performed a visually guided tracking task. If their visual target was blanked briefly from the screen, they could continue tracking with only slightly increased errors. This implies that they had no difficulty in predicting the target's movement. However, if the joystick-controlled cursor was blanked off briefly, their movements became significantly less accurate; this was not the case for control subjects. This suggests that the cerebellar damage had interrupted an internal prediction of the arm movement and that they were able to track successfully only when provided with visual feedback of arm position.

Regarding the control problems implicit here, note that the force required to follow a desired trajectory can be computed either by an inverse dynamics model or by a forward model embedded in a fast feedback loop (with little or no delay). A forward model is a neural representation of the transformation from motor commands to the resultant behavior of the controlled object. Long delays in feedback make it difficult to provide proper control of a motor system in fast movements. A predictive model of the motor apparatus can enhance its performance. The Smith Predictor (Smith 1959) is an engineering method that adopts this approach. The predictor consists of a fast negative feedback loop with an internal forward model of the controlled object and a positive feedback loop with the same internal forward model and an estimate of the time delay from motor command to receipt of sensory signals concerning the

outcome. The role of the second loop is to cancel the command generated by an external feedback loop with long delays.

Miall, Weir, and Stein (1993a) and Miall et al. (1993b) hypothesized that the cerebellum forms both types of internal model: a forward model of the motor apparatus and a model of the delays in the control loop (due to receptor and effector delays, axonal conductance, and cognitive processing delays). The second model delays the copy of the prediction made by the first model, so that it can be compared in temporal registration with sensory feedback from the movement. These authors simulated a Smith Predictor to demonstrate its advantage in assisting motor control and coping with long feedback delays.

Actually, Miall et al. (1993) viewed the cerebellum as providing two controllers for different aspects of the one action. They argued for at least two different Smith Predictors implemented in the cerebellum, with the more medial parts of the cerebellum involved at the limb-muscle level, whereas the more lateral parts are more involved in higher-level planning of movements in space.

The lateral cerebellum forms a link between visual association areas, especially the posterior parietal cortex, and the motor and premotor cortices. The authors suggest that the lateral cerebellum here acts as a Smith Predictor, transforming a movement command specified by the posterior parietal cortex in visual, egocentric coordinates into a motor control signal for the motor cortex. Interaction between the cerebellar cortex and the cerebellar nuclei would form the inner and outer control loops of the Smith Predictor.

A second Smith Predictor resides in the intermediate cerebellar cortex, which accepts corticospinal and corticobulbar inputs and projects back to the motor cortex or to the red nucleus. This predictor is to predict the limb kinematics based on descending motor commands.

Both the dynamics and time-delay models in a Smith Predictor are hypothesized as predictive neural networks. The former gives a forward prediction of the consequence of the action, whereas the latter makes a backward prediction of a delayed copy of the action. The familiar elements of a cerebellar learning model are invoked but have not been tested by simulation. Climbing fiber input from the IO acts as reinforcement, signaling a mismatch between the predicted and actual feedback. LTD caused by the coincidence of climbing fiber and parallel fiber inputs to Purkinje cells could allow modification of the dynamic model, with diffuse noradrenergic and serotinergic inputs from the locus coerulus and raphe nucleus providing the training signal to the time-delay model.

Although Miall et al. (1993) argued how the Smith Predictor model can be fitted into a cerebellar framework, the lack of a working neural network model based on behavioral, anatomical, and neurophysiological data raises problems, such as how the credit assignment problem can be resolved in learning both the dynamics and time-delay models simultaneously.

9.4.4 Adaptation and Eligibility

This section extends our analysis of the role of microcomplexes in the discussion of VOR (sec. 9.3.3) and applies them to models of both the adaptation of saccade metrics and the adaptation of throwing to a visual target that follows donning a pair of prisms. Although not presented here, recent work also has applied this microcomplex model in a variant model of the classic conditioning reviewed in section 9.3.4. Thus, this work lays the basis for the development of a universal cerebellar module that (when appropriately tuned and embedded within the appropriate input and output pathways) can explain much, if not all, the variety of cerebellar functions. (On a coarser scale, see the variety of cerebellar modules diagrammed in figure 9.19.)

The Cerebellar Role in Saccade Adaptation

We already have studied brainstem mechanisms for saccade generation (sec. 3.3) and cortical mechanisms for their "higher control" (sec. 8.4.2). We now look at data showing how the metrics of saccades can change through adaptive mechanisms that appear to involve the cerebellum. In a target perturbation experiment, a nontrained monkey (Goldberg et al. 1993) or a human subject (Albano and King 1989) has to make a saccadic eye movement toward a target, though during the saccade, the target is shifted to a new position. This shift is not perceived by the subject during the movement: We speak of "saccadic suppression." As the first saccade does not end at the new target position, it appears incorrect, and a second, corrective, saccade is generated with a latency comparable to the latency of the first saccade (Albano and King 1989). In fact, small errors nullified by a following corrective saccade or two appear to be a part of the normal human or monkey strategy (Optican 1982). This is because the brainstem saccade generator uses a noisy integrator, so completion of the saccade does not guarantee that the eye is on target. However, over a few hundred trials, the amplitude and direction of the initial saccade change, and the amplitude of the corrective saccade decreases until the trained animal can saccade, with little error, directly to the displaced tar-

get. The gain changes gradually and recovers gradually, and the gain for similar directions and amplitudes also is changed (Goldberg et al. 1993). The learning curve shows an exponential time course for the adaptation, with recovery apparently faster than learning.

The influence of the cerebellum and its associated structures on the execution of saccades can be observed in cerebellar patients and monkeys. Ritchie (1976) made symmetrical lesions of lobes VI and VII of cerebellar cortex and found that large saccades made toward the primary position (centripetal) were grossly hypermetric, whereas those made away from primary position (centrifugal) were hypometric. Goldberg et al. (1993) found that learning was abolished in the target perturbation experiment for monkeys after lesions of the interpositus and fastigial nuclei. Moreover, due to the loss of the modulation supplied by the cerebellum, the saccades have a greater amplitude than do those before the adaptation runs in the normal monkey, and taken as the variance around the mean curve, the performance is poorer after than before the lesion. These results suggest that the adaptation occurs in a system that includes the cerebellum and that performance is somewhat degraded by cerebellar lesions even when no adaptation is required.

As noted by Ito (1984), the contribution of the vermis may be to *modify* central command signals executing a saccade, and Noda, Sugita, and Ikeda (1990) showed that the cerebellum indeed is not the primary domain of the signal processing. Cerebellar impulses are projected downstream to saccade-programming circuits wherein visual information already has been converted into motor-commanding signals. The cerebellar eye movement map does not provide the total saccade command for a given frontocollicular eye movement command but rather provides the *correction* that modulates the command issued by the superior colliculus and other regions in response to the retinal input.

This distinction supports the hypothesis that the cerebellum adjusts an MPG rather than being the MPG. Later, we argue further that coordination of MPGs also is required for successful saccade adaptation.

The Structure of the Model

Figure 9.21a shows the overall structure of our model of saccade adaptation (Schweighofer, Arbib, and Dominey 1996a). Goldberg et al. (1993) found that stimulation of the superior colliculus (SC), known to provide a retinotopic control surface for saccades, produces saccades that are not adapted to target perturbations. This result suggests that the path concerned with target location

(a)

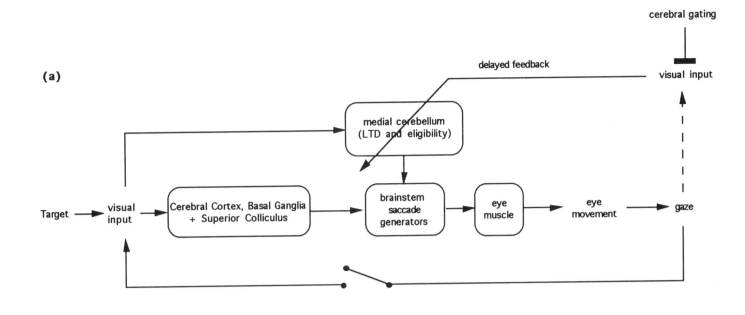

(b)

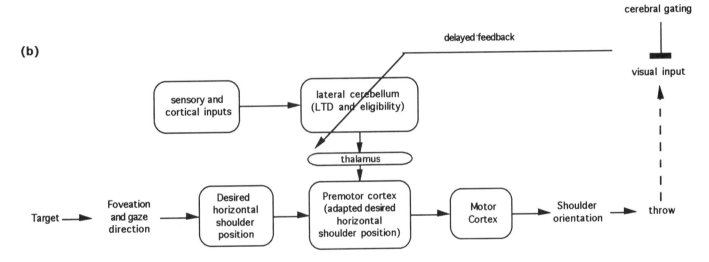

Figure 9.21
System views of cerebellar modulation of the saccadic system and in the adaptation of the throw to deviating prisms. (a) The saccadic system must be adaptive. Note that "delayed feedback," which is relayed via the inferior olive (not shown), is a form of visual input, but it is segregated from that which serves as input to the nonadaptive pathway. (b) Putative mechanisms of adjustment between eye position and synergy of the muscles in the trunk and arm involved in throwing. Af-

ferent information on eye position arriving in intermediate zone lobulus simplex is carried over parallel fibers to Purkinje cells that project to cells in the dentate nucleus and control eye, neck, arm, and hand muscle synergies. As in the saccade model, the cerebellum provides a correction to the main pathway, but here the correction is further "upstream", via premotor cortex. (Reprinted with permission from Arbib, Schweighofer, and Thach 1995.)

and involving the cerebellum comes from higher up than SC colliculus. It could come from the frontal eye fields (FEF) of the cerebral cortex, the posterior parietal cortex, or even the visual cortex or the lateral geniculate nucleus. Schweighofer, Arbib, and Dominey (1996a) assume that the cerebropontovermal side path for saccade adaptation starts from the FEF, goes through a pontine nucleus, then through the lobules VIc or VII of the vermis to the FOR (fastigial oculomotor region),

ending up in the parapontine reticular formation wherein the brainstem saccade generators reside (at least for horizontal movements).

From Goldberg et al.'s 1993 experiments, we infer the existence of one or several neural maps wherein adaptation occurs at specific spatial positions, based on the positions of the first target; indeed, the adaptation is selective to a set of saccades with similar amplitude and direction. To account for the crude "correction map" found in the cerebellar cortex, we will keep the major thesis of the Dominey-Arbib model (sec. 8.4.2), that a functional topography that preserves saccade direction and amplitude is maintained through multiple projections between brain regions until finally it is transformed into a temporal pattern of activity that drives and holds the eyes onto the target. The preserved topography is a map coding for amplitude and direction of an eye movement vector that, when combined with the current eye location, will center the eye on the target. The Schweighofer model (Schweighofer, Arbib, and Dominey 1996a) adds an adaptive component, postulating (in line with the experimental data) that saccadic gain change for a particular region of space around the target will be accomplished within the functional topography of the granule cell layer and the Purkinje cell layer. We present here the essential features of the model but refer the reader to the original study for the equations and parameter settings that constitute the formal description of the model.

A retinotopic map is sent via the pontine nucleus to a set of mossy fibers called *mfret*. To simplify, we assume that the pontine nucleus cells from which the retinotopic mossy fibers arise are mere relays in which the precise target map is blurred somewhat by divergence-convergence. The spread of activity is modeled by a gaussian distribution of weights to form a "blurry" topographical connection from the motor layer of the FEF. This "coarse coding" speeds up adaptation (Albus 1981), allowing one to update a group of cells that are "close" to the selected cell so that learning thus is extended to saccades of similar amplitude and direction, as seen in Goldberg et al.'s (1993) experiments.

In the model, another set of mossy fibers carries eye position. The position-coding cells receive proprioception signals from the oculomotor muscles. Another factor to be taken into account is the correlation observed between firing of cells of the FOR and the saccade duration as well as the anatomical connections from the brainstem SGs back to the vermis (Yamada and Noda 1987). These fibers carry a temporal signal, such that the firing of the FOR neurons (and Purkinje cells) will be synchronized somewhat with the SG's activities.

The model represents three types of cerebellar neurons: granule cells, Purkinje cells, and FOR (cerebellar nucleus) cells, but no cerebellar interneurons are taken into consideration. The granule cells generate a statistical distribution of combinations of mossy fibers carrying retinotopical signals, two position signals, and a temporal signal. Each Purkinje cell receives inputs from all the parallel fibers. The parallel fiber → Purkinje cell weights

are modifiable. For the present study, we make the following simplifying assumption: As the climbing fibers send collaterals to the deep nuclei on the way to the cerebellar cortex, the excitation of the fastigial neurons by these collaterals will nullify the strong inhibition caused by the complex spikes, which are the response of the Purkinje cells to the climbing fiber firing. Thus, the present model omits the real-time (as distinct from the training) role of the climbing fibers. This assumption may be useful as a first approximation but must be removed in future modeling. The Purkinje cell axons then converge to the FOR, the cells of which they inhibit. Collaterals of the mossy fibers also converge to nuclear cells and give an excitatory projection. It is the output of the nuclear cells that provides the correction signal to the saccadic generators. We must demonstrate that it can be adapted in the right direction (i.e., corresponding to the corrective saccade) as long as the initial saccade requires correction.

We assume that the postsaccadic information available to correct an erroneous motor command is an encoding of the motor activity (or corollary discharge) for a visually guided corrective saccade. Thus, we posit that the IO, the source of climbing fibers, receives both sensory and motor information: The error detector system comprises three neurons: a "goal" neuron, a "memory" cell, and a "pre-IO" neuron. The motivation for having a goal neuron is the need for a signal that continues until target acquisition is complete. Thus, this cell starts firing as soon as the target is not on the fovea and continues firing until the eye acquires the target; it encodes the goal of the saccadic system. Moreover, when a saccade is generated, some SG signals are sent to a movement memory cell. These two neurons project to the pre-IO neuron. The pre-IO neuron receives visual and motor inputs and has the role of an error detector: an error will be detected if a target is on the retina but not on the fovea and a saccade has just been completed. If these three conditions are fulfilled, the output of this neuron "ungates" the saccadic IO cells. Therefore, the corrective saccade will send an error signal to the appropriate microcomplex (i.e., direction of the error) with some amplitude information. (The IO fires with a higher probability for a large saccade.)

Adaptation: Problems and Solutions

Error information is delayed relative to the efferent signal because the error can be assessed only after the movement has been completed. If, after the first saccade, the absence of a target on the fovea and the presence of a target nearby signals an error, adaptation changes the gain of the agonist-antagonist pair of muscles responsible for the first (erroneous) saccade. This implies the need for a short-term memory system capable of retaining the appropriate parameters of the first saccade (position on the retina and corresponding eye position). Moreover, the climbing fiber error signal corresponding to the erroneous first saccade reaches the cerebellar cortex after the signal carried by the parallel fibers corresponding to the second saccade. The problem is to associate the learning not with the second saccade but with the first.

To address these temporal problems, we assume that synapse *eligibility*—which determines the degree of plasticity of a synapse and which we assume is coded by the concentration of some second messenger in the synapse—should tend to be largest for synapses involved in the initial saccade. As noted in section 6.3.5, we therefore introduced the concept of a time window of eligibility, with the concentration, denoted by [2nd], of the second messenger that adjusts the degree of synaptic plasticity having the response of a second-order system. Ideally, the concentration matches in time the occurrence of the error signal, and the concentration decays relatively rapidly to ensure a minimum of interference with the next saccade.

In the model, there are two 1000-element weight vectors w_{ltd}, one for each Purkinje cell, as each parallel fiber makes a synaptic contact with each Purkinje cell. With the assumption that the rise in calcium concentration is rapid compared to the second-messenger dynamics, the weight update rule is that at each time step, the strength w_{ltdi} of the ith synapse on a Purkinje cell is adjusted by

$$\Delta w_{ltdi} = -\alpha IO[2\text{nd}]_i.$$

Here, α is the learning coefficient, IO is the binary climbing fiber error signal, and $[2\text{nd}]_i$ is the concentration of messenger that signals the eligibility of synapse i. We also apply the constraint $w_{max} > w_{ltdi} \geq 0$. To avoid having all the weights tend to zero, we implemented a weight normalization that can be thought of as providing nonspecific long-term potentiation of synaptic strength so as to maintain constant the sum of synaptic weights for each Purkinje cell. (The normalization adopted is a subtractive normalization. In simulations, we also tried a multiplicative normalization; however, this gave a learning curve somewhat different from the data.) Each weight receives the additional increment:

$$\frac{\sum \Delta w_{ltdi}}{1,000}$$

where the sum is over all the weights of one Purkinje cell, 1000 being the total number of synapses per Purkinje cell. This potentiation has no direct functional role as far as the behavior is concerned, except that it degrades the performance of the entire system somewhat. This effect is reduced by the large number of synapses.

In the nonadaptive pathway, a light in the upper half of the retina does not elicit a downward movement, because the corresponding signals are not transmitted to the "downward" generator. However, to correct for errors, this constrained access is not possible for the adaptive system. For instance, suppose that the first target falls on the upper sector of the map and the second falls on the lower half. In this case, the first saccade amplitude should be decreased, as it is hypermetric. To compensate for this error, a decrease of the agonist innervation pulse and an increase of the antagonist pulse are needed. Therefore, the adaptive saccadic system requires that simple gain control be augmented by adaptation of coordination between the different saccade generators. Consequently (as is indeed seen in microstimulation experiments), each microcomplex should be able to influence the SGs of the antagonist and agonist muscle. In other words, restricting ourselves here to vertical eye movements so that we may concentrate on a single pair of eye muscles, for each direction for the first saccade there are two degrees of freedom: Either adaptation occurs in the same direction or in the opposite direction. *Adaptation requires coordination.*

Modeling the Role of Cerebellum in Adaptation of Dart Throwing

As already exemplified in our model of saccade adaptation, our theory of cerebellar function posits that the cerebellar output affects motor repertoires resident in movement generators located elsewhere and that this effect is both modulatory, controlling the gain of these MPGs, and combinatorial, mixing motor elements within and across generators so as to adapt old and develop new synergies of multiple body parts. Now we note that a similar model can be applied to the data of Martin et al. (1994) in Thach's laboratory, on the adjustment of eye, head (gaze), arm, and hand in humans throwing a dart or ball at a target while wearing wedge prism spectacles. In throwing, the eyes and head fixate the target and serve as reference aim for the arm. If wedge prism spectacles are placed over the eyes with the base to the right, the optic path is bent to the subject's right, and the eyes and head move to the left to see the target as a result of which the arm, calibrated to the line of sight, will throw to the left of the target. However, with repeated throws, the calibration will change, and the arm will throw closer to (and finally on) target. After adaptation, when the prisms are first removed, the eyes are now on-target, but the eye-head-arm calibration for the previously left-bent gaze persists; the arm throws to the right of target by an amount almost equal to the original leftward error. With repeated throws, eye-head position and arm synergy are recalibrated: Each throw moves closer to (and finally on) target.

Is the adaptation visual and global, motor and specific for the trained body parts, or somewhere in between? To address these questions, Martin et al. (1994) asked subjects to make both right-hand and left-hand throws, with and without prisms, to see whether there was carryover of adaptation from one task to the other. They found that prism adaptation occurred in the throwing arm, did not affect (or abate) with throws by the other arm, and readapted only during throws by the first arm. Therefore the adaptation could not be considered generally to be of vision but instead to be to some extent specific for the trained body parts.

Given this result, how specific is the adaptation to the task? Does the adaptation of the trained body parts carry over to their use in other tasks, or is it specific for the use of those body parts during the one task only? To address these questions, Martin et al. (1994) asked subjects to use the same arm to make underhand and overhand throws, with and without prism adaptation. On wearing prisms, all subjects adapted the overhand throw. For two subjects, the subsequent underhand throw showed absolutely no effect of prior overhand adaptation. In these subjects, prior overhand adaptation persisted in subsequent overhand throws despite intervening underhand throws and readapted with repeated overhand throws. In four subjects, the results were similar except for an apparent carryover of the overhand prism adaptation to the first subsequent underhand throw. Nevertheless, this effect disappeared with the second throw, and therefore it is unclear to what extent this represented an adaptive change. In these as in the first two subjects, the prior overhand adaptation survived the intervening underhand throws, persisting undiminished in subsequent overhand throws and readapting only after repeated overhand throws. Two subjects showed persistent carryover from prior overhand adaptation to underhand throws, but only one showed carryover of overhand adaptation to the underhand throws, which then readapted without any apparent adaptation left in the final overhand throw.

To test if one can learn to store more than the one gaze-throw calibration simultaneously, Martin et al. (1994) asked subjects to make 200 throws while wearing the prisms and 250 without the prisms each day, 4 days per week for 7 weeks. They measured the progress on the fifth day of each week with 25 throws before, 100 throws during, and 75 throws after wearing the prisms. This made a total of 900 throws with prisms and 1,100 throws without prisms each week for 7 weeks. Over time and with practice, the first throw with the prisms worn landed closer to the target, and the first throw without the prisms worn (aftereffect) also landed closer to the target. By 7 weeks, throws were on-target for the first trial while wearing and the first trial after removing the "known" prisms. This suggests that two adaptations (no-prisms and known-prisms) may be stored simultaneously and separately. A subject who had adapted to one prism behaved as if naive when presented with a novel prism. Both nonprism and known prism calibrations were affected; both had to be readapted independently.

Prism adaptation in macaques is abolished by cerebellar lesion (Baizer and Glickstein 1974). Weiner, Hallet, and Funkenstein (1983) reported more detailed results in patients with cerebellar disease and showed that adaptation was not impaired by disease of corticospinal or basal ganglia systems. Martin et al. (1994) also applied their paradigm to patients with cerebellar disease. In a cerebellar patient who had multiple sclerosis, with tremor and ataxia (and no other deficits), no adaptation was seen after donning and doffing the prisms. In a patient with right cerebellar hemisphere infarct, tremor, and ataxia, little adaptation was seen after donning and doffing the prisms. Martin et al. (1994) also found that two patients with magnetic resonance imaging—documented IO hypertrophy (a degenerative disease of the IO, the exclusive source of the cerebellar climbing fibers) could not adapt, despite otherwise normal performance. Both patients had ataxia of gait (damage leads immediately to malfunction and ultimately to atrophy of the cerebellum (Strata 1987; Murphy and O'Leary 1971)), but the upper extremity movements were relatively normal. This suggests that the adaptation mechanism could be dissociated at least in degree from those of coordination and performance. Finally, Martin et al. (1994) studied patients who had lesions presumed to involve mossy fibers of the middle cerebellar peduncle and also showed impaired adaptation (cases of ataxic hemiparesis, with contralateral lesions of the basis pontis involving leg corticospinal and arm pontocerebellar fibers).

This is not to say that the cerebellar cortex, the IO, and the mossy fibers are equivalent in their control of learning, but only that all are necessary. Their roles are quite different, but the differences are only to be revealed by integrated modeling and experiments that ask questions about each.

In our model of the adaptation of throwing to wearing prisms, the essential adjustment is proposed to be between eye position and synergy of the muscles in the trunk and arm involved in throwing. The target is seen, and the eye foveates and fixates the center of the target. Afferent information on eye position not necessarily excluding the visual arrives in the visual and "face" tactile receiving areas in intermediate zone lobulus simplex (see Snider and Stowell 1944; Snider and Eldred 1952). Information is carried over parallel fibers to Purkinje cells that are located more laterally in the hemisphere and that project to dentate nucleus cells that control eye, neck, arm, and hand muscle synergies.

The structure of the model is shown in figure 9.21b (Schweighofer, Arbib, and Thach 1994); the model of the cerebellar microcomplex adopted is that of the saccade adaptation model. The essential change is not in the cerebellar corticonuclear circuitry and its plasticity but in the circuit in which it is embedded. After repeated throws, adjustments are made in the strength of the parallel fiber input to Purkinje cells such that the changing output produced by the Purkinje cells in response to the eye position and visual input modulates the throw sufficiently for it to hit the target. Adjustments are possible in cortical interneurons—basket, stellate and Golgi cells—but they are not included in the present model.

The system (human + dart) is an open loop system because the error in dart throwing is available only after the movement, so the error cannot be used to correct the given movement; however, over trials, the correct match between gaze and throw is learned. Before throwing, the subject foveates the target; therefore, the internal representation of gaze and hence of the desired shoulder position before it undergoes adaptation is changed. This information is coded in a distributed manner, providing robustness to lesion and noise. A signal distributed over many noisy nonlinear channels may be summed to yield an accurate signal. This system has been modeled by using leaky integrator neurons in our NSL simulation environment (see Appendix A). To reproduce all the experiments, the mossy fiber inputs that we consider are as follows:

1. *Desired arm configuration at the end of aiming:* the position calculated from eye position muscles or from a cor-

ollary discharge for the control of gaze. Before aiming, proprioceptive inputs of the end point are not available. Instead, a desired vertical shoulder position should be available to the cerebellum via mossy fibers (this is coherent with fact that there are no direct inputs from the periphery to the lateral cerebellum). This desired position is well learned and cerebellar patients can throw well if no adaptation is required.

2. *Desired vertical shoulder position:* to distinguish underarm from overarm throws.

3. *Cortical projections for some form of mental set:* not explicitly coding knowledge for the present purpose but differing depending on whether the subject is or is not wearing prisms and whether the prisms are known or unknown. This input is necessary to explain the ability of highly practiced subjects to switch "gain" immediately when donning or removing known prisms. The cortical input to the cerebellar cortex is known to be large. Indeed, the corticopontine fibers form a very large group that arises from the entire cerebral cortex. The data show that "prism knowledge" has a large influence on the response and that this knowledge has an orthogonal representation at the parallel fiber level; orthogonality of the inputs is an important issue in this model.

In this model, adaptation acts by coding a rotation of the shoulder vector rather than providing a correction vector that is to be added. The algorithm we use to perform this rotation was developed by Hoff (unpublished work 1987); Burnod et al. (1991) reached a similar result by using cortical columns whose output is a combination of sums and product of the inputs. With Flanders et al. (1992), we assume that the target location and arm position share the same coordinate system, with error "in register" with the shoulder position. A leftward error activates a leftward group of IO cells. These cells receive a weighted retinotopic projection from the retina so that a large error will give rise to several spikes. Therefore, the climbing fibers fire to give the direction and amplitude of the error given by a visual projection to the IO, which retains some retinotopy. A large error will activate (with a certain probability) Purkinje cells different from those activated by a smaller error. However, there is a gradient of climbing fiber firing activities within each microzone. In a more complete model, vertical shoulder position also should be able to undergo adaptation (e.g., to vertical prisms, muscle lesions, aging, and the like). Therefore, the same parallel fiber set would overlap four microzones instead of the two in the present model, and the IO would encode horizontal as well as vertical errors.

The purely feedforward nature of the movement and the delay between motion generation and error detection require again the concept of eligibility, especially because the throw is made between the aiming and the receipt of the error signal. (The error is not corrected during the movement, as the error is not known before the dart hits the wall holding the target.) Therefore, the eligibility model developed for saccadic adaptation is used also in the present case.

Both forgetting and relearning are present in the system. Forgetting is included in the learning rule and is due to normalization. If there is no climbing fiber activity at a particular site, the weights are increased very slowly. As the error signal carried by the climbing fibers decreases the weights, there is forgetting of the previously learned patterns. By contrast, readaptation to the nonprism situation after adaptation to prisms is due to learning rather than to forgetting, as can be seen in figure 9.22c. In the Purkinje cell layer, there is a large depression after complete readaptation.

In the overhand-underhand experiments, the vertical shoulder position is different for the two throwing strat-

egies. The model reproduced the experimental data reported by Martin et al. There is some transfer from overhand to underhand in the prism adaptation, though in some subjects there is no transfer, whereas in others the transfer is total. We adopted a middle ground, with some overlap in the mossy fiber inputs between the two positions and a not-too-large mossy fiber input for the vertical shoulder position.

9.4.5 Adaptation and Coordination of MPGs

The proposed model for both saccade adaptation and dart throwing embeds the cerebellum in a very general framework. Even though the direct mapping from sensory to motor output is somewhat plastic, adaptation to novel context does not occur reliably without the cerebellum. The model uses the same cerebellar model for two different types of adaptation, with a similar coding of the error, but in the dart-throwing model, the cerebellum projects upstream to the premotor cortex instead of downstream to the brainstem. The microcomplex concept holds in both cases. The unification of

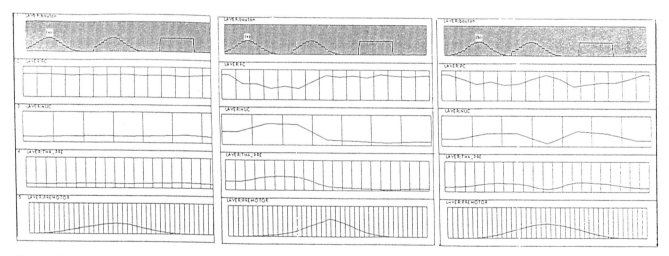

Figure 9.22

These three simulations show the spatial behavior of the cerebellar neurons in the course of adaptation to 25-degree prisms and underhand throwing with a known prism. Each row graphs the activity of a layer of cells just prior to the throw. (Reprinted with permission from Arbib, Schweighofer, and Thach 1994.) First row, the mossy fiber input; second row, the firing rates of 15 Purkinje cells (vertical scale, 0–110 spikes/sec, as in the following groups of neurons); third row, the nuclear cells' firing rates. The nuclear cells are inhibited by the Purkinje cells, and are driven by a high background rate; fourth row, the response of the 20 thalamic neurons; last row, the 40 premotor neuron activities. The shoulder position is derived from the premotor layer activity by the population vector transformation. (a) Situation before the first throw with prism on. The apparent uniform background rate of the Purkinje cells is due to random connections from the parallel fibers with initial random weights. The background firing rate in the nucleus pro-

vides facilitation to the premotor activity, which is deviated from the middle due to the gaze input. The premotor activity corresponds to a 25-degree angle between the shoulder and the forward direction. (Note that the activity peak does not represent the shoulder direction, as the latter is given by the "center of mass.") (b) End of adaptation to a prism. The depressed Purkinje cell activities (on the left) release activity in the nuclear cells and in the thalamic neurons. The premotor distributed activity is pushed back in the middle (the corresponding shoulder position is 0 degrees). (c) After readaptation to the nonprism situation. The Purkinje cell layer shows another depression on the right side: It is not forgetting but relearning that occurs. Also note the quasi-constant thalamic total activity (during adaptation) due to the negative feedback achieved by the reticular thalamic complex, which results in contrast enhancement and, consequently, in a better shift of the premotor "hump." The shoulder angle is 0 degrees again.

diverse information—from sensory signals to cerebral codes for mental set—is made possible by the large number of granule cells, each of which forms a sample of diverse mossy fiber signals.

Thach, Goodkin, and Keating (1992) argue that coordination of the modulation of different MPGs is made possible by the long length of the parallel fibers, overlapping different microzones. We have now seen a number of models which assert that the cerebellum is "hierarchically above" pathways to spinal cord from motor cortex, red nucleus, and basal ganglia, each with their own function generators. Thach et al. (1992) add that the cerebellum is responsible for the coordination of body parts, not just for the tuning of downstream events. This approach to cerebellar function is based on two observations.

First, cerebellar output occurs via the replicative representation of body maps in each of the cerebellar nuclei, with each coding a different type and context of movement and each appearing to control movement of multiple body parts more than of single body parts. Second, the newly assessed long length of the parallel fibers (Mugnaini 1983): By virtue of its connection through Purkinje cells to the deep nuclei, the parallel fiber appears optimally designed to combine the actions at several joints and to link the modes of adjacent nuclei into more complex coordinated acts.

Because the parallel fibers are connected to the nuclear cells by Purkinje cells, a coronal "beam" of parallel fibers would control through inhibitory modulation the nuclear cells that influence a wide range of synergistic muscles. Thach looked at effects of inactivating cerebellum by injections of muscimol into the deep cerebellar nuclei. He saw no change in single-joint tasks with fastigial injection; some tremor, but satisfactory endpoint control, with interpositus and dentate injections. This might suggest at most a role of cerebellum in fine tuning. However, *natural tasks* yielded dramatic deficits. The animal with a fastigial injection could not get up from a chair and walk without falling over; it could elicit locomotor patterns but not combine these with antigravity control. Reversible lesions of the interpositus yielded a fast tremor. Those in dentate yield major overshoots in reaching (see Holmes 1939 on compounding of single-joint errors), yet the animal still made the movement. The animal could not make a precision pinch to extract an object from a food well (failing to get other fingers out of the way) and instead used single-finger strategies to winkle food out from the well. This suggests the need for a multicausal view of how different areas *cooperate* and suggests that it is the role of the cerebellar cortex to

mediate this cooperation. The key idea is that the length of the parallel fibers allows Purkinje cells involved in the modulation of distinct MPGs via the cerebellar nuclei to adapt to overlapping sets of contexts and thus come to recognize how multiple MPGs should be coordinated in diverse situations. A model of multijoint coordination in reaching, based on this approach to cerebellum and addressing the Holmes data, has been developed recently by Schweighofer et al. (1997).

9.5 The Cerebellum and Mental Activity

In introducing this chapter, we noted that there is much debate about the functions actually performed by cerebellum, and we stressed that our focus in sections 9.4.3 and 9.4.4—on modeling the cerebellar role in adaptation of motor control—did not endorse the exclusion of other cerebellar functions from future modeling. Clearly, we still have much to learn; we close this chapter with a very brief look at the evidence, still in its early days, that cerebellum plays a cognitive role as well as a sensorimotor role. In doing so we contribute to the argument (developed further in chapter 11) that the approach to neural organization taken in this book has much to offer in the future development of cognitive neuroscience.

The lateralmost parts of the human cerebellum are enlarged dramatically in parallel with the development of cerebral association cortices. On the basis of this comparative anatomical finding, Leiner, Leiner, and Dow (1986, 1987, 1989, 1991) proposed that the cerebellum plays a role in certain mental activity. Indeed, activation of the cerebellum in noninvasive measurement of human cerebellar activity suggests involvement of the cerebellum in silent counting, imaginary tennis playing, or language activity (e.g., see Roland 1993).

The role proposed by Ito (1982) for the flocculus in controlling the VOR conforms to the modern concept of an adaptive feedforward control system. VOR lacking feedback is a typical feedforward system, able to be controlled precisely only when the flocculus adaptively regulates it by referring to retinal error signals. If the control is perfect, the output of the VOR (eye velocity) should become equivalent to the input of the VOR (head velocity), with signs reversed. In this situation, the dynamic characteristics of the adaptive controller composed of the flocculus and VOR relay neurons reciprocally should be equal to that of the control object (i.e., the oculomotor system). The role of a corticonuclear microcomplex thus would be specified as generating dynamics inversely equivalent to the dynamics of a control object.

Thus, Ito (1993) argues that the proposed contribution of the cerebellum to mental activity can be explained by the same control system scheme for voluntary movement if an eye, arm, or leg is replaced with a part of the cerebral cortex. This cerebral cortical area would be a control object on which another cortical area acts as a controller. Such a corticocortical system initially would operate in a feedback mode but, after learning, the cerebellum would develop a model that replaces the role of the controller cerebral area, as proposed by Leiner, Leiner, and Dow (1986). However, just as we (and Ito) have argued against a "takeover role" for cerebellum in visuomotor coordination and motor control, so would we argue against such a role for the cerebellum in cognition. Thach (1996) provided a much fuller discussion of the clues from positron emission tomography activation and lesion studies in humans as to the specific role of the cerebellum in motor learning and cognition; his study is supplemented by numerous commentaries and the author's reply. Thach's article is part of a special issue of *Behavioral and Brain Sciences* titled "Controversies in Neurosciences IV: Motor Learning and Synaptic Plasticity," which contains a wealth of material relevant to this chapter.

Basal Ganglia

We describe the structure of the basal ganglia (BG) in terms of its components and the circuits in which it participates (sec. 10.1). In section 10.1.1, we present the major subdivisions of the BG: the striatum (caudate and putamen), the globus pallidus (GP) (internal [GPi] and external [GPe]), substantia nigra (pars reticulata [SNr] and pars compacta [SNc]), and the subthalamic nucleus (STN). The striatum, serving as the prime recipient of input to the BG, consists mainly of medium spiny neurons (MSP); it is described in some detail. The GP and SNr are the main output nuclei of the BG and project to the thalamus, which in turn projects to the prefrontal cortex, the premotor cortex (PMC), the supplementary motor cortex, and the motor cortex. In section 10.1.2, we show the BG as embedded in four disjoint loops that embed them in reciprocal interactions with cortex. These four loops are the oculomotor circuit, the motor circuit, the "cognitive" (dorsolateral prefrontal) circuit, and the limbic (lateral orbitofrontal) circuit.

Section 10.1.3 contains a twofold examination of the structure of the striatum: looking at the two pathways (direct and indirect) whereby it acts on the output pathways of the BG and looking at the division of the striatum into "patches" embedded in a "matrix." Also, we discuss the crucial role of the dopaminergic input from SNc in regulating the activity and plasticity of the striatum. The models presented in this chapter focus on the direct pathway, ignoring the patch-matrix division of striatum, but the distinctive roles of the direct and indirect pathways do contribute to our understanding of diseases of the BG (sec. 10.2). The distinct movement disorders seen in Huntington's disease—hyperkinetic and hypotonic—and in Parkinson's disease (PD)—hypokinetic and hypertonic—are associated with decreased BG output in Huntington's disease and a marked increase of this output in PD. Recent clinical studies have shown further that sequencing of movements is impaired in PD and that the intact BG may help to generate internal cues for releasing successive stages of a predefined movement sequence, acting cooperatively with a variety of cortical areas.

Section 10.3 is a discussion of self-reorganization of the striatum, and in section 10.3.1 we discuss the self-organizing character of the pattern formation for striatal compartments. (It seems likely that migration and adhesion are the primary processes that compartmentalize the striatum.) In section 10.3.2, we discuss modular remapping, binding, and sensorimotor learning, analyzing the relationship between the modular remapping architecture, the tonic firing of certain striatal neurons, and their role in coordinated motor behavior. Tonically active neurons (TANs), the presumptive inhibitory interneurons of striatum, may contribute to temporal binding during behavioral learning by undergoing dopamine sensitive changes.

Section 10.4 presents a model of the role of the oculomotor loop of the BG in generating saccades. Section 10.4.1 contains models of the interactions between the basal ganglia and the working memory systems of prefrontal cortex to complete the Dominey-Arbib model of saccade control (chapters 3 and 8). Absence of SNr inhibition allows reciprocal connections between frontal eye fields (FEF) and mediodorsal thalamus (MD) to generate a spatial working memory cycle or loop. In section 10.4.2, we suggest that if the FEF and direct visual input do not yield the encoding of a unique target, then experience based on inferotemporal or prefrontal information may provide contextual, learned information to bias activity in the BG to help decide which target is appropriate. Our visuomotor conditioning model, including spatial generalization, is based on a form of reinforcement learning in which dopamine released by the SNc acts as the reinforcement signal to toggle between hebbian learning (positive reinforcement: long-term potentiation [LTP]) and antihebbian learning (negative reinforcement: long-term depression [LTD]). In section 10.4.3, we return to the notion of eligibility introduced in our discussion of cerebellar learning (chap. 9). We suggest that the shaping of the eligibility signal may be task dependent, setting an important goal for neuroscience to bridge from this systems level of neural analysis to that of synaptic neurochemistry.

Section 10.5 is an examination of the still somewhat discordant views of the roles of the BG in motor coordination and learning. We emphasize the view that the BG receive rich contextual information and then "release" components of motor programs through disinhibition. To exemplify this view of the role of BG in sequencing movements, in section 10.5.1 we present a model of sequential behavior model based on the strong hypothesis that this learning is mediated by corticostriatal plasticity (as is the visuomotor conditioning model of sec. 10.4.2). Section 10.5.2 is an attempt to distinguish between the role of BG and cerebellum, suggesting that BG are in-volved in combining explicitly the "pieces" that make up a skilled behavior, whereas the cerebellum serves to turn a procedure into a skill, adjusting parameters to adapt and coordinate components of the movement so as to yield a seamless whole. Among other things, we suggest that BG neuronal responses are task-dependent, with the current responsiveness of a neuron possibly determined by the state of behavioral experience or learning and temporarily maintained until the relevant memory is formed in premotor cortices. Thus, we stress the importance of the supplementary motor area (SMA) and other areas of cerebral cortex in sequential behavior.

10.1 Structure of the Basal Ganglia

10.1.1 Components of the BG

The BG comprise a number of subcortical nuclei: the striatum, the GP, the substantia nigra (comprising a pars reticulata SNr and a pars compacta SNc), and the STN.

The *striatum*, comprising the *caudate nucleus (CD) and putamen*, is the largest component of the BG and receives most (but not all) of the BG's input, primarily from the cerebral cortex and the intralaminar nuclei of the thalamus. In nonhuman primates and humans, the CD and putamen form separate nuclei divided posteriorly by the internal capsule. The corticostriate projection contains fibers from the entire cerebral cortex, including motor, sensory, association, and limbic areas. These cortical inputs are excitatory, mediated by glutamatergic neurons and terminating on the MSPs (see sec. 10.1.3), which are the principal cells of the striatum. The motor cortex also can influence BG via the path motor cortex → centromedian nucleus of the thalamus → intralaminar nuclei of the thalamus → putamen. Each part of the striatum projects to specific parts of the GP and the substantia nigra.

The GP is derived from the diencephalon and lies medial to the putamen and lateral to the internal capsule. It is divided into internal and external segments: GPi and GPe, respectively. The *substantia nigra* lies in the midbrain and has a ventral pale zone, the SNr, which resembles the GP cytologically, and another part, the SNc. The GP and the SNr can be considered as a single structure arbitrarily divided by the internal capsule, much like the CD and putamen. They are major output nuclei of the BG and project to three nuclei in the thalamus: the ventrolateral, the ventroanterior, and the mediodorsal nuclei. The internal segment of the GP has an additional projection to the centromedian nucleus of the thalamus. The portions of the thalamus that receive input from the

BG project to the prefrontal cortex, the PMC, the SMA, and the motor cortex.

The STN lies below the thalamus at its junction with the midbrain. It receives the output of GPe and has topographically organized projections to both segments of the GP and to SNr. The STN also receives direct, topographically organized inputs from the motor cortex and premotor cortices, providing the motor cortex another means for modulating the output of the BG.

10.1.2 Four Circuits of the BG

In discussing the connections of the striatopallidal complex of the BG with the thalamic system (sec. 7.3.2), we noted that there are multiple circuits of the following form that embed the BG in reciprocal interactions with cortex.

A, B, C in cortex → striatum → SNr → thalamus → prefrontal A

The Oculomotor Circuit

The FEF and several other cortical areas (e.g., dorsolateral prefronted cortex, DLPC) project to the body of the CD, which projects to the SNr. Then the SNr projects to both the SC and the FEF via MD.

The Motor Circuit

The SMA, the parietal and premotor areas, the cingulate cortex, the motor cortex, the somatosensory cortex, and the superior parietal lobule project to the motor portion of the putamen, which then projects to the output nuclei, SNr and GPi. The output of this pathway is directed primarily back to the SMA and premotor cortex via thalamus [the ventroanterior (VA) and ventrolateral (VL$_o$) nuclei]. These cortical areas are interconnected reciprocally and with the motor cortex, and all have direct descending projections to brainstem motor centers and to the spinal cord.

The "Cognitive" (Dorsolateral Prefrontal) Circuit

The dorsolateral prefrontal cortex and several other areas of association cortex project to the dorsolateral head of the CD, which in turn projects back to the dorsolateral prefrontal cortex via the thalamus.

The Limbic (Lateral Orbitofrontal) Circuit

This circuit links the lateral orbitofrontal cortex with the ventromedial caudate.

This view of distinct loops marked a radical departure from classic views, which saw the BG as providing a single, unstructured integration of input from many regions. Rolls (1994) reviewed supporting data on the activity of neurons in different parts of the striatum of primates:

- *In much of the putamen:* It receives inputs from the sensorimotor cortex, and the neurons have activity related to limb movements.

- *In the CD:* It receives inputs from the association cortex, and the neurons have activity related, for example, to environmental stimuli that signal preparation for, or initiation of, behavioral responses.

- *In the tail of the CD:* It receives strong inputs from the inferior temporal visual cortex, and the neurons respond when a patterned visual stimulus changes.

- *In the posterior ventral putamen:* It receives inputs from the inferior temporal visual cortex and the prefrontal cortex, and the neurons respond in a visual short-term memory task (delayed matching to sample). The neurons respond in the delay period, differentially to match and nonmatch stimuli. These neurons do not respond in an auditory delayed match-to-sample task, so that their activity is not related to movement per se, but instead is related more closely to visual inputs relevant to the memory task (sec. 10.4.1).

- *In the ventral striatum (including the nucleus accumbens):* It receives inputs from limbic structures, such as the amygdala and hippocampus, and the neurons respond to stimuli associated with reinforcement or to novel stimuli.

We provide a detailed model of the oculomotor circuit (sec. 10.4) as the basis for further analysis of the role of the BG in the motor system, but do not treat the cognitive or limbic circuits further in this volume.

10.1.3 Organization of the Striatum

The structure of the striatum can be viewed in two ways: by looking at the two pathways, direct and indirect, whereby it acts on the output pathways of the BG, and by looking at the division of the striatum into patches embedded in a matrix.

We shall look also at two major classes of cells in striatum: the MSPs and the TANs. We examine the crucial role of the dopaminergic input from SNc in regulating the activity and plasticity of the striatum.

The Medium Spiny Neurons of the Striatum

MSPs are the main neurons of the striatum (Groves et al. 1995; Wilson 1995). Spiny cells fall into two categories: one with approximately 50 dendritic tips (approximately 24,000 spines) and the other with approximately 25 dendritic tips (approximately 12,000 spines). Each cortical afferent makes only one or two synapses on a given MSP, which thus may act as a pattern recognition element, trained by the separate dopamine input. In the 1970s, MSPs were viewed as forming a lateral inhibitory network with neighbors inhibiting each other, but Wilson's thesis showed that the MSP was *not* an interneuron: even though it has extensive axon collaterals around the cell it has an axon leaving the striatum. (We will later discuss the TANs, which are considered to be interneurons.) MSP axons wander "aimlessly" before moving in the direction of the GP (which is why Ramón Cajal thought the MSP was an interneuron). The MSP has local collaterals, making synapses on dendritic shafts and necks of spines of other MSPs—and these cells are activated by γ-aminobutyric acid (GABAergic)—but there is little physiological evidence of effects of one MSP on another. The MSP cell body and first 20 μm of dendrites are smooth, but thereafter dendrites are laden heavily with spines. Inputs end in two ways on MSP neurons: on the head of a dendritic spine and on a dendritic shaft. The latter inputs are few. There is no evidence of (even rare) excitatory output from striatum.

Most synapses on MSPs come from cerebral cortex. Electrical stimulation of cortex (a glutamatergic projection) shows MSPs responding with alternation of bursts and silences that may last for a second or more (three or four cycles) after a shock. However, spontaneous activity in a urethane-anesthetized rat sees cells toggling between −46 mV and −80 mV (both subthreshold; see the model of a Purkinje cell posited in sec. 9.2.4, regarding loops and motor learning). This is *not* the result of inhibitory interneurons. Thus, Wilson (1995) spoke of an up-state and a down-state and suggested that synaptic input is effective in the up-state. Extrinsic afferents cause the up-state (one can remove it by inducing spreading depression in cortex). Aspiny cells (the main class of non-MSP neurons in striatum) do not show this effect. Wilson could not find effects on firing of MSP collaterals, so he sought another organizing principle for striatal activity, analyzing the currents involved in these states, the sharp transitions between them, and the generation of action potentials. The up-state is noisier than is the down-state. The sharp transition is intrinsic; the timing of the transition depends on the synaptic inputs.

Corticostriatal cells show a similar up-state and down-state, with similar statistics (Cowan and Wilson 1994). A pyramidal cell with collaterals to striatum may show firing at 35 Hz, with ripples in membrane potential lining up with a 35-Hz oscillation in phase with the up-state

and out of phase with the down-state. Thus, it provides appropriate input to induce the striatal up-state.

Different pyramidal tract neurons have a small arbor making collaterals into a specific place in striatum. The cortical site and the striatal site seem to co-vary, with approximately 20–25 boutons in striatum for such an arbor. With a corticocortical cell, Wilson found 900 boutons in its collateral to striatum; these filled a large volume. An MSP probably will see one branch at most of this latter collateral, and Wilson thought that there will be only one synapse at most (though there will be 10 synapses along the traverse shared by that MSP dendrite with other dendrites).

With all these properties, MSPs have become an attractive target for compartmental modeling. Kotter and Wickens (1995) used bicompartmental models, discriminating between the soma and a dendritic compartment. A network of these simplified neurons connected by GABAergic inhibitory coupling was simulated in studying the effects of the glutamatergic corticostriatal synapses and of the dopaminergic nigral afferents. Among other things, it was demonstrated that increased dopamine concentrations could compensate for the effects of reduced glutamatergic input. However, in later sections we use only single-compartment models of neurons, as part of large-scale models designed to illuminate the overall role of the striatum in motor control and sensorimotor coordination.

Direct and Indirect Pathways

BG output cells have a fast tonic discharge (70–80 Hz) that is modulated by two major pathways through the BG (figure 10.1). The two pathways have opposite effects on SNr and thus on the thalamus.

The *direct* pathway is the striatal projection to GPi and SNr, which then project to the thalamus. The direct pathway from striatum to the output nuclei is mediated by GABA and substance P. This pathway is inhibitory, as is the pathway from the output nuclei to the thalamus, mediated by GABA. Corticostriate inputs excite striatal neurons, which inhibit the inhibitory cells in the BG output nuclei, releasing the thalamic cells from tonic inhibition. The resulting phasic disinhibition of thalamocortical neurons is thought to facilitate movement by exciting premotor areas and SMA and thus activating their projections to the motor cortex, the brainstem, and the spinal cord.

The *indirect* pathway is the circuit from the striatum to GPe, which projects to the STN. The STN, in turn, projects back to both pallidal segments and to the substantia

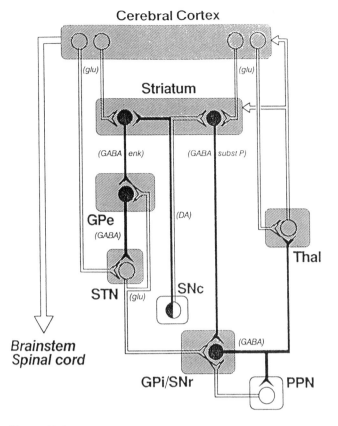

Cerebral Cortex

(glu) *(glu)*

Striatum

(GABA enk) *(GABA subst P)*

GPe

(GABA)

STN *(glu)* **SNc**

**Brainstem
Spinal cord**

Thal

(DA)

(GABA)

GPi/SNr **PPN**

Figure 10.1
A schematic view of the direct and indirect pathways. Shown are inhibitory (black) and excitatory cells and pathways and identified neurotransmitters. (Reprinted with permission from Alexander and Crutcher 1990.) glu, glutamate; subst P, substance P; DA, dopamine; enk, enkephalin; Thal, thalamus; PPN, parapontine nucleus. For other abbreviation, see text.

nigra. Most BG pathways are inhibitory, except for STN projections. Corticostriatal excitation results in inhibition of the GPe (mediated by GABA and enkephalin) and disinhibition of the STN (mediated by GABA), which excites the output nuclei (mediated by glutamate). This activity inhibits the thalamus and decreases the excitation of the SMA.

SNc is Dopaminergic

The striatum receives an important dopaminergic projection from the neurons of the dorsal, darkly pigmented zone of the substantia nigra, the SNc. The dopaminergic projection from SNc has several effects on neurons in the striatum. Dopamine is thought to have a dual action, loss of dopamine strengthens the indirect pathway and weakens the direct pathway. Dopamine excites the direct pathway, the striatal neurons that send GABA and substance P projections to the output nuclei. In contrast, dopamine inhibits the indirect pathway, the striatal neu-

rons that send GABA and enkephalin projections to GPe. Because in the motor loop the direct pathway appears to facilitate movement by exciting the SMA whereas the indirect pathway has the opposite effect, dopamine appears to facilitate movement by its action on both pathways.

Houk, Adams, and Barto (1995) hypothesized that dopamine signals useful contexts, singling out new representations to be sent back to cortex. Thalamic neurons have low-threshold calcium currents, so removal of pallidal inhibition could give a thalamic burst that sets off a reverberation between thalamus and cortex to constitute a working memory. (See secs. 10.3, 10.6 for models of the role of the BG in working memory and of the role of dopamine in the BG, respectively.) In the view of Houk, Adams, and Barto (1995), a burst in striatal spinal neurons leads to a pause in pallidal output neuron, which leads to sustained discharge in thalamic and frontal cortical neurons that persists until the information is "used." This view is very close to that of their model of the cerebellum (sec. 5.7.2; Berthier et al. 1993). This process raises the general issue: What distinguishes the circuitry and function of different brain regions? (For more on this subject, see sec. 10.5.6.)

Patch-Matrix Organization of Striatum

Inputs to the striatum from cortex and thalamus end in two kinds of neurochemically specialized compartments with the smaller *patches* (also called *striosomes*) embedded in the *matrix* (Gerfen 1989, 1992). The striatum also receives inputs from thalamic sites implicated in rhythmic firing in the forebrain (Graybiel et al. 1994). It is believed now that cells in different layers of the cortex project to patch and matrix, rather than that some regions of cortex project to patches and others to matrix. Most cortical projections to the striatum that are concerned with sensation and movement or with carrying information critical for motor or cognitive behavior terminate in the matrix, which projects in turn to the pallidum and SNr. The limbic projections terminate in the striosomes, which project to the dopaminergic neurons of SNc. During passive movements of a single joint, the cells in certain compartments become active, whereas during active movements of the same joint, cells of other compartments become active.

The mapping from cortex to putamen shows a nice separation of foot, arm, and face area. Yet, no matter how small the injection, there is a patchiness of the input that is separate from the patchiness of the striosomes. Why are these inputs dispersed? Injecting homologous areas in motor and somatosensory cortex shows strong overlap in striatal projection. Inputs from these different areas converge in small zones of striatum (Flaherty and Graybiel 1994). There are similar clusters elsewhere in striatum, including recipients of prefrontal cortex.

MSPs receive many en passant fibers (somewhat reminiscent of the parallel fibers in cerebellum), so the coincidence of similar inputs from other areas might be the key to bringing cells to threshold (perhaps from downstate to up-state). Why have divergence to different patches? Perhaps it is to allow different arrangements of neighbors in striatum to detect novel combinations, as a basis for some forms of plasticity.

We saw that the direct pathway involves substance P and the indirect pathway involves enkephalin. Probably no one knows the differential role of enkephalin and substance P at present. Given the heterogeneity of dopamine receptors, these substances affect the receptors in different ways. Enkephalin patches in cat CD, thought to correspond to the striosomal compartments form a highly organized three-dimensional lattice, whereas substance P patches are better attractors for cholinergic fibers, and these cross the patch-matrix boundaries (see Groves et al. 1995 for a review).

Tonically Active Neurons of Striatum

Apicella, Scarnati, and Schultz (1991) found that in monkeys already trained to perform a behavioral task, tonically discharging neurons in the striatum responded with short-lasting depressions or activations to stimuli significant to performing the task. On the basis of the firing characteristics, it is believed that this TAN is the large aspiny cholinergic interneuron in the striatum. Kimura, Aosaki, and Graybiel (1993) found that the number of TANs in both CD and putamen, firing in response to the performance of a task, gradually increased from 10%–20% to 60%–70% as the task was learned. These authors also found that the TANs developed a pause in their firing often flanked by short excitatory pulses. This pause occurred shortly after the conditioned stimulus was presented. Aosaki, Kimura, and Graybiel (1995) have shown that these neurons become coordinated temporally across large regions of the striatum during sensorimotor learning. When monkeys were given extinction training, this pause response diminished and eventually disappeared.

When Kimura et al. (1993) removed the supply of dopamine via the injection of the neurotoxin MPTP, the number of TANs firing was reduced to 13% in putamen and 18% in caudate. Then they injected the dopamine agonist apomorphine and found that after 10–15 minutes, the response rate to the conditioned stimulus recovered. Response rates of dopamine-depleted TANs did not increase, even during 3 months of additional training. These authors proposed that the supply of dopamine by the nigrostriatal system is essential for the maintenance of conditioned responses of TANs in the striatum. Last, they found that these TANs, though only a small percentage of the number of neurons in the striatum, tend to lie along the striosome-matrix borders. Approximately one-half of the neurons lie along the striosomal borders, and one-half lie in the matrix (Aosaki et al. 1995). Thus, many of these neurons are in a position to communicate a primary reward signal (e.g., food or juice) from the striosomes, carried via dopamine to the surrounding matrix containing MSPs that synapse onto the output structures in the BG. This signal then would be used to facilitate the execution of motor behaviors selected by higher cortical centers involved in motor planning.

10.2 Diseases of the Basal Ganglia

Diseases of the BG characteristically produce involuntary movements. We concentrate here on Parkinson's disease (PD), which is hypokinetic, and Huntington's disease, which is hyperkinetic, and do not discuss hemiballismus and tardive dyskinesia.

10.2.1 Learning from the Contrast Between Parkinson's and Huntington's Diseases[1]

PD symptoms include a rhythmical tremor at rest (3–6 beats/sec), cogwheel rigidity (an increase in muscle tone or rigidity that often is ratchetlike), difficulty in the initiation of movement and paucity of spontaneous movements (akinesia), and slowness in the execution of movement (bradykinesia) These are evident in the way a patient gets up from a bed or chair and in the characteristic shuffling gait and postural reflex impairment.

The pathological hallmark of PD is loss of dopamine neurons in the SNc that results in a loss of more than 80% of the dopamine content of the striatum. Some 80% of the dopamine in the brain is localized in the BG, even though the BG make up less than 0.5% of the total weight of the brain (Carlsson 1959). Hornykiewicz

---

1. The treatment in this section follows that of Côté and Crutcher (1991).

(1966) found that in addition to dopamine, the levels of such other neurotransmitters as norepinephrine and serotonin were low in the brains of patients with PD. The severity of cell loss in the SNc varies between patients with PD but parallels the reduction of dopamine in the striatum. Dopaminergic neurons from the ventral tegmental area project to the limbic system, cortex, and striatum. In patients with PD, the akinesia, often associated with rigidity and postural abnormalities, results from destruction or blockade of the ascending dopamine pathways and may be attributable in part to dopamine depletion in the limbic system, especially in the nucleus accumbens. Cognitive deficits of the disease may be due to loss of dopamine from nerve endings in the cortex. Although recent evidence suggests that the loss of striatal dopamine alone accounts for most of the symptoms, in PD there also are losses of noradrenergic neurons in the locus ceruleus and losses of noradrenergic and serotonergic neurons in the raphe nuclei. Parkinsonian-like symptoms can be produced in experimental animals more easily by altering specific transmitter systems, such as dopamine, which causes an abnormal output from the BG, than by lesions in the BG, which eliminate the output.

Parkinsonian patients have difficulty in performing two motor acts simultaneously. Dopamine may play a critical role in the coordination (antagonistic suppression, coactivation, and general suppression) of different motor signals.

Output from GPi may increase from 80 Hz to 100 Hz, and this may account for the hypokinesia. Increased activity in the *indirect* pathway seems to be responsible. Dyskinesia (wild disoriented movements of the contralateral limbs) induced by lesion of STN yields opposite effects, with decreased GPi output.

There are limited areas in the STN in which small injections of muscimol—lowering the BG output—can ameliorate specific defects, such as arm akinesia (Bergman, Wichmann, and DeLong 1990), and so the presence of dopamine is not essential for BG function.

Huntington's disease is characterized by heritability, chorea, and dementia. Death usually occurs 15–20 years after onset. The first signs of the disorder are subtle: absentmindedness, irritability, and depression accompanied by fidgeting, clumsiness, or sudden falls. Uncontrolled movements (chorea, from the Greek *choreia*, dance or dancing movements), a prominent feature of the disease, gradually increase. Speech is slurred at first, then incomprehensible, and finally stops altogether as facial expressions become distorted and grotesque. Cognitive functions also deteriorate, and eventually the ability to

reason disappears. The disease is characterized by degeneration of GABAergic neurons in the striatum, cell loss in the cortex, and reduction in choline acetyltransferase, glutamic acid decarboxylase, and GABA. Nerve cell death (up to 90%) in the striatum is thought to cause the chorea.

The impaired cognitive functions and eventual dementia may be due either to the concomitant loss of cortical neurons or to the disruption of normal activity in the cognitive portions of the BG: the dorsolateral prefrontal and lateral orbitofrontal circuits.

Huntington's disease (hyperkinetic and hypotonic) and PD (hypokinetic and hypertonic) are associated with almost opposite alterations in BG output (decreased in Huntington's disease and increased in PD). Moreover, in both disorders, the STN is implicated strongly in mediating the abnormal BG output. Normally, a balance is maintained among the activities of three biochemically distinct but functionally interrelated systems: the nigrostriatal dopaminergic system, the intrastriatal cholinergic neurons, and the GABAergic system, which projects from the striatum to the GP and substantia nigra.

In PD, reduction of the dopaminergic system causes an increase in the output of the BG to the thalamus, leading to tremor, rigidity, and bradykinesia. In Huntington's disease, the GABAergic projection neurons are destroyed. The loss of striatal neurons in Huntington's disease is selective, first involving the population of GABAergic neurons projecting to the GPe and GABA neurons that project to the SNr. This loss releases the inhibition of the GPe and thus suppresses subthalamic activity as a result of the increased GABAergic input.

10.2.2 Role of BG in Sequential Movement

Further studies have investigated PD for more insight into the role of BG in sequential movement. Morris et al. (1988) studied planning ability in a group of medicated PD patients and in a group of matched control subjects, using a computerized version of Shallice's Tower of London task. The PD group was unimpaired on measures of the ability to execute a given plan of action or to generate low-level strategies required for efficient searching and in spatial working memory capacity, all of which contribute to performance on the planning task. The patients also were unimpaired in terms of the average number of moves required to solve a Tower of London problem. Of course, the fact that the patients were medicated reduces the significance of these negative findings. However, a specific planning deficit was evident when "thinking" times were analyzed, which occurred after the confounding influence of motor initiation and execution times had been extracted carefully from total performance times. It is suggested that an attention-switching problem accounts for this planning deficit.

This notion of an attention-switching problem may be related to the finding that external cues appear to enhance performance in PD patients by replacing defective, internally generated cues (discharges) of the BG (see the primate studies of Schultz and Romo 1992). Kritikos et al. (1995) studied the effect of contingent and noncontingent auditory cueing. PD patients and their normal controls performed two experiments involving a sequential movement task, depressing a series of buttons at choice points along a response board. Visual or auditory cues were presented prior to each move according to various contingencies. PD typically manifests with poor execution of motor sequences. External cueing facilitated motor sequencing in PD patients. In particular, auditory cues which occurred late in the movement cycle maximally facilitated switching between subcomponents of a sequence. Georgiou et al. (1994) also examined the extent of reliance by PD patients on external cues. Eighteen patients with idiopathic PD and their matched controls performed a series of button presses at sequential choice points along a response board. The illuminated pathway to be followed was extinguished successively ahead of each move according to three levels of reduction of external cues. Patients with PD were particularly disadvantaged with high levels of reduction of external cueing in terms both of movement preparation time (button down time) and movement execution time (movement time between buttons). Moreover, with high levels of reduction of external cueing, patients with PD were particularly subject to progressive slowing (movement time, not down time) further down the sequence.

Dominey et al. (1995b) found that motor imagery of a lateralized sequential task is slowed asymmetrically in hemi-parkinsonian patients. They compared right-handed, asymmetrical (right side affected) PD patients with age-matched controls in a manual finger-sequencing test using left and right hands in vision, no-vision, and motor imagery conditions. All patients favored the left hand and even displayed *motor imagery asymmetry*, mentally simulating movement more slowly with the right, affected hand than with the left hand. These data support the hypotheses that motor sequence imagery and execution share common neural structures and that the frontostriatal system is among these shared structures.

Because we are on the topic of sequential movement, we depart from diseases of the BG in the rest of this section to examine other human motor behavior studies that show us that, in mediating sequential behavior, the BG act cooperatively with (at least) lateral premotor cortex, the SMA, and the adjacent anterior cingulate area. A skilled typist can type accurately from a text while holding a conversation. The task of copy typing has become automatic; this means that the person can attend to another task at the same time. Jenkins et al. (1994) used positron emission tomography (PET) imaging to measure brain activity changes that occur when a task becomes automatic, with scans performed at different times during learning. The subjects learned sequences of key presses by trial and error using auditory feedback, and both the timing of their responses and their errors in sequence were measured. Two groups of subjects were scanned by using the same paradigm. The subjects were scanned with their eyes closed under three different conditions: during the process of acquiring new motor sequences, while performing a motor sequence that they had practiced until they could perform it automatically, and at rest.

The areas in which the activation during performance of the prelearned task was greater than the activation during rest include the cerebellar hemispheres bilaterally (with a significant activation) and posterior lobes of the vermis. Also, there were foci of activation that appear to lie in the cerebellar nuclei. There was activation of the left putamen, and there was also a focus of activation on the right border between the striatum and claustrum. The ventral thalamus was activated bilaterally. The activated cortical areas include left sensorimotor cortex, left lateral premotor cortex, SMA, and the adjacent anterior cingulate area. Compared with the rest condition, there was a significant depression in activation in both temporal lobes, including both the left and right hippocampus.

The areas in which there was a greater activation in new learning than during rest include both cerebellar hemispheres and the anterior and posterior lobes of the vermis. There were also foci of activation that appeared to lie in the cerebellar nuclei. A separate increase in regional cerebral blood flow (rCBF) was found in the midbrain near the midline, in the region of the red nucleus. The left putamen was activated, and there was also a focus of activation near the claustrum between the right striatum and insula. Compared with the rest condition, there was a significant depression extending to the temporal lobes and the hippocampus on both sides. Decreases also were found in several other cortical areas.

On the basis of these data and data on areas in which activation differed between new learning and the prelearned task, Jenkins et al. (1994) hypothesized that the cerebellum plays some role in the process by which learned tasks become automatic, the putamen either performs the same function in new learning and in performance of the prelearned sequence task or different subpopulations of cells are active to the same extent in these two situations, but that motor learning need not engage the hippocampal system. Reduced activity of areas concerned with visual processing (particularly during new learning) suggested that selective attention may involve depressing the activity of cells in modalities that are not engaged by the task. When subjects learn new sequences of motor actions, prefrontal cortex is activated, but when a motor task has become automatic, the prefrontal cortex no longer is engaged. However, our initial attempts to relate neural firing to PET activity (sec. 8.4.3) show that the lack of significant PET activity does not preclude sparse but computationally significant synaptic activity in a given region.

Seitz and Roland (1992) offered further evidence that the BG are involved critically in the learning phase of a movement sequence, establishing the final motor program. Cerebral structures participating in learning of a manual skill were mapped with rCBF measurements and PET in nine healthy volunteers. The task was a complicated right-hand finger-movement sequence. The subjects were examined at three stages: during initial practice of the finger-movement sequence, in an advanced stage of learning, and after they had learned the finger-movement sequence. Quantitative evaluation of videotapes and electromyographic records of the right forearm and hand muscles demonstrated that the finger movements significantly accelerated and became more regular. Significant mean rCBF increases were induced in the left motor hand area, the left premotor cortex, the left SMA, the left sensory hand area, the left supplementary sensory area, and the right anterior lobe of the cerebellum. During the learning process, significant depressions of the mean rCBF occurred bilaterally in the superior parietal lobule, the anterior parietal cortex, and the pars triangularis of the right inferior frontal cortex. The mean rCBF increases in these structures during the initial stage of learning were related to somatosensory feedback processing and internal language for the guidance of the finger movements. These activations disappeared when the subjects had learned the finger-movement sequence. Conversely, the mean rCBF significantly rose during the course of learning in the midsector of the putamen and GP on the left side.

Halsband et al. (1993) focused on the role of premotor cortex (PMC) and the SMA in the temporal control of movement in humans. Temporal control of movement

was analyzed systematically in patients with unilateral lesions of the lateral or medial PMC or SMA and in age-matched controls. The ability to learn new temporal adjustments was evaluated by examining rhythm reproduction that used either the left or right hand or both hands in an alternating manner. A severe impairment in rhythm reproduction was found after lateral or medial PMC lesions; the deficit was most pronounced when patients were required to use both hands in an alternating manner. The impairment occurred in the absence of difficulties in manual dexterity or impairments in discriminating the rhythm patterns. A second series of experiments examined the contribution of the SMA in organizing movements in the time domain. In this series, two patients with left-sided lesions (including the SMA but sparing tissue from the lateral hemispheric surface) and seven age-matched controls were requested to reproduce rhythm constellations both in the presence of a sound signal and from memory. Results revealed that patients with left medial lesions involving the SMA had most severe difficulties to produce any rhythms from memory, though they were able to produce the rhythms under auditory pacing (reminiscent of the way in which BG mediates internal cueing). This deficit in programming sequential patterns from memory in the time domain should be interpreted in the context of a decline in the ability to benefit from previous stimulus presentation, which prevents an effective later programming of these sequences when they have to be rehearsed from memory. It was found that patients with left SMA lesions had an increase in reaction time on a sequential digit task when sequences had to be produced under delayed conditions; by contrast, the controls showed a decrease of reaction time after previous stimulus presentation. In summary, both PMC and SMA play an important role in temporal organization of movements, but SMA seems more crucial in internally remembered motor sequences (though not in sensory-guided sequential activities).

Pascualleone et al. (1996) studied the role of the dorsolateral prefrontal cortex in procedural learning. Normal subjects completed several blocks of a serial reaction time task, using only one hand without or with concurrent noninvasive repetitive transcranial magnetic stimulation. To disrupt their function transiently, stimulation was applied at low intensity over the SMA or over the dorsolateral prefrontal cortex contralateral or ipsilateral to the hand used for the test. Stimulation to the contralateral dorsolateral prefrontal cortex markedly impaired procedural implicit learning, as documented by the lack of significant change in response times during the task. Stimulation over the other areas did not interfere with learning. These results support the notion of a critical role of contralateral dorsolateral prefrontal structures in learning of motor sequences.

10.3 Self-Reorganization of the Striatum

Self-organization is ubiquitous in the nervous system, as we have seen in different parts of the book. This section deals with the self-organizing aspects of the BG. We address first the self-organizing character of the pattern formation of striatal compartments. Then, we focus on the relationship between the modular remapping architecture, the tonic firing of certain striatal neurons, and their role in coordinated motor behavior.

10.3.1 Pattern Formation of Striatal Compartments

Patch and matrix compartments are the fundamental units in the mammalian striatum (sec. 10.1.3) but only in the mammal: The compartmentalization of striatum may be an emergent evolutionary phenomenon in the mammalian line. The development of striatal compartments to patches was analyzed by van de Kooy et al. (1987). Their questions are related to self-organizing pattern formation: How do group of cells aggregate to form functional units? What are the steps of the developmental mechanism leading to multicellular aggregates?

Because several striatal markers are compartmentalized prenatally, important events that establish the compartment must occur embryonically. Specifically, neurons in the striatal patch compartment are connected to the substantia nigra embryonically. How do the embryonic patch neurons physically aggregate into patches? It seems likely that migration and adhesion are the primary processes that compartmentalize the striatum. A selectively adhering patch population provides one possible mechanism for compartmentalizing the striatum during late embryogenesis. Cepeda et al. (1989) and Walsh et al. (1989) found that electrotonic coupling between neurons occurs between neostriatal neurons and that the incidence of interneuronal coupling declines with age. The high incidence of coupling in early development might reflect intercellular communication that contributes to cell differentiation and pattern formation.

Pattern formation (the aggregation of groups of cells into functional units) should be distinguished from phenotypic differentiation. Though the latter is related to a rigid program of phenotypic expression, the former could be considered as a self-organization phenomenon.

10.3.2 Modular Remapping, Binding, and Sensorimotor Learning

Graybiel et al. (1994) analyzed the relationship between the architecture of the BG and the BG's role in adaptive motor control. Modular remapping occurs in the BG; the input-output architecture of the striatum has a modular structure that remaps cortical inputs onto distributed local modules of striatal projection neurons. The remapping shows general topographical organization, which is broken by local constraints to focus inputs into special modules. Divergence from the cortex to the striatum is followed by reconvergence from the striatum to the pallidum. Though the information is parceled into distributed modules in the striatum, it can be brought together again at the next stage of processing. Within individual modules, there is a local spatiotemporal coherence, whereas across the modules there is diversity, which could allow plasticity in striatal processing. Organized local processing is the key feature of the remapping in the striatum. How can the activities in different constellations of modules be coordinated? One answer might be an analogy between the module coordination process and the binding problem assumed to be solved in the visual system (sec. 4.5.2) and hypothesized also in the motor system.

TANs, the presumptive inhibitory interneurons of striatum, may contribute to temporal binding across such modular networks during behavioral learning by undergoing dopamine-sensitive changes. Learning is accompanied by changes in neuronal firing patterns of TANs (Aosaki et al. 1994). TAN responses are distributed broadly and are coordinated temporally and may have a special functional role in coordinating the distributed modular circuitry of cortical–basal ganglia channels. Graybiel et al. (1994) suggested that the motor analog of the binding problem could be solved by the striatal modular architecture, the divergent input structure, and the coordination of loop activities by distributed sets of TANs. TAN responses also are reward-related and DOPA-dependent: Nigrostriatal dopaminergic input plays the role of the "teacher." (See sec. 10.6 for reinforcement learning in the BG.)

It has been found that midbrain dopamine-containing neurons that project to the striatum fire in response to novel and reward-reinforced stimuli. Also, it has been found that as time progresses, a sufficiently trained monkey's TAN activity eventually disappears. This finding indicates that learning has taken place and that the influence of these neurons on the striatum no longer is necessary. TANs gradually develop a response to conditioned stimuli. In an experiment conducted on a monkey, clicks or light flashes were paired with a reward (conditioning). The TANs started firing in response to the CS. Initially, a very small percentage (10–15%) fired for the CS independent of the reward. Following 3 weeks of training, roughly two-thirds of the TANs fired in response to the CS. It was found that the TANs had retained their responsiveness to the CS even after a 4-week hiatus. It appears that learning had taken place initially, was put into storage, and was retrieved from storage on resumption of the task. The CRs of the TANs were stored somewhere in memory.

Both the TANs and the dopamine-containing neurons of the midbrain appear to code for reinforcement or incentive stimuli. However, there are two major differences between them: TANs did not fire for novel or initial offerings of rewarded stimuli even though later they were active for such stimuli, and once the TANs acquired a responsiveness to a particular stimulus, they continued to maintain that responsiveness, whereas the midbrain neurons' firing activity gradually disappeared with time. This decreased responsiveness after overtraining was interpreted by Schultz et al. (Ljungberg, Apicella, and Schultz 1992; Schultz et al. 1993) as paralleling the animal's reduced attention to the conditioned stimulus as the task became merely a "temporal reference" for the automatic execution of behavior. Thus, nigrostriatal dopamine-containing neurons code for the incentive value of stimuli. Their projections onto the TANs in the striatum could condition the TANs to acquire this responsiveness gradually. The TANs in turn could modulate striatal projections to other regions, which ultimately would result in the initiation of learned behaviors and the storage of these behaviors (sequences). By placing the nigrostriatal dopamine-containing neurons as the bridge between the limbic system and the striatum, this model provides a mechanism by which the limbic system can interact with the motor system. The excitatory projection from the striatum to the SMA also would initiate movement. Thus, as was seen in our study of the oculomotor system, the BG could contribute to the initiation of movement in a behaviorally context-dependent manner, either directly promoting the occurrence of a particular behavior as a sequence of multiple movements or indirectly contributing to them by inhibiting competing movements or postures (Kimura, Aosaki, and Ishida 1993).

10.4 Role of Basal Ganglia in Saccade Control

We now focus on the "oculomotor loop" of the BG, presenting a model of the role of the entire loop in generating the fast eye movements known as *saccades* and paying particular attention to the interactions between the BG and the working memory systems of prefrontal cortex (Fuster 1995). In section 10.4.1, we complete the exposition of the Dominey-Arbib (1992) model of saccade control. In section 10.4.2, we extend this model by looking at a possible role of corticostriatal plasticity in learning how a visual cue can determine which of multiple potential targets will be chosen as actual target for a saccade. Especially interesting is that this extended model exhibits spatial generalization.

10.4.1 Basal Ganglia and Working Memory

The SC influences the brainstem saccade generator, with the topographical code of target position transformed into the appropriate time course of burst neuron activity to move the eyes to the target (chapter 3). Cortical systems play down on this collicular-brainstem system to yield an increasingly rich pattern of oculomotor behaviors, an activity that emphasizes the role of working memory in delay saccades (chap. 8; fig. 8.28, 8.29). The output of the retina travels through various waystations to the posterior parietal cortex (PP). Dynamic remapping of visual information is controlled by corollary discharge to PP, with PP projecting to the quasi-visual cells in SC, yielding a model of the double-saccade paradigm. PP then sends target information (whether relayed from current visual input or remapped) to the FEF. FEF do project to the brainstem (thus allowing generation of eye movements even after lesion of SC), but here we emphasize (1) the FEF projection to SC, focusing on two types of cells, the FOn ("fovea on") cells active when a target occupies the fovea and FEFsac (FEF cells coding saccades) that code the loci of possible targets and (2) the reciprocal interaction with MD thalamus that is posited to underlie working memory during the delay period for a memory saccade.

As is seen in figure 8.29, two inhibitory nuclei of the BG, CD and SNr, are arranged in series and provide an additional link between the FEF and SC. This link allows FEF selectively to modulate the tonic inhibition of SNr on SC and thalamus through CD (Deniau and Chevalier 1985; Alexander, Delong, and Strick 1986). In addition, the BG pathways provide a mechanism for the initiation of corticothalamic interactions via the removal of SNr inhibition on MD.

In our model of these functions of the BG, the FEF has an excitatory projection to CD—a topographical projection that preserves saccade amplitude and direction—that can regulate SNr's inhibition of SC (Bruce and Goldberg 1984; Segraves and Goldberg 1987; Stanton, Goldberg, and Bruce 1988a). Hikosaka, Sakamoto, and Usui (1989a–c) found a large number of caudate neurons that were responsive to visual saccade targets and to remembered targets. To provide cortical control while a target is foveated, foveal cells in FEF could gate activity in CD and SC, preventing saccades while a target is fixated. Target fixation is signaled by the activity of so-called FOn cells in FEF, which serve to reduce the likelihood that SC will generate a saccade. This tends to keep the system stable when targets are foveated by preventing peripheral targets from exciting CD and SC (Bruce and Goldberg 1984; Segraves and Goldberg 1987).

Figure 10.2 shows the data and a simulation for FEF-mem memory cells based on the model in section 8.4.2, and figure 10.3 introduces the role of the BG. The majority of saccade-related cells found in the CD are phasically active before and during saccades (Hikosaka, Sakamoto, and Usui 1989a). Roughly one-third of these cells had presaccadic activity for both visual and memory-guided saccades. This phasic activity is attributable to the corticostriatal projection (Stanton, Goldberg, and Bruce 1988a), so we simply model saccade-related cells of caudate (CDsac) as driven by saccade-related cells of FEF (FEFsac). In addition, CD has sustained memory response cells that are tonically active following the presentation of a target that is to be remembered for a subsequent saccade until the offset of the fixation point (Hikosaka, Sakamoto, and Usui 1989c). Thus, the model simulates two types of task-dependent CD cells, CDsac and CD-sustained memory response cells (CDmem), attributing their activity to the corticostriatal projection (Stanton, Goldberg, and Bruce 1988a), with CDmem cells driven by the FEFmem memory cells (i.e., the FEF cells with maintained activity during the delay period for a memory saccade). Continuing the equations to describe the model (sec. 8.4.2), we model the CD saccade response as being driven solely by FEFsac:

$$\tau_{CDsac} = 10 \text{ msec}$$

$$S_{CDsac} = FEFsac \tag{1}$$

and the CD memory response as driven solely by FEFmem:

$$\tau_{CDmem} = 10 \text{ msec}$$

$$S_{CDmem} = FEFmem \tag{2}$$

CD inhibits SNr via the direct pathway, controlling SNr inhibition of SC. (The indirect pathway is not included in the present model.) Hikosaka and Wurtz (1983a–d) showed that the SNr provides a tonic (50–100 spikes/sec) inhibitory topographical projection to the SC, preventing SC from generating saccade signals and thus forming an *inhibitory mask* on SC. Visual and memory-related decreases of SNr firing rate release collicular inhibition and facilitate initiation of saccades. Again, we simulate two classes of cells, related to saccade and memory responses. The tonic activity of SNsac and SNmem cells is inhibited by a topographical projection from the CDsac and CDmem cells, respectively. This dual inhibition (CD on SNr and SNr on SC) allows cortex to manage selectively the inhibitory mask on SC via the FEF-to-CD pathway. By managing the SNr inhibitory mask on SC via CD, the FEF can control the targets for saccades selectively, overriding collicular attempts to initiate saccades to distracting peripheral targets. Thus, we model SNr by two layers, SNRsac and SNRmem, each with a tonic activity level that can be lowered by inhibition from the corresponding layer of CD:

$$\tau_{SNRsac} = 40 \text{ msec}$$

$$S_{SNRsac} = 100 - CDsac \tag{3}$$

$$\tau_{SNRmem} = 40 \text{ msec}$$

$$S_{SNRmem} = 100 - CDmem \tag{4}$$

Cortical control over thalamocortical interactions provides the basis for spatial memory. In the nigrothalamocortical system of the rhesus monkey, Ilinsky, Jouandet, and Goldman-Rakic (1985) found a topographical pathway from SNr to VA magnocellular and MD paralaminar nuclei of the thalamus, and from these thalamic nuclei to the FEF. The MD projection to FEF is topographical and reciprocal. In addition, MD neurons show a sustained activity during the delay period of a delayed-response task, and cooling the prefrontal cortex in the principal sulcal area causes a reversible disruption of the sustained response in the MD neurons during the delay period (Alexander and Fuster 1973). On the basis of similar deficits in memory saccade and delayed-response tasks from prefrontal lesions, the model follows the assumption that the memory saccade task and the delayed-response tasks employ at some level the same thalamocortical mechanism for storage of visuospatial targets (Goldman-Rakic 1987).

The activity of this spatial memory could be regulated by the inhibitory topographical projection from SNr to MD (see figure 10.3). Absence of SNr inhibition allows

a)

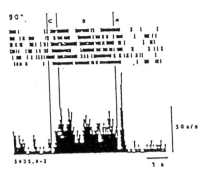

b)

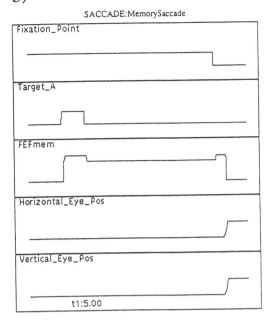

c)

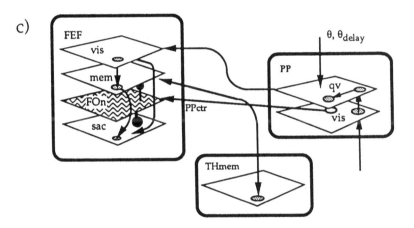

Figure 10.2

Frontal eye fields (FEF) sustained response during memory saccade task. (a) Response of a directionally sensitive sustained response FEF cell. The top six traces show the "raster" of spikes generated by the cell in six separate trials, one per line. The bottom trace shows the histogram obtained by summing an entire set of such spike trains. The vertical lines labeled *C* indicate the presentation of the target. The portion labeled *D* represents the delay period, and *R* indicates the response period signaled by the offset of the fixation point. This neuron had significant excitatory tonic activity during the delay period of the memory saccade when the target was presented in its visual field and was suppressed when the target was away from the cell's visual field. (Reprinted with permission from Funahashi, Bruce, and Goldman-Rakic 1989). (b) Simulation of the sustained response in the delay task. The upper trace shows the fixation point, the second trace shows the target, the third shows the sustained FEF cell (FEFmem), and the last two traces show the horizontal and vertical eye displacement. Note that though there is fluctuation in the activity of the FEF cell in (a), our FEFmem cell shows fairly constant activation. The spike at the end of the delay period is not captured by our simulation; we model only average firing rates, not individual spike generation. Further, our cell represents the average activity over a population of cells, rather than a single cell. (c) A model of cortical and thalamic structures involved in the sustained response. See figure 8.29 for further details. (Reprinted with permission from Dominey and Arbib 1992.)

a)

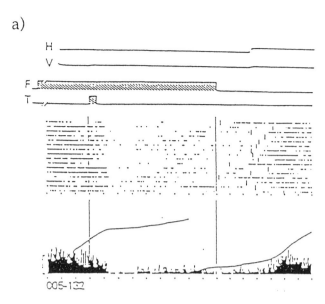

```
H  _____  ___
V  _____
F _▨▨▨▨▨▨▨▨▨▨▨▨▨▨▨▨▨▨▨▨▨_____
T _/▨_____
```

005-132

c)

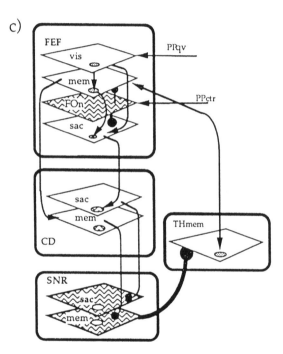

b)

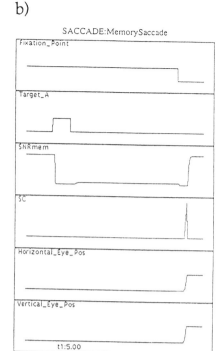

SACCADE:MemorySaccade

Fixation_Point

Target_A

SNRmem

SC

Horizontal_Eye_Pos

Vertical_Eye_Pos

t1:5.00

Figure 10.3

Extension of the model shown in figure 10.2. The extension brings in the role of caudate (CD) and substantia nigra pars reticulata (SNR) in providing a memory-contingent sustained response. (a) This cell shows sustained decrease in firing in response to a target in the contralateral visual field that is to be memorized for the delay saccade task. (See the caption to figure 10.2a for an explanation of the raster graph and histogram.) The decrease usually follows the target presentation and remains until the saccade onset. (Reprinted with permission from Hikosaka and Wurtz 1983c). (b) Simulation of the memory-contingent sustained response (SNRmem). The sustained suppression of SNr allows the medio-dorsal thalamus to participate in the reciprocal activity with frontal eye fields (FEF) that instantiates a spatial memory. This SNRmem is inhibited by CDmem, which in turn is excited tonically by FEFmem in the delay period of the memory saccade. (c) Model of cortico-striato-nigro-thalamo-cortical path subserving spatial memory. See figure 8.29 for further details. (Reprinted with permission from Dominey and Arbib 1992.)

reciprocal connections between FEF and MD to generate a spatial "memory" cycle or loop (Hikosaka 1989). Once a saccade has been made to a remembered target, the memory trace must be erased to prevent generation of further saccades of equal magnitude and direction. The SC projects to the dorsal thalamus (Ilinsky, Jouandet, and Goldman-Rakic 1985). The model uses an inhibitory path from SC to MD so that when a saccade is elicited, it will erase the FEF ↔ MD trace of the remembered target location. In the memory saccade task, while the fixation point is still present and the target briefly appears, the memory-contingent sustained SNr cell (SNRmem) reduces its inhibition on the thalamus to allow the initiation of the thalamus ↔ FEF cyclical excitation that embodies the memory function. The CD participates by inhibiting SNr, setting up the conditions for the thalamocortical memory to be instantiated. As seen in section 8.4.2 (equation 17), Dominey and Arbib proposed that reciprocal connection between FEF and MD thalamus implements the spatial memory

$$\tau_{FEFmem} = 8 \text{ msec}$$

$$S_{FEFmem} = 8 * THmem + FEFvis - 0.25 * FOn \quad (5)$$

where FEFvis initiates storage, the interaction with THmem sustains it, and the FOn term yields an increase in activity at removal of the fixation point. In bringing in the role of the BG in target memory, we now posit that in addition to its reciprocal interaction with FEFmem, THmem receives input SNRmem from substantia nigra and SC_Delay:

$$\tau_{THmem} = 100 \text{ msec}$$

$$S_{THmem} = 2.0 * FEFmem - 2.0 * SNRmem - 8 * SC\_Delay \quad (6)$$

10.4.2 Another Model of Visuomotor Conditioning

The apparent redundancy of the two pathways from FEF to SC presents a paradox: FEF both signals the locus of a saccade by direct excitation to SC and disinhibits the corresponding SC locus via the BG. This duplicity might suggest that the BG are unnecessary and play a completely redundant role in relaying the FEF command to SC. However, Dominey, Arbib, and Joseph (1995) suggest an answer to this paradox in the use of corticostriatal plasticity to allow the BG to modulate the FEF pattern on the basis of experience. We thus turn from the question of working memory to that of long-term memory and, in particular, to issues of visuomotor conditional learning and of sequential behavior.

Dominey and Arbib (1992) hypothesized that if the FEF and direct visual input do not yield the encoding of a unique target in the deep layers of SC, a WTA mechanism will choose one of the targets. To remove the paradox, we argue that experience based on inferotemporal (IT) or prefrontal information may provide contextual, learned information to bias activity in the BG and thereby "tip the balance" to one "winner" or another. Dominey, Arbib, and Joseph (1995) make the strong hypothesis that this learning is mediated by corticostriatal plasticity (figure 10.4). Later versions can look at alternative sites (see following discussion) once we see how to marshal the data appropriately. We first illustrate this for a model of visual-motor conditional learning. The next section treats sequence learning.

The paradigm for visuomotor conditional learning here is to present to a monkey two visual targets on either side of the fixation point, now a patterned stimulus such as a red circle or a blue triangle. First, we present the fixation point, which is also the cue for the appropriate response; then, we present both targets with the cue; and finally, when the fixation point goes off (there being no delay in this paradigm), the monkey is to saccade to one of the two targets. Each cue codes for a particular direction (e.g., when the cue is the blue triangle, the monkey will always and only be rewarded for a saccade to the right-hand target). In both experimental data and model simulation, we see in the monkey's behavior a transition from a random response to a consistent response to the target associated with the current cue, with other cues reliably associated with the opposite response.

The basic idea of the model is illustrated in figure 10.5a. If we have twin peaks in the FEF activity playing on SC and we feed them into a WTA circuit with a little noise added, then it would be random as to which one of the peaks would be selected, and thus to which target the system will saccade. This effect occurs in the Dominey-Arbib model if we add a little bit of noise as the visual input passes through PP and FEF. However, if we add disinhibition to, say, the rightmost peak, the WTA will select the rightmost target. What we would like is to have a learning process that pairs disinhibition with the appropriate cue (figure 10.6).

Using the FEF as the center of the figure, the left side of the figure can be recognized as a restructuring of figure 8.29, with PP driving FEF, which commands SC both monosynaptically and via CD and SNr. The new parts of the model are shown at right. Though information about target location continues to be available via PP, information about the shape and color of the fixated

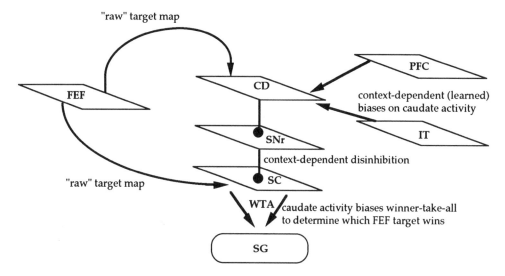

Figure 10.4
Simplified illustration of the model of corticostriatal plasticity for selective disinhibition. When multiple targets are represented in the frontal eye fields (FEF) command to caudate (CD) and superior colliculus (SC), the choice between these targets (the winner-take-all [WTA] activity between SC and the saccade generator [SG]) can be made as a result of additional corticostriatal influences that will favor one of the targets. Corticostriatal projections from inferotemporal cortex (IT) and prefrontal cortex (PFC) are modified by learning to bias caudate—and thus, via substantia nigra pars reticulata (SNr), SC—in favor of the correct one of multiple saccade targets dependent on the association or sequence context. (Reprinted with permission from Dominey, Arbib, and Joseph 1991.)

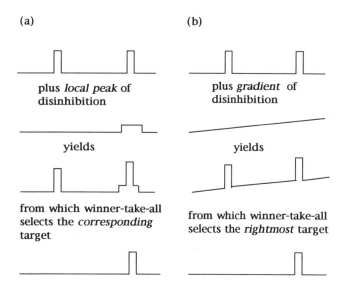

Figure 10.5
Basic concept of visuomotor conditional learning of preferred target location. The second line of each diagram shows the peak of disinhibition that can tilt the balance in a winner-take-all mechanism to select (a) the peak that is in the corresponding position or (b) the rightmost of two peaks, whatever its position. (Reprinted with permission from Dominey, Arbib, and Joseph 1995.)

cue travels via V4 to IT and thence projects onto the same CD cells as those influenced by FEF. At present, we assume no structure to these connections, only that each distinctive cue will yield a distinctive pattern of IT input to CD and that the synapses carrying these patterns are distributed uniformly across CD.

If the monkey is correct, it gets rewarded with a squirt of juice. We know from the work of Schultz, Apicella, and Ljunberg (1993) that the effect of reward is that dopamine is released from SNc to striatum. We hypothesize that this helps to modify the IT → CD synapses according to a reinforcement learning rule that says that at active CD cells, when dopamine is released, synapses from active IT cells will be strengthened (LTP), whereas those for other IT cells will be weakened (LTD), to yield a normalization effect with overall synaptic strength remaining the same. Formally, this is expressed by the equations:

$$w_{ij}(t + 1) := w_{ij}(t)$$

$$+ \text{DA\_Modulation} * (\text{RewardContingency}$$

$$- 1) * C1 * F_i * F_j \tag{7}$$

$$w_{ij}(t + 1) := w_{ij}(t + 1) * \frac{\sum_j w_{ij}(t)}{\sum_j w_{ij}(t + 1)} \tag{8}$$

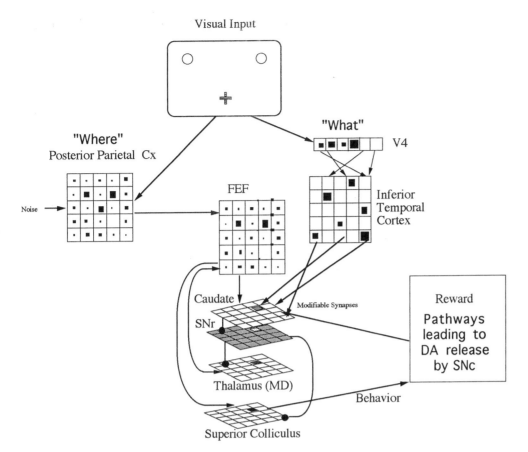

Visual Input

"Where"
Posterior Parietal Cx

"What"

V4

Noise →

FEF

Inferior
Temporal
Cortex

Caudate

Modifiable Synapses

SNr

Reward
Pathways
leading to
DA release
by SNc

Thalamus (MD)

Behavior

Superior Colliculus

Figure 10.6
Schematic of visuomotor conditional learning model. Cue-related activity in inferotemporal cortex (IT) is produced from features extracted from visual cue input in visual area V4. IT influences saccade production via its projections to caudate. Random noise added to the visual input in PP breaks the symmetry between the two targets, providing a form of guessing. On correct cue-guided saccades, a reward contributes to strengthening synapses between IT cells activated by the cue and caudate cells participating in the saccade. After training, cue-driven activity in IT preferentially will drive the caudate cells involved in the correct saccade to overpower the noise in the posterior parietal cortex (Cx), yielding correct performance. FEF, frontal eye fields; SNc, substantia nigra pars compacta; SNc, substantia nigra pars reticulata; MD, mediodorsal thalamus. (Reprinted with permission from Dominey, Arbib, and Joseph 1991.)

where the ":=" denotes assignment rather than equality. F_i and F_j are the firing rates of the IT and CD cells, respectively, whereas w_{ij} is the strength of the synapse from IT cell i to CD cell j. We simulate reward-related modulation (which we regard as mediated by dopamine release from SNc) by the term *RewardContingency*, which is 1.5 for correct trials, 0.5 for incorrect trials, and 1 when no reward or punishment is applied, corresponding to the increases and decreases in SNc activity seen for reward and error trials, respectively (Schultz 1989). The term $DA\_Modulation * (RewardContingency - 1)$ will be positive on rewarded trials and negative on error trials. C1 is a constant that specifies the learning rate.

Weight normalization conserves the total synaptic weight that each IT cell can distribute to its striatal synapses (equation 8). If, after learning has occurred, one synapse from cell i to cell j was increased, because the total synaptic weight from cell i is conserved, the result of this increase is a small decrease in all other synapses from i. Similarly, when a weight is decreased owing to an incorrect response, the other synapses from i are increased. Via this normalization, postsynaptic cells compete for influence from presynaptic cells, producing cue discrimination. Especially in the case of rewarded trials, equations 7 and 8 approximate how LTP may occur in the most active postsynaptic cells (via equation 7), and LTD in the others (via normalization, equation 8).

The term $DA\_Modulation$ expresses a role of dopamine complementary to its role in learning in a feedback loop that regulates the excitability of CD. Release of dopamine in striatum decreases the excitability of striatal cells by corticostriatal afferents and thus attenuates corticostriatal activity, allowing striatum once again to detect the effect of IT's bias. In our model, when

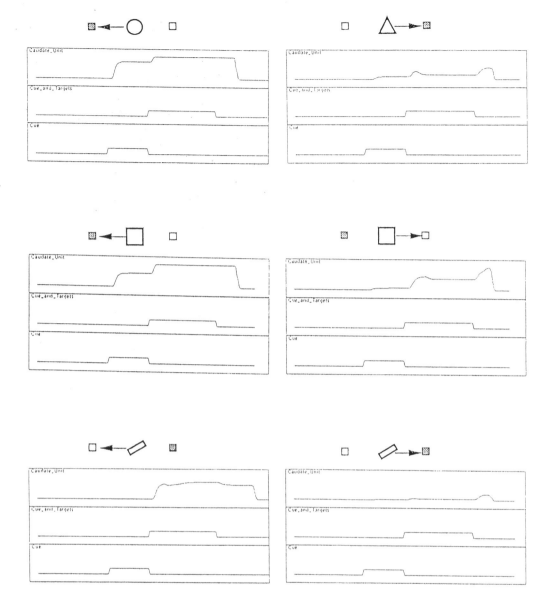

Figure 10.7
Simulated saccade preparation cell. Arrow indicates direction of saccade; dark square indicates correct direction. In each window, the lower trace indicates when the cue alone appears, the middle trace show when the cue and target overlap, and the upper trace shows the cell activity. All traces are from a cell that has preference for leftward saccades. (Left column) Responses to cued leftward saccades. In the first and second rows, the cues are associated with a leftward saccade. The cell discharges with the cues and increasingly with the targets through the saccade. This response demonstrates the task-related activity and the equivalence of two cues associated with the same saccade. In the bottom row, an incorrect saccade is made to the left with a cue associated with a rightward saccade. The cell still discharges for its preferred direction. In the right column, rightward saccades are made both in correct and in incorrect situations, and in neither case is there significant activity. (Reprinted with permission from Dominey, Arbib, and Joseph 1991.)

strong cortical inputs overstimulate striatum, SNr is inhibited strongly. This inhibition of SNr leads to the *dis*inhibition of SNc (Carlsson and Carlsson 1990). The resulting increase in activity of SNc (dopaminergic) cells leads to the increased release of dopamine in striatum, which attenuates the corticostriatal signal (Calabresi et al. 1993) (bringing the most active cells back to the maximum input capacity of striatum) and reducing the activity of the less active *surrounding* striatal cells, thus increasing the signal-to-noise ratio. (See Dominey, Arbib, and Joseph 1995 for further details). Figure 10.7 shows the successful simulation of learning affecting a saccade preparation cell.

The foregoing model hypothesizes that corticostriatal connections provide the crucial substrate for the kind of visuomotor conditional learning under study. However, where does plasticity really reside? The model posits the plasticity of a projection from IT cortex to CD. The existence of such a projection is shown by Selemon and Goldman-Rakic (1985), but this projection is sparse, and the confluence might involve PP (rather than FEF) and IT cortex. This alternative is functionally equivalent for the present model of activity in CD, SNr, and SC, but does require experimental resolution.

We now consider spatial generalization in visuomotor conditional learning. Figure 10.5a showed that a "bump" of cue-related activity placed by IT input in CD activity could cause the model to yield a saccade to a *specific* target associated with the fixation cue by reinforcement learning. However, where do we put the "bump" if we want a given cue to signal that the animal should choose, for example, the rightmost of two targets *regardless of where the two targets are located*? The theoretical answer (figure 10.6b) is to use not a bump but a gradient sloping upward to the right, so that when it is added to twin peaks, the one on the right will become higher than the one on the left and thus the WTA always will choose the rightmost one. Pleasingly, the reinforcement learning model "discovered" this solution rather than having it inserted as a constraint of the model. If we present pairs of targets in many positions but always reward, say, a saccade to the rightmost target when the cue is a blue triangle, the incremental effect is that those IT → CD synapses active for the blue triangle cue will be increasingly larger for those CD cells associated with saccades increasingly far to the right.

10.4.3 Eligibility

In reinforcement learning, the reward signal does not specify anything about the correct response. When a reward is given, our model asserts that Hebbian learning occurs; that is, IT → CD synapses that actively participate in the generation of the rewarded response are strengthened. However, when we change the sign of the reinforcement, we get an anti-hebbian rule according to which the synapses that were actively involved in generating an incorrect response are weakened.

However, note that equations 7 and 8 are set up on a trial-by-trial basis; they specify how synaptic weights are adjusted after each trial. In future, we will need to address the real-time issue, namely that the release of dopamine by SNc occurs after the animal is rewarded, which occurs after the animal has acted, which occurs after the activity in the IT → CD synapses that assisted the generation of the response. How then does such a synapse "know" that it should respond with LTD or LTP when the dopamine finally affects it? In the context of models of classic conditioning by Klopf (1982) and Sutton and

Barto (1981), the answer offered was the notion of an *eligibility trace*: A synapse "remembers" that it was activated recently. The use of second-messenger systems could mediate this eligibility so that the reward will affect just those synapses wherein eligibility is above zero. In equation 7, then, the time scale would become much finer (say millisecond by millisecond rather than trial by trial) and the term $F_i^*F_j$ would be replaced by the eligibility of the synapse w_{ij}.

We offered an interesting approach to eligibility in our study (sec. 9.4.4) of the role of the cerebellum in metric adaptation of saccades. As we have seen, in such adaptation the monkey's incorrect saccade is followed immediately by a corrective saccade. How, then, does the error signal affect those synapses involved in the incorrect saccade rather than those involved in the corrective saccade? Our answer was to shape the eligibility trace so that it peaks only after a delay of approximately 200 msec. This adjustment ensures that when the error signal (climbing fiber input to a Purkinje cell) arrives, those plastic synapses (from parallel fibers to Purkinje cells) involved in the first saccade are at the peak of their eligibility, whereas those involved in the corrective saccade are not yet eligible.

This work suggests that the shaping of the eligibility signal may be task-dependent. Thus, it has become an important goal for neuroscience to bridge from this systems level of neural analysis to that of synaptic neurochemistry (see sec. 6.3) by trying to match behavioral constraints on the dynamics of the eligibility trace with the pharmacokinetics of the secondary messengers and the like, which may mediate it. For example, Borisyuk, Wickens, and Kotter (1994) have pursued the hypothesis that calcium concentrations in dendritic spines may constitute an eligibility trace such as is used by reinforcement learning mechanisms for solving the credit assignment problem. They used a simple network model of the BG to determine the efficency of three different eligibility functions in producing and maintaining movement sequences followed by reinforcement.

10.5 Roles of the Basal Ganglia in Motor Coordination and Learning

10.5.1 Models of Sequential Behavior

As an example of the learning of new "motor programs" (see sec. 8.5.1), consider the sequence-learning paradigm studied by Barone and Joseph (1989a,b). A monkey faced three keys displayed in a triangle around the fixation point. The monkey is trained repeatedly—in

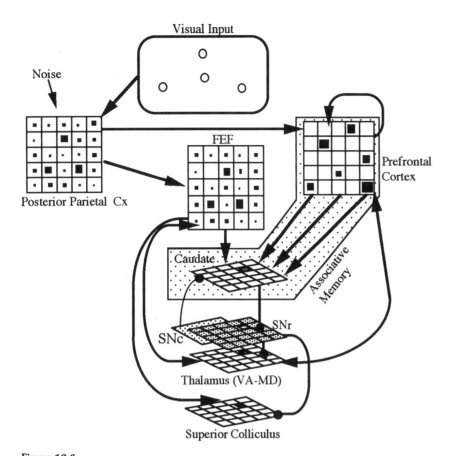

Figure 10.8

Schematic of sequencing model. Caudate saccade-related cells are influenced not only by frontal eye fields (FEF) but also by modifiable, non-topographical projections from prefrontal cortex. Prefrontal cortex combines visual, saccade-efferent copy, and self-input to generate a time-varying sequence of internal states for each presaccade period in the sequence reproduction task. These states or patterns of activity be-

come associated with caudate activity for the correct saccade by learning. Noise in posterior parietal cortex (Cx) provides initial guessing, which is dominated after learning modifies PFC-to-caudate synapses. SNr, substantia nigra pars reticulata; VA and MD, ventroanterior and mediodorsal nuclei of thalamus. (Reprinted with permission from Dominey, Arbib, and Joseph 1991.)

sequences of one, then two, then three targets—to respond to seeing the targets illuminated in a particular sequence while the fixation point is on (the fixation point itself having no cue properties) by pressing the targets in the same sequence in response to three successive "go" stimuli after the offset of the fixation point. This involves immense shaping. The monkey never "clicks" with the general idea of a sequence. Unlike a human, it cannot see a novel sequence and immediately repeat it; rather, it must be trained again and again with a specific sequence before its visual presentation can act as the cue for its manual repetition. In fact, one monkey successfully learned to repeat five of the six possible three-element sequences, yet never achieved as low an error rate with the sixth.

The Dominey, Arbib, and Joseph (1995) model for such sequence learning (figure 10.8) has a structure similar to that for visuomotor conditional learning in figure 10.6, but now the context dependence is provided by

the input from prefrontal cortex rather than IT. The self-loops in prefrontal cortex ensure that prefrontal cortex activity changes as the visual inputs are received and as subsequent saccades are triggered. Thus, prefrontal cortex input to CD is sufficiently diverse for an animal eventually to learn a set of sequences (but, as we have seen, not necessarily all the sequences).

Again, we have a model that hypothesizes that corticostriatal connections provide the crucial substrate for learning under study. Alternatives must be evaluated. Unfortunately, anatomical evidence militates against the convergence of prefrontal cortex inputs (part of the prefrontal loop) with the region of CD involved in the oculomotor loop as hypothesized in our model. An alternative would be to incorporate the known cortico-cortical connections from prefrontal cortex (PFC) to FEF. Plastic PFC → FEF synapses then could bias the target representation in FEF, so that changes in CD then would be the expression of FEF input rather than the expression of corticostriatal plasticity. (Dopamine plays a role in cortical plasticity also.)

Wickens (1993; Wickens, Hyland, and Anson 1994) outlined the form of a model in which the striatum is not a site at which motor programs are stored. Instead, he posits that motor programs are stored in the cerebral cortex, especially in areas that receive input from the striatum via the GP and thalamus. Here, a motor program is conceptualized as a cell assembly, which is stored in the form of strengthened synaptic connections between cortical pyramidal neurons. These connections constrain the combinations of movements and the sequence that will result when the cell assembly is activated. By taking into account the parallel, reentrant loops between the cerebral cortex and BG, this model of cortical cell assemblies suggests a mechanism for motor plans that involve longer sequences.

Whatever the mechanism for change, new studies from the Joseph laboratory inspired in part by the aforementioned modeling have indeed shown sequence-related activity in the caudate. Kermadi et al. (1993) and Kermadi and Joseph (1995) examined neural activity in the caudate nucleus of monkeys while the animals executed motor and oculomotor sequences based on memorized information. In each trial, the monkeys had to remember the illumination order of three fixed spatial targets. After a delay, the animals had to press the targets in the same sequence. The "task-related" cells were activated by onset of the targets and on execution of saccades or arm movements. In a majority of cells, activation depended not only on the retinal position of the stimuli or on the spatial parameters of gaze and arm movements but was contingent on the particular sequence in which the targets were illuminated or the movements were performed. During central fixation, a number of cells showed anticipatory activity preceding onset of specific events. Four groups were considered: neurons anticipating offset of the central fixation point, neurons anticipating the illumination of any target (regardless of its spatial position or order of presentation or rank), neurons anticipating the illumination of the first target (regardless of its spatial position), and neurons anticipating the illumination of a given target, regardless of its rank. Phasic visual responses to target onset also were observed, and in a majority of these, visual responses were modulated by the rank of the target(s). Many cells responded only if the corresponding target were first; other cells responded only if the target were second or if it had complex time relationships with the other targets. Cells were also observed which had postsaccadic activation, or activity associated with target pressing. Taken together, the data are compatible with the hypothesis that the CD would select the successive targets for the oculomotor apparatus as sequences progress. It would participate in the execution of the saccades and arm movements and would control the environmental changes that action generates.

10.5.2 Basal Ganglia and Motor Programs

In studying models for the learning of coordinated behaviors (sec. 8.5), we paid special attention to the role of cerebral cortex, then built on that role, primarily in schema-theoretical terms (sec. 8.6), to gain some insights into how "higher cognitive functions" of cerebral cortex might build on (and yet differ from) the mechanisms of action-oriented perception that have dominated much of our discussion of function in this volume. In chapter 9, we discussed how the cerebellum may serve to tune and coordinate motor pattern generators, with some parts of cerebellum exercising this role through interaction with cerebral cortex and other parts acting "downstream" on brainstem and spinal cord. We even examined recent suggestions that the lateralmost parts of cerebellum may refine the more cognitive processes of cerebral cortex. Like the cerebellum, the BG are part of the major corticosubcortical feedback loops of the motor system. We learn more about the BG by contrasting it explicitly with the cerebellum. Both receive major projections from the cerebral cortex and both project back to the cortex via the thalamus, but differences in their anatomical connections suggest they have different functions.

First, the BG receive inputs from the entire cerebral cortex. In contrast, the cerebellum receives input only from that part of the cortex directly related to sensorimotor functions. Also, the output of the cerebellum is directed back to the premotor and the motor cortex, whereas the output of the BG is directed not only to the premotor and the motor cortex but also to the prefrontal association cortex. Additionally, the cerebellum receives somatosensory information directly from the spinal cord and has major afferent and efferent connections with many brainstem nuclei directly connected with the spinal cord. In contrast, the BG have relatively few connections to the brainstem and have no direct connections at all to the spinal cord.

These differences suggest that the cerebellum directly regulates execution of movement, whereas the BG are involved in higher-order, cognitive aspects of motor control: the planning and execution of complex motor strategies. We studied the role of the cerebellum in saccadic adaptation—wherein the concern is with the metric scaling of saccades (chapter 9)—rather than the BG role of sequencing or working memory for target location. In that model, when a saccade does not reach its target, there is an immediate corrective saccade, and it is the magnitude of this corrective saccade that supplies an "error signal" routed via inferior olive climbing fibers to that part of the cerebellum the job of which it is to modulate and coordinate the various saccade generators of the brainstem.

Thus, we hypothesize that BG are involved in combining explicitly the "pieces" that make up a skilled behavior, whereas the cerebellum serves to turn a procedure into a skill, adjusting parameters to adapt and coordinate components of the movement to yield a seamless whole.

With this general perspective, we now turn to neurophysiological data and related theorizing on the role of BG in complex movements. In a number of visually guided tracking tasks, the cells in the BG selective for movement fire later than do cells in the cortical motor areas, and neurons in the putamen are more likely to be selective for the direction of limb movement than for the activation of specific muscles. This tendency has suggested to some workers that the BG do not play a significant role in the initiation of stimulus-triggered movements. However, Kimura (1995) argued that this lag between the neuronal activity of the prime mover muscle and movement-related BG activity in certain tasks was observed only because the behavioral tasks in these studies were simple movements. Kimura showed that if a monkey is trained in using more complex, sequential, movements, a burst of activity in the BG motor zone can be observed up to 100 milliseconds before neuronal activity in the prime mover muscle. This activity in the putamen would be indicative of initiation of a movement sequence (see clinical observations, sec. 10.2). There are two reasons why a sequential task was needed to trigger the early activity in the BG.

Both GPi and SNr output are mediated by GABA. They receive input from putamen and CD, which also are GABAergic and inhibitory in function, consistent with the hypothesis of disinhibition as the mode of BG function. This process has been demonstrated and modeled for CD → SNr → SC (and thalamus) in oculomotor function (sec. 10.4). Putamen → GPi → thalamus may play a similar role for other types of movement. Thus, just as was seen in our study of the oculomotor system, the BG could contribute to the initiation of movement in a behaviorally context-dependent manner, either directly promoting the occurrence of a particular behavior as a sequence of multiple movements or indirectly contributing to them by inhibiting competing movements or postures (Kimura, Aosaki, and Ishida 1993). However, future modeling also must bring in the role of the indirect pathway, which was ignored in the model of the oculomotor system in section 10.4. Chemical blockade of GABAergic outputs from SNr (by injection of muscimol) induces continuous locomotion in the cat (perhaps via the pathway SNr → PPN [pedunculopontine nucleus]), but continual forced saccades in the monkey. All this discussion suggests that the midbrain contains a variety of motor stations controlled by the BG, which could be evoked by BG disinhibition even in absence of cerebral cortex, perhaps SC for oculomotor ≈ PPN for locomotor. This supposition probably is true also for the crude arm and hand movements that can be obtained without cortical involvement (Lawrence and Kuypers 1968) but not true for the more precise forms of grasping for which the cortical pathways were reviewed (sec. 8.4.3).

We argue that the BG weights the current context with the "activation" and "deactivation" commands in a coordinated control program to facilitate some movements and suppress others selectively. Hikosaka (1991) hypothesized that the BG have an instrumental-instructive function, guiding the storage of motor memories in, say, premotor cortex and complementing its gating-coordinative function. BG neuronal responses are task-dependent; the current responsiveness of a neuron could be determined by the state of behavioral experience or learning and could be maintained temporarily perhaps until the relevant memory is formed in premotor cortices. Motor cortex "loads up" the motor command prior to the release allowed by BG disinhibition. Recall (sec. 10.4) that even within the oculomotor loop, we do not see the role of the BG as monolithic. Rather, we emphasize two "channels," one involved in working memory and the other involved in initiation of movement. Thus, activity in cortex during the delay period is preparatory to movement but awaits BG "permission" (disinhibition) to enter into the elicitation of a movement.

Our discussion of saccade control (sec. 10.2) introduced the notion of inhibitory masks to model the possible role of BG in gating movements. A learning model for this system (sec. 10.6) supports the notion that BG's inhibitory influences are used in the selection of movement. It gives one example of how BG might represent different components of behavior and how these elements are (re)organized to yield new combinations of movement via complex cortical loops as evidenced in the model of double saccades. On this view, selection of a movement is akin to release of BG inhibition.

STN is thought to provide SNr and GPi (the output elements of BG, which are inhibitory) with an excitatory drive. We hypothecate that STN enables cerebral cortex to suppress movements through direct connections to STN or via striatum and GPe. A major group of STN neurons shows a sustained discharge while an animal is fixating a target and anticipating a reward, maintaining high SNr activity to suppress saccades. Preparation and suppression of a movement go hand in hand. If not, initiation, sequencing, and termination of movements are devastated, as seen in Parkinsonism (sec. 10.2).

Mushiake and Strick (1995) examined the activity of neurons in the GP while two monkeys performed sequential pointing movements under two task conditions: visually guided (track task) and remembered (rem task). Almost two-thirds of the task-related neurons in GP were considered task-dependent because they displayed exclusive or enhanced changes in activity for one of the two task conditions. More than 65% of the task-dependent neurons were termed *rem neurons* because either they displayed changes in activity that occurred only during the rem task or they displayed changes that were more pronounced during the rem task than during the track task. Nearly half of the rem neurons in GP displayed activity changes limited to a single phase of the rem task (i.e., phase-specific). Phase-specific neurons varied in the extent to which their activity depended on the particular sequence of movements performed. Some displayed a change in activity for all of the eight different movement sequences. Others displayed a change in activity during only one of the eight different sequences (i.e., phase- and sequence-specific). The authors speculate that an ensemble of GP neurons with phase-specific responses could be used to encode the detailed spatio-temporal characteristics of a sequential movement.

Hikosaka (1991) posited that GPe and STN provide a shared suppression system for the otherwise separate disinhibitory systems for limb movement and eye movement (figure 10.9). Activating putamen can disinhibit STN to increase SNr inhibition so that limb movements can be antagonistic to eye movements, and vice versa, whereas direct excitation or inhibition of STN can yield temporal coordination of the activity of the two systems. The segregation-of-channels view (sec. 10.1.2) thus may be contrasted with the convergence view espoused by Hikosaka. Percheron et al. (1984) noted that in the path cortex → putamen → GP, there is a reduction in size and that the axonal arborization suggests pooling, and Hikosaka sees strong evidence of pooling in STN and

GP. Of course, figure 10.9 is a simplification of the complete circuitry. (1) Figure 10.9 excludes SNc; later, it is posited to play a major role in learning. (2) Part of SNr receives input from the putamen; part of GPi receives input from the caudate. (3) Putamen projects mainly to the ventral part of GPe; CD projects to its dorsal part. However, the segregation is not absolute.

The BG may compare movement commands from the precentral motor fields with proprioceptive feedback from the evolving movement, regulating a movement or monitoring its consequences. The BG also may be involved in the initiation of internally generated movements. This is consistent with the akinesia—the inability to initiate movement—of Parkinsonian patients (sec. 10.2). Possible functions of BG-induced suppressions may include the following (Hikosaka et al. 1993):

• *Focusing:* suppression of inappropriate movements

• *Sequencing:* suppression of forthcoming movement during preparation

• *Simulation:* switching between overt and covert behaviors.

Simulation in the foregoing sense refers to the idea that BG may play a role in suppressing motor areas to allow activity in association cortex to be "disconnected," yielding covert "mental" processes without immediate overt motor consequences. Because some sequential behavior survives BG lesion, it may be that if a sequence is overlearned, it can be stored elsewhere and then not require BG.

In purely behavioral experiments, Hikosaka et al. (1995) addressed the issue of motor sequence acquisition and motor memory in training two monkeys to carry out motor-sequencing tasks. The monkeys were seated in a monkey chair and were presented with a 4 × 4 matrix of light-emitting diodes (LEDs). They were given a ready signal, after which two of sixteen LEDs would light up. The monkeys had to press the LED keys in a specific order, which they would learn by trial and error. If the monkeys pressed the keys in the wrong sequence, a warning tone would sound, the LEDs would randomly flash, and the sequence would start over again. Each pair of LEDs presented was called a *set*. Five consecutive sets were known as a *hyperset*. To work through the five sets, the monkeys had to perform all the previous responses correctly; if a mistake were made in, say, the third or fourth set, the warning tone would sound, the LEDs would flash randomly, and the first set was presented again. In this way, the monkeys were learning 10 key strokes in a manner that was much easier than learning

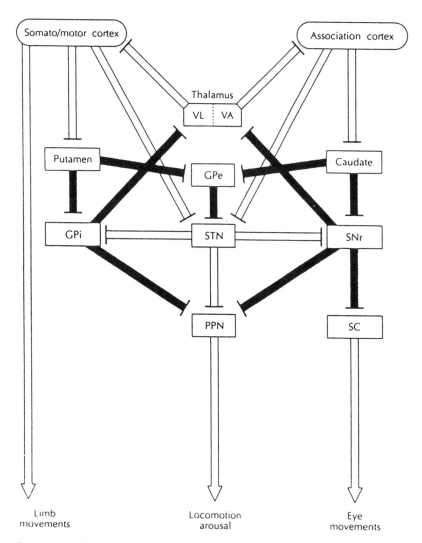

Figure 10.9

The provision by GPe and STN of a shared suppression system for the otherwise separate disinhibitory systems for limb movement and eye movement. VL, VA, ventrolateral and ventroanterior nuclei of thalamus; GPe and GPi, external and internal path of globus pallidus; STN, subthalamic nucleus; PPN, parapontine nucleus; SNr, substantia nigra pars reticulata; SC, superior colliculus. (Reprinted with permission from Hikosaka 1991.)

them all at once. This task was known as the *2 × 5 task* (two LEDs in a set, five sets in a hyperset). Compare this with the discussion of the neuralization of coordinated control programs (sec. 8.5.1).

There were two criteria for measurement of the task: procedural accuracy and speed. As a measure of procedure, the numbers of trials were counted until 10 consecutively successful trials were reached. For example, if 15 trials passed before 10 successful trials in a row, this measure would be 25. As a measure of speed, the time required for pressing the 10 keys was measured. In this manner, the performance of motor systems versus sequential representation was differentiated.

On the basis of this experimental paradigm, several interesting results and conclusions emerged. The mon-

keys were given hypersets on which to train every day. Over the course of numerous days (more than 300), two decidedly different forms of learning were evident. The first of these was the acquisition of short-term memory, in which a given sequence of keystrokes was learned from one trial to the next. However, this knowledge did not transfer to the consecutive day(s). The second form of learning was learning not specific to any sequence, which could be observed over a period of more than 300 days in which a general trend was seen which eased the learning of any sequence in general. This type of learning indicated a familiarity with the experimental paradigm as a whole, and it was seen that even novel sequences were learned at a rate faster than before.

After the monkeys had learned six hypersets sufficiently, they received no more training for a month. After a month, when presented with the learned hypersets, the monkeys did make some mistakes in the beginning of the sequences but quickly relearned the sequences, learning them much more quickly than they learned novel sequences. This was the procedural performance. As for the motor-speed performance, initially the speed was worse than before the 1-month hiatus, but still it was much faster than that manifested for novel sequences. However, as the trials went on, the speed performance also matched the earlier performance before the hiatus, suggesting that the motor memory had not been lost.

After a 6-month gap in the practice, the procedural performance for the previously learned hypersets was just as poor as for novel stimuli. However, the speed criterion was comparable to that before the gap, and it definitely was faster than that of new hypersets. This finding seems to suggest that even though the procedural memory had deteriorated, the motor memory was still intact.

Thus, Hikosaka et al. (1995) differentiate three distinct mechanisms of learning.

1. *Short-term and sequence-selective learning:* This activity occurred when, during a block of trials, the monkeys successfully acquired a memory for the correct key sequences.

2. *Long-term and sequence-selective learning:* This process occurred when the monkeys acquired the correct sequence for hypersets and could retain it over days.

3. *Long-term and sequence-unselective learning:* This activity occurred when there was an improvement in both the procedure and speed criteria for acquiring novel hypersets over the course of days. This improvement could be due to the monkeys' learning not to press the same key first if they caused an error last time or the monkeys' being more comfortable in the experimental environment.

In studying such learning, we must recall the viewpoint that holds that cerebellum acts to tune and coordinate motor pattern generators located elsewhere in the nervous system (chapter 9; sec. 10.5.2). However, what can be said of the "learned pattern generators" that we have characterized as coordinated control programs? We hold that they are acquired by the cerebral cortex but that their execution relies on the BG both to suppress and to release the constituent motor schemas. (Much more experimental support is needed.) However, we argue further (sec. 10.6) that BG are involved not only in

selection of movements but also in learning new coordinated control programs. BG have their main influence via thalamus and cortex for skilled movement, such as those involving coordinated use of hand and fingers, and to midbrain motor centers for innate movements, such as those involved in saccades, locomotion, and mastication.

Selective modification of BG pathways by slowly acting transmitters (e.g., dopamine) may underlie motor coordination. The combination of motor signals so created may act as a neural template for motor learning, which takes place in the premotor cortical areas. Learned limb movements are controlled by the BG through their access (via thalamus) to motor memories stored in cerebral cortex.

A portion of the current coordinated control program must occupy our working memory, but not necessarily the whole coordinated control program, and that portion (sec. 8.4.4) need involve the activation of only some of the motor schemas at a given time. Sensory outcomes of the movement also must be embedded in the working memory so that the next movement(s) can be prepared in a predictive manner. Cortical, thalamic, limbic, and brainstem signals fed into BG are used for the control of behavior either directly (via projections to the midbrain) or indirectly (via projections to the thalamic nuclei), BG would either withhold ongoing thalamocortical activity or allow it to proceed on the basis of stored motor memory. BG may be selective or preferential for movements that are planned internally, guided by memory, or triggered by sensory stimuli. Sensory responses are common but usually are dependent on the behavioral outcome predicted by the sensory stimulation. Responses correlated with prediction or expectation commonly are seen in the CD. Preparatory and movement-related activity in putamen may be selective for the direction of the target or the direction of movement as seen in the motor and supplementary motor cortices.

We stress that the BG work not in isolation but in cooperation with cerebral cortex. Already we have noted the work of Kermadi et al. (1993) (sec. 10.5.1) implicating the CD of monkeys in the performance of motor and oculomotor sequences based on memorized information. Data show that the BG-thalamocortical loop involving the SMA plays an important role in the processing of sequential movements. Tanji and Shima (1994) examined the role of SMA cells in planning several movements ahead. To achieve a volitional goal, one needs to execute multiple movements in a specific temporal order. After repetitive performance of a particular sequence of movements, one is able to memorize the entire sequence (not necessarily consciously) and execute it without external guidance. Tanji and Shima trained a monkey to listen for a tone signaling that it should perform from memory one of four different sequences (SEQ1, SEQ2, SEQ3, or SEQ4). Each movement was composed of three operations (push, pull, and turn) and was signaled by a movement-onset tone. These authors found a group of cells in the SMA (but not in the primary motor cortex) of monkeys whose activity is related exclusively to a sequence of multiple movements performed in a particular order. For example, they found an SMA neuron that appears to code specifically for the execution of SEQ4 from memory. The cell does not seem to code for the execution of a turn (or a turn at the beginning of a sequence) because it is quiescent during the execution of SEQ3 (which begins with a turn), and likewise the neuron does not fire when SEQ4 is guided visually instead of being executed from memory. They propose that such cells contribute a signal about the order of forthcoming multiple movements and are useful for planning and coding of several movements ahead.

In a related study, Halsband, Matsuzaka, and Tanji (1994) examined neuronal activity in the primate SMA, pre-SMA (the motor area immediately rostral to the SMA), premotor cortex (PMC), and primary motor cortex while the monkey performed a conditional sequential motor task that ensures sequencing of multiple movements to the same manipulandum. (Recall the related study by Halsband et al. (1993) of the role of PMC and the SMA in the temporal control of human movement.) Neuronal activity during the following periods was analyzed: instruction (300 msec following the onset of an auditory instruction signal); delay (interval between the end of the instruction period or the termination of the previous movement and the movement trigger); premovement (interval between the trigger signal and the movement onset); movement (interval between the mechanically sensed movement onset and the completion of the movement); and reward (500-msec period centered at the time of reward delivery). Pre-SMA neurons generally were more active during the delay and premovement as compared to the movement, instruction, and reward periods. Activity in the pre-SMA was more related to externally triggered movements during the premovement period but exhibited a preferential relationship to internally generated movements in the movement period. SMA neurons were more active when the sequential motor task was generated internally. By contrast, PMC neurons were more active when the sequence was guided· visually. Such preferential activity rarely was found in primary motor cortex neurons.

In conclusion, we see that the BG-thalamocortical loop crucially involves the SMA and other regions of cerebral cortex in the processing of sequential movements. Once again, we see the theme of cooperative computation playing a crucial role in our analysis of neural organization. In chapter 11, we argue that this principle (as well as other principles, such as that of the action-perception cycle) has a key role to play in the future development of cognitive neuroscience.

Prospects for a
Neuroscience of Cognition

In this chapter, we provide a summary of what we have covered, a philosophical perspective on our approach to neuroscience, and a proposal for future work in cognitive neuroscience.

In section 11.1, Following the Threads: The Book in Perspective, we provide the symmetrical parenthesis to the introduction provided in chapter 1. We single out a number of key threads that we have woven in and out of various chapters. By summarizing the course of each thread section by section, we hope to aid the reader in seeing the overall contributions of the book more clearly.

In section 11.2, Multiple Levels, Multiple Methodologies, and The Need for Their Integration, we review our progress in integrating multiple styles and levels of analysis to chart the contributions of different brain regions in action-oriented perception, control of action, rhythmogenesis, and various memory systems. Also, we delineate the processes of self-organization and learning that underlie these abilities. Moreover, we place our review of progress in a methodological and philosophical perspective.

Finally, in section 11.3, Implications and Outlook for Cognitive Neuroscience, we argue that the methodologies exemplified in this volume can be extended to provide an account of the neural mechanisms underlying cognitive function.

11.1 Following the Threads: The Book in Perspective

In summarizing the contributions made by this volume, we examine threads associated with our three overarching themes: structure, function, and dynamics.

Section 11.1.1 is an examination of the following threads for structure: (1) phylogeny and ontogeny, (2) the architectonic basis for analysis of function and dynamics of circuitry, and (3) the embedding of the region in loops and pathways that integrate it with other regions. We note that the transition from structure to function rests crucially (but not only) on "filling in the signs" in the structure as the basis for the interplay of excitation and inhibition.

Im section 11.1.2, we study the threads of behavior: (1) the place of schema theory in neuroscience, (2) high-level constraints on system modeling afforded by the study of behavior, and the use of (3) the saccadic system and (4) reaching and grasping to challenge the creation of models of function and learning at the level of both schemas and neural networks.

Section 11.1.3 is a a review of the threads woven into our study of dynamics: (1) the basic dynamic concepts of fixed points, rhythmogenesis and synchronization, and chaos; (2) self-organization; (3) plasticity and the modeling of learning; and, finally, dynamics considered at the increasingly fine levels of (4) compartmental modeling; and (5) neurochemistry.

11.1.1 Structure

Phylogeny and Ontogeny

In section 2.1, we introduced the idea that the embryology of a structure may make clear crucial relationships that may be obscured in the adult form. We used the segmented part of the neuraxis (i.e., the spinal cord and the lower brainstem) to ground discussion of the progressive loss of segmentation in the upper brainstem, including the diencephalon. Moreover, we showed that the embryonic nervous system is able to generate movement before it is able to respond to sensory stimuli, thus supporting the action-oriented view of brain function (chapter 3). We addressed also the evolution of the mammalian brain, showing how (as the brain evolves) basic structures become overlaid with more and more complex structures than can both inhibit and coordinate what has evolved before. This evolutionary theme was taken up from a functional point of view in section 3.2, wherein we showed how brain function can be analyzed in a process of evolutionary refinement in which basic systems serve as the substrate for the designed "evolution" of more refined systems. We posited that new schemas often arise as "modulators" of existing schemas rather than as new systems with independent functional roles.

Section 7.1 was a study of an intermediate embryonic stage to illuminate the relationship between the diencephalon and the telencephalic vesicles. The two developmentally different structures are welded together by the progressive emergence of fiber tracts (white matter) formed by the axonal processes of neurons—both ascending and descending—that have the tendency to gather in, and to occupy, the outer surface areas of the original neural tube (as in the formation of the spinal cord and the lower brainstem). Again, the structural

overview of cerebral cortex began with a view of its development (sec. 8.1), and in section 8.2, we analyzed the development of two striking examples of modular architectonics in primary visual cortex: ocular dominance columns and orientation columns. Finally, our structural view of the cerebellum was initiated (sec. 9.1) by a review of its phylogeny and ontogeny; we showed how the relative size of different parts of cerebellum may vary from species to species and traced the delicate mechanisms of cell growth, migration, and interaction yielding the quasi-crystalline structure of the mature cerebellar cortex.

The Architectonic Basis for the Analysis of Function and Dynamics

In section 2.2, we approached a hierarchy of levels of structural analysis—neurons, networks, an integrated system—by presenting data supporting the *modular architectonic principle*: Neuronal connectivity in a typical neural center is sufficiently specific to permit disassembly of the entire network into neuronal modules of characteristic internal connectivity, and the larger structure can be reconstituted by repetition of these modules. We analyzed the spinal gray matter and the lower brainstem in these terms. Then we showed that the upper diencephalic and telencephalic parts of the brainstem do not retain the quasi-segmental arrangement of the lower neuraxis but that elements of the basic architectural principle of the neuraxis are preserved. We noted further the importance in many structures of local circuit neurons and of the complex synaptic arrangements called *glomeruli*, with their synaptic triads in, for example, the cerebellar cortex, the olfactory bulb, and some of the anterior thalamic nuclei.

We applied the modular architectonics principle to the cerebral cortex, linking observations of anatomical regularities to Mountcastle's observations on physiological "columns" in somatosensory cortex and to Hubel and Wiesel's analysis of visual cortex. Section 2.3's title, Multiple Models of Modularity, stressed that the search for a hierarchy in levels of neuronal, network, and integrated systems is not confined to the columnlike structures of cerebral sensory cortex. We introduced both the quasi-crystalline structure of the cerebellar cortex and the basic lamellar structure of the hippocampus.

In section 5.1, we reviewed the layers, cell types, and synaptic organization of the olfactory bulb and continued the investigation into the olfactory cortex. On that subject, we stressed how its laminar structure relates to the afferent fibers from the olfactory bulb. Also we analyzed reexcitatory connections that may be the anatomical substrate for olfactory associative memory; commissural fiber systems connecting the two halves of the cortex; and neurochemically varied centrifugal inputs from different brain areas. Section 6.1 contained a structural view of the hippocampus; we treated in turn the intrinsic organization (cells and circuits) of the hippocampus; both the cortical and subcortical hippocampal afferents and efferents; and basic quantitative data regarding cell numbers and the convergence and divergence of connections. Special attention was paid to the synaptic matrices revealed in lamellae orthogonal to the long axis of the hippocampus, thus establishing a basic circuit for the analysis of hippocampal function.

In section 7.1, we advanced the theme of modular architectonics by noting that frontally oriented successive discs of the cortex (from front to back) have a relationship with close to sagittal discs of the thalamus. Section 8.1 was an analysis of the synaptic connectivity of cortical neurons; we noted the interplay of excitation and inhibition and the role of neuronal chains in cortical function, then returned to the modular architectonics principle with Szentágothai arguing for the modular *structural* organization of the cortex, but questioning the functional role of such units. In section 8.2, we offered two striking examples of modular architectonics seen in primary visual cortex: ocular dominance columns and orientation columns.

In section 9.2, we studied the quasi-crystalline structure and the "space economy" of the cerebellar cortex in some quantitative detail. The only output cells of the cerebellar cortex are Purkinje cells, and these inhibit nuclear cells. Thus, we stressed the integration of the circuitry of the cerebellar cortex into a "microcomplex" that unites a microzone of cortex with the region of nucleus to which it projects and with which it shares afferents. In this way, we established a "basic circuit" for the analysis of cerebellar function.

Section 10.1 was an examination of the structure of the striatum, the region of the basal ganglia that receives most of its input pathways. We looked at the two pathways, direct and indirect, whereby it acts on the output pathways of the basal ganglia, and we looked at the division of the striatum into "patches" embedded in a "matrix."

The Embedding of Regions in Loops and Pathways

In section 2.3, we emphasized that many regions of the brain are best thought of as embedded within even larger systems integrated by loops traversing many brain regions. Consider, for example, the links of the cerebellar system—"upstream" with the cerebral cortex and "downstream" with the spinal cord—that are closed in the cerebellar nuclei to which the output cells of cerebellar cortex project. The fact that the output of cerebellar cortex is purely inhibitory ties into our theme that the passage from structure to function often is based on understanding the patterns of interplay of excitation and inhibition. In this case, the inhibition from cerebellar cortex serves to modulate the activity in the cerebellar nuclei, which serve in turn to tune and coordinate motor pattern generators (MPGs) located elsewhere in the nervous system.

The role of the thalamus as the chief relay for sensory input to cerebral cortex is only a small fraction of the crucial role of the thalamus in all kinds of pathways. Thus, we devoted section 7.3 to thalamocortical loops and cooperative computation, reviewing the descending control of sensory systems in the lateral geniculate nucleus of mammals; and thalamocortical oscillations. Also, we reviewed the thalamocortical loops involving the basal ganglia and cerebellum. In section 9.3, we stressed that the microcomplexes integrate cerebellar cortex into a cerebellar system that modulates MPGs. In section 10.1, we showed the basal ganglia to be embedded in four disjoint loops of the form "cortex → basal ganglia → thalamus → cortex": the oculomotor circuit, the motor circuit, the "cognitive" (dorsolateral prefrontal) circuit, and the limbic (lateral orbitofrontal) circuit.

11.1.2 Function

The Place of Schema Theory in Neuroscience

In chapter 3, we presented schema theory as a framework for the rigorous analysis of behavior that requires no prior commitment to hypotheses on the localization of each schema (or unit of functional analysis) but can be linked to a structural analysis as and when this becomes appropriate. Section 3.1 introduced an approach to schema theory that emphasizes action-oriented perception, with the paradigm of the *action-perception cycle* replacing the stimulus-response paradigm. However, in a number of later sections, we have made clear that schema theory and the action-perception cycle (and our approach to functional neuroscience in general) are not limited to those forms of, say, sensorimotor coordination for which extensive neural data are available and which we have treated at length in part II. These sections include section 3.1.5. (Visual Scene Interpretation), section 6.5 (Hippocampal Function and Human Memory), and section 8.6. (From Action-Oriented Perception to Cognition). The discussion continues later in, for instance, sections 11.3.2. (Schema Theory and the Construction of Reality) and 11.3.3 (Language).

In section 3.1, we explored the constraints imposed by linking schema theory to functional neuroscience and provided a quasi-formal introduction to perceptual and motor schemas, coordinated control programs (illustrated with an introduction to the visual control of reaching and grasping), cooperative computation, and schema assemblages (the basis for a schema-based model of visual perception that provided a perspective on short-term and long-term memory). A simple account of approach and avoidance behavior in frogs illustrated the use of perceptual and motor schemas, showing how they may be linked and illustrating the issues involved in making a schema-based account of a function into a neural model.

Behavioral Constraints

In section 3.2, we presented *Rana computatrix*, a set of models of visuomotor coordination in frog and toad. Therein, we addressed approach, avoidance, and detour behavior to show how perception may demand the mutual refinement of one perceptual schema by another, how multiple motor schemas may act together to yield complex motor behaviors, and how brain function can be analyzed in a process of evolutionary refinement. Also, we looked at neural mechanisms of avoidance behavior to provide our first example of how neural modeling can be used to replace schemas with neural networks of equivalent functionality.

Sections 3.3 and 3.4 were an introduction to schemas for looking, reaching, and grasping; we demonstrated that much is to be learned at the level of schema analysis prior to, or in concert with, the analysis of neural circuitry. In chapters 8 and 10, these schemas were shown to be distributed across cerebral cortex and basal ganglia, and in chapter 9, we showed the role of cerebellum in their adaptation and coordination.

Section 6.4 was a combination of a functional view of the hippocampus—its role in the cognitive maps underlying navigation and spatial behavior in rats—and a dynamic view of how synaptic plasticity may enable hippocampal cells to learn to encode different "places" in a cognitive map. We offered a general framework for the study of spatial representation and cognitive maps in rats, including the general idea of world graphs as cognitive maps for motivated behavior. Then we reviewed the neurophysiology of spatial representation, with spe-

cial emphasis on the "place cells" of hippocampal regions CA3 and CA1. We offered two contrasting systems views of the role of the hippocampus in navigation, in each case emphasizing that the representation of current place in CA3 and CA1 is insufficient for a cognitive map which underlies navigation. In section 6.5, we viewed the role of hippocampal function in human memory, introducing the crucial dichotomies of procedural and declarative memory and of skill versus episodic learning. The data suggest that the hippocampus is involved in declarative rather than in procedural memory and in episodic rather than in skill learning. We closed the chapter by discussing the unanswered question: Is there a commonality of mechanism between the two main functions attributed to the hippocampus, cognitive mapping in rats and declarative memory in humans? Because learning is a crucial aspect of adaptive behavior, a number of the issues discussed here overlap those discussed later in section 11.1.3 (Plasticity: Modeling Learning) under Dynamics.

In section 8.2, we looked briefly at how primary visual cortex provides input to a variety of visual processes. We introduced psychophysical and neurophysiological data on spatial visual perception and addressed the role of long-range horizontal connections in the integration of information. In section 8.4, we discussed cortical mechanisms for using vision in the control of movement. In that section, we focused on frontal-parietal interactions in cortex, but many other brain regions are involved in the integration of vision with action. Section 8.5 was focused on the theme of learning of coordinated behaviors and provided both a schema-level analysis of motor set and the neuralization of coordinated control programs and a specific neural network model of visuomotor conditional learning. Foreshadowed in the study of rat spatial learning (chapter 6), this theme was developed further in our study of cerebellum (chapter 9) and basal ganglia (chapter 10). In section 8.6, we charted basic processes underlying cognitive functions from a high-level, schema-theoretical viewpoint.

Section 9.3 was a focus on the issue of how skills are acquired, viewing the cerebellum as a learning machine, stressing the idea that cerebellar nuclei modulate MPGs whereas the cerebellar cortex learns how best to modulate the cerebellar nuclei—modulating the modulator. First we studied the role of the cerebellum in the vestibulo-ocular reflex, wherein data strongly support the notion of a functional role of an adaptive microcomplex in modulating the gain of eye movements that compensate for head movements and in the classical conditioning of the rabbit eyeblink response. In section 9.4, we presented models of how the cerebellum adapts the metrics of movement to changing circumstances. We showed how the detailed circuitry of the cerebellar cortex and of various nuclei with which it interacts could modulate activity in MPG-related loops on a short-term basis (i.e., one appropriate to the current circumstances, as in adjusting to step height in climbing a flight of stairs). The remaining subsections contained a review of approaches to modeling adaptation of motor control wherein the adaptation persists on a long-term basis involving synaptic plasticity. We presented feedback-error learning whereby the cerebellum could "take over" motor control from other parts of the brain, but we argued that the cerebellum "works" by modulating and coordinating multiple MPGs rather than by replacing them.

In addition to behavior in normal subjects, we can learn much about neural function and dynamics by studying their fate in subjects with a variety of diseases. In section 9.3, we noted clinical data on the role of the cerebellum in skilled movements as a basis for our study of how these skills are acquired, viewing the cerebellum as a learning machine. In section 10.2, we focused on diseases of the basal ganglia, showing that the distinct movement disorders seen in Huntington's disease (hyperkinetic and hypotonic) and Parkinson's disease (hypokinetic and hypertonic) are associated with decreased basal ganglia output in the former and a marked increase in the latter.

The Saccadic System

Section 3.3 was an introduction to schemas for controlling the rapid eye movements called *saccades*; we focused on the homology between the tectum in frog and toad and the superior colliculus in primates—the whole-body movement of the frog toward its prey corresponding to the orienting of gaze toward a visual target in the monkey. We showed how schemas for working memory and for dynamic remapping may extend the monkey's saccadic repertoire to include saccades to remembered targets or to two targets in succession.

In later sections, we showed how circuitry in various regions of the brain may contribute to these and other schemas. In section 8.4, we presented a detailed model of corticothalamic systems for saccade control and paid particular attention to the roles of posterior parietal cortex, frontal eye fields, and thalamus in providing mechanisms for dynamic remapping and working memory. Section 9.4 contained models of the cerebellar role in saccade adaptation, refining the corticothalamic model

by adjusting the metrics of saccades, a feat of learning that is impossible in animals or humans lacking certain portions of the cerebellum. In section 10.4, we completed our model of saccade control by focusing on the "oculomotor loop" of the basal ganglia, presenting a model of the role of the entire loop in generating saccades and modeling the interactions between the basal ganglia and the working memory systems of prefrontal cortex. Interruption of SNr inhibition allows reciprocal connections between frontal eye fields and thalamus to generate a spatial "memory" cycle or loop. Once a saccade has been made to a remembered target, the memory trace must be erased to prevent generation of further saccades of equal magnitude and direction. We posit that the activity of this spatial working memory could be regulated by the inhibitory topographical projection from SNr to thalamus.

In section 10.4.2, we suggested that if the frontal eye field and direct visual input do not yield the encoding of a unique target in the deep layers of superior colliculus, a winner-take-all mechanism will "choose" one of the targets. Then we argued that experience based on inferotemporal or prefrontal information may provide contextual, learned information to bias activity in the basal ganglia and thereby "tip the balance" to one "winner" or another, presenting models of visuomotor conditioning, including spatial generalization and sequential behavior based on the strong hypothesis that this learning is mediated by corticostriatal plasticity.

Reaching and Grasping

In studying the role of perception in mediation of behavior, we stressed that in general, no complete and objective "percept" of an object exists. Rather, there is a set of partial characterizations (including parameters that we may not be able to represent symbolically in any explicit fashion) related to the current set of goals and motivations of the observer, and they may continue to unfold as interaction with, or contemplation of, the object continues. Section 3.4 was an illustration of this concept, using the schemas involved in reaching and grasping. We presented the concepts of virtual fingers and opposition space to offer a precise but compact description of the degrees of freedom involved in a number of grasping movements. Then we analyzed a series of experiments that motivated the design of a new coordinated control program explicitly involving a coordinating schema as well as perceptual and motor schemas.

We devoted section 8.4 to cortical systems for reaching and grasping. After showing that visual input to parietal cortex is processed for "where and how" information, whereas visual input to inferotemporal cortex is processed for "what" information, we analyzed data for "neural codes" in parietal lobe and premotor cortex in relation to schema-based analysis of hand movements (chapter 3). Section 9.4 contained a model of the role of cerebellum in adapting a particular class of arm movements: the adaptation of dart throwing in the wearing of prisms.

Section 10.5 was an examination of the still somewhat discordant views on the roles of the basal ganglia in motor coordination and learning, emphasizing the view that the basal ganglia receive rich contextual information and then "release" components of motor programs through disinhibition. We suggested that basal ganglia neuronal responses are task-dependent, with the current responsiveness of a neuron possibly determined by the state of behavioral experience or learning and temporarily maintained until the relevant memory is formed in premotor cortices. We emphasized "channels" involved in working memory and in initiation of movement. The basal ganglia were seen, in part, as controlling a kind of working memory for coordinated control programs of motor schemas. Roles for basal ganglia inhibition may include focusing (suppression of inappropriate movements), sequencing (suppression of forthcoming movement during preparation), and simulation in the sense of suppressing motor areas to allow activity in association cortex to be "disconnected," yielding covert mental simulation without immediate overt movement. We distinguished the roles of basal ganglia and cerebellum, suggesting that basal ganglia are involved in explicitly combining the "pieces" that make up a skilled behavior, whereas the cerebellum serves to turn a procedure into a skill, adjusting parameters to adapt and coordinate components of the movement to yield a seamless whole.

11.1.3 Dynamics

Fixed Points, Rhythmogenesis and Synchronization, and Chaos

In chapter 4, we stressed that neural systems can be studied at different levels, such as the molecular, membrane, cellular, synaptic, network, and system levels. Moreover, we noted two main neurodynamical problems: study of the dynamics of activity spreading through a network with fixed wiring and the study of the dynamics of the connectivity of networks with modifiable synapses—both in normal ontogenetic development and in learning as a network is tuned by ex-

perience. We introduced the key dynamical concept of an attractor, a pattern of activity that "captures" nearby states of an autonomous system. An attractor may be an equilibrium point, a limit cycle (oscillation), or a strange attractor (chaotic behavior). We looked also at the structure-function problem: For which overall patterns of connectivity will a network exhibit a particular pattern of dynamical behavior? Unfortunately, the results given were qualitative rather than directly applicable to biologically realistic models of neural networks. The introduction of Hopfield networks (sec. 4.5) showed work on neural networks motivated by statistical mechanics, including ideas of "energy," "temperature," and the statistical distribution of patterns in relation to an attractor-based model of pattern recognition. We gave a critique of "computation with attractors."

In section 4.2, we introduced the topic of oscillatory behavior in neural systems: single-cell oscillations resulting from the interplay of a few currents, and central pattern generators in which network of neurons can produce rhythmic behavior in the absence of sensory input. Bifurcation analyses were used to show a transition from equilibrium point to small amplitude oscillation or from oscillation to chaos, as some control parameter passes through a critical value. We analyzed phase lags in chains of oscillators (mimicking data on the spinal cord of the lamprey), the importance of long-range coupling in the synchronization of more fully coupled networks (as in models of cortical structures), and bifurcation analysis of gait transitions in locomotion.

Section 4.3 was a study in chaotic behavior in the nervous system. Chaotic systems are characterized by sensitivity to initial conditions. We showed that the structural conditions of chaos occur at different hierarchical levels of neural organization. Neurochemical synaptic transmission often is characterized as a random process, but the dripping-faucet model may be adapted to explain this apparent randomness as a case of deterministic chaos. We found that global cortical dynamics, as seen at the global level in the electroencephalogram, also may exhibit chaotic behavior. We discussed "dynamical diseases," introducing the diagnosis and also the control of chaos associated with normal and pathological brain functions. Further, we discussed the possibly controversial but intriguing functional roles of chaos in normal brain activity, including perception and memory formation.

We focused on the dynamics of activity in the olfactory system (sec. 5.2), contrasting slow oscillations (~ 5 Hz) that the respiratory nuclei may impose on the olfactory bulb with fast oscillations with frequency 35–90 Hz in different parts of the olfactory bulb. We addressed these data with the methods of our dynamical overview so as to model oscillation and chaos in the olfactory bulb, offering a bifurcation analysis of a simple network model (with single-compartment models of the neurons) using the parameter c, which controls the strength of lateral connections in the mitral layer as control parameter. Also we modeled rhythmical activity in the olfactory cortex. Similarly, we gave a dynamic analysis of electrical activity patterns in the hippocampus (sec. 6.2), addressing data on the normal electrical activity patterns known as *theta rhythms* and *sharp waves* and the abnormal electrical activity exhibited in epileptic seizures. Also, we compared the hippocampus with the olfactory system, giving special attention to the neural mechanisms of rhythm generation and synchronization.

Thalamus and cortex are interconnected highly by reciprocal projections, which gives rise to characteristic dynamic patterns. High-frequency rhythms are associated with the waking state, whereas low-frequency rhythms are associated with sleeping. In section 8.3, we analyzed the balance between oscillations intrinsic to single neurons and network properties in the generation of thalamocortical oscillations. We analyzed the intrinsic electrophysiological properties of thalamic neurons, thalamocortical neurons, and reticular thalamic neurons, then addressed the dynamics of spindle oscillations and of delta and slow-sleep oscillations. We analyzed the role of brainstem control and cellular mechanisms in thalamocortical activation and closed by using a number of models to explore the role of single-cell dynamics versus emergent network properties.

Self-Organization: Modeling Development

Both ontogenetic development of neural structures and their plastic behavior often are considered as dynamic processes in the state space of synaptic connections. The self-organization of the nervous system in general is a broader process, including both addition and removal of synapses and the modification of synaptic strengths. Self-organizing mechanisms are related to normal ontogenetic development (this subsection) and learning (see the next subsection).

Section 4.4 was a focus on retinotectal connections. We discussed the following issues: specificity versus plasticity; genetically prespecified versus environmentally controlled wiring; marker theories versus activity-dependent mechanisms; decrease of synaptic strength by normalization rule only versus selective mechanisms;

deterministic versus stochastic models; sets of discrete nerve cells versus continuous neural fields; and positional information.

In section 8.2, we showed that modular architectonics may be seen as a pattern of organization resulting from the dynamics of self-organization rather than as being laid down completely in the genome. In particular, we provided models of the development of two examples of modular architectonics in primary visual cortex: ocular dominance columns and orientation columns.

Section 10.3 was centered on a discussion of self-reorganization of the striatum, both the self-organizing character of the pattern formation for striatal compartments and the relationship between the modular remapping architecture, the tonic firing of certain striatal neurons, and their role in coordinated motor behavior.

Plasticity: Modeling Learning

Whatever the model of the individual neuron, neural tissues may be modeled as networks of intricately connected neurons in which strengths w_{ij} of the synaptic connections themselves may be described by differential (or difference) equations. These "learning rules" (sec. 4.5) included hebbian learning and its variations, which incorporate means to avoid saturation of synaptic strengths, ways to accommodate various time delays, differential learning mechanisms, and "anti-Hebbian" rules to describe features of dissociations of patterns. We analyzed synaptic matrix models of associative memory but also saw how invariant pattern recognition may be modeled by using the dynamic link architecture in which Hebbian plasticity is invoked on a fast time scale.

In section 5.3, we reviewed learning and plasticity in the olfactory bulb and olfactory cortex. Building on the relation of different attractor regions to different lateral connection strengths, we showed how synaptic modification can induce transitions between these regions. Another study of the olfactory bulb modeled associative memory, and showed that incomplete input patterns due to lower odor concentrations also can be identified as proper stimuli if a suitable learning rule is used to modify the lateral connections between mitral cells. We presented two scenarios for learning and memory in the olfactory cortex. One was based on the observation that the sniffing rhythm of 5 Hz may be optimal for inducing long-term potentiation (LTP) in olfactory cortex; therein, we described a hierarchical clustering of input stimuli. The other scenario was based on the argument that the mechanism of object recognition in the olfactory cortex is close to those offered by abstract associative memory models; we emphasized that the incoming (bulbar) information has a complex, distributed representation, whereas the intrinsic excitatory connections between pyramidal cells are spatially extensive, overlapping, and modifiable.

To ground a dynamic view of synaptic plasticity (sec. 6.4) we used the role of the hippocampus in the cognitive maps underlying navigation and spatial behavior in rats to show how hebbian-like plasticity may enable hippocampal cells to learn to encode different "places" in a cognitive map. We reviewed various neural network models of place-cell training, allocentric location, and navigation, one model of which paid special attention to data relating place-cell activity to the theta rhythm (i.e., relating the dynamics of rhythmogenesis to the synaptic dynamics of learning).

We explored the learning of coordinated behaviors (sec. 8.5), providing therein both a schema-level analysis of motor set and neuralization of coordinated control programs and a specific neural network model of visuomotor conditional learning.

In section 9.3, we focused on models of the cerebellum as a machine for learning motor skills. We started with the Marr-Albus model, which views the Purkinje cell (the output cell of cerebellar cortex) as a perceptron, and noted that data on long-term depression (LTD) support the Albus version of the model, namely that "coincidence" of climbing fiber and parallel fiber activity on a Purkinje cell *depresses* the efficacy of the synapses of parallel fibers active during the conjunction. We reviewed approaches to modeling adaptation of motor control (sec. 9.4) wherein the adaptation persists on a long-term basis and involves synaptic plasticity (with the emphasis remaining on LTD of parallel fiber → Purkinje cell synapses).

In section 10.4.2, we argued that experience based on inferotemporal or prefrontal information may provide contextual, learned information to bias activity in the basal ganglia. We posited that this learning is mediated by corticostriatal plasticity, using a form of reinforcement learning in which dopamine released by the substantia nigra pars compacta acts as the reinforcement signal to toggle between Hebbian and anti-Hebbian learning.

Compartmental Modeling

We introduced some of the specific formalisms used to treat neurons and neural networks as dynamic systems (sec. 4.2). The framework for the detailed treatment of the membrane potential dynamics of a neuron patch is provided by both the neuronal cable equation and the Hodgkin-Huxley equation and its relatives. An entire neuron may be modeled in either of two ways: by a multicompartment model with compartments chosen to take into account the location of the entering synaptic currents or the geometry of dendritic branching or as a single-compartment model characterized by a single membrane potential. The leaky integrator neuron is a popular model for the single-compartment case. In section 8.4.1, we provided the formalism for large-scale models of the nervous system (for more detail, see Appendix A) used in many of the previously described models based on simple (single-compartment) models of neurons. Both periodic and chaotic temporal patterns can be generated at the single neuron level (sec. 4.3). Basic phenomena can be modeled with membrane equations involving two functionally distinct currents, the slow and fast currents, in which a series of complex patterned activities (simple slow oscillation, bursting, bursting-chaos, beating-chaos and beating) can be generated by changing the time constant of inactivation of the slow current.

In addition to modeling a network built from "integrate-and-fire" elements, we offered multicompartmental models for the mitral and granule cells: six and four compartments were taken into account, respectively (sec. 5.2.2). They demonstrated specific effects of the individual ionic conductances on the overall performance of the compartment; signal propagation through the compartments; and synchronization in small networks. The Wilson-Bower-Hasselmo model of temporal patterns in the piriform cortex was presented in section 5.2.3. It uses a five-compartment model for each pyramidal cell and explicit delays for transmission and axonal activity to clarify the assumptions leading to near 40-Hz cortical oscillations. By contrast, the Liljenström-Hasselmo model is designed to simulate modulatory cholinergic effects. Their network is built from relatively simple units whose output depends on a factor Q designed to be influenced by the level of acetylcholine. Depending on the values of Q, the system may exhibit convergence to a fixed point, limit cycle oscillation, or at least transient chaotic behavior. Moreover, the strengths of the synaptic connections also can influence the dynamic behavior drastically.

In section 6.2, we presented multicompartmental neuronal models of pyramidal cells and (to much less extent) interneurons of the CA3 region of hippocampus based on the Traub-Miles approach. These models served as a basis for the study of large networks of CA3 neurons, enabling us to see how variations in key parameters can switch the network between normal and epileptiform activity.

We used a number of models to explore the role of single-cell dynamics versus emergent network properties in thalamocortical oscillations (see 8.3).

In section 9.2, we analyzed the simulation of a single Purkinje cell as a very detailed compartmental model with realistic ion conductances and synaptic currents in each compartment. Because massive computing resources are needed to simulate a single cell, the models of cerebellar function in sections 9.3 and 9.4 used simpler, single-compartment models. However, we pointed the way to future multilevel modeling that will relate system behavior to the fine details of neuronal function.

Neurochemistry

Finally, we recall material assessing the biological grounding of learning rules (in Plasticity: Modeling Learning). In section 6.3, we looked at one of the best-studied forms of dynamics at the synaptic level: namely long-term potentiation. We showed its implication in experimental studies of hebbian synaptic modification and analyzed models of potentiation based on AMPA and NMDA receptors. We linked this back to dynamics at the activity level by studying the role of NMDA receptors in the generation of oscillations at the cellular level. Also, we discussed the need for LTD in hebbian synapses.

We modeled the cerebellar role in saccade adaptation (sec. 9.4), extending our view of LTD by stressing the notion of a "window of eligibility" to constrain the timing relation between the parallel fiber "context" and the climbing fiber "training signal." In section 10.4.2, we discussed corticostriatal plasticity and posited a form of reinforcement learning in which dopamine released by the substantia nigra pars compacta acts as the reinforcement signal to toggle between hebbian learning (positive reinforcement, long-term potentiation) and anti-hebbian learning (negative reinforcement, LTD). We suggested also that shaping of the eligibility signal may be task-dependent, thereby setting an important goal for neuroscience to bridge from this systems level of neural analysis to that of synaptic neurochemistry.

11.2 Multiple Levels, Multiple Methodologies, and the Need for Their Integration

We view the themes of this book now from a more philosophical, methodological perspective. We start with a discussion of the implications of a nonmonolithic approach to the brain involving multiple views and multiple theories. We examine general issues of brain theory and examine the transition from the cartesian reflex paradigm to the paradigm of the self-directed, self-organizing brain and conclude by listing a number of principles of neural organization.

11.2.1 Multiple Views, Multiple Theories

Our ability to perceive, act, plan, learn, and remember can be traced to the incredible intricacies of the hundreds of billions of neurons whose networks constitute a single human brain. The search for understanding has taken many neuroscientists deeper and deeper into the microworld wherein even a single neuron is too large for study. A neuron may have tens of thousands of synapses; yet for some neuroscientists, even the synapse is too large, and they focus their energies on the analysis of patches of membrane or minute chemical machines within the cell or the synapse. Thereby, they seek to understand the chemical and genetic engines that enable the neuron to develop, to function, and to change. Deep in the microworld, researchers can make many important discoveries that lead directly back to the macroworld of human health; learning how genetic abnormalities are expressed in neural circuitry and how drugs can act on neurons to rectify some diseases of the brain. Yet, for all this, these wonderful advances in the study of neurochemistry and subcellular mechanisms seem at times to be taking us far from our basic questions about the mind. Admittedly, we need to probe the brain's most detailed components, but for a real understanding of the human mind, we need to know how the pieces fit together into a functional whole.

How can the human mind come to grips with the complexity of the very brain that embodies it? The answer offered here is to view the brain at many different levels of analysis. In seeking to understand a world of five billion people, we need the vocabularies of geography and history and economics to describe the patterns within which we can make sense of the fates and plans of individuals. In this same way, in seeking to understand a brain of hundreds of thousands of billions of synapses, we need new vocabularies from the language of mind to the language of neurochemistry. In the 1940s, cybernetics was created for the comparative study of communication and control in the animal and the machine (Wiener 1948). The 1960s and 1970s saw the development of artificial intelligence, brain theory, and cognitive science. This evolution brings us to the present day, when new types of computers and new experimental techniques offer fresh challenges to our understanding of the brain. However, no unified theory exists. Instead, there is a constellation of minitheories, each providing more or less successful explanations of a limited range of phenomena. Thus, our challenge (an exciting one) is twofold: to provide increasingly accurate understanding of limited areas of the mind and brain and to seek unifying patterns that allow us to combine a number of minitheories into more powerful concepts.

11.2.2 Brain Theory

The work of the nineteenth century neurologists led us to think of the brain in terms of large interacting regions each with a more or less specified function. This localization was reinforced by the work of the turn-of-the-century anatomists who were able to subdivide the cerebral cortex on the basis of cell characteristics (cytoarchitectonics). At this same time, the discoveries of neuroanatomist Ramón y Cajal and neurophysiologist Sherrington helped to establish the neuron doctrine, leading us to view the functions of the brain in terms of discrete units—the neurons—interacting via excitatory and inhibitory synapses. The issue for the brain theorist, then, is to map complex functions, behaviors, and patterns of thought either on the interactions of these rather large entities (anatomically defined brain regions) or on these very small and numerous components (the neurons). This issue has led many neuroscientists to look for structures intermediate in size and complexity between brain regions and neurons to provide stepping stones in an analysis of how neural structures subserve various functions. Thus, the notion of the brain as an interconnected set of modules, intermediate in complexity between neurons and brain regions, was established with the module as a *structural* entity. This notion provides the basis for the "modular architectonics" that we used to anchor the structural overview (chapter 2).

Top-down brain theory is essentially functional in nature: It starts with the isolation of some overall function, such as some pattern of behavior or linguistic performance or type of perception, and seeks to explain it by decomposing it into the interaction of a number of subsystems. What makes this exercise brain theory as distinct from cognitive psychology or almost all of current connectionism is that the choice of subsystems is biased in part by what we know about the function of different parts of the brain. Whether obtained by analysis of the effects of brain lesions, imaging, or neurophysiology,

that knowledge fuels an attempt to map the subsystems onto anatomical regions.

In a *bottom-up* brain theory, the emphasis tends to be on single neurons, plastic synapses, and neural networks built from these elements. With a given set of neurons interconnected by excitatory and inhibitory synapses, the theory allows us to answer the question whether, how, and with what involvement of self-organization or plasticity the network is able to implement a given function. In the spirit of our dynamic overview, the general method is to build network models to describe spatiotemporal activity patterns and their change with synaptic modifiability to explain development, learning, and function. The refinement of anatomical tracing techniques combined with new physiological methods (e.g., dual intercellular recording) have allowed us to build and test very detailed single-cell models incorporating biophysical, physiological, and pharmacological properties of cells, the types and kinetics of channels, the connectivity patterns and synaptic distributions between cells, and so on. We have seen a number of such detailed compartmental models. However, in general we argue that these detailed models will yield greater insights when embedded into more global frameworks. On the one hand, we have the schema theory of our functional overview, which has framed many of the detailed, physiologically and anatomically grounded studies of neural networks in the chapters that followed. On the other hand, incorporation of results of detailed single-cell modeling into statistical population models may result in a methodological breakthrough in brain modeling.

11.2.3 From the Cartesian Reflex Paradigm to the Self-Directed, Self-Organizing Brain

For 300 years, understanding of neural actions was (and to a great extent still is) under the spell of the reflex principle. It would be ridiculous to question the crucial importance, the germane nature, and the heuristic value of this concept. Few ideas in the history of civilization were pronounced as explicitly and with such clarity as was this theory by René Descartes, more remarkably because of its basis on such meager factual information. Nerve cells were identified under the microscope only some two and a half centuries later. The only thing known about nerves in Descartes's time were certain tube-like structures (myelin sheaths) that could be seen by the early microscopists. Yet, Descartes correctly foresaw the principle of neural inhibition that was assumed to occur and later was observed directly in reciprocal innervation. The reflex principle and the view of animal behavior as that of a kind of reflex robot led to the belief that human cognitive behavior had to be interpreted by assuming as its substrate another fundamentally different kind of "substance." Hence, it was logically necessary to introduce two fundamentally different substances: *res extensa*, matter with extension, and *res cognitans*, thinking substance lacking in the physical properties of matter. This view of neural organization was quite satisfactory in the earlier period of modern experimental research into the structure, functions, and (even) the chemistry of neural systems. However, when the higher, especially cognitive functions of the neural systems came into the orbit of exact scientific study, the inadequacy of the traditional dualistic view became increasingly apparent.

The observations of neuropsychology—of brain and behavior—do not seem to support the idea of the existence of the mind (*res cognitans*) as an ontologically different substance. More importantly, there is no need for such an assumption, which is an idea ex vacuo (i.e., without any evidence from the field of natural science). All the arguments in this book militate against the still widely held notion that the *res cognitans* is a separate element that must be added to a brain to endow it with the capability for perception, thought, and action. We note two specific factors that contribute to the monism that informs the present volume: self-organization and the action-perception cycle.

Self-Organization

If all neural functions, from the simplest elementary reflexes to complex global functions of the entire organism, have at their very origins spontaneous activities arising, in part randomly, in individual nerve cells, and if all neural functions are integrated by self-organization into various activity patterns, our entire understanding of neural organization has to undergo rather fundamental changes. If the reflex paradigm of neural systems is to be abandoned for the new concept of "self-organization" of spontaneous (random or other) activity, this would be an entirely new challenge for "brain-mind philosophy." As long as the original cartesian reflex paradigm of the nervous system held sway, there simply was no way to accept the "downward causation" (i.e., a causal chain from emergent mental phenomena downward on the physiological functions of neural structures) within the framework of our classic views on the physical world. (Some philosophical arguments have been suggested by Szentágothai 1984.) On the basis of the relationship between information-theoretical and thermodynamic entropy, it was suggested (Érdi 1983; Szentágothai and Érdi 1989)

that information related to higher cognitive functions may help to establish neural order.

The Action-Perception Cycle and the Self-Directedness of the Organism

As was stressed in chapter 3, the behavior of an organism is to be analyzed in terms of an action-perception cycle rather than in stimulus-response terms. The organism uses an internal model of the world to provide partial information to predict (though not infallibly) the result of interacting with the environment in various ways. The repertoire of present actions helps to determine the most appropriate representations for perceptual information. Though an animal may perceive many aspects of its environment, only a few of these at any time can become the primary locus of interaction. Planning is required to determine the plan of action on the basis of current goals and the environmental model. Models have the advantages of allowing efficiency of recognition, prediction of outcomes in new situations, and the exploitation of similarities but have the disadvantages that they may lead to the overlooking of crucial differences and may mislead when the environment changes rapidly. We distinguish short-term memory as holding the model of the organism's current situation from long-term memory as the repository of the organism's knowledge of the world. Both classes of model must adapt.

11.2.4 The Brain-Mind-Computer Trichotomy

Often, the term *brain* is associated with the notions of *mind* and of *computer*. The brain-mind-computer problem has been treated within the framework of three separate dichotomies.

First, the brain-mind problem is related to the age-old philosophical debate among monists and dualists. Attempts to solve the brain-mind problem can be classified into two basic categories: (1) materialistic monism, leading in its ultimate consequences to some kind of reductionism, and (2) interactionist dualism, which is more or less some type of neo-cartesian philosophy.

The classification is an obviously crude oversimplification. A wide spectrum of monistic theories exists from Skinner's (1971) radical behaviorism and Patricia Churchland's (1986) eliminative materialism through Smart's (1981) physicalism to Bunge's (1980) emergent materialism. Interactionist dualism always has been an influential viewpoint since Descartes defined the interaction between the spatially extended body and a noncorporeal mind. Though its modern version was elaborated by two intellectual heroes of the twentieth century (Popper and Eccles 1977), still it has been criticized or even ignored by the representatives of the main stream of the philosophy of mind (mostly functionalists) and by biologically oriented thinkers. Érdi (1996) argued that the philosophical tradition of hermeneutics (i.e., the art of interpretation) which is a priori neither monist nor dualist, can be applied to the brain. Even more is stated: On one side, the brain is an "object" of interpretation; on the other side, it is itself an interpreter. Both natural science as "objective analyzer" and (post)modern art reiterate the old philosophical question, What is reality? The human brain is not only capable of perceiving what is called objective reality, but also of creating new reality. It is a hermeneutic device. In a similar vein, Arbib (1989) argued in *The Metaphorical Brain 2* (see also sec. 11.3.2) that our theories of the brain are metaphors, whereas the brain itself represents the world through schemas, which may themselves be viewed as metaphors. (See Arbib and Hesse 1986 for the role of hermeneutics in a schema-based epistemology.)

Second, the problem of the brain-computer analogy-disanalogy was a central issue of early cybernetics, in a sense revived by the neurocomputer boom. More precisely, the two sides of the metaphor (computational brain versus neural computer) merit a brief discussion. There are several different roots of the early optimism related to the power of the brain-computer analogy. First, both elementary computing units and neurons were characterized as digital input-output devices, suggesting an analogy at even the elementary hardware level. Second, the (more or less) equivalence had been demonstrated between the mathematical model of the "control box" of a computer as represented by the state-transition rules for a Turing machine and of the nervous system as represented by the McCulloch-Pitts model. Binary vectors of 0s and 1s represented the states of elementary components of both computer and brain, and the temporal behavior of computer and brain was described by the updating of these vectors. In his posthumously published book, *The Computer and the Brain*, John von Neumann (1958) emphasized the particular character of "neural mathematics": "... The logics and mathematics in the central nervous system, when viewed as languages, must structurally be essentially different from those languages to which our common experience refers..."

Arguments for the computer-brain *dis*analogy were listed by Conrad (1989). Digital computers are programmed from outside; are structurally programmable; have low adaptability; and work by discrete dynamics.

Their physical implementation is irrelevant in principle; they exhibit sequential processing; and the information processing happens mostly at network level. Brains are self-organizing devices; they are structurally nonprogrammable; they work by both discrete and continuous dynamics; their functions depend strongly on the physical (i.e., biological) substrate; the processing is parallel; and processing occurs for both network and intraneuronal information.

Inspiration from the brain leads away from emphasis on a single universal machine toward a device composed of different structures, just as the brain may be divided into cerebellum, hippocampus, motor cortex, and so on. Thus, we can expect to contribute to neural computing as we come to chart more fully the special power of each structure. The brain may be considered as a metaphor for sixth generation computing, wherein the latter is characterized by cooperative computation, perceptual robotics, and learning (Arbib 1994).

Third, the computational theory of mind holds that the computational metaphor is the final explanation of mental processes (e.g., Johnson-Laird 1988). Connectionism (Rumelhart and McClelland 1986) is an ambitious conceptual framework for a would-be general brain-mind-computer theory movement, but it is based on principles of brain-style computation that ignore many of the real-brain data that have occupied much of the present volume. Thus, the connectionist movement is directed more to the engineers of near-future-generation computer systems and to cognitive psychologists. Connectionist models in general are dynamic systems (e.g., Farmer 1990), and in this respect do offer useful concepts for brain theory. When the structure and function of the brain are studied by using theoretical methods, two concepts have to be emphasized: hierarchy and dynamics. The brain is considered as a prototype of hierarchical structures and can be studied at different levels (e.g., molecular, membrane, cellular, synaptic, network, and system).

However, the study of networks relevant to brain theory is not limited to connectionism. The theory of networks with large numbers of nodes constituting very complex structures offers, at least in principle, a common model of natural and synthetic information-processing systems. Though research motivated by statistical physics adopts elementary units (e.g., neurons or computing elements) as nodes, the neoconnectionist school defines networks with intermediate level computational-cognitive elements. Schemas provide even more sophisticated building blocks for network models of "parallel distributed processing."

11.2.5 Principles of Neural Organization

The *modular architectonics* principle states that the nervous system is composed of building blocks of repetitive structures. Columnar structure has been demonstrated in different parts of the cerebral cortex by anatomical and physiological techniques. Though the functional significance of cortical columns is not clear, it seems to be accepted that many neural and even perceptual phenomena can be explained in terms of dynamic intercolumnar interactions. More generally, we have traced a variety of modular structures (e.g., the hippocampal lamella and the cerebellar microcomplex) that allow us to bridge from individual neurons to overall functions.

Sensory information is represented in primary sensory cortices and a number of other structures in a *topographically ordered* way. This principle ensures that mapping between areas preserves spatial relationship. Skin surface and retina are mapped into the cortex topographically. However, available data coupled with our models of self-organization support the view that these topographical mappings are not determined genetically *in detail* and that the detailed properties of the map are generated by activity-dependent self-organizing mechanisms. Of course, once we move far from the periphery, the *action-perception cycle*, rather than topographical organization, predominates, and the emphasis shifts to the melding of information from disparate sources (both internal and external) to determine a course of action. However, even here, we expect most of the necessary connectivity to be generated by processes of activity-dependent self-organization.

Behavior of neural systems may be studied by concepts of population theories. As collective properties emergent in physical systems made from a large number of elementary components (spins, molecules, and the like) are treated by statistical mechanics, so (analogously) have *statistical dynamic theories* of neural populations been established. Specifically, both the determinism-randomness dilemma and the problem of neural ordering by noise-induced transition have been treated.

Though one characteristic aspect of neural organization is its hierarchical nature, it is at least as important to note the prevalent occurrence of *recurrent connections*. The overwhelming majority of all connections of the cerebral cortex are corticocortical; thus, reentry may have an important role in cortical integration (Tononi 1994). Moreover, the cortex is embedded in loops, whether returning to sensory thalamic nuclei; involving basal ganglia, cerebellum, and hippocampus; executing cooperative computation; or implementing perceptual and motor schemas.

Self-organization is considered as a mechanism for generating emergent structures. Neurodynamic phenomena (e.g., ontogeny, development, normal performance, learning, and plasticity) can be treated by coherent concepts within the formalism of neurodynamic system theory.

11.3 Implications and Outlook for Cognitive Neuroscience

Our studies of structure, function, and dynamics are located in a broad sweep running all the way from the motility of the embryo to the learning of visually guided behavior. In concluding, we turn from retrospect to prospect, suggesting ways in which the ideas developed in this volume may contribute to future work in cognitive neuroscience. This prospectus embodies a strong philosophical position: Mind (at least that aspect of it known as *cognition*) can be explained in terms of the workings of matter (especially that structured as neural systems). This concept raises a methodological challenge, because the categories of "mindtalk" and "brain talk" do not map directly one onto the other. Szentágothai and Arbib (1975) confronted this by providing two introductory overviews, functional and structural, for their study of *Conceptual Models of Neural Organization* and then analyzing both a question about the structures for a function—How is stereopsis implemented in the brain?—and a question about the functions of a structure—What does the cerebellum do? In the years since 1975, neuroscience has made immense progress in delimiting structure, whether in the functional neuroanatomy that has, for example, used double labeling techniques to subdivide and chart the terra hitherto incognita of the primate association cortices or in the studies in neurochemistry and molecular neurobiology that reveal more and finer structures within the individual neuron. We also have seen conceptual advances in the study of large networks of somewhat simplified neurons, ranging from studies of low-level vision to the statistical mechanics of self-organization emphasizing the matching of a single function to a single network. Chapter 3 emphasized work at a different level, in which a network of functions (schemas and schema assemblages) must be mapped to a network of neural networks. We now discuss the implications of this for cognitive neuroscience.

11.3.1 Memory, Perception, and Intelligence

The reader may object that much of human behavior is verbal rather than involving activity of the body and limbs, and may regret that our emphasis on perception as preparation to interact would seem to exclude from study most of people's more intelligent behavior, in particular the use of language for "internal thought" as distinct from external communication. However, human brains have evolved from the brains of animals that interacted in a complex fashion with their environments without the aid of language. Thus, we believe that language in both its external and internal forms can be understood best as a device that refines an already complex system. The evolutionary history of brains gives brain theory its biological character, for whereas in brain theory, language is to be explained as a recently evolved refinement of an underlying ability to interact with the environment, robotics starts from computers that are primarily linguistic (or at least symbol-manipulating) devices and tries to evolve better programs to guide robot behavior.

Certain properties contribute importantly to intelligence.

Possession of a modifiable model of the world, with its attendant adaptability. To act intelligently, a system must be able to take properties of its environment into account and be able to update its record of these properties to take account of new observations and changing relationships.

Flexibility and generality. An intelligent system must use past experience to act adaptively and be able to apply its past experience to situations not superficially similar to those encountered before. Again, techniques that have been developed to solve one type of problem should be recognized as applicable even when a very different domain of problems is involved.

Dynamic planning. An intelligent system should use its model to plan and evaluate alternative courses of action before committing itself to one of them. For a symbol-manipulation system, there may be little real distinction between planning and action, but for a robot or an animal, the distinction is very real and very important—it pays to recognize a precipice in advance and plan to avoid it rather than to recognize one's mistake after going over the edge. However, it is crucial that the plan be dynamic (i.e., rapidly and effectively updatable when new data reveal unexpected obstacles or make sought-for information available).

Perception of an event, thought, voluntary movement, and the like, (i.e., "elementary" events taking place during at most a few seconds) are accompanied by fast transient changes in the activity of the brain. Roland's monograph (1993) is an attempt to integrate knowledge on the bio-

chemical machinery of neurons and glial cells obtained mostly from in vitro experiments and results of in vivo physiological experiments made on invertebrates, vertebrates, and (mostly) on mammals. The development of methods measuring regional biochemical and physiological changes (as regional blood flow) accompanying brain activation, such as positron emission tomography (PET), make it possible to image functional mechanisms (sensation and perception, general and selective attention, motor function, language, thinking, and learning and memory) in the human brain and attempt to discover its functional dissection. In contrast to another technique (magnetic resonance imaging, MRI), which provides static images of brain anatomy), PET is appropriate to follow dynamic changes, and seems to be an important device for near-future cognitive neuroscience; functional MRI (fMRI) promises to combine advantages of both methods.

A large class of models of memory employed by cognitive psychologists is based on the assumption that knowledge structures stored in a semantic memory system can be identified with a network of nodes representing concepts connected by edges expressing relations between them (Quillian 1968; Collins and Quillian 1969). The spreading-activation hypothesis (Collins and Loftus 1975; Anderson 1983) offers a mechanism for the dynamics of the retrieval process. A node is activated by "priming" a concept (seeing, hearing, and the like). Activation of a node implies the activation of adjacent nodes, and so on. Gröbler, Marton, and Érdi (1991) presented a dynamic model of free recall and explained the relationship between the structure and performance of the network.

One important form of working memory is obtained by holding a particular pattern of firing during a delay task. Such neurons have been found in dorsolateral prefrontal cortex and in hippocampus. What distinguishes these two systems? The answer still is far from clear, but (see sec. 6.5) we assert that a full analysis of the procedural-declarative distinction in humans requires a theory of consciousness that distinguishes conscious-declarative from nonconscious-procedural access to schemas. The fact that a schema may be activated without conscious awareness emphasizes the notion that different neural processes must be involved in *monitoring* the use of a schema as distinct from the *use* per se of the schema. The "what"-"how" distinction (chap. 8) shows that some schemas are instantiated on paths to conscious awareness and that others are not. One patient may be able to "declare" the size of an object yet not be able to preshape the hand appropriately to grasp it; another patient may exhibit the opposite. Moreover, at least some of the working memory systems of prefrontal cortex are coupled tightly to specialized areas of parietal cortex and thus are tightly integrated into the procedural "how" system rather than into the conscious-declarative "what" system. Thus, the loop of explanation must be closed back from the theory of consciousness. As we have already noted (Hippocampal Function and Human Memory, sec. 6.5), this requirement is consistent with Rozin's view (1976) that procedural learning may be phylogenetically old, having developed as a collection of encapsulated special-purpose abilities of specific neural systems to register cumulative changes in their functioning. By contrast, the capacity for declarative learning reaches its full development only with the elaboration of medial temporal areas in mammals, especially the hippocampus and related cortical areas.

Perception provides access to motor schemas so as to control interaction with the object but does not necessarily entail execution of even one of these motor schemas. Although an animal may perceive many aspects of its environment, only a few of these at any time can become primary loci of interaction. *Planning* is the process whereby the system combines an array of relevant knowledge to determine a course of action suited to current goals. In its fullest subtlety, planning can involve the refinement of knowledge structures and goal structures and action per se. Novel inputs (e.g., coming on an unexpected obstacle) can alter the elaboration of high-level structures into lower-level tests and actions that in turn call on the interaction of motor and sensory systems (see the notion of dynamic planning). We seek to study programs that are part of the internal state of the system and that flexibly can guide ongoing action in terms of internal goals or drives and external circumstances. Note that we do not imply that planning is a conscious process and that planning goes beyond mere choice. In *choice*, we suggest that a decision (whether conscious or not) must be made between a few clearly delimited alternatives. In planning, by contrast, solutions to many possibly conflicting subproblems will have to be constructed to yield a possibly quite novel course of action. Already we have provided an evolutionary view of how visual perception may evolve into a distributed capability for planning (sec. 8.6, From Action-Oriented Perception to Cognition).

Because learning the salient features in the environment is so crucial to the acquisition of skills, one may suggest that in some learning situations, what we learn is not what a sensory input pattern is but rather what is the most appropriate feature to attend to. For example, a rat

in a maze is not simply pairing a response with a stimulus, it is executing complex muscular activity while being bombarded with a mass of sensory input. A rat might remember perfectly well how it got to the food on a certain trial yet still fail at the next because it does not know whether it was a subtle smell, the texture of the floor, a direction, a patterning of its muscular activity, or a mark on a door that was significant. Thus, even with "perfect" recall of what happened at each trial, the rat might require many, many trials to learn to disregard irrelevant stimuli and consistently to focus on the experimenter's cue to locate the reward. An animal's behavior in a learning experiment shows periods of little progress followed by a sudden jump in performance, as if the animal had hit on a new strategy or learned to pay attention to some relevant feature of the experimental situation. Thus, one may imagine learning progressing by a cumulative procedure in which the learner saves time by learning to apply the current strategy to fewer of the irrelevant features, to construct new features within the current strategy, and to change strategy. Anything that could tell the rat which aspect of its stimulation mattered would lead to almost instant learning— by directing attention rather than by conveying a specific message as to the location of food. Much of the most basic usefulness of language resides in its ability to direct (or misdirect) the attention of the listener.

11.3.2 Schema Theory and the Construction of Reality

To what extent can cognitive science give a theory of the person? Cognitive science is a loose federation of work in artificial intelligence, linguistics, psychology, and neuroscience. We use it as an umbrella term to unite several areas: artificial intelligence ("the attempt to program computers to do things that you would swear require intelligence until you know that a computer has been programmed to do them"); cognitive psychology, which uses the language of information processing to design models that can be run on computers to emulate the overt behavior of a human performing some intelligent task; and, at the finest grain of detail, brain theory, which must not only explain behavior patterns of animals and humans but must incorporate data on brain function and neural circuitry. What these have in common is that they yield models of cognition and intelligence that can be run on the computer. Thus, to the extent that cognitive science succeeds, we will have theories of mind that are operative.

Schema theory designates an approach to cognitive science based on the schema as the basic functional unit of action and perception (chap. 3). It gives an account of the embodied mind, transcending mind-body dualism by integrating an account of our mental representations with an account of the way in which we interact with the world. The brain "models" the world so that when we recognize something, we "see" in it things that will guide our interaction with it. There is no claim of infallibility, no claim that the interactions always will proceed as expected, but the point is that we recognize things not as linguistic animals, merely to name them, but as embodied animals.

In this volume, we have used schemas to provide a functional level of analysis of what occurs in the brain of an animal during sensorimotor coordination. Other studies (e.g., Arbib, Conklin, and Hill 1986) have used schemas in computational models of language acquisition and production. We have seen that to make sense of any given situation, we call on hundreds of schemas in our current "schema assemblage" (short-term memory) and that our lifetime of experience, our skills, our general knowledge, our recollection of specific episodes, might be encoded in a personal "encyclopedia" of hundreds of thousands of schemas (long-term memory), enriched from the verbal domain to incorporate the representations of action and perception, of motive and emotion, of personal and social interactions, of the *embodied self*. In terms of these hundreds of thousands of schemas, we would offer a naturalistic account of the self embodied in space and time. Nonetheless, for many people, this raises the question: Could hundreds of thousands of schemas— or billions of neurons—cohere to constitute a single personality, a self, a personal consciousness? This question motivated the title *In Search of the Person: Philosophical Explorations in Cognitive Science* (Arbib 1985).

The brain theorist seeks to instantiate schemas in terms of neural networks; and the cognitive psychologist analyzes, in information-processing terms, schemas for basic pattern recognition or memory tasks. To move from these levels of analysis to an understanding of the human individual, we need to study the coherence and conflicts within a schema network that constitutes a personality, with all its contradictions, as when we look at Freud's concept of identification as providing person-schemas and at the holistic nets of social reality, of custom, language and religion (Arbib and Hesse 1986). The following points summarize and extend our understanding of schema theory as an open-ended subject, responding to (but changing) our concepts of the reality of our personal and social worlds.

1. There is an everyday reality of persons and things. When cut, we bleed. If we drop a hot kettle, boiling water may scald us. Love can turn to jealousy. How can we come to know this reality?

2. Schema theory answers that our minds comprise a richly interconnected network of schemas. An assemblage of some of these schemas represents our current situation; planning then yields a coordinated control program of motor schemas that guide our actions. As we act, we perceive; as we perceive, so we act.

3. Perception is not passive, like a photograph; rather, it is active, as our current schemas determine what we take from the environment. If we have perceived someone as a friend, we may perceive their remark as a pleasing joke; yet the same words uttered by someone we dislike, even if intended as a joke, may be perceived as an insult that elicits a vicious response.

4. As a unit of interaction with, or representation of, the world, a schema is partial and approximate. It provides us not only with abilities for recognition and guides to action but also with expectations about what will happen. These may be wrong. Sometimes we learn from our mistakes. Our schemas, and their connections within the schema network, change. Piaget gave us some insight into these processes of schema change with his talk of assimilation and accommodation.

5. There is no single set of schemas imposed on all persons in a uniform fashion. Even young children have distinct personalities. Each of us has very different life experiences, on the basis of which our schemas change over time. Thus, each of us has our knowledge embodied within a different schema network, and thus, each of us has constructed a different world-view that each of us takes for reality.

Schemas may rest on individual style yet be shaped by the social milieu. A network of schemas—be it an individual personality, a scientific paradigm, an ideology, or a religious symbol system—can itself constitute a schema at a higher level. Such a great schema certainly can be analyzed in terms of its constituent schemas, but (the crucial point) once we have the overall network, these constituents can find their full meaning only in terms of this network of which they are a part.

This hierarchical view of schemas is very close to the views of C. S. Peirce regarding what he calls *habits* (see Burks 1980). For Peirce, a habit was any set of operative rules embodied in a system. He emphasized (anticipating Piaget) that they possess both stability and adaptability. He had in mind an evolutionary metaphor: Species form a stable unit for our analysis of the present state of the animal world, yet we know that these units are subject to evolutionary change. Thus Peirce's habits, like our schemas, can serve as building blocks in a hierarchy of personal rules, of society, science and evolution, and yet may themselves change over time.

In this way, we view knowledge as inseparable from an evolving schema network. There is then no such thing as sure knowledge, and we must reject the philosopher's definition of knowledge as true belief. Certainly, there are schemas that embody what we now take to be true, but schemas also include false but useful models; there are ideals as given by schemas for the beautiful, the true, and the good, and they are very real as determinants of the way in which we behave, whether or not we believe that they represent some external reality.

An important gap in most computational analyses of the mind comes about because few neuroscientists think about the social nature of being a human (see Brothers and Ring 1992, 1993, for an entry point to that small body of literature that does begin to link neural activity to social cognition). To be human is not just to have in the head a sophisticated "computer" called the *brain*. It is also to have grown up as a member of society and to have learned the nuances of that society. Neuroscientists and cognitive scientists emphasize what they can measure objectively (e.g., language wherein we analyze a string of symbols, or vision wherein there are particular patterns to which we can see how people or animals or neurons respond). *In Search of the Person* (Arbib 1985) emphasized that much of human experience (or, if you will, person-reality, of being a member of society, being aware, and having experience of love, hate, and anguish) normally is not addressed at all within the framework of brain research or cognitive science. The point was not to reduce these elements to current brain theory or cognitive science but rather to show how the science and the personal experience might be thought about in a unified framework in which understanding of each reality could come to shape that of the other (a hermeneutic process).

People differ as to the limits of this understanding. Seeing that we understand more and more of what it is to be a person in terms of our understanding of the brain, some people will believe that everything in due course can be shown to be a function of the brain (though our understanding of the brain will be enriched greatly in the process, this being a *two-way* reductionism). Others will emphasize, rather, that much of person-reality has not been explained and will espouse a dualist faith that some aspects of mental life *never* can be explained in these terms. However, at least we may set the debate in terms of a program of understanding how we could narrow the apparent gap between our personal awareness and our present day cognitive science (although for the authors

of this book, monism has been a better guide to science than dualism has been).

11.3.3 Language

We can end on a more concrete note by discussing the controversial issue of whether the study of language can be illuminated by approaches to neural organization of the kind presented in this volume. Elsewhere, Szentágothai and Érdi (1989) have argued that "... [t]he deep logical structures of the specifically human ability of speech acquisition are wired genetically into the upper surface of the human left (to much less degree into the right) temporal lobe, exactly as the neuronal mechanisms for moving a limb are wired (Székely and Czéh 1971) into the limb-innervating segments of the medullary tube..." However, Arbib and Hill (1988) urged a more cautious view. The problem is to decide whether parts of the brain may be specialized to cooperatively acquire "the deep logical structures" of language or whether these structures themselves are "wired genetically." To clarify this distinction, we recall that the traditional grounding of linguistics is in *grammar*, a systematic set of rules for structuring the sentences of a particular language. From the 1960s on, *generative linguistics*, which provides formal specifications for generating the grammatically well-formed sentences of a language, has been dominated by the ideas of Noam Chomsky. His ideas have gone through successive stages in which the formulation of grammars has changed radically [e.g., from the "aspects" theory of Chomsky (1965) to the theory of government and binding (see van Riemsdijk and Williams 1986 for an introduction) with other theories before, between, and after]. However, even if one accepts the descriptive power of generative grammar, one may or may not choose also to accept two of Chomsky's theses about language that between them constitute a very influential version of the claim that the deep logical structures of language are wired genetically: (1) There is a universal grammar that defines what makes a language human, and each human language has a grammar that is a parametric variation of the universal grammar, and (2) language is too complicated for a child to learn from scratch; instead, a child has universal grammar as an "innate mental capacity." Hearing example sentences of a language, a child sets parameters in the universal grammar to allow for acquiring the grammar of the particular language.

Connectionist linguists (see Elman 1995) attack these claims on two fronts. First, they say that language processing is understood more fully in terms of connectionist processing. As a *performance* model (i.e., a model of behavior distinct from a *competence* model that gives a static representation of a body of knowledge), this processing can give an account of errors, as well as regularities, in language use. Second, they say that it provide powerful learning tools that Chomsky has chosen to ignore. With these tools, connectionists can model how children could acquire language on the basis of far less specific mental structures than those posited by Chomsky in his universal grammar.

Note that one may accept the claim that connectionism provides a better account of language acquisition than one based on parameter setting in universal grammar while still accepting that generative grammar gives a better account of the structure of adult language. For example, "The dog ate the rat" and "The rat was eaten by the dog" both convey the same meaning. In his government and binding theory, Chomsky explains the relation between these different forms by postulating that the syntactical structure contains a trace $[t_i]$, as in "The rat$_i$ was eaten $[t_i]$ by the dog," to indicate where the noun phrase with the same index (i in this case) would fit into the thematic role. Most connectionist models lack the tools for analyzing such relationships.

Neurolinguistics is the branch of psycholinguistics that seeks to link the processes underlying language performance to the activity of specific regions of the brain. Much work in neurolinguistics is based on the study of aphasia, the correlation of forms of language disorder with localized damage to the brain, but the field now is gaining new insights from functional brain imaging of normal, as well as impaired, activity. *Computational neurolinguistics* is the branch of brain theory that seeks to build on computational models of brain function (such as those we have sampled in many of the preceding chapters), connectionist models of language processing, neurology, and psycholinguistics. We review two kinds of models: those constrained by neurological data and connectionist models that reproduce aspects of language performance without structural constraints on their inner workings. In either case, processes are to be modeled in terms of the interaction of neural (biological or artificial) subsystems (neurons or brain regions); lesion deficits then are to be modeled via the interaction of residual subsystems.

Many psycholinguists choose to work in a chomskian paradigm, seeking, for example, to structure parsers that embody a generative grammar yet exhibit processing properties that represent certain aspects of psycholin-

guistic data. Frazier (1990) had a parser that exhibited "minimal attachment" and "late closure" to explain why, in reading the sentence, "Because Jennifer always reads a book is never far from her," a preliminary misanalysis yields the temporary interpretation that "Jennifer always reads a book." In Frazier's analysis, grammatical parsing forms a relatively isolated module. Other workers argue for interactive models in which semantical, syntactical, and pragmatic information interact throughout sentence comprehension (McDonald and MacWhinney 1989). However, few of the details of syntactical processing survive into the analysis of aphasic data. For example, "Broca's aphasics" may be characterized loosely as exhibiting agrammatism: They tend to simplify syntactical structures and omit closed class items (e.g., prepositions and grammatical markers).[1] Bradley, Garrett, and Zurif (1980) used a computational account of the distinction between open and closed class items to account for the syntactical deficits in Broca's aphasia, with psycholinguistical studies that suggested that normal access to closed class items was destroyed by lesions of Broca's area (though other access paths remained). Subsequent data suggest that this analysis is too simple (see Zurif 1984 for a review).

Arbib, Caplan, and Marshall (1982) placed neurolinguistics in a historical perspective, starting with the classic work of Broca (1861) and Wernicke (1874) and its synthesis by Lichtheim (1885) as background to the twentieth century development of holist and process models. Arbib and Caplan (1979) contrasted the *faculty approach* to neurolinguistics (typified by Lichtheim's one-faculty-per-region codification of the data from Broca and Wernicke up to his day) with the *process* approach of Luria, which saw localization as a dynamic process, with any faculty embodied in the interaction of a multiplicity of brain regions so that, in particular, a single region might enter into numerous overall types of psychological behavior. Arbib and Caplan (1979) analyzed Luria's 1973 survey of the effects of brain damage on different aspects of language function (naming of objects, verbal expression of motives, speech understanding, and speech repetition). (Figure 11.1 is an improved version of their figures summarizing this analysis.) Given the great variability of localization for aphasia (Caplan 1995), let alone other aspects of language performance, much research needs to be done both clinically and theoretically to update the analysis radically. The points to stress here

---

1. We note in warning that as exemplified by the study of Vanier and Caplan (1990) discussed later, Broca's aphasia is at best a cluster of symp-

toms rather than an effect unequivocally characteristic of a lesion to Broca's area of the human brain and to Broca's area alone.

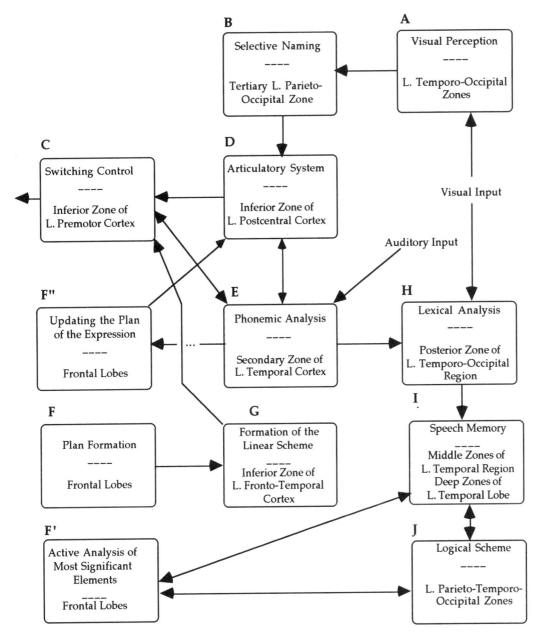

Figure 11.1

A diagram synthesizing Luria's (1973) survey of the effects of brain damage on different aspects of language function. These aspects include naming of objects, verbal expression of motives, speech under-standing, and speech repetition. (Adapted from Arbib and Caplan 1979.)

are that each of the foregoing functions involves the interaction of many brain regions; that many of the brain regions are involved in multiple functions; and that normal language behavior probably invokes all the functions (and thus all the brain regions) in constantly shifting combinations. In other words, the cooperative computation style of brain modeling developed in these pages, with special attention to visuomotor coordination, provides tools for language processing, one of the highest of cognitive functions.

Vanier and Caplan (1990) found immense variability in the site of lesions in 20 patients with agrammatism and found cases in which lesions spared Broca's area. Indeed, if sentence analysis involves cooperative computation, removal of many different subsystems may yield effects that are agrammatical, a classification broad enough to gloss over the subtleties required to discriminate between the behavioral effects of different lesions. If we accept at face value Caplan's (1995) argument that the construction of syntactic forms "is accomplished by quite different areas of the association cortex in the peri-sylvian area in different individuals," it seems strongly prejudicial to the chomskian view of universal grammar as an innate structure of the human brain, a view which rejects the notion that learning plays a major role in language acquisition. Lability of localization seems a more likely result of a process of self-organization than of a rigid, genetically specified program for the brain's syntactical processor (Arbib and Hill 1988).

Connectionist modelers distinguish two main architectures for their networks. In a layered feedforward network, the "neurons" are arranged in a series of layers, with the only connections being from neurons in one layer to neurons in the next layer. Because there are no loops, there is no possibility of a reverberating memory, and thus, after a suitable propagation delay, each input pattern yields a unique output pattern. By contrast, a network with loops acts as a dynamic system; for each fixed input pattern, patterns of activity may move around the network, creating dynamic sequences of internal states. In many studies, the behavior of such a network is not characterized in terms of input-output pairs but rather in terms of settling into a steady state, such as a *point attractor*, a *limit cycle* (yielding a sustained oscillation), or even a *strange attractor* (deterministic chaos). Thus, networks studied from this point of view often are referred to as *attractor networks* (sec. 4.5.4, Computation with Attractors: Scope, Limits, and Extensions). Recent studies of lesioned attractor networks (e.g., Hinton and Shallice 1991; Plaut and Shallice 1993) provided further insights into the clinical observations of neuropsychology. Simulated damage to attractor networks can mimic qualitatively some of the deficits seen following human brain damage. In particular, such studies suggest how there may be an appearance of functional modularity (i.e., two functions may be impaired differentially by network damage) even when the functions are implemented by a single network. Horn and Ruppin (1995) suggested an attractor neural network model of schizophrenia. They showed that memory performance may be preserved to a certain limit by strengthening the synaptic connectivity. However, this compensatory mechanism may imply spontaneous, stimulus-independent retrieval of stored patterns.

Despite their real contributions, such studies make little progress in explaining the contributions of specific brain regions to language capabilities. Recent work on "mirror" neurons (di Pellegrino et al. 1992) provides promise in this direction by suggesting a new path for integration between the study of human language and the study of detailed neural mechanisms of visuomotor coordination. These mirror neurons are a subset of the grasp-related neurons of the F5 region of premotor cortex (sec. 8.4.3). They discharge when a monkey observes meaningful hand movements made by the experimenter (e.g., placing objects on or taking objects from a table, grasping food from another experimenter, or manipulating objects). There is always a link between the effective observed movement for a mirror neuron and the effective executed movement.

These data suggest that area F5 is endowed with an observation-execution matching system and led Fadiga et al. (1995) to seek evidence for an observation-execution matching system in humans. In a PET study of brain activation of humans observing hand gestures, they found a highly significant activation of the posterior part of the left inferior frontal gyrus—the rostral part of Broca's area. Though homologies between cortical areas of different species are always difficult, a good case can be made that Broca's area is in part homologous with F5. In man, the frontal region related to speech (Broca's area) as outlined by electrical stimulation studies (Penfield and Roberts 1959) is formed by areas 44 and 45 of Brodmann. Area 44 corresponds to area FCBm of von Economo (1929), whereas area 45 corresponds to his area FDγ. Von Bonin (1944) compared the premotor cortex of human, chimpanzee, and macaque monkey brains and recognized an area similar in architecture to FCBm in both chimpanzees and monkeys; in the macaque monkey, this homolog of FCBm is basically coextensive with F5 as defined by Matelli, Luppino, and Rizzolatti (1985).

These data have led Rizzolatti et al. (1996) to a bold hypothesis: The functional specialization of human Broca's area derives from an ancient mechanism related to the production and understanding of motor acts. To this we would add that this specialization may correspond to verbs or verb phrases but seems separate from the functions of naming and of noun phrases more generally. This view is concordant with our emphasis that language, like other functions studied in this volume, is to be seen more as a distributed function (cooperative computation in the spirit of figure 11.1) than as being a "unitary faculty." Rizzolatti et al. argued more specifically that the sophisticated capacity of action analysis shown by mirror cells is at the basis of the evolutionary prevalence of the lateral motor system over the medial (emotion-related) system in becoming the main communication channel in higher primates and man. Currently, much work is under way to turn this hypothesis into a rigorous neurolinguistical model subject to coherent testing that integrates monkey neurophysiology and human brain mapping within a framework offered by the current debate over language evolution (Pinker and Bloom 1990; Wilkins and Wakefield 1995). The point for our current claim—that this book provides powerful tools for cognitive neuroscience—is that we see here an approach to language that does not treat it in grand isolation in the style of Chomsky but instead (without denying the special character of these higher mental functions) sees language and other cognitive processes within the framework of neural organization that we have charted in these pages.

Appendixes

Many tools have been built to aid in the task of modeling and simulating neural networks at different levels of detail. The more detailed neuronal models, such as the Hodgkin-Huxley model and compartmental models, permit the modeling of only a few neurons at a time and are supported by simulation systems such as GENESIS or NEURON (De Schutter 1992; Hines 1993). The coarser neural models, such as the leaky-integrator model, permit the modeling of thousands of neurons and are supported by such simulation systems as Neural Simulation Language (NSL) (Weitzenfeld 1991). Appendix A focuses on the NSL simulation of large neural networks.

A number of models described in this book and a growing number of other models besides (many of them implemented in NSL) now are available on the World Wide Web (WWW), as part of the materials placed there by the University of Southern California Brain Project (USCBP). This database of models is called Brain Models on the Web (BMW). Appendix B tells readers how they may interact with the models via the Internet and may import them onto their own computers. The BMW home page provides access to a growing range of neural models and explains how to get access to an NSL tutorial and how to ftp the code.

Neural Simulation Language

In the Neural Simulation Language (NSL; Weitzenfeld 1991), the basic neural model is the single-compartment model, having one output and many inputs. The internal state of the neuron is described by a single scalar quantity—its membrane potential m—which depends on the neuron's inputs and its history. The output is described by another single scalar quantity—its firing rate M—and may serve as input to many other neurons, including itself. As the input to a neuron varies, the membrane potential and firing rate also vary.

The membrane potential for m is described by the differential equation

$$\tau_m \frac{dm(t)}{dt} = f(m(t), S_m(t), t)$$

which depends on the neuron's input S_m, previous values of m, and time parameter t. τ_m is the time constant. The choice of f defines the particular neural model that is used. In particular, the leaky-integrator model is described by

$$f(S_m, m, t) = -m(t) + S_m(t), \text{ or}$$

$$\tau_m \frac{dm(t)}{dt} = -m(t) + S_m(t).$$

The *firing rate* M, the output of the neuron, is obtained by applying a *threshold function* to the neuron's membrane potential,

$$M(t) = \sigma(m(t))$$

where σ usually is a nonlinear function. Some of the most common threshold functions are *ramp, step, saturation,* and *sigmoidal.*

The most common formula for the input to a neuron v is

$$S_v = \sum_{i=1}^{n} w_i M_i(t)$$

where $M_i(t)$ is the firing rate of the neuron the output of which is connected to the ith input of neuron v, and w_i is the weight on that link.

In NSL, two DATA structures are required to represent a neuron: one structure corresponding to the membrane potential and the other to the firing rate. However, as we see later, it is common to *extend* these data structures to represent entire arrays of similar neurons rather than single neurons. The notation is as follows (with a semicolon at the end of each statement):

DATA m;

DATA M;

The membrane potential m is represented by a differential equation

$\text{DIFF}(m, t_m) = f(S_m, m)$;

where DIFF defines a first-order differential equation for m with time decay t_m (time parameter t is implicit in the equation). The leaky-integrator model corresponds to

$\text{DIFF}(m, \tau_m) = -m + S_m.$

The firing rate M is represented simply by

$M = \sigma(m)$

where σ represents the choice of threshold function.

In modeling thousands of neurons and their interconnections, it becomes extremely difficult to name every single one of them. Because in the brain we often find neural networks structured into two-dimensional homogeneous neural arrays, with regular connection patterns between them, NSL extends the basic neuron abstraction into neural arrays and connection masks. The computational advantage is that neural arrays and interconnection masks then can be described concisely as higher-level data structures and, similarly, the connections between arrays can be described by a mask storing synaptic weights. An interconnection among neurons then would be processed by computing a spatial convolution of a mask and a layer. For example, if A represents an array of outputs from one array of neurons, B represents the array of inputs to another layer, and the mask $W(k, l)$ (for $-d \leqslant k$, $l \leqslant d$) represents the synaptic weight from the $A(i + k, j + l)$ (for $-d \leqslant k, l \leqslant d$) elements to $B(i, j)$ element for each i and j, we have

$$B = \sum_{k=-d}^{d} \sum_{l=-d}^{d} W(k, l)A(i + k, j + l)$$

which can be described by a simple expression

$B = W * A$

To support arrays and masks, the basic DATA structure in NSL is extended with two arrays types, VECTOR and MATRIX, which are one- and two-dimensional, respectively.

The main challenge in the development of NSL and with other simulation tools is to provide a general purpose user-friendly simulation environment and at the same time to be as efficient as possible in the time-consuming process of neural network simulation. As NSL evolves, it will offer a distributed and parallel framework for the simulation of neural networks (Weitzenfeld and Arbib 1991), integrating with schema models (as described in abstract schema language ASL, Weitzenfeld 1993). It will facilitate the development of hierarchical and distributed neural networks in which code may be re-used in developing one model on the basis of another. The foregoing description applies to NSL versions 2.1 and 2.5. As of mid-1997, a new version of NSL, incorporating features of ASL, was under development with implementations in both C++ and Java. As these become available, details will be posted in Brain Models on the Web.

Brain Models on the Web

Brain Models on the Web (BMW), a growing database of exemplary neural models, may be found at:

http://www-hbp.usc.edu/HBP/models/

BMW is being developed as a framework for the electronic publication of computational models of neural systems. It also offers linkages to databases of empirical data and an environment for the analysis of the strengths and weaknesses of current models in the light of available data, all in the context of developing new models of greater validity in part by re-usage of components of existing models (Arbib 1995). This Appendix is based on the state of BMW as of mid-1997. The state of BMW is changing rapidly, and readers are invited to log in to view our progress and offer their comments on how to advance it. In any case, readers will be able to learn more about many of the models described in this book and to track models that build on them.

BMW is part of the University of Southern California Brain Project (USCBP), the key goal of which is to build a federation of databases that catalyze the integrated development of experiment and modeling in the neuroscience community. The goal includes providing databases that link data from several levels of analysis (molecular, cellular, network) with functional models, whether mathematical or not, all in the context of an anatomical framework.

Models currently available in BMW include a number described in this volume, such as studies of the role of basal ganglia in saccade control and of cerebellum in prism adaptation in dart throwing, and models of the role of cerebellum in classic conditioning, of basal ganglia in arm movements, and of hippocampus in spatial navigation. BMW allows users to view, via the World Wide Web, tutorials, code, and sample simulations of models; ftp then may be used to bring a model to a local site for detailed testing. Future work will expand the database and develop tools that will allow users around the world to comment on models, develop new versions, and contribute new models to BMW.

Already (mid-1997), we have developed Brain Models on the Web as a set of models written in NSL with a tutorial, NSL code, and interfaces designed to ease simulation of standard experiments, all coded in html hypertext for WWW access. In addition, a number of Java applets were already available. BMW's future development will include models formulated at a variety of levels and written in a variety of simulation languages. Here are the four choices offered the user by the BMW Home Page for the Dominey-Arbib model, our example for control of saccadic eye movements (chapters 3, 8, 9, and 10):

Theoretical background. This tool provides a tutorial for the model, with hypertext links to relevant data used in designing the model or in setting criteria for what the model is to contain.

Computer code. In this case, the code is in NSL, but BMW will not be limited to this language.

Run. This element provides help in starting to use the model. It gives step-by-step instructions on how to run the model, explains the output, and provides examples of parameters that could be adjusted.

Project diary. This component provides a description of what was needed to place the model in BMW.

An important aspect of BMWfication (pronounced "beamerfication," the process of placing the model in BMW) addressed the needs of users who are not modelers and thus want to be able to conduct "experiments" that test whether the model's performance matches or predicts experimental data without knowing the particular modeling language (in this case, NSL). Thus, we created an interface for each significant class of experiments addressed by the model. It allows the user to set up the conditions of an experiment by, say, clicking on an array (to specify the position of a visual target) and typing in a few numbers (e.g., to specify the onset and offset times for various stimuli).

Our plans for development of BMW emphasize the need for explicit links between models and the biological data that *support* them and explicit links between simulation results and data that *test* their predictions.

Four elements comprise a BMW model: a narrative describing the model, a formal description of the model, the commented code that implements the model, and simulation resources for running the simulation. Appropriate material in these four collections are to be linked to databases containing both empirical data and simulation results. Development of BMW addresses the following points:

• Laboratory data mean little unless they are stored in the database with information about the protocol used to obtain them.

• Much of our access to such data will be indirect, via empirical generalizations and summary tables and figures.

• Such summaries should be linked to laboratory data from which they are derived or to journal articles in which they have been published.

• Tools are needed to summarize laboratory data for publication.

• Tools are needed to contrast and compare experimental results, generalizations, and the predictions of models of neural activity.

In mid-1997, most the BMW models were based on large networks composed of a number of arrays, each of multiple neurons (with the entire model coded in NSL). In this version, all biological data were contained in a tutorial coded as HTML hypertext for WWW access, whereas other work in the USCBP had generated a preliminary database of legacy data, also coded as HTML hypertext. Work during 1996–7 included placement of legacy data in an Illustra database, with links to the "lab-based" databases of physiological and other data. Currently, the tutorial, code, and instructions for running simulation experiments are accessible on most WWW platforms. Sample simulation results are made available without rerunning the model. To exercise more fully those models that prove to be sufficiently interesting, the user may transfer NSL and the programs of interest by ftp to their local site. We are developing Java code to ease use of code on the client machine.

A current effort is to extend BMW to include compartmental models and even more detailed synaptic-neurochemical models. We are working with colleagues who are developing a variety of simulation languages (e.g., NEURON and GENESIS as well as NSL) to design standards for structuring models to be related to data and embedded in BMW; then we will design the next generation of NSL, NSL 3.0, to be a language (but, it is hoped, not the only language) to meet those standards. The resultant framework will provide the user with access to a variety of neurosimulators, exploiting the strengths of each, depending on the modeling task at hand.

Experimental data in the USC neuroscience databases (and the broader federation of databases of which they will eventually be a part) will be supplemented by synthetic data linking experimental results to alternative models, documenting the extent to which the models fit empirical data of interest or make predictions that can guide new experiments. Thus, part of the work in progress is designed to provide

users of BMW with tools to enter shortcomings of the model—or novel properties revealed by new simulations—into a database relating these results to model, parameter set, and "experimental details." Also, the design aims to provide versioning tools to aid in the preparation of revised models yielding better performance in a biologically consistent way. This goal will involve linkages between biological data, simulation results approximating or contradicting them, and the underlying model and details.

The full development of the USCBP will provide an environment that makes it easy for the user to pass from empirical data to related models and back again. If successful, BMW-based standards activity will provide modelers using a variety of simulation languages (not just NSL) with tools to develop interfaces that make it easy for nonprogrammers to run basic "experiments" with the models and to add to the database comments on the comparison of simulation results with available empirical data. Also, users will be able to install models, create versions of both models and parameter sets, and freeze models in various "interesting" states for later analysis under varying conditions. A crucial aspect in all this development is to catalyze a truly cumulative style of modeling in neuroscience by facilitating the *reusability* of modules within current neural models, with the pattern of re-usage fully documented and tightly constrained by the linkage with a federation of databases of empirical neuroscientific data.

References

Abbott, L. F. 1994. Single neuron dynamics: An introduction. In *Neural modeling and neural networks*, ed. F. Ventriglia, 57–78. Oxford: Pergamon Press.

Abeles, M. 1991. *Corticonics: Neural circuits of the cerebral cortex.* London: Cambridge University Press.

Ádám, A. 1968. Simulation of rhythmic nervous activities. II. Mathematical models for the function of networks with cyclic inhibition. *Kybernetik* 5:103–109.

Adrian, E. D. 1941. Afferent discharges to the cerebral cortex from peripheral sense organs. *J. Physiol. (Lond.)* 100:159–191.

Adrian, E. D. 1942. Olfactory reactions in the brain of hedgehog. *J. Physiol.* 10:459–473.

Adrian, E. D. 1950. Sensory discrimination with some recent evidence from the olfactory organ. *Br. Med. Bull.* 6:330–331.

Ahissar, E., and Vaadia, E. 1990. Single cell cortical oscillators in a somatosensory cortex of awake monkey. *Proc. Natl. Acad. Sci. U.S.A.* 87:8935–8939.

Aihara, K. 1990. Chaotic neural networks. In *Bifurcation phenomena in nonlinear systems and theory of dynamical systems*, ed. H. Kawakami, 143–161. Singapore: World Scientific.

Albano, A. M., and Rapp, P. E. 1993. On the reliability of dynamical measures of EEG signals. In *Proceedings of the Second Annual Conference on Nonlinear Dynamical Analysis of the EEG*, eds. B. H. Jansen and M. E. Brandt, 117–139. Singapore: World Scientific.

Albano, J. E., and King, W. M. 1989. Rapid adaptation of saccadic amplitude in humans and monkeys. *Vis. Sci.* 30:1883–1893.

Albeck, Y. 1995. Sound localization and binaural processing. In *The handbook of brain theory and neural networks*, ed. M. A. Arbib, 891–895. Cambridge, MA: Bradford Books/MIT Press.

Albus, J. 1981. *Brains, behavior and robotics.* Peterborough, NH: BYTE Books.

Albus, J. S. 1971. A theory of cerebellar function. *Math. Biosci.* 10:25–61.

Alexander, G. E., and Crutcher, M. D. 1990. Functional architecture of basal ganglia circuits: Neural substrates of parallel processing. *Trends Neurosci.* 13:266–271.

Alexander, G. E., Delong, M. R., and Strick, P. L. 1986. Parallel organization of functionally segregated circuits linking basal ganglia and cortex. *Annu. Rev. Neurosci.* 9:357–381.

Alexander, G. E., and Fuster, J. M. 1973. Effects of cooling prefrontal cortex on cell firing in the nucleus medialis dorsalis. *Brain Res.* 61:93–105.

Alger, B. E., and Nicoll, R. A. 1982. Pharmacological evidence for two kinds of GABA receptors on rat hippocampal cells studies in vitro. *J. Physiol.* 328:125–141.

Alonso, J. R., and Frotscher, M. 1989. Hippocampo-septal fibers terminate on identified spiny neurons in the lateral septum: A combined Golgi/electron microscopic and degeneration study in the rat. *Cell Tissue Res.* 258:243–246.

Altman, J. 1982. Morphological development of the rat cerebellum and some of its mechanisms. In *The cerebellum: New vistas*, eds. S. Palay and V. Chan-Palay. Berlin: Springer-Verlag.

Amaral, D. G. 1978. A Golgi study of cell types in the hilar region of the hippocampus of the rat. *J. Comp. Neurol.* 182:851–914.

Amaral, D. G. 1987. Memory: Anatomical organization of candidate brain regions. In *Handbook of physiology—the nervous system*, eds. V. B. Mountcastle, F. Blom, and S. P. Geier, 211–294. Bethesda, MD: American Physiological Society.

Amaral, D. G., Ishizuka, N., and Claiborne, B. 1990. Neurons, numbers and the hippocampal network. *Prog. Brain Res.* 8:1–11.

Amaral, D. G., and Kurz, J. 1985. An analysis of the origins of the cholinergic and noncholinergic septal projections to the hippocampal formation of the rat. *J. Comp. Neurol.* 240:37–59.

Amaral, D. G., and Witter, M. P. 1989. The three-dimensional organization of the hippocampal formation: A review of anatomical data. *Neuroscience* 31:571–591.

Amari, S. 1974. A method of statistical neurodynamics. *Kybernetik* 14:201–215.

Amari, S. 1980. Topographic organization of nerve fields. *Bull. Math. Biol.* 42:339–364.

Amari, S. 1982. Competitive and cooperative aspects in dynamics of neural excitation and self-organization. In *Competition and cooperation in neural nets. Vol. 45, Lecture notes in biomathematics*, eds. S. Amari and M. Arbib, 1–28. Berlin: Springer-Verlag.

Amari, S. 1983. Field theory of self-organizing neural nets. *I.E.E.E. Trans. Syst. Man. Cybern.* 13:741–748.

Amari, S., and Arbib, M. A. 1977. Competition and cooperation in neural nets. In *Systems neuroscience*, ed. J. Metzler, 119–165. New York: Academic Press.

Ambros-Ingerson, J., Granger, R., and Lynch, G. 1990. Simulation of paleocortex performs hierarchical clustering. *Science* 247:1344–1348.

Amit, D. J. 1989. *Modeling brain function*. London: Cambridge University Press.

Andersen, P., and Andersson, S. A. 1968. *Physiological basis of the alpha rhythm*. New York: Appleton-Century-Crofts.

Andersen, P., Bliss, T. V. P., and Skrede, K. K. 1971. Lamellar organization of hippocampal excitatory pathways. *Exp. Brain Res.* 113:222–238.

Andersen, P., Silfvenius, H., Sundberg, S. H., and Sveen, P. 1980. A comparison of distal and proximal dendritic synapses of CAI pyramids in hippocampal slices in vitro. *J. Physiol. (Lond.)* 307:273–299.

Andersen, R., Snowden, R., and Graziao, M. 1991. Hierarchical processing of motion in the visual cortex of monkey. *Cold Spring Harb. Symp. Quant. Biol.* 55:741–748.

Andersen, R. A., Asanuma, C., Essick, G., and Siegel, R. M. 1990. Corticocortical connections of anatomically and physiologically defined subdivisions within the inferior parietal lobule. *J. Comp. Neurol.* 296:65–113.

Anderson, C. H., Olshausen, B. A., and Van Essen, D. 1995. Routing networks in visual cortex. In *The handbook of brain theory and neural networks*, ed. M. A. Arbib. Cambridge, MA: Bradford Books/MIT Press.

Anderson, J. A. 1968. A memory storage model utilizing spatial correlation functions. *Kybernetik* 5:113–119.

Anderson, J. R. 1983. *The architecture of cognition*. Cambridge, MA: Harvard University Press.

Andrade, R., Malenka, R. C., and Nicoll, R. A. 1986. A G protein couples serotonin and GABA receptor to the same channels in hippocampus. *Science* 234:1261–1265.

Angulo, A. W. 1951. A comparison of the growth and differentiation of the trigeminal ganglia with the cervical spinal ganglia in albino rat embryos. *J. Comp. Neurol.* 75:53–71.

Anninos, P. A., Beek, B., Csermely, T. J., Harth, E., and Pertile, G. 1970. Dynamics of neural structures. *J. Theor. Biol.* 26:121–148.

Aosaki, T., Tsubokawa, H., Ishida, A., Watanabe, K., Graybiel, A. M., and Kimura, M. 1994. Responses of tonically active neurons in the primate's striatum undergo systematic changes during behavioral sensorimotor conditioning. *J. Neurosci.* 14(6):3969–3984.

Apicella, P. E., Scarnati, E., and Schultz, W. 1991. Tonically discharging neurons of monkey striatum respond to preparatory and rewarding stimuli. *Exp. Brain Res.* 84:672–675.

Aradi, I., Barna, G., Érdi, P., and Gröbler, T. 1995. Chaos and learning in the olfactory bulb. *Int. J. Intell. Syst.* 10:89–117.

Aradi, I., and Érdi, P. 1996a. Signal generation and propagation in the olfactory bulb: Multicompartmental modeling. *Computers Math. Applic.* 32:1–27.

Aradi, I., and Érdi, P. 1996b. Multicompartmental modeling of neural circuits in the olfactory bulb. *Int. J. Neural Syst.* 7:519–527.

Arbib, M. A. 1972. *The metaphorical brain: An introduction to cybernetics as artificial intelligence and brain theory*. New York: Wiley Interscience.

Arbib, M. A. 1975. Artificial intelligence and brain theory: Unities and diversities. *Ann. Biomed. Eng.* 3:238–274.

Arbib, M. A. 1981. Perceptual structures and distributed motor control. In *Handbook of physiology in the nervous system: II. Motor control*, ed. V. B. Brooks, 1449–1480. Bethesda, MD: American Physiological Society.

Arbib, M. A. 1985. *In search of the person: Philosophical explorations in cognitive science*. Amherst: University of Massachusetts Press.

Arbib, M. A. 1987. Levels of modelling of visually guided behavior (with peer commentary and author's response). *Behav. Brain Sci.* 10: 407–465.

Arbib, M. A. 1989. *The metaphorical brain: 2. Neural networks and beyond*. New York: Wiley Interscience.

Arbib, M. A. 1990a. *Brains, machines,and mathematics*, 2d ed. Berlin: Springer-Verlag.

Arbib, M. A. 1990b. Programs, schemas, and neural networks for control of hand movements: Beyond the RS Framework. In *Attention and* performance: XIII. Motor representation and control, ed. M. Jeannerod, 111–138. Hillsdale, NJ: Lawrence Erlbaum Associates.

Arbib, M. A. 1991a. Interaction of multiple representations of space in the brain. In Brain and space, ed. J. Paillard, 379–403. London: Oxford University Press.

Arbib, M. A. 1991b. Neural mechanisms of visuomotor coordination: The evolution of Rana computatrix. In Visual structures and integrated functions. Vol. 3, Research notes in neural computing, eds. M. A. Arbib and J.-P. Ewert, 3–30. Berlin: Springer-Verlag.

Arbib, M. A. 1992. Schema theory. In The encyclopedia of artificial intelligence, ed. S. Shapiro, 1427–1443. New York: Wiley Interscience.

Arbib, M. A. 1994. The brain as a metaphor for sixth generation computing. In Computing with biological metaphors, ed. R. Paton, 105–123. London: Chapman and Hall.

Arbib, M. A. 1995. Brain models on the web. In Computational intelligence: A dynamic systems perspective, ed. M. Palaniswami, Y. Attikouzel, R. J. Marks II, D. Fogel, and T. Fukuda, 219–231. New York: I.E.E.E. Press.

Arbib, M. A., Bischoff, A., Fagg, A. H., and Grafton, S. T. 1995. Synthetic pet: Analyzing large-scale properties of neural networks. Human Brain Mapping 2:225–233.

Arbib, M. A., Boylls, C. C., and Dev, P. 1974. Neural models of spatial perception and the control of movement. In Cybernetics and bionics, eds. W. D. Keidel, W. Handler, and M. Spreng, 216–231. Munich: Oldenbourg Verlag.

Arbib, M. A., and Caplan, D. 1979. Neurolinguistics must be computational. Behav. Brain Sci. 2:449–483.

Arbib, M. A., Caplan, D., and Marshall, J. C., eds. 1982. Neural models of language processes. New York: Academic Press.

Arbib, M. A., Conklin, E. J., and Hill, J. C. 1987. From schema theory to language. London: Oxford University Press.

Arbib, M. A., and Didday, R. L. 1971. The organization of action-oriented memory for a perceiving system: I. The basic model. J. Cybernet. 1:3–18.

Arbib, M. A., and Hesse, M. B. 1986. The construction of reality. London: Cambridge University Press.

Arbib, M. A., and Hill, J. C. 1988. Language acquisition: Schemas replace universal grammar. In Explaining language universals, ed. J. A. Hawkins, 56–72. Basel: Blackwell.

Arbib, M. A., and House, D. H. 1987. Depth and detours: An essay on visually guided behavior. In Vision, brain, and cooperative computation, eds. M. A. Arbib and A. R. Hanson, 129–163. Cambridge, MA: Bradford Books/MIT Press.

Arbib, M. A., Iberall, T., and Lyons, D. 1985. Coordinated control programs for control of the hands. In Hand function and the neocortex (Exp. Br. Res. Suppl. 10), ed. A. W. Goodwin and I. Darian-Smith, 111–129. Berlin: Springer-Verlag.

Arbib, M. A., and Liaw, J.-S. 1995. sensorimotor transformations in the worlds of frogs and robots. Artif. Intell. 72:53–79.

Arbib, M. A., and Lieblich, I. 1977. Motivational learning of spatial behavior. In Systems neuroscience, ed. J. Metzler, 221–239. New York: Academic Press.

Arbib, M. A., Schweighofer, N., and Thach, W. T. 1994. Modeling the role of cerebellum in prism adaptation. In From animals to animats: 3. Proceedings of the Third International Symposium on Simulation of Adaptive Behavior, eds. D. Cliff, P. Husbands, J.-A. Meyer, and S. W. Wilson, 36–44. Cambridge, MA: MIT Press.

Arbib, M. A., Schweighofer, N., and Thach, W. T. 1995. Modeling the cerebellum: From adaptation to coordination. In Motor control and sensory-motor integration: Issues and directions, eds. D. J. Glencross and J. P. Piek, 11–36. Amsterdam: Elsevier North-Holland.

Arkin, R. C. 1995. Reactive robotic systems. In The handbook of brain theory and neural networks, ed. M. A. Arbib. Cambridge, MA: Bradford Books/MIT Press.

Armstrong, D. M., Harvey, R. J., and Schild, R. F. 1973a. Cerebello-cerebellar responses mediated by climbing fibres. Exp. Brain Res. 18:19–39.

Armstrong, D. M., Harvey, R. J., and Schild, R. F. 1973b. The spatial organisation of climbing fibers branching in the cat cerebellum. Exp. Brain Res. 18:1–18.

Arnold, L. 1973. Stochastic differential equations. Munich: Oldenbourg Verlag.

Artola, A., and Singer, W. 1987. Long-term potentiation and NMDA receptors in rat visual cortex. Nature 330:649–652.

Ashby, W. R. 1962. Principles of the self-organizing systems. In Principles of self-organization, eds. H. von Foerster and G. W. Zopf. Oxford: Pergamon Press.

Assad, J. A., and Maunsell, J. H. R. 1995. Neuronal correlates of inferred motion in primate posterior parietal cortex. Nature 373:518.

Atmanspacher, H. 1992. Categorical and acategorical representation of knowledge. Cogn. Syst. 3:25–288.

Attardi, D. G., and Sperry, R. W. 1963. Preferential selection of central pathways by regenerating optic fibers. Exp. Neurol. 7:46–64.

Atyia, A., and Baldi, P. 1989. Oscillations and synchronization in neural networks: An exploration of the labeling hypothesis. Int. J. Neural Syst. 1:103–124.

Babloyantz, A. 1992. From the single neuron to the cortical networks: A coherent model of EEG. In Artificial neural networks, Vol. 2, eds. I. Alexander and J. Taylor, 385–390. Amsterdam: Elsevier.

Babloyantz, A., and Destexhe, A. 1986. Low-dimensional chaos in an instance of epilepsy. Proc. Natl. Acad. Sci. U.S.A. 83:3513–3517.

Babloyantz, A., Salazar, J. M., and Nicolis, C. 1985. Evidence of chaotic dynamics of brain activity during the sleep cycle. Phys. Lett. 111A:152–156.

Baird, B. 1990. Bifurcation and category learning in networks models of oscillating cortex. Physica D 42:365–384.

Baizer, J. S., and Glickstein, M. 1974. Role of the cerebellum in prism adaptation. J. Physiol. (Lond.) 236:34–35.

Baizer, J. S., Ungerleider, L. G., and Desimone, R. 1991. Organization of visual inputs to the inferior temporal and posterior parietal cortex in macaques. J. Neurosci. 11:168–190.

Barkai, E., Bergman, E., Horwitz, G., and Hasselmo, M. E. 1994. Modulation of associative memory function in a biophysical simulation of rat piriform cortex. J. Neurophysiol. 72:659–677.

Barkai, E., and Hasselmo, M. E. 1994. Modulation of the input/output function of rat piriform cortex pyramidal cells. *J. Neurophysiol.* 72:644–658.

Barker, L. A., and Mittag, T. W. 1975. Comparative studies of substrates and inhibitors of choline transport and choline acetyltransferase. *J. Pharmacol. Exp. Ther.* 192:86–94.

Barlow, H., and Foldiak, P. 1989. Adaptation and decorrelation in the cortex. In *The computing neuron*, eds. R. Durbin, C. Miall, and G. Mitchison, 54–72. Reading, MA: Addison-Wesley.

Barlow, H. B. 1969. Pattern recognition and the responses of sensory neurons. *Ann. N. Y. Acad. Sci.* 156:872–881.

Barna, G., and Érdi, P. 1986. Pattern formation in neural systems: II. Noise-induced selective mechanisms for the ontogenetic formation of ocular dominance columns. In *Cybernetics and systems '86*, ed. R. Trappl, 343–350. Dordrect: D. Reidel.

Barna, G., and Érdi, P. 1988. "Normal" and "abnormal" dynamic behavior during synaptic transmission. In *Computer simulation in brain science*, ed. R. J. Cotterill, 293–301. London: Cambridge University Press.

Barna, G., and Tsuda, I. 1993. A new method for computing Lyapunov exponents. *Phys. Lett.* 175A:421–427.

Barone, P., and Joseph, J.-P. 1989a. Prefrontal cortex and spatial sequencing in macaque monkey. *Exp. Brain Res.* 78:447–464.

Barone, P., and Joseph, J.-P. 1989b. Role of dorsolateral prefrontal cortex in organizing visually guided behavior. *Brain Behav. Evol.* 33:132–135.

Barrow, H. G. 1987. Learning receptive fields. *Proc. I.E.E.E. First Annu. Conf. Neural Networks* IV:115–121.

Bartha, G. T. 1992. A computer model of oculomotor and neural contributions to conditioned blink timing. Ph.D. diss., University of Southern California.

Bartha, G. T., and Thompson, R. F. 1992. Control of rabbit nictitating membrane movements: II. Analysis of the relation of motoneuron activity to behavior. *Biol. Cybern.* 68:145–154.

Bartha, G. T., and Thompson, R. F. 1995. Cerebellum and conditioning. In *The handbook of brain theory and neural networks*, ed. M. A. Arbib, 169–172. Cambridge, MA: Bradford Books/MIT Press.

Bartlett, F. C. 1932. *Remembering.* Cambridge: Cambridge University Press.

Barto, A. G., and Sutton, R. S. 1981. Landmark learning: An illustration of associative search. *Biol. Cybern.* 42:1–8.

Basar, E. 1990. *Chaos in brain function.* Berlin: Springer-Verlag.

Baudry, M., and Davis, J. L. 1991. *Long-term potentiation: A debate of current issues.* Cambridge, MA: Bradford Books/MIT Press.

Bear, M. F., and Abraham, W. C. 1996. Long-term depression in hippocampus. *Annu. Rev. Neurosci.* 19:437–462.

Bear, M. F., Cooper, L. N., and Ebner, F. F. 1987. The physiological basis of a theory for synapse modification. *Science* 237:42–48.

Bear, M. F., Press, W. A., and Connors, B. W. 1992. Long-term potentiation of slices of kitten visual cortex and the effects of NMDA receptor blockade. *J. Neurophysiol.* 67:841–851.

Bell, C. C., Caputi, A., Grant, K., and Serrier, J. 1993. Storage of a sensory pattern by anti-Hebbian synaptic plasticity in an electric fish. *Proc. Natl. Acad. Sci. U.S.A.* 90:4650–4654.

Bell, C. C., and Kawasaki, T. 1972. Relations among climbing fiber responses of nearby Purkinje cells. *J. Neurophysiol.* 35:155–169.

Berger, T. W., Semple-Rowland, S., and Bassett, J. L. 1981. Hippocampal polymorph neurons are the cells of origin for ipsilateral association and commissural afferents to the dentate gyrus. *Brain Res.* 215:329–336.

Bergman, H. T., Whitman, T., and DeLong, M. R. 1990. Reversal of experimental parkinsonism by lesions of the subthalamic nucleus. *Science* 249:1436–1438.

Berlin, R. 1858. *Beiträge zur Struktur der Grosshirnwindungen.* Erlangen.

Bernard, C. 1878. *Lecons sur les phénomènes de la Vie.* Paris: Bailliére.

Bernstein, N. A. 1967. *The coordination and regulation of movement.* Trans. from the Russian. New York: Pergamon Press.

Berthier, N. E., Singh, S. P., Barto, A. G., and Houk, J. C. 1993. Distributed representation of limb motor programs in arrays of adjustable pattern generators. *J. Cogn. Neurosci.* 5:56–78.

Bhalla, H. S., and Bower, J. 1993. Exploring parameter space in detailed single neuron models: Simulations of the mitral and granule cells of the olfactory bulb. *J. Neurophysiol.* 69:1948–1965.

Biedenbach, M. A. 1966. Effects of anesthetics and cholinergic drugs on prepyriform electrical activity in cats. *Exp. Neurol.* 16:464–479.

Bienenstock, E. 1985. Dynamics of the central nervous system. In *Dynamics of macrosystems*: *Lecture notes in economics and mathematical systems*, eds. J. P. Aubin, D. Saari, and K. Sigmund, 3–20. Berlin: Springer-Verlag.

Bienenstock, E., and von der Malsburg, C. 1987. A neural network for invariant pattern recognition. *Europhysics Lett.* 4:121–126.

Bienenstock, E. L., Cooper, L. N., and Munro, P. W. 1982. Theory for the development of neuron selctivity: Orientation specificity and binocular interaction in visual cortex. *J. Neurosci.* 2:32–48.

Bisiach, E., Perani, D., Vallar, G., and Barti, A. 1986. Unilateral neglect: Personal and extra-personal. *Neuropsychologia* 24:759–767.

Blackstad, T. W. 1956. Commissural connections of the hippocampal region in the rat, with special reference to their mode of termination. *J. Comp. Neurol.* 105:417–537.

Blasdel, G., and Salama, G. 1986. Voltage-sensitive dyes reveal a modular organization in monkey striate cortex. *Nature* 321:579–585.

Bliss, T. V. P., and Collingridge, G. L. 1993. A synaptic model of memory: Long-term potentiation in the hippocampus. *Nature* 361:31–39.

Bliss, T. V. P., and Lømo, T. 1973. Long-lasting potentiation of synaptic transmission in the dentate area of the anaesthetized rabbit following stimulation of perforant path. *J. Physiol.* 232:331–356.

Bloedel, J. R. 1992. Functional heterogeneity with structural homogeneity: How does the cerebellum operate? *Behav. Brain Sci.* 15:666–678.

Bloedel, J. R., and Bracha, V. 1995. On the cerebellum, cutaneomuscular reflexes, movement control and the elusive engrams of memory. *Behav. Brain. Res.* 68:1–44.

Bloedel, J. R., Bracha, V., and Larson, P. S. 1993. Real time operations of the cerebellar cortex. *Can. J. Neurol. Sci.* 20 (suppl. 3):S7–S18.

Blum, E. K., Khademi, P. M., Leung, P. K., Lavond, D., Thompson, R. F., Krupa, D. J., and Tracy, J. 1993. Modeling and simulation of compartmental cerebellar networks for conditioning of rabbit eyeblink response. In *Computation and neural systems 1992*, eds. J. Bower and F. Eeckman. Norwell, MA: Kluwer Academic Publishers.

Bodian, D. 1952. Introductory survey of neurons. *Cold Spring Harb. Symp. Quant. Biol.* 17:1–13.

Bolhuis, J. J., Stewart, C. A., and Forest, E. M. 1994. Retrograde amnesia and memory reactivation in rats with ibotenate lesions to the hippocampus or subiculum. *Q. J. Exp. Psychol.* 47B:129–150.

Borisysuk, R. M., and Kyrillov, A. B. 1992. Bifurcation analysis of a neural network model. *Biol. Cybern.* 66:319–325.

Borisyuk, R. M., Wickens, J. R., and Kötter, R. 1994. Reinforcement learning in a network model of the basal ganglia. In *Cybernetics and system '94*, Vol. 2, ed. R. Trappl, 1681–1686. Singapore: World Scientific.

Bostock, E., Muller, R. U., and Kubie, J. L. 1991. Experience dependent modifications of hippocampal place cell firing. *Hippocampus* 1:193–205.

Boussaoud, D., Ungerleider, L. G., and Desimone, R. 1990. Pathways for motion analysis: Cortical connections of the medial superior temporal and fundus of the superior temporal visual areas in the macaque. *J. Comp. Neurol.* 296:462–495.

Bower, J. M. 1990. Reverse engineering the nervous system: An anatomical, physiological, and computer-based approach. In *An introduction to neural and electronic networks*, eds. S. Zornetzer, J. Davis, and C. Lau, 3–24. New York: Academic Press.

Bower, J. M. 1991. Piriform cortex and olfactory object recognition. In *Olfaction: A model system for computational neuroscience*, eds. J. L. Davis and H. Eichenbaum, 265–285. Cambridge, MA: MIT Press.

Bower, J. M., and Beeman, D. 1994. *The book of GENESIS: Exploring realistic neural models with the GEneral NEural SImulation System*, TELOS. New York: Springer-Verlag.

Boylls, C. C. 1975. A theory of cerebellar function with applications to locomotion: I. The physiological role of climbing fiber inputs in anterior lobe operation. Tech. rep. no. 75C 6. Amherst, MA: Computer and Information Science Department, University of Massachusetts at Amherst.

Boylls, C. C. 1978. Prolonged alterations of muscle activity induced in locomoting premamillary cats by microstimulation of the inferior olive. *Brain Res.* 159:445–450.

Boylls, C. C. 1980. Contributions to locomotor coordination of an olivo-cerebellar projection to the vermis in cat: Experimental results and theoretical proposals. In *The inferior olivary nucleus: Anatomy and physiology*, eds. J. Courville, C. de Montigny, and Y. Lamarre, 321–348. New York: Raven Press.

Braak, H. 1971. Über das Neurolipofuscin in der unteren Olive und dem Nucleus dentatus cerebelli des Menschen, Z.f.Zellforsch.u.mikrosk. Anatomie 121:573–592.

Braak, H. 1984. Architectonics as seen by lipofuscin stains. In *Cerebral cortex*, Vol. 1, eds. A. Peters and E. G. Jones. New York: Plenum.

Bradley, D. C., Garrett, S. L., and Zurif, E. B. 1980. Syntactic deficits in Broca's aphasia. In *Biological studies of mental capacities*, ed. D. Caplan. Cambridge, MA: MIT Press.

Bradley, P., and Berry, M. 1976. The effects of reduced climbing and parallel fibre input on Purkinje cell dendritic growth. *Brain Res.* 109:133–151.

Bragin, A., Jandó, G., Nádasdy, Z., Hetke, J., Wise, K., and Buzsáki, G. 1995. Gamma (40–100 Hz) oscillation in the hippocampus of the behaving rat. *J. Neurosci.* 15:47–60.

Braitenberg, V. 1965. Taxis, kinesis, decussation. *Prog. Brain Res.* 17:210–222.

Braitenberg, V. 1978. Cortical architectonics: General and areal. In *Architectonics of the cerebral cortex*, eds. M. A. B. Brazier and H. Petsche, 443–465. New York: Raven Press.

Braitenberg, V. 1984. *Vehicles: Experiments in synthetic psychology*. Cambridge, MA: Bradford Books/MIT Press.

Braitenberg, V. 1985. Charting the visual cortex. In *Cerebral cortex*, Vol. 3, eds. A. Peters and E. G. Jones, 379–414. New York: Plenum Press.

Braitenberg, V., and Braitenberg, C. 1979. Geometry of orientation columns in visual cortex. *Biol. Cybern.* 33:179–186.

Braitenberg, V., and Onesto, N. 1961. The cerebellar cortex as a timing organ. *Proc. 1st Int. Conf. on Med. Cybern.* 239–255.

Braitenberg, V., and Preissl, H. 1992. Why is the output of the cerebellum inhibitory? *Behav. Brain. Sci.* 15:715–717.

Braitenberg, V., and Schüz, A. 1991. *Anatomy of the cortex: Statistics and geometry*. Berlin: Springer-Verlag.

Brand, S., Dahl, A.-L., and Mugnaini, E. 1976. The length of parallel fibers in the cat cerebellar cortex: An experimental light and electron microscope study. *Exp. Brain Res.* 26:39–58.

Brändle, K., and Székely, G. 1973. The control of alternating coordination of limb pairs in the newt (*Triturus vulgaris*). *Brain Behav. Evol.* 8:366–385.

Breese, C. R., Hampson, R. E., and Deadwyler, S. A. 1989. Hippocampal place cells: Stereotopy and plasticity. *J. Neurosci.* 9:1097–1111.

Bremer, F. 1938. Effets de la déafferentation complète d'une région de lcore cérébrale sur son activité électrique spontaneé. *C.R. Soc. Biol. (Paris)* 127:355–359.

Brennan, P., Kaba, H., and Keverne, E. B. 1990. Olfactory recognition: A simple memory system. *Science* 250:1223–1226.

Brennan, P., and Keverne, E. B. 1989. Impairment of olfactory memory by local infusions of non-selective excitatory amino acid receptor antagonists into accessory bulb. *Neuroscience* 33:463–468.

Bressler, S. 1984. Spatial organization of EEGs from olfactory bulb and cortex. *Electroencephalogr. Clin. Neurophysiol.* 57:270–276.

Bressler, S., and Freeman, W. 1980. Frequency analysis of olfactory system EEG in cat, rabbit and rat. *Electroencephalogr. Clin. Neurophysiol.* 56:19–24.

Bressler, S. L. 1987a. Relation of olfactory bulb and cortex: I. Spatial variation of bulbocortical interdependence. *Brain Res.* 409:285–293.

Bressler, S. L. 1987b. Relation of olfactory bulb and cortex: II. Model for driving of cortex by bulb. *Brain Res.* 409:294–301.

Brinkman, J., and Kuypers, H. G. J. M. 1972. Split brain monkey: Cerebral control of ipsilateral and contralateral arm, hand, and finger movements. *Science* 176:536–539.

Broca, P. 1861. Nouvelle observation d'aphémie produite par une lésion de la moitié posterieure des deuxième et troisième circonvolutions frontales. *Bull. Soc. Anat.* 6:398–407.

Brodal, A., Lacerda, A. M., Destombes, J., and Anguat, R. 1972. The pattern in the projection of the intracerebellar nuclei onto the nucleus reticularis tegmenti pontis in the cat: An experimental anatomical study. *Exp. Brain Res.* 16:140–160.

Brodal, A., and Szikla, G. 1972. The termination of the brachium conjunctivum descendens in the nucleus reticularis tegmenti pontis: An experimental anatomical study in the cat. *Brain Res.* 39:337–351.

Brodin, L., Traven, H., Lansner, A., Wallén, P., Ekeberg, Ö and Grillner, S. 1991. Computer simulations of *N*-methyl-D-aspartate (NMDA) receptor induced membrane properties in a neuron model. *J. Neurophysiol.* 66:473–484.

Brodmann, K. 1908. Beitrage zur histologischen Lokalisation der Grosshirnrinde, die Cortexgliederung des Menschen. *J. Psychol. Neurol.* 6:231.

Brodmann, K. 1912. Neue Ergebnisse uber die vergleichende histologische Lokalisation der Grosshirnrinde mit besonderer Berucksichtigung des Stirnhirns. *Anat. Anz. Suppl.* 41:157–216.

Brodmann, K. 1914. Physiologie des Gehirns. In *Neue Deutsche Chirurgie*, Vol. IX, ed. P.v. Brun, 85–462. Stuttgart.

Brooks, R. A. 1986. A robust layered control system for a mobile robot. *I.E.E.E. J. Robotics Autom.* RA-2:14–23.

Brothers, L., and Ring, B. 1992. A neuroethological framework for the representation of minds. *J. Cogn. Neurosci.* 4:107–118.

Brothers, L., and Ring, B. 1993. Mesial temporal neurons in the macaque monkey with responses selective for aspects of social stimuli. *Behav. Brain Res.* 57:53–61.

Brown, T. G. 1911. The intrinsic factors in the act of progression in the mammal. *Proc. R. Soc. Lond. [B]* 84:308–319.

Brown, T. G. 1914. On the nature of the fundamental activity of the nervous centres, together with an analysis of the conditioning of rhythmic activity in progression, and a theory of evolution of function in the nervous system. *J. Physiol. Lond.* 48:18–46.

Brown, T. H., Chapman, P. F., Kairiss, E. W., and Keenan, C. L. 1988. Long-term synaptic potentiation. *Science* 242:724–728.

Brown, T. H., and Chattarji, S. 1994. Hebbian synaptic plasticity: Evolution of the contemporary concept. In *Models of neural networks*, Vol. 2, ed. L. van Hemmen. New York: Springer-Verlag.

Brown, T. H., and Chattarji, S. 1995. Hebbian synaptic plasticity. In *The handbook of brain theory and neural networks*, ed. M. A. Arbib, 454–459. Cambridge, MA: Bradford Books/MIT Press.

Brown, T. H., Kairiss, E. W., and Keenan, C. L. 1990. Hebbian synapses: Biophysical mechanisms and algorithms. *Annu. Rev. Neurosci.* 13:475–511.

Bruce, C. J., and Goldberg, M. E. 1984. Physiology of the frontal eye fields. *Trends Neurosci.* November: 436–441.

Buchholtz, F., Golowasch, J., Epstein, I. R., and Marder, E. 1992. Mathematical model of an identified stomatogastric ganglion neuron. *J. Neurophysiol.* 67:332–340.

Buck, L. B. 1996. Information coding in the vertebrate olfactory system. *Annu. Rev. Neurosci.* 19:517–544.

Buck, L., and Axel, R. 1991. A novel multigene family may encode odorant receptors: A molecular basis for odor recognition. *Cell* 65:175–187.

Buckmaster, P. S., and Schwartzkoin, P. A. 1995. Interneurons and inhibition in the dentate gyrus of the rat in vivo. *J. Neurosci.* 15:774–789.

Buhl, E. H., Malasy, K., and Somogyi, P. 1994. Divergent sources of hippocampal unitary inhibitory postsynaptic potentials and the number of synaptic release sites. *Nature* 368:823–828.

Buhmann, J. 1989. Oscillations and low firing rates in associative memory neural networks. *Physiol. Rev. [A].* 40:4145–4148.

Buhmann, J., Divko, R., and Schulten, K. 1989. Associative memory with high information content. *Physiol. Rev. [A]* 39:2689–2692.

Buhmann, J., Lange, C., and von der Malsburg, C. 1989. Distortion invariant object recognition by matching hierarchically labeled graphs. In *Int. Joint Conf. on Neural Networks*, Washington, 1:155–159.

Bullock, D. 1995. Motoneuron recruitment. In *The handbook of brain theory and neural networks*, ed. M. A. Arbib. Cambridge, MA: Bradford Books/MIT Press.

Bunge, M. 1980. *The mind-body problem.* New York: Pergamon Press.

Burgess, N., O'Keefe, J., and Recce, M. 1993. Using hippocampal "place cells" for navigation: Exploiting phase coding. In *Advances in Neural information processing systems*, Vol. 5, eds. S. J. Hanson, C. L. Giles, and J. D. Cowan, 929–936. San Mateo, CA: Morgan Kaufmann.

Burgess, N., Recce, M., and O'Keefe, J. 1994. A model of hippocampal function. *Neural Networks* 7:1065–1081.

Burks, A. W. 1980. Enumerative induction vs. eliminative induction. In *Applications of inductive logic*, eds. L. J. Cohen and M. B. Hesse. London: Oxford University Press.

Burnod, Y., Grandguillaume, P., Otto, I., Ferraina, S., Johnson, B. P., and Caminiti, R. 1991. Visuomotor transformations underlying arm movements toward visual targets: A neural network model of cerebral cortical operations. *J. Neurosci.* 4:1435–1453.

Bushnell, M. C., Goldberg, M. E., and Robinson, D. L. 1981. Behavioral enhancement of visual responses in monkey cerebral cortex: I. Modulation in posterior parietal cortex related to selective attention. *J. Neurophysiol.* 46:755–772.

Buzsáki, G. 1984. Feed-forward inhibition in the hippocampal formation. *Prog. Neurobiol.* 22:131–153.

Buzsáki, G. 1986. Hippocampal sharp waves: Their origin and significance. *Brain Res.* 398:242–252.

Buzsáki, G. 1989. Two-stage model of memory trace formation: A role for "noisy" brain states. *Neuroscience* 31:551–570.

Buzsáki, G. 1991. The thalamic clock: Emergent properties. *Neuroscience* 2/3:351–364.

Buzsáki, G. 1996. The hippocampo-neocortical dialogue. *Cerebral Cortex* 6:81–92.

Buzsáki, G., Bragin, A., Chrobak, J. J., Náasdy, Z., Sík, A., Hsu, M., and Ylinen, A. 1994. Oscillatory and intermittent synchrony in the hippocampus: Relevance to memory trace formation. In *Temporal coding in the brain*, eds. G. Buzsáki, R. Llinás, W. Singer, A. Berthoz, and Y. Chrisen, 145–172. Berlin: Springer-Verlag.

Buzsáki, G., and Chrobak, J. 1995. Temporal structure in spatially organized neuronal ensembles: A role for interneuronal networks. *Curr. Biol.* 5:504–510.

Buzsáki, G., Grastáyn, E., Tveritskaya, I. N., and Czopf, J. 1979. Hippocampal evoked potentials and EEG changes during classical conditioning in the rat. *Electroencephalogr. Clin. Neurophysiol.* 47:67–74.

Buzsáki, G., Horváth, Z., Urioste, R., Hetke, J., and Wise, K. 1992. High-frequency network oscillation in the hippocampus. *Science* 256:1025–1027.

Buzsáki, G., Leung, L.-W. S., and Vanderwolf, C. H. 1983. Cellular bases of hippocampal EEG in the behaving rat. *Brain Res. Rev.* 6:139–171.

Buzsáki, G., Llinás, R., Singer, W., Berthoz, A., and Christen, Y. 1994. *Temporal coding in the brain*. Berlin: Springer-Verlag.

Calabresi, P., Maj, R., Pisani, A., Mercuri, N. B., and Bernardi, G. 1992a. Long-term synaptic depression in the striatum: Physiological and pharmacological characterization. *J. Neurosci.* 12:4224–4233.

Calabresi, P., Pisani, A., Mercuri, N. B., and Bernardi, G. 1992b. Long-term potentiation in the striatum is unmasked by removing the voltage-dependent magnesium block of NMDA receptor channels. *Eur. J. Neurosci.* 4:929–935.

Campbell, F. W., and Robson, J. G. 1968. Application of Fourier analysis to the visibility of gratings. *J. Physiol. (Lond.)* 197:551–566.

Canavier, C. C., Baxter, D. A., Clark, J. W., and Byrne, J. H. 1994. Multiple models of activity in a model for the effects of neuromodulators. *J. Neurophysiol.* 72:872–882.

Cannon, W. B. 1929. Organization for physiological homeostasis. *Physiol. Rev.* 9:399–431.

Caplan, D. 1995. The cognitive neuroscience of syntactic processing. In *The cognitive neurosciences*, ed. M. Gazzaniga, 871–879. Cambridge, MA: Bradford Books/MIT Press.

Carlsson, A. 1959. The occurrence, distribution, and physiological role of catecholamines in the nervous system. *Pharmacol. Rev.* 11:490–493.

Carlsson, M., and Carlsson, A. 1990. Interactions between glutamatergic and monoaminergic systems within the basal ganglia—implications for schizophrenia and Parkinson's disease. *Trends Neurosci.* 13(7):272–276.

Carpenter, G., and Grossberg, S., 1987. A massively parallel architecture for a self-organizing neural pattern recognition machine, *Comp. Vision, Graphics and Image Proc.* 37:54–115.

Carpenter, G. A. 1979. Bursting phenomena in excitable membranes. *S.I.A.M. J. Appl. Math.* 36:334–372.

Castiello, U., Paulignan, Y., and Jeannerod, M. 1991. Temporal dissociation of motor responses and subjective awareness: A study in normal subjects. *Brain* 114:2639–2655.

Cavada, C., and Goldman-Rakic, P. S. 1989. Posterior parietal cortex in rhesus monkey: I. Parcellation of areas based on distinctive limbic and sensory corticocortical connections. *J. Comp. Neurol.* 287:393–421.

Cepeda, C., Walsh, J. P., Hull, C. D., Howard, S. G., Buchwald, N. A., and Levine, M. S. 1989. Dye-coupling in the neostriatum of the rat: I. Modulation by dopamine-depleting lesions. *Synapse* 4:229–237.

Changeux, J.-P. 1985. *Neuronal man*. New York: Oxford University Press.

Changeux, J.-P., Courrege, O., and Danchin, A. 1973. A theory of epigenesis of neuronal networks by selective stabilization of synapses. *Proc. Natl. Acad. Sci. U.S.A.* 70:2974–2978.

Changeux, J.-P., and Danchin, A. 1976. Selective stabilization of developing synapses as a mechanism for the specification of neuronal networks. *Nature* 264:705–712.

Changeux, J.-P., Heidmann, T., and Patte, P. 1984. Learning by selection. In *The biology of learning*, eds. P. Marler and H. S. Terrace, 115–133. Berlin: Springer-Verlag.

Chan-Palay, V. 1977. *Cerebellar dentate nucleus*. Berlin: Springer-Verlag.

Chay, T. R. 1984. Abnormal discharges and chaos in a neuronal model system. *Biol. Cybern.* 52:301–311.

Chay, T. R. 1985. Chaos in a three-variable model of an excitable cell. *Physica D* 16:233–242.

Chay, T. R., and Lee, Y. S. 1990. Bursting, beating, and chaos by two functionally distinct inward current inactivations in excitable cells. *Ann. N. Y. Acad. Sci.* 591:328–350.

Chay, T. R., and Rinzel, J. 1985. Bursting, beating and chaos in an excitable membrane model. *Biophys. J.* 47:357–366.

Chen, E. W., and Chiu, A. Y. 1992. Early stages in the development of spinal motor neurons. *J. Comp. Neurol.* 320:291–303.

Cherjnavsky, A., and Moody, J. 1990. Spontaneous development of modularity in simple cortical models. *Neural Computation* 2:334–354.

Chevalier, G., Vacher, S., Deniau, J. M., and Desban, M. 1985. Disinhibition as a basic process in the expression of striatal functions: I. The striato-nigral influence on the tecto-spinal/tecto-diencephalic neurons. *Brain Res.* 334:215–226.

Choi, D. W. 1988. Glutamate neurotoxicity and diseases of the nervous system. *Neuron* 1:623–634.

Chomsky, N. 1965. *Aspects of the theory of syntax*. Cambridge, MA: MIT Press.

Chrobak, J. J., and Buzsáki, G. 1996. High-frequency oscillations in the output networks of the hippocampal-entorhinal axis of the freely behaving rat. *J. Neurosci.* 16:3056–3066.

Churchland, P. S. 1986. *Neurophilosophy: Toward a unified science of the mind-brain. Cambridge*, MA: MIT Press.

Claiborne, B. Y., Amaral, D. G., and Cowan, W. M. 1986. A light and electron microscopic analysis of the mossy fibers of the rat dentate gyrus. *J. Comp. Neurol.* 246:435–458.

Clark, J. W., Rafelski, J., and Winston, J. V. 1985. Brain without mind: Computer simulation of neural networks with modifiable neuronal interactions. *Phys. Rep.* 123:215–273.

Clarke, P. G. H. 1981. Chance, repetition and error in the development of normal nervous systems. *Persp. Biol. Med.* 25:2–19.

Cliff, D. 1995. Neuroethology: Computational. In *The handbook of brain theory and neural networks*, ed. M. A. Arbib. Cambridge, MA: Bradford Books/MIT Press.

Cobas, A., and Arbib, M. 1992. Prey-catching and predator-avoidance in frog and toad: Defining the schemas. *J. Theor. Biol.* 157:271–304.

Cohen, M., and Grossberg, S. 1983. Absolute stability of global pattern formation and parallel memory storage by competitive neural networks. *I.E.E.E. Trans. Syst. Man Cybern.* SMC-13:815–826.

Cohen, N. J. 1984. Preserved learning capacity in amnesia: Evidence for multiple memory systems. In *The neuropsychology of memory*, ed. N. Butters and L. R. Squire, 83–103. New York: Guilford Press.

Cohen, N. J., and Eichenbaum, H. 1993. *Memory, amnesia, and the hippocampal system*. Cambridge, MA: MIT Press.

Cohen, N. J., and Squire, L. R. 1980. Preserved learning and retention of a pattern-analyzing skill in amnesia: Dissociation of knowing how and knowing that. *Science* 210:207–210.

Collett, T. 1982. Do toads plan routes? A study of the detour behaviour of *Bufo viridis*, bv. *J. Comp. Physiol.* 146:261–271.

Collett, T. S., Cartwright, B. A., and Smith, B. A. 1986. Landmark learning and visuospatial memories in gerbils. *J. Comp. Physiol. [A]* 158:835–851.

Collins, A. M., and Loftus, E. F. 1975. A spreading activation theory of cognitive processing. *Psychol. Rev.* 82:407–428.

Collins, A. M., and Quillian, M. R. 1969. A spreading-activation theory of semantic processing. *Psychol. Rev.* 82:45–73.

Collins, J. J., and Stewart, I. 1993a. Coupled nonlinear oscillators and the symmetries of animal gaits. *J. Nonlinear Sci.* 3:349–392.

Collins, J. J., and Stewart, I. 1993b. Hexapodal gaits and coupled nonlinear oscillator models. *Biol. Cybern.* 68:287–298.

Collins, J. J., and Stewart, I. 1994. A group-theoretic approach to rings of coupled biological oscillators. *Biol. Cybern.* 71:95–103.

Colonnier, M. 1966. The structural design of the neocortex. In *Brain and conscious experience*, ed. J. C. Eccles, 1–29. Berlin: Springer-Verlag.

Conrad, M. 1989. The brain-machine disanalogy. *BioSystems* 22:197–213.

Constanti, A., and Sim, J. A. 1987. Muscarinic receptors mediating suppression of the M-current in guinea-pig olfactory cortex neurones may be of the M2-subtype. *Br. J. Pharmacol.* 90:3–5.

Constantine-Paton, M., Cline, H. T., and Debski, E. 1990. Patterned activity, synaptic convergence, and the NMDA receptor in developing visual pathway. *Annu. Rev. Neurosci.* 13:129–154.

Corbacho, F. J., and Arbib, M. S. 1995. Learning to detour. *Adap. Behav.* 4:419–468.

Costa, L. F. 1994. Topographical maps of orientation selectivity. *Biol. Cybern.* 71:537–546.

Côté, L., and Crutcher, M. D. 1991. The basal ganglia. In *The principles of neural science*, eds. E. R. Kandel, J. H. Schwartz, and T. M. Jessell, 647–659. New York: Elsevier.

Cotman, C. W., Nieto-Sampedro, M., and Harris, E. W. 1981. Synapse replacement in the nervous system of adult vertebrates. *Physiol. Rev.* 61:684–784.

Cottrell, M., and Fort, J. C. 1986. A stochastic model of retinotopy: A self-organizing process. *Biol. Cybern.* 53:405–411.

Cowan, J. D. 1991. Stochastic neurodynamics. In *Advances in Neural information processing systems*, Vol. 3, eds. M. P. Lippmann, J. E. Moody, and D. S. Touretzky, 62–69. San Mateo, CA: Morgan Kaufmann.

Cowan, J. D. 1995. Fault tolerance. In *The handbook of brain theory and neural networks*, ed. M. A. Arbib. Cambridge, MA: Bradford Books/MIT Press.

Cowan, J. D., and Friedman, A. E. 1990. Development and regeneration of eye-brain maps: A computational model. In *Advances in neural information processing systems*, Vol. 2, ed. D. S. Touretzky, 92–99. San Mateo, CA: Morgan Kaufmann.

Cowan, J. D., and Friedman, A. E. 1991. Studies of a model for the development and regeneration of eye-brain maps. In *Advances in neural information processing systems*, Vol. 3, ed. D. S. Touretzky, 3–10. San Mateo, CA: Morgan Kaufmann.

Cowan, R. L., and Wilson, C. J. 1994. Spontaneous firing patterns and axonal projections of single corticostriatal neurons in the rat medial agranular cortex. *J. Neurophysiol.* 71:17–32.

Cragg, B. G., and Temperley, H. N. V. 1954. The organization of neurons: A cooperative analogy. *Electroencephalogr. Clin. Neurophysiol.* 6:85–92.

Cragg, B. G., and Temperley, H. N. V. 1955. Memory: The analogy with ferromagnetic hysteresis. *Brain* 78(2):304–316.

Craik, K. J. W. 1943. *The nature of explanation*. Cambridge: Cambridge University Press.

Crain, S. M. 1973. Tissue culture models of developing brain functions. In *Studies on the development of behavior and the nervous system: Vol. 2, Aspects of neurogenesis*, ed. G. Gottlieb, 69–114. New York: Academic Press.

Crepel, F., and Audinat, E. 1991. Excitatory amino acid receptors of cerebellar Purkinje cells: Development and plasticity. *Prog. Biophys. Mol. Biol.* 55:31–46.

Crick, F. 1984. Function of the thalamic reticular complex: The searchlight hypothesis. *Proc. Natl. Acad. Sci. U.S.A.* 81:4586–4590.

Crick, F., and Koch, C. 1990. Towards a neurobiological theory of consciousness. *Semin. Neurosci.* 2:263–275.

Crick, F. H. C. 1970. Diffusion in embryogenesis. *Nature* 225:420–422.

Crutchfield, J. P., Farmer, J. D., Packard, N. H., and Shaw, R. S. 1986. Chaos. *Sci. Am.* 255:38–49.

Csillik, B., and Knyihár, E. 1986. *The protean gate*. Budapest: Akadémiai Kiadó.

Cunningham, M. 1972. *Intelligence: Its origins and development*. New York: Academic Press.

Darian-Smith, C., and Gilbert, C. D. 1994. Axonal sprouting accompanies functional reorganization in adult striate cortex. *Nature* 368:737–740.

Dawkins, R. 1976. *The selfish gene*. Oxford: Oxford University Press.

Dean, J., and Cruse, H. 1995. Motor pattern generation. In *The handbook of brain theory and neural networks*, ed. M. A. Arbib. Cambridge, MA: Bradford Books/MIT Press.

Decety, J., Perani, D., Jeannerod, M., Bettinardi, V., Tadary, B., Woods, R., Mazziotta, J. C., and Fazio, F. 1994. Mapping motor representations with positron emission tomography. *Nature* 371:600–602.

Deiters, O. 1865. *Untersuchungen über Gehirn und Rückenmark des Menschen und Saugetiere.* Braunschweig.

Del Castillo, J., and Katz, B. 1954. Quantal components of the end-plate potential. *J. Physiol. (Lond.)* 124:560–573.

DeLong, M. R., Georgopoulos, A. P., and Crutcher, M. D. 1983. Cortico-basal ganglia relations and coding of motor performance. In Neural coding of motor performance, eds. J. Massion, J. Paillard, M. Schultz, and M. Wiesendanger, 30–40. Berlin: Springer-Verlag.

Deniau, J. M., and Chevalier, G. 1985. Disinhibition as a basic process in the expression of striatal functions: II. The striato-nigral influence on thalamocortical cells of the ventromedial thalamic nucleus. *Brain Res.* 334:227–233.

DeRoberties, E., and Bennett, H. S. 1957. Some features of the submicroscopic morphology of synapses in frog and earthworm. *J. Biophys. Biochem. Cytol.* 1:47–58.

De Schutter, E. 1992. A consumer guide to neuronal modeling software. *Trends Neurosci.* 15(11):462–464.

De Schutter, E., and Bower, J. M. 1993. Sensitivity of synaptic plasticity to the Ca^{2+} permeability of NMDA channels: A model of long-term potentiation in hippocampal neurons. *Neural Comput.* 5:681–694.

De Schutter, E., and Bower, J. M. 1994a. An active membrane model of the cerebellar Purkinje cell: I. Simulation of current clamps in slice. *J. Neurophysiol.* 71:375–400.

De Schutter, E., and Bower, J. M. 1994b. An active membrane model of the cerebellar Purkinje cell: II. Simulation of synaptic responses. *J. Neurophysiol.* 71:401–419.

Desimone, R., Wessinger, M., Thomas, L., and Schneider, W. 1990. Attentional control of visual perception: Cortical and subcortical mechanisms. *Cold Spring Harb. Symp. Quant. Biol.* 55:963–971.

Destexhe, A., and Babloyantz, A. 1991. Pacemaker-induced coherence in cortical networks. *Neural Comput.* 3:145–154.

Destexhe, A., Contreras, D., Sejnowski, T. J., and Steriade, M. 1994. A model of spindle rhythmicity in the isolated thalamic reticular nucleus. *J. Neurophysiol.* 72:803–818.

Dev, P. 1975. Perception of depth surfaces in random-dot stereograms: A neural model. *Int. J. Man-Mach. Stud.* 7:511–528.

DeValois, R. L., and DeValois, K. K. 1988. *Spatial vision.* London: Oxford University Press.

Devor, M. 1995. Pain networks. In The handbook of brain theory and neural networks, ed. M. A. Arbib. Cambridge, MA: Bradford Books/MIT Press.

Diamond, D. M., Dunwiddie, T. V., and Rose, G. M. 1988. Characteristics of hippocampal primed burst potentiation in vitro and in the awake rat. *J. Neurosci.* 8:4079–4088.

Dichiara, G. 1995. The role of dopamine in drug-abuse viewed from the perspective of its role in motivation. *Drug and Alcohol Dependence* 38:95–137.

Didday, R. L. 1970. The simulation and modelling of distributed information processing in the frog visual system. Ph.D. diss., Stanford University.

Didday, R. L. 1976. A model of visuomotor mechanisms in the frog optic tectum. *Math. Biosci.* 30:169–180.

Didday, R. L., and Arbib, M. A. 1975. Eye movements and visual perception: "Two visual systems" model. *Int. J. Man-Mach. Stud.* 7:547–569.

Diener, H. C., Hore, J., Ivry, R., and Dichgans, J. 1993. Cerebellar dysfunction of movement and perception. *Can. J. Neurol. Sci.* 20 (suppl. 3):S62–S69.

Dominey, P. F., and Arbib, M. A. 1992. A cortico-subcortical model for generation of spatially accurate sequential saccades. *Cerebral Cortex* 2:153–175.

Dominey, P. F., Arbib, M. A., and Joseph, J.-P. 1995. A model of cortico-striatal plasticity for learning associations and sequences. *J. Cogn. Neurosci.* 7:311–336.

Dominey, P. F., Decety, J., Broussolle, E., Chazot, G., and Jeannerod, M. 1995. Motor imagery of a lateralized sequential task is asymmetrically slowed in hemi-parkinson s patients. *Neuropsychologia* 33:727–741.

Donegan, N. H., and Wagner, A. R. 1987. Conditioned diminution and facilitation of the UCR: A sometimes-opponent-process interpretation. In Classical conditioning: II. Behavioral, neurophysiological, and neurochemical studies in the rabbit, eds. I. Gormezano, W. Prokasy, and R. F. Thompson. Hillsdale, NJ: Lawrence Erlbaum Associates.

Draper, B. A., Collins, R. T., Brolio, J., Hanson, A. R., and Riseman, E. M. 1989. The schema system. *Int. J. Comput. Vis.* 2:209–250.

Drescher, G. L. 1989. A mechanism for early Piagetian learning. In Proceedings of the International Joint Conference on Artificial Intelligence, 290–294.

Droulez, J., and Berthoz, A. 1991. A neural network model of sensoritopic maps with predictive short-term memory properties. *Proc. Natl. Acad. Sci. U.S.A.* 88:9653–9657.

Duchamp-Viret, P., and Duchamp, A. 1993. GABAergic control of odor-induced activity in the frog olfactory bulb: Possible GABAergic modulation of granule cell inhibitory action. *Neuroscience* 56:905–914.

Duchamp-Viret, P., Duchamp, A., and Chaput, M. 1993. GABAergic control of odor-induced activity in the frog olfactory bulb: Electrophysiological study with picrotoxin and bicuculline. *Neuroscience* 53:111–120.

Dudek, S. M., and Bear, M. F. 1992. Homosynaptic long-term depression in area CA1 of hippocampus and the effects on NMDA receptor blockade. *Proc. Natl. Acad. Sci.* 89:4363–4367.

Du Lac, S., Raymond, J. L., Sejnowski, T. J., and Lisberger, S. G. 1995. Learning and memory in the vestibulo-ocular reflex. *Annu. Rev. Neurosci.* 18:409–441.

Dunant, Y., Israel, M., Lesbats, B., and Manaranche, R. 1977. Oscillation of acetylcholine during nerve activity in the Torpedo Electric Organ. *Brain Res.* 125:123–140.

Durand, J. 1993. NMDA actions on rat abducens motoneurons. *Eur. J. Neurosci.* 3:621–633.

Durbin, R., and Mitchison, G. 1990. A dimension reduction framework for understanding cortical maps. *Nature* 343:644–647.

Durbin, R., and Willshaw, D. 1987. An analog approach to the travelling salesman problem using an elastic net method. *Nature* 326:689–691.

Dvořak, I., and Holden, A. V. 1991. *Mathematical approaches to brain functioning diagnostics*. Manchester, UK: Manchester University Press.

di Pellegrino, G., Fadiga, L., Fogassi, L., Gallese, V., and Rizzolatti, G. 1992. Understanding motor events: A neurophysiological study. *Exp. Brain Res.* 91:176–180.

Ebner, T. J., and Bloedel, J. R. 1984. Climbing fiber action on the responsiveness of Purkinje cells to parallel fiber inputs. *Brain Res.* 309:182–186.

Eccles, J. C. 1964. *The physiology of synapses*. Berlin: Springer-Verlag.

Eccles, J. C. 1973a. The cerebellum as a computer: Patterns in space and time. *J. Physiol.* 229:1–32.

Eccles, J. C. 1973b. *The understanding of the brain*. New York: McGraw-Hill.

Eccles, J. C., Ito, M., and Szentágothai, J. 1967. *The cerebellum as a neuronal machine*. New York: Springer-Verlag.

Eckhorn, R., Bauer, R., Jordan, W., Brosch, M., Kruse, W., Munk, M., and Reitboek, H. J. 1988. Coherent oscillations: A mechanism of feature linking in the visual cortex? *Biol. Cybern.* 60:121–130.

Eckhorn, R., Frien, A., Bauer, R., et al. 1994. Oscillation frequencies (40–90 Hz) in monkey visual cortex depend on stimulus size and velocity. *Eur. J. Neurosci. Suppl.* 7:90.04.

Edelman, C. M. 1984. Cell-surface modulation and marker multiplicity in neural patterning. *Trends Neurosci.* 7:78–84.

Edelman, G. M. 1987. *Neural darwinism*. New York: Basic Books.

Edelman, G. M., and Finkel, H. H. 1984. Neuronal group selection in the central cortex. In *Dynamic aspects of neocortical function*, eds. G. M. Edelman, W. E. Gall, and W. M. Cowan, 653–695. New York: Wiley.

Eichenbaum, H., Kuperstein, M., Fagan, A., and Nagode, J. 1986. Cue sampling and goal-approach correlates of hippocampal unit activity in rats performing an odor discrimination task. *J. Neurosci.* 7:16–732.

Eichenbaum, H., Otto, T. A., Wible, C. G., and Piper, J. M. 1991. Building a model of the hippocampus in olfaction and memory. In *Olfaction: A model system for computational neuroscience*, eds. J. L. Davis and H. Eichenbaum, 167–210. Cambridge, MA: MIT Press.

Eigen, M., and Schuster, P. 1979. *The hypercycle: A principle of natural self-organization*. Heidelberg: Springer-Verlag.

Eisenfeld, J., and DeLisi, C. 1985. On conditions for qualitative instability of regulatory circuits with applications to immunological control loops. In *Mathematics and computers in biomedical applications*, eds. J. Eisenfeld and C. DeLisi, 39–53. New York: Elsevier.

Elbert, T., Ray, W. J., Kowalik, Z. J., Skinner, J. E., Graf, K. E., and Birbaumer, N. 1994. Chaos and physiology. *Physiol. Rev.* 74:1–47.

Elman, J. L. 1995. Language processing. In *The handbook of brain theory and neural networks*, ed. M. A. Arbib, 508–513. Cambridge, MA: Bradford Books/MIT Press.

Engel, A. K., König, P., Kreiter, A. K., Schillen, T. B., and Singer, W. 1992. Temporal coding in the visual cortex: New vistas on integration in the nervous system. *Trends Neurosci.* 15:218–226.

Epstein, S. 1979. Vermin users' manual. Unpublished M. S. thesis, Department of Computer and Information Science, University of Massachusetts at Amherst.

Érdi, P. 1983. Hierarchical thermodynamic approach to the brain. *Int. J. Neurosci.* 20:193–216.

Érdi, P. 1991. Self-organization in the nervous system: Network structure and stability. In *Mathematical approaches to brain functioning diagnostics*, eds. I. Dvořak and A. V. Holden, 31–43. Manchester, UK: Manchester University Press.

Érdi, P. 1994. Noise and chaos in neural systems. In *Neural modeling and neural networks*, ed. F. Ventriglia, 163–184. Oxford: Pergamon Press.

Érdi, P. 1996a. The brain as a hermeneutic device. *BioSystems* 38:179–189.

Érdi, P. 1996b. Levels, models, and brain activities: Neurodynamics is pluralistic. *Behav. Brain Sci.* 19:296–297.

Érdi, P., Aradi, I., and Grőbler, T. 1997. Rhythmogenesis in single cells and pupulation models: Olfactory bulb and hippocampus. *BioSystems* 40:45–53.

Érdi, P., and Barna, G. 1984. Self-organizing mechanism for the formation of ordered neural mappings. *Biol. Cybern.* 51:93–101.

Érdi, P., and Barna, G., 1985. Self-organization of neural networks: Noise-induced transition. *Phys. Lett.* 107A:287–290.

Érdi, P., and Barna, G. 1987. Self-organization in the nervous system: Some illustrations. In *Mathematical topics in population biology, morphogenesis and neuroscience. Vol. 71, Lecture notes in biomathematics*, eds. E. Teramoto and M. Yamaguti, 301–317. Berlin: Springer-Verlag.

Érdi, P., and Barna, G. 1991. "Neural" model for the formation of the ocularity domains. In *Artificial neural networks*, Vol. 1, eds. T. Kohonen, K. Mäkisura, U. Simala, and J. Kongas, 513–518. Amsterdam: Elsevier North-Holland.

Érdi, P., Grőbler, T., Barna, G., and Kaski, K. 1993. Dynamics of the olfactory bulb: Bifurcations, learning, and memory. *Biol. Cybern.* 69:57–66.

Érdi, P., Grőbler, T., and Tóth, J. 1992. On the classification of some classification problems. In *Proceedings of the International Symposium on Information Physics*, 110–117. Iizuka, Japan: Kyushu Institute of Technology.

Érdi, P., and Szentágothai, J. 1985. Neural connectivies: Between determinism and randomness. In *Dynamics of macrosystems*, eds. J.-P. Aubin, D. Saari, and K. Sigmund, 21–29. Berlin: Springer-Verlag.

Érdi, P., and Tóth, J. 1988. Anomalous stochastic kinetics. In *chemical reactivity in liquids: Fundamental aspects*, eds. M. Moreau and P. Turq, 511–516. New York: Plenum Press.

Érdi, P., and Tóth, J. 1989. *Mathematical models of chemical reactions*. Pinceton: Princeton University Press.

Érdi, P., and Tóth, J. 1990. What is and what is not stated by the May-Wigner theorem? *J. Theor. Biol.* 145:137–140.

Erdős, P., and Rényi, A. 1960. On the evolution of random graphs. *Publ. Math. Inst. Hung. Acad. Sci.* 5:17–61.

Ericson, J., Thor, J., Edlund, S., Jessell, T. M., and Yamada, T. 1992. Early stages of motor neuron differentiation revealed by expression. *Science* 256:1555–1560.

Ermentrout, G. B. 1986. The behavior of rings of coupled oscillators. *J. Math. Biol.* 23:55–74.

Ermentrout, G. B. 1994. An introduction to neural oscillators. In *Neural modeling and neural networks*, ed. F. Ventriglia, 79–110. Oxford: Pergamon Press.

Ermentrout, G. B. 1995. Phase-plane analysis of neural activity. In *The handbook of brain theory and neural networks*, ed. M. A. Arbib, 732–738. Cambridge, MA: Bradford Books/MIT Press.

Ermentrout, G. B., and Cowan, J. D. 1979. Temporal oscillations in neuronal nets. *J. Math. Biol.* 29:571–585.

Ermentrout, G. B., and Kopell, N. 1984. Frequency plateaus in a chain of weakly coupled oscillators. *S.I.A.M. J. Math. Anal.* 15:215–237.

Evarts, E. V., Shinoda, Y., and Wise, S. P. 1984. *Neurophysiological approaches to higher brain functions*. New York: Wiley.

Evarts, E. V., and Tanji, J. 1976. Reflex and intended responses in motor cortex pyramidal tract neurons of monkey. *J. Neurophysiol.* 39:1069–1080.

Ewert, J.-P. 1987. Neuroethology of releasing mechanisms: Prey-catching in toads. *Behav. Brain Sci.* 10:337–405.

Ewert, J.-P. 1989. The release of visual behavior in toads: Stages of parallel/hierarchical information processing. In *Visuomotor coordination: Amphibians, comparisons, models, and robots*, eds. J.-P. Ewert and M. A. Arbib, 39–120. New York: Plenum Press.

Fadiga, L., Fogassi, L., Pavesi, G., and Rizzolatti, G. 1995. Motor facilitation during action observation: A magnetic stimulation study. *J. Neurophysiol.* 73:2608–2611.

Fagg, A. H. 1996. A computational model of the cortical mechanisms involved in primate grasping. Ph.D. diss., University of Southern California.

Fagg, A. H., and Arbib, M. A. 1992. A model of primate visual-motor conditional learning. *Adap. Behav.* 1:1–37.

Fagg, A. H., and Arbib, M. A. to appear. *Modeling parietal-premotor interactions in primate control of grasping*.

Fagg, A. H., Arbib, M. A., and Grafton, S. T. to appear. *Linking PET imaging in humans to a model of neural mechanisms of grasping*.

Fagg, A. H., Grafton, S. T., and Arbib, M. A. to appear. *PET study of neural mechanisms of grasping*.

Fan, Y. S., and Chay, T. R. 1994. Generation of periodic and chaotic bursting in an excitable cell model. *Biol. Cybern.* 71:417–431.

Farmer, J. D. 1990. A Rosetta stone for connectionism. *Physica D* 42:153–187.

Farah, M. 1990. *Visual agnosia*. Cambridge, MA: MIT Press.

Fatt, P., and Katz, B. 1952. Spontaneous subthreshold activity of motor nerve endings. *J. Physiol. (Lond.)* 117:109–128.

Ferster, D., and LeVay, S. 1978. The axonal arborization of lateral geniculate neurons in the striate cortex of the cat. *J. Comp. Neurol.* 182:923–944.

FitzHugh, R. 1961. Impulses and physiological states in theoretical models of nerve membrane. *Biophys. J.* 1:445–466.

Flaherty, A. W., and Graybiel, A. M. 1994. Input-output organization of the primate sensorimotor system. *J. Neurosci.* 14:599–610.

Flanders, M., Helms Tillery, S. I., and Soechting, J. F. 1992. Early stages in sensorimotor transformation. *Behav. Brain Sci.* 309–362.

Flash, T., and Hogan, N. 1985. The coordination of arm movements: An experimentally confirmed mathematical model. *J. Neurosci.* 5:1688–1703.

Földiak, P. 1990. Forming sparse representations by local anti-Hebbian learning. *Biol. Cybern.* 64:165–170.

Forssberg, H., and Grillner, S. 1973. The locomotion of the acute spinal cat injected with clonidine I. V. *Brain Res.* 50:184–186.

Foster, T. C., Castro, C. A., and McNaughton, B. L. 1988. Spatial selectivity of rat hippocampal neurons: Dependence on preparedness for movement. *Science* 244:1580–1582.

Frank, P. M. 1978. *Introduction to system sensitivity theory*. New York: Academic Press.

Frazier, L. 1990. Exploring the architecture of the language-processing system. In *Cognitive models of speech processing: Psycholinguistic and computational perspectives*, ed. G. T. M. Altmann, 409–433. Cambridge, MA: Bradford Books/MIT Press.

Frederiks, J. A. M. 1969. Disorders of the body schema. In *Handbook of clinical neurology: 4. Disorders of speech perception and symbolic behavior*, eds. P. J. Vinken and G. W. Bruyn, 207–240. Amsterdam: Elsevier North-Holland.

Freeman, W. J. 1975. *Mass action in the nervous system*. New York: Academic Press.

Freeman, W. J. 1978. Spatial properties of an EEG event in the olfactory bulb and cortex. *Electroencephalogr. Clin. Neurophysiol.* 44:585–605.

Freeman, W. J. 1979. Nonlinear gain mediating cortical stimulus-response relations. *Biol. Cybern.* 35:237–247.

Freeman, W. J. 1987. Simulation of chaotic EEG patterns with a dynamic model of the olfactory system. *Biol. Cybern.* 56:139–150.

Freeman, W. J. 1991. Nonlinear dynamics in olfactory information processing. In *Olfaction: A model system for computational neuroscience*, eds. J. L. Davis and H. Eichenbaum, 225–249. Cambridge, MA: MIT Press.

Freeman, W. J. 1992. Predictions on neocortical dynamics derived from studies in paleocortex. In *Induced rhythms of the brain*, eds. E. Basar and T. H. Bullock, 183–199. Cambridge, MA: Birkhauser.

Freeman, W. J., and Barrie, J. M. 1994. Chaotic oscillations and the genesis of meaning in cerebral cortex. In *Temporal coding in the brain*, eds. G. Buzsáki, R. Llinás, W. Singer, A. Berthoz, and Y. Christen, 13–37. Berlin: Springer-Verlag.

Freeman, W. J., and Schneider, W. 1982. Changes in spatial patterns of rabbit olfactory EEG with conditioning to odors. *Psychophysiology* 19:44–56.

Freeman, W. J., and Skarda, C. A. 1985. Spatial EEG patterns, nonlinear dynamics and perception. The neo-Sherringtonian view. *Brain Res. Rev.* 10:47–175.

Freund, F. F., Martin, K. A. C., Somogyi, P., and Whitteridge, D. 1985. Innervation of cat visual areas 17 and 18 by physiologically identified X- and Y-type afferents: II. Identification of postsynaptic targets by GABA immunocytochemistry and Golgi impregnation. *J. Comp. Neurol.* 242:275–291.

Freund, T. F., and Antal, M. 1988. GABA-containing neurons in the septum control inhibitory interneurons in the hippocampus. *Nature* 336:170–173.

Freund, T. F., Gulyás, A. I., Acsádi, L., Görcs, T., and Tóth, K. 1990. Serotoninergic control of the hippocampus via local inhibitory interneurons. *Proc. Natl. Acad. Sci. U.S.A.* 87:8501–8505.

Frisby, J. P. 1995. Stereo correspondence and neural networks. In *The handbook of brain theory and neural networks*, ed. M. A. Arbib, 937–941. Cambridge, MA: Bradford Books/MIT Press.

Fromherz, P. 1988. Self-organization of the fluid mosaic of charged channel proteins in membranes. *Proc. Natl. Acad. Sci. U.S.A.* 85:6353–6357.

Frotscher, M., and Zimmer, J. 1983. Lesion-induced mossy fibers to the molecular layer of the rat fascia dentata: Identification of postsynaptic granule cells by the Golgi-EM technique. *J. Comp. Neurol.* 215:299–311.

Fuchs, A. F., Kaneko, C. R. S., and Scudder, C. A. 1985. Brainstem control of saccadic eye movements. *Annu. Rev. Neurosci.* 8:307–337.

Fujita, M. 1982a. Adaptive filter model of the cerebellum. *Biol. Cybern.* 45:195–206.

Fujita, M. 1982b. Simulation of adaptive modification of the vestibulo-ocular reflex with an adaptive filter model of the cerebellum. *Biol. Cybern.* 45:207–214.

Fukai, T. 1994. A model of cortical memory processing based on columnar organization. *Biol. Cybern.* 70:427–434.

Fukai, T. 1995. Bulbocortical interplay in olfactory information processing via synchronous oscillations. *Biol. Cybern.* 34:209–217.

Fukushima, K. 1975. Cognitron: A self-organizing multilayered neural network. *Biol. Cybern.* 20:121–136.

Fukushima, K. 1988. Neocognitron: A hierarchical neural network capable of visual pattern recognition. *Neural Networks* 1:119–130.

Fukushima, K. 1994. Pattern recognition with neural networks. In *Neural modeling and neural networks*, ed. F. Ventriglia, 283–308. Oxford: Pergamon Press.

Fukushima, K., and Wake, N. 1992. An improved learning algorithm for the neocognitron. In *Artificial neural networks*, Vol. 2, eds. I. Alexander and J. Taylor, 497–505. Amsterdam: Elsevier North-Holland.

Fulton, J. F., ed. 1938. *Physiology of the nervous system*. London: Oxford University Press.

Funahashi, S., Bruce, C. J., and Goldman-Rakic, P. S. 1989. Mnemonic coding of visual space in monkey's dorsolateral prefrontal cortex. *J. Neurophysiol.* 61:331–349.

Fuster, J. M. 1989. *The prefrontal cortex: Anatomy, physiology, and neuropsychology of the frontal lobe*, 2d ed. New York: Raven Press.

Fuster, J. M. 1995. *Memory in the cerebral cortex: An empirical approach to neural networks in the human and nonhuman primate*. Cambridge, MA: Bradford Books/MIT Press.

Fuster, J. M., Bauer, R. H., and Jervey, J. P. 1982. Cellular discharge in the dorsolateral prefrontal cortex of the monkey in cognitive tasks. *Exp. Neurol.* 77:679–694.

Gaál, Gy. 1995. Relationship of calculating the Jacobian matrices of nonlinear systems and population coding algorithms in neurobiology. *Physica D* 84:582–600.

Gähwiler, B. H. 1980. Excitatory action of opioid peptides and opiates on cultured hippocampal pyramidal cells. *Brain Res.* 104:193–203.

Gähwiler, B. H. 1981. Development of acute tolerance during exposure of hippocampal explants to an opioid peptide. *Brain Res.* 217:196–200.

Gähwiler, B. H. 1988. Das kultivierte Gehirn. *Neue Zuricher Zeitung* 256:73.

Gallez, D., and Babloyantz, A. 1991. Predictability of human EEG: A dynamic approach. *Biol. Cybern.* 64:381–391.

Gao, J.-H., Parsons, L. M., Bower, J. M., Xiong, J., Li, J., and Fox, P. T. 1996. Cerebellum implicated in sensory acquisition and discrimination rather than motor control. *Science* 272:545–547.

Gardner, M. R., and Ashby, W. R. 1970. Connectance of large dynamic (cybernetic) systems: Critical values for stability. *Nature* 228:784.

Garfinkel, A., Spano, M. L., Ditto, W. L., and Weiss, J. N. 1992. Controlling cardiac chaos. *Science* 257:1230–1235.

Gehring, W. J. 1987. Homeoboxes in the study of development. *Science* 239:170–175.

Gel'fand, I. M., Gurfinkel, V. S., Fomin, S. V., and Tsetlin, M. L., eds. 1971. *Models of the structural functional organization of certain biological systems*. Translated by C. R. Beard. Cambridge, MA: MIT Press.

Gellman, R., Gibson, A. R., and Houk, J. C. 1985. Inferior olivary neurons in the awake cat: Detection of contact and passive body displacement. *J. Neurophysiol.* 54:40–60.

Gennari, F. 1782. *De peculiari structura cerebri nonnulisque eius morbis*. Parma.

Georgiou, N., Bradshaw, J. L., Iansek, R., Phillips, J. G., Mattingley, J. B., and Bradshaw, J. A. 1994. Reduction in external cues and movement sequencing in parkinson's disease. *J. Neurol. Neurosurg. Psychiatry* 57:368–370.

Georgopoulos, A. P., Kalaska, J. F., and Massey, J. T. 1981. Spatial trajectories and reaction times of aimed movements: Effects of practice, uncertainty, and change in target location. *J. Neurophysiol.* 46:725–743.

Georgopoulos, A. P., Kettner, R. E., and Schwartz, A. B. 1988. Primate motor cortex and free arm movements to visual targets in three-dimensional space: II. Coding of the direction of movement by a neuronal population. *J. Neurosci.* 8:2928–2937.

Gerfen, C. R. 1989. The neostriatal mosaic: Striatal patch-matrix organization is related to cortical lamination. *Science* 246:385–388.

Gerfen, C. R. 1992. The neostriatal mosaic: Multiple levels of compartmental organization in the basal ganglia. *Annu. Rev. Neurosci.* 15:285–320.

Gerstein, G. L., and Mandelbrot, B. 1964. Random walk models for the spike activity of a single neuron. *Biophys. J.* 4:41–68.

Gerstner, W., Ritz, R., and van Hemmen, J. L. 1993. A biologically motivated and analytically soluble model of collective oscillations in the cortex: I. Theory of weak coupling. *Biol. Cybern.* 68:363–374.

Getchell, T. V., and Shepherd, G. M. 1978. Responses of olfactory receptor cells to step pulses of odour at different concentrations in the salamander. *J. Physiol. (Lond.)* 282:521–540.

Ghez, C. 1991. The cerebellum. In *Principles of neural science*, 3d ed, eds. E. Kandel, J. Schwartz, and T. Jessel, 626–646. New York: Elsevier.

Gibson, G. E., and Blass, J. 1976a. Inhibition of acetylcholine synthesis and of carbohydrate utilization by maple-syrupine disease metabolites. *J. Neurochem.* 26:1073–1078.

Gibson, G. E., and Blass, J. 1976b. Impaired synthesis of acetylcholine in the brain accompanying mild hypoxia and hypoglycemia. *J. Neurochem.* 27:37–42.

Gierer, A. 1981. Development of projections between areas of the nervous system. *Biol. Cybern.* 42:69–78.

Gilbert, C. D. 1985. Horizontal integration in the neocortex. *Trends Neurosci.* 8:160–165.

Gilbert, C. D. 1993. Circuitry, architecture, and functional dynamics of visual cortex. *Cerebral Cortex* 3:373–386.

Gilbert, C. D., and Wiesel, T. N. 1979. Morphology and intracortical projections of functionally identified neurons in cat visual cortex. *Nature* 280:120–125.

Gilbert, C. D., and Wiesel, T. N. 1983. Clustered intrinsic connections in cat visual cortex. *J. Neurosci.* 3:1116–1133.

Gilbert, C. D., and Wiesel, T. N. 1989. Columnar specificity of intrinsic horizontal and corticocortical connections in cat visual cortex. *J. Neurosci.* 9:2432–2442.

Gilbert, P. F. C., and Thach, W. T. 1977. Purkinje cell activity during motor learning. *Brain Res.* 128:309–328.

Glass, L. 1995. Chaos in neural systems. In *The handbook of brain theory and neural networks*, ed. M. A. Arbib, 186–189. Cambridge, MA: Bradford Books/MIT Press.

Glass, L., and Young, R. E. 1979. Structure and dynamics of neural network oscillators. *Brain Res.* 179:207–218.

Gleick, J. 1987. *Chaos.* New York: Viking.

Glenn, L. L., Hada, J., Roy, J. P, Deschenes, M., and Steriade, M. 1982. Anterograde tracer and field potential analysis of the neocortical layer I projection from nucleus ventralis medialis of the thalamus in cat. *Neuroscience* 7:1861–1877.

Glickstein, M., and Sperry, R. W. 1960. Intermanual somesthetic transfer in split brain rhesus monkeys. *J. Comp. Physiol. Psychol.* 53:322–327.

Gluck, M. A., Goren, O. A., Myers, C. E., and Thompson, R. F. 1996. A higher-order recurrent network model of the cerebellar substrates of response timing in motor-reflex conditioning. *J. Cog. Neurosci.* [[Au: Pls update.]]

Gluck, M. A., and Granger, R. 1993. Computational models of the neural bases of learning and memory. *Annu. Rev. Neurosci.* 16:667–706.

Gnadt, J. W., and Andersen, R. A. 1988. Memory-related motor planning activity in posterior parietal cortex of macaque. *Exp. Brain Res.* 70:216–220.

Goetz, K. G. 1987. Do "d-blub" and "l-blub" hypercolumns tesselate the monkey visual cortex? *Biol. Cybern.* 56:107–109.

Goetz, K. G. 1988. Cortical templates for self-organization of orientation-specific D- and L-hypercolumns in monkey and cats. *Biol. Cybern.* 58:213–223.

Goldberg, M. E., and Bruce, C. J. 1990. Primate frontal eye fields: III. Maintenance of a spatially accurate saccade signal. *J. Neurophysiol.* 64:489–508.

Goldberg, M. E., Colby, C. L., and Duhamel, J.-R. 1990. The representation of visuomotor space in the parietal lobe of the monkey. *Cold Spring Harb. Symp. Quant. Biol.* 55:729–739.

Goldberg, M. E., Musil, S. Y., Fitzgibbon, E. J., Smith, M., and Olson, C. R. 1993. The role of the cerebellum in the control of saccadic eye movements. In *Role of the cerebellum and basal ganglia in voluntary movement*, eds. N. Mano, I. Hamada, and M. R. DeLong, 203–211. Amsterdam: Excerpta Medica.

Goldberger, A., and West, B. 1986. Chaos in physiology. In *Chaos in biological systems*, eds. A. V. Holden, H. Degn, and L. F. Olsen, 1–5. New York: Plenum Press.

Goldman, P. S., and Nauta, W. J. H. 1977. Columnar distribution of cortico-cortical fibers in the frontal association, limbic, and motor cortex of the developing rhesus monkey. *Brain Res.* 122:393–413.

Goldman-Rakic, P. S. 1987. Circuitry of primate prefrontal cortex and regulation of behavior by representational memory. In *Handbook of physiology: Sec. 1. The nervous system. Vol. 5, Higher functions of the brain (part 2)*, eds. V. B. Mountcastle, F. Plum, and S. R. Geiger, 373–417. Bethesda, MD: American Physiological Association.

Goldman-Rakic, P. S. 1991. Parallel systems in the cerebral cortex: The topography of cognition. In *Natural and artificial computation*, eds. M. A. Arbib and J. A. Robinson, 155–176. Cambridge, MA: MIT Press.

Goldman-Rakic, P. S., and Schwartz, M. L., 1982. Interdigitation of contralateral and ipsilateral columnar projections to frontal association cortex in primates. *Science* 216:755–757.

Golgi, C. 1873. Sulla struttura della sostanza grigia del cervello. *Gazz. Med. Lombarda* 33:244–246.

Golgi, C. 1875. Sulla fina struttura del bulbi olfattori. In *Opera omnia: Vol. 1, Istologia normale*, 113–132. Milano: Ulrico Hoepli, 1903.

Golgi, C. 1883. Recherches sur l'histologie des centres nerveux. *Arch. Italiennes de Biol.* 3:285–317.

Golomb, D., Wang X.-J., and Rinzel, J. 1994. Synchronization properties of spindle oscillations in a thalamic reticular nucleus model. *J. Neurophysiol.* 53:899–904.

Golowasch, J., Buchholz, F., Epstein, I. R., and Marder, E. 1992. Contribution of individual ionic currents to activity of a model stomatogastric ganglion neuron. *J. Neurophysiol.* 67:341–349.

Gomi, H., and Kawato, M. 1992. Adaptive feedback control models of the vestibulocerebellum and spinocerebellum. *Biol. Cybern.* 68:105–114.

Goodale, M. A. 1993. Visual routes to knowledge and action. *Biomed. Res.* 14(suppl. 4):113–123.

Goodale, M. A., and Milner, A. D. 1992. Separate visual pathways for perception and action. *Trends Neurosci.* 15:20–25.

Goodale, M. A., Milner, A. D., Jakobson, L. S., and Carey, D. P. 1991. A neurological dissociation between perceiving objects and grasping them. *Nature* 349:154–156.

Goodale, M. A., Pelisson, D., and Prablanc, C. 1986. Large adjustments in visually guided reaching do not depend on vision of the hand or perception of target displacement. *Nature* 320:748–750.

Goodhill, G. 1992. Correlations, competition, and optimality: Modelling the development of topography and ocular dominance. *Cog. Sci. Res. Papers* 226. Brighton: University of Sussex.

Goodhill, G. J., and Willshaw, D. J. 1990. Application of the elastic net algorithm to the formation of ocular dominance stripes. *Network* 1:41–49.

Goodwin, B. C., and Cohen, M. H. 1969. A phase shift model for the spatial and temporal organization of developing systems. *J. Theor. Biol.* 29:99–107.

Gormezano, I., Kehoe, E. K., and Marshall, B. S. 1983. Twenty years of classical conditioning with the rabbit. *Prog. Psychobiol. Physiol. Psychol.* 10:197–275.

Gould, S. J. 1995. Ontogeny and phylogeny. Cambridge, MA: Harvard University Press.

Grafton, S. T., Fagg, A. H., Woods, R. P., and Arbib, M. A. 1996a. Functional anatomy of pointing and grasping in humans. *Cerebral Cortex* 6:226–237.

Grafton, S. T., Arbib, M. A., Fadiga, L., and Rizzolatti, G. 1996b. Localization of grasp representation in humans by PET: 2. Observation compared with imagination. *Exp. Brain Res.* 112:103–111.

Granger, R., Ambros-Ingerson, J., and Lynch, G. 1989. Derivation of encoding characteristics of layer II cerebral cortex. *J. Cogn. Neurosci.* 1:61–87.

Granger, R., Staubli, U., Ambros-Ingerson, J., and Lynch, G. 1991. Specific behavioral predictions from simulations of the olfactory system. In *Olfaction: A model system for computational neuroscience*, eds. J. L. Davis and H. Eichenbaum, 251–264. Cambridge, MA: MIT Press.

Granit, R., and Phillips, C. G. 1965. Excitatory and inhibitory processes acting upon individual Purkinje cells of the cerebellum in cats. *J. Physiol.* 133:520–547.

Grassberger, P., and Procaccia, I. 1983. Characterization of strange attractors. *Physiol. Rev. Lett.* 50:346–349.

Gray, C. M. 1994. Synchronous oscillations in neuronal system: Mechanisms and functions. *J. Comp. Neurosci.* 1:11–38.

Gray, C. M., König, P., Engel, A. K., and Singer, W. 1989. Oscillatory response in cat visual cortex exhibits intercolumnar synchronization which reflects global stimulus properties. *Nature* 338:334–337.

Gray, C. M., and McCormick, D. A. 1996. Chattering cells: Superficial pyramidal neurons contributing to the generation of synchronous oscillations in the visual cortex. *Science* 274:109–113.

Gray, C. M., and Singer, W. 1989. Stimulus-specific neuronal oscillations in orientation columns of cat visual cortex. *Proc. Natl. Acad. Sci. U.S.A.* 86:1698–1702.

Gray, C. M., and Viana di Prisco, G. 1993. Properties of stimulus-dependent rhythmic activity of the visual cortical neurons in the alert cat. *Soc. Neurosci. Abstr.* 16:359.8.

Graybiel, A. M., Aosaki, T., Flaherty, A. W., and Kimura, M. 1994. The basal ganglia and adaptive motor control. *Science* 265:1826–1831.

Graziao, M., Andersen, R., and Snowden, R. 1991. Tuning of MST neurons to spiral motions. *J. Neurosci.* 14:54–67.

Graziao, M. S. A., Andersen, R. A., and Snowden, R. J. 1994. Selectivity of area MST neurons for expansion, contraction, and rotation motions. *Invest. Ophthalmol. Vis. Sci.* 32:823–82.

Green, J. D., and Arduini, A. A. 1954. Hippocampal electrical activity in arousal. *J. Neurophysiol.* 17:533–557.

Greene, P. H. 1972. Problems of organization of motor systems. *Prog. Theor. Biol.* 2, eds. R. Rosen and F. M. Snell, 303–338. New York: Academic Press.

Gregory, R. L. 1969. On how so little information controls so much behavior. In *Towards a theoretical biology: 2. Sketches*, ed. C. H. Waddington. Edinburgh: Edinburgh University Press.

Grillner, S. 1985. The central nervous system utilizes a simple control strategy to generate the synergy used to control locomotion. In *Complex systems—operational approaches*, ed. H. Haken, 150–155. Berlin: Springer-Verlag.

Grillner, S., Wallén, P., Brodin, L., and Lansner, A. 1991. Neuronal network generating locomotor behavior in lamprey: Circuitry, transmitters, membrane properties, and simulation. *Annu. Rev. Neurosci.* 14:169–199.

Grillner, S., and Zangger, P. 1974. Locomotor movements generated by the deafferented spinal cord. *Acta Physiol. Scand.* 91:38A 39A.

Grinvald, A., and Malach, R. 1994. Functional architecture and connection rules in primary visual cortex of macaque monkey. In *Structural and functional organization of the neocortex: Proceedings of a symposium in the memory of Otto D. Creutzfeldt, May 1993*, eds. B. Albowitz, K. Albus, U. Kuhnt, H.-C. Nothdurft, and P. Wahle, 291–304. Berlin: Springer-Verlag.

Grőbler, T., and Barna, G. 1996. A statistical model of the CA3 region of the hippocampus. In *Cybernetics and System Research '96*, 503–507. Vienna: Austrian Society for Cybernetic Studies.

Grőbler, T., Marton, P., and Érdi, P. 1991. On the dynamic organization of memory. A mathematical model of associative free recall. *Biol. Cybern.* 65:73–79.

Grossberg, S. 1976. Adaptive pattern classification and universal recording: I. Parallel development and coding of neural feature detectors. *Biol. Cybern.* 23:121–134.

Grossberg, S., ed. 1988. *The adaptive brain*, Vols. 1, 2. Amsterdam: Elsevier North-Holland.

Groves, P. M., Garcia-Munoz, M., Linder, J. C., Manley, M. S., Martone, M. E., and Young, S. J. 1995. Elements of the intrinsic organization and information processing in the neostriatum. In *Models of information processing in the basal ganglia*, eds. J. C. Houk, J. L. Davis, and D. G. Beiser, 51–96. Cambridge, MA: Bradford Books/MIT Press.

Guigon, E., and Burnod, Y. 1995. Short-term memory. In *The handbook of brain theory and neural networks*, ed. M. A. Arbib, 867–871. Cambridge, MA: Bradford Books/MIT Press.

Gulyás, A. I. 1993. Local connections and subcortical innervation of neurochemically characterized subpopulations of hippocampal interneurons [in Hungarian]. Unpublished thesis, Hungarian Academy of Science, Budapest.

Gulyás, A. I., Görcs, T. J., and Freund, T. F. 1990. Innervation of different peptide-containing neurons in the hippocampus by GABAergic septal afferents. *Neuroscience* 37:31–44.

Gulyás, A. I., Miettinen, R., Jacobowitz, D. M., and Freund, T. F. 1992. Calretinin is present in nonpyramidal cells of the rat hippocampus: I. A new type of neuron specifically associated with the mossy fibre system. *Neuroscience* 48:1–27.

Gulyás, A. I., Miles, R., Hájós, N., and Freund, T. F. 1993a. Precision and variability in postsynaptic target selection of inhibitory cells in the hippocampal CA3 region. *Eur. J. Neurosci.* 5:1729–1751.

Gulyas, A. I., Miles, R., Sik, A., Tóth, K., Tamamaki, M., and Freund, T. F. 1993b. Hippocampal pyramidal cells excite inhibitory neurons through a single release site. *Nature* 366:683–687.

Gulyás, A. I., Tóth, K., Dános, P., and Freund, T. F. 1991. Subpopulation of GABAergic neurons containing parvalbumin, calbindin-D28k and cholecystokinin in the rat hippocampus. *J. Comp. Neurol.* 312:371–378.

Gulyas, B., Ottoson, D., and Roland, P. C., eds. 1982. *Functional organization of the human visual cortex.* Oxford: Pergamon Press.

Haberly, L. 1985. Neuronal circuitry in olfactory cortex: Anatomy and functional implications. *Chem. Senses* 10:219–238.

Haberly, L., and Bower, J. M. 1989. Olfactory cortex: Model circuit for study of associative memory. *Trends Neurosci.* 17:258–264.

Hajdú, F., Somogyi, G., and Tömböl, T. 1974. Neuronal and synaptic arrangement in the lateralis posterior-pulvinar complex of the thalamus in the cat. *Brain Res.* 73:89–104.

Haken, H. 1977. *Introduction to synergetics: Nonequilibrium phase transitions and self-organizations in physics, chemistry and biology.* Berlin: Springer-Verlag.

Haken, H. 1996. *Principles of brain functioning: A synergetic approach to brain activity, behavior and cognition.* Berlin: Springer-Verlag.

Halasy, K., and Somogyi, P. 1993a. Subdivision in the multiple GABAergic innervation of granule cells in the dentate gyrus of the rat hippocampus. *Eur. J. Neurosci.* 5:411–429.

Halasy, K., and Somogyi, P. 1993b. Distribution of GABAergic synapses and their targets in the dentate gyrus of rat: A quantitative immunoelectron microscopic analysis. *J. Hirnforsch.* 34:299–308.

Halász, N. 1990a. *The vertebrate olfactory system.* Budapest: Akadémiai Kiadó.

Halász, N. 1990b. Morphological basis of information processing in the olfactory bulb. In *Chemosensory information processing*, NATO ASI Series, Vol. H 39, ed. D. Schild, 175–190. Berlin: Springer-Verlag.

Halsband, U., Ito, N., Tanji, J., and Freund, H. J. 1993. The role of premotor cortex and the supplementary motor area in the temporal control of movement in man. *Brain* 116:243–266.

Halsband, U., Matsuzaka, Y., and Tanji, J. 1994. Neuronal activity in the primate supplementary, pre-supplementary and premotor cortex during externally and internally instructed sequential movements. *Neurosci. Res.* 20:149–155.

Hamburger, V. 1977. The developmental history of the motor neuron. *Neurosci. Res. Prog. Bull.* 15(Sept):1–13.

Hamburger, V., and Hamilton, H. L. 1951. A series of normal stages in the development of the chick embryo. *J. Morphol.* 88:49–92.

Hamburger, V., Wenger, E., and Oppenheim, R. 1966. Motility in the duck embryo in the absence of sensory input. *J. Exp. Zool.* 162:133–160.

Hámori, V., and Mezey, É. 1977. Serial and triadic synapses in the cerebellar nuclei of the cat. *Exp. Brain Res.* 30:259–273.

Han, Z.-S., Buhl, E. H., Lörinczi, Z., and Somogyi, P. 1993. A high degree of spatial selectivity in the axonal and dendritic domains of physiologically identified local-circuit neurons in the dentate gyrus of the rat hippocampus. *Eur. J. Neurosci.* 5:395–410.

Harnad, S. 1987. Categorial perception: A critical overview. In *Categorial perception. The groundwork of perception*, ed. S. Harnad. New York: Cambridge University Press.

Harth, E., Csermely, T. J., Beek, B., and Lindsay, R. D. 1970. Brain functions and neural dynamics. *J. Theor. Biol.* 26:93–120.

Harth, E., Unnikrishnan, K. P., and Pandya, A. S. 1987. The inversion of sensory processing by feedback pathways: A model of visual cognitive functions. *Science* 237:184–187.

Hassard, B. 1978. Bifurcation of periodic solutions of the Hodgkin-Huxley model for the squid giant axon. *J. Theor. Biol.* 71:401–420.

Hasselmo, M. E. 1994. Runaway synaptic modification in models of cortex: Implications for Alzheimer's disease. *Neural Networks* 7:13–40.

Hasselmo, M. E., Anderson, B. P., and Bower, J. M. 1992. Cholinergic modulation of cortical associative memory function. *J. Neurophysiol.* 67:1230–1246.

Hasselmo, M. E., and Bower, J. M. 1992. Cholinergic suppression specific to intrinsic, not afferent, fiber synapses in rat piriform (olfactory) cortex. *J. Neurophysiol.* 67:1222–1229.

Hasselmo, M. E., and Schnell, E. 1994. Laminar selectivity of the cholinergic suppression in rat hippocampal region CA1: Computational modeling and brain slice physiology. *J. Neurosci.* 14:3898–3914.

Hastings, H. M., Juhász, F., and Schreiber, M. A. 1992. Stability of structured random matrices. *Proc. R. Soc. Lond. [B]* 249:223–225.

Haussler, A. F., and von der Malsburg, C. 1983. Development of retinotopic projections: An analytic treatment. *J. Theor. Neurobiol.* 2:47–73.

Hayashi, H., and Ishizuka, S. 1990. Chaotic activity in hippocampus neural network and intracranial self-stimulation. In *Proceedings of the International Conference on Fuzzy Logic and Neural Networks*, Vol. 2, 583–586. Kyushu Institute of Technology.

Hayashi, H., and Ishizuka, S. 1992. Chaotic nature of bursting discharges in the *Onchidium* pacemaker neuron. *J. Theor. Biol.* 156:169–191.

Hayashi, H., Ishizuka, S., Ohta, M., and Hirakawa, K. 1982. Chaotic behavior in *Onchidium* giant neuron under sinusoidal stimulation. *Phys. Lett.* 88A:435–438.

Head, H., and Holmes, G. 1911. Sensory disturbances from cerebral lesions. *Brain* 34:102–254.

Hebb, D. O. 1949. *The organization of the behavior.* New York: Wiley.

Heidmann, T., and Changeux, J.-P. 1982. A molecular model for the regulation of synapse efficacy at the postsynaptic level. *Compt. Rendus Acad. Sci. Paris*, Ser. 2. 295:665–670.

Hepp-Reymond, M. C., Husler, E. J., Maier, M. A., and Qi, H. X. 1994. Force-related neuronal activity in two regions of the primate ventral premotor cortex. *Can. J. Physiol. Pharmacol.* 72:571–579.

Hesse, M. B. 1980. *Revolutions and reconstructions in the philosophy of science.* Bloomington, IN: Indiana University Press.

Hikosaka, O. 1991. Basal ganglia—possible role in motor coordination and learning. *Curr. Opin. Neurobiol.* 1:638–643.

Hikosaka, O., Matsumara, M., Kojima, J., and Gardiner, T. W. 1993. Role of basal ganglia in initiation and suppression of saccadic eye movements. In *Role of the cerebellum and basal ganglia in voluntary movement*, eds. N. Mano, I. Hamada, and M. R. DeLong, 213–219. Amsterdam: Excerpta Medica.

Hikosaka, O., Rand, M. K., Miyachi, S., and Miyashita, K. 1995. Learning of sequential movements in the monkey: Process of learning and retention of memory. *J. Neurophysiol.* 74:1652–1661.

Hikosaka, O., Sakamoto, M., and Usui, S. 1989a. Functional properties of monkey caudate neurons: I. Activities related to saccadic eye movements. *J. Neurophysiol.* 61:780–798.

Hikosaka, O., Sakamoto, M., and Usui, S. 1989b. Functional properties of monkey caudate neurons: II. Visual and auditory responses. *J. Neurophysiol.* 61:799–813.

Hikosaka, O., Sakamoto, M., and Usui, S. 1989c. Functional properties of monkey caudate neurons: III. Activities related to expectation of target and reward. *J. Neurophysiol.* 61:814–832.

Hikosaka, O., and Wurtz, R. 1983a. Visual and oculomotor functions of monkey substantia nigra pars reticulata: I. Relation of visual and auditory responses to saccades. *J. Neurophysiol.* 49(5):1230–1253.

Hikosaka, O., and Wurtz, R. 1983b. Visual and oculomotor functions of monkey substantia nigra pars reticulata: II. Visual responses related to fixation of gaze. *J. Neurophysiol.* 49(5):1254–1267.

Hikosaka, O., and Wurtz, R. 1983c. Visual and oculomotor functions of monkey substantia nigra pars reticulata: III. Memory-contingent visual and saccade responses. *J. Neurophysiol.* 49(5):1268–1284.

Hill, J. C. 1983. A computational model of language acquisition in the two-year-old. *Cogn. Brain Theory* 6:287–317.

Hindmarsh, J. L., and Rose, R. M. 1982. A model of the nerve impulse using two first-order differential equations. *Nature* 296:162–164.

Hines, M. 1984. Efficient computation of branched nerve equations. *J. Biomed. Comp.* 15:69–74.

Hines, M. 1993. NEURON—a program for simulation of nerve equations. In *Neural systems: Analysis and modeling*, ed. F. Eeckman, 127–136. Norwell, MA: Kluwer Academic.

Hinton, G. 1989. Connectionist learning procedures. *Artif. Intell.* 40:185–234.

Hinton, G. E., and Shallice, T. 1991. Lesioning an attractor network: Investigations of acquired dyslexia. *Psychol. Rev.* 98:74–95.

Hirai, Y. 1980. A new hypothesis for synaptic modification: An interactive process between postsynaptic competition and presynaptic regulation. *Biol. Cybern.* 36:41–50.

Hirsch, M. W. 1991. Network dynamics: Principles and problems. In *Neurodynamics*, eds. F. Pasemann and H. D. Doebner, 3–29. Singapore: World Scientific.

Hirsch, M. W. 1984. The dynamical systems approach to differential equations. *Bull. Am. Math. Soc.* 11:1–64.

Hirsch, M. W. 1987. Convergence in neural nets. *Proc. I.E.E.E. First Int. Conf. Neural Networks* II:115–125.

Hirsch, M. W. 1989. Convergent activation dynamics in continuous time networks. *Neural Networks* 2:331–349.

Hochman, S., Jordan, L. M., and MacDonald, J. F. 1994. N-methyl-D-aspartate receptor mediated voltage oscillations in neurons surrounding the central canal in slices of rat spinal cord. *J. Neurophysiol.* 72:565–577.

Hodgkin, A. L., and Huxley, A. F. 1952. A quantitative description of membrane current and its application to conduction and excitation in nerve. *J. Physiol. (Lond.)* 117:500–544.

Hoff, B., and Arbib, M. A. 1992. A model of the effects of speed, accuracy, and perturbation on visually guided reaching. *Exp. Brain Res.* 22:285–306.

Hoff, B., and Arbib, M. A. 1993. Simulation of interaction of hand transport and preshape during visually guided reaching to perturbed targets. *J. Motor Behav.* 5:175–192.

Hogan, N. 1984. An organizing principle for a class of voluntary movements. *J. Neurosci.* 4:2745–2754.

Hogg, T., and Huberman, B. A. 1985. Attractors on finite sets: The dissipative dynamics of computing structures. *Phys. Rev.* 32A:2338–2346.

Hogg, T., Huberman, B. A., and McGlade, J. M. 1989. The stability of ecosystems. *Proc. R. Soc. Lond. [B]* 237:43–51.

Holden, A. V. 1976. *Models of stochastic activity of neurones: Vol. 12, Lecture notes in biomathematics.* Berlin: Springer-Verlag.

Holden, A. V. 1985. Why the nervous system is not as chaotic as it should be. In *Dynamic phenomena in neurochemistry and neurophysics: Theoretical aspects*, ed. P. Érdi. Budapest: KFKI.

Holden, A. V. 1986. *Chaos.* Manchester: Manchester University Press.

Holden, A. V., Hyde, J., and Muhamed, A. 1991. Equilibria, periodicity, bursting and chaos in neural activity. In *Neurodynamics*, eds. F. Pasemann and H. D. Doebner, 96–128. Singapore: World Scientific.

Holden, A. V., Winlow, W., and Haydon, P. G. 1982. The induction periodic and chaotic activity in molluscan neurone. *Biol. Cybern.* 43:169–173.

Holmes, G. 1939. The cerebellum of man. *Brain* 62:1–30.

Holmes, W. R., and Levy, W. 1990. Insights into associative long-term potentiation from computational models of NMDA receptor-mediated calcium influx and intracellular calcium concentration changes. *J. Neurophysiol.* 63:1148–1168.

Holmes, W. R., and Rall, W. 1995. Dendritic spines. In *The handbook of brain theory and neural networks*, ed. M. A. Arbib, 289–292. Cambridge, MA: Bradford Books/MIT Press.

Hooper, S. L., and Moulins, M. 1989. Switching of a neuron from one network to another by sensory-induced changes in membrane properties. *Science* 244:1587–1589.

Hope, R. A., Hammond, B. J., and Gaze, F. R. S. 1976. The arrow model: Retino-tectal specificity and map formation in the goldfish visual system. *Proc. R. Soc. Lond. [B]* 194:447–466.

Hopfield, J. J. 1982. Neural networks and physical systems with emergent collective computational abilities. *Proc. Natl. Acad. Sci. U.S.A.* 79:2554–2558.

Hopfield, J. J. 1984. Neurons with graded response have collective computational properties like those of two-state neurons. *Proc. Natl. Acad. Sci. U.S.A.* 1:3088–3092.

Horn, D., and Ruppin, E. 1995. Compensatory mechanisms in an attractor neural network model of schizophrenia. *Neural Comput.* 7:182–205.

Horn, D., Sagi, D., and Usher, M. 1991. Segmentation binding and illusory conjunctions. *Neural Comput.* 3:510–525.

Horn, D., and Usher, M. 9991. Parallel activation of memories in an oscillatory neural network. *Neural Comput.* 3:31–43.

Hornykiewicz, O. 1966. Metabolism of brain dopamine in human parkinsonism: Neurochemical and clinical aspects. In *Biochemistry and pharmacology of the basal ganglia*, eds. E. Costa, L. J. Côté, and M. D. Yahr, 171–185. New York: Raven Press.

Horsthemke, W., and Lefever, R. 1984. *Noise-induced transition. Theory and application in physics, chemistry and biology.* Berlin: Springer-Verlag.

Horton, J. C., and Hubel, D. H. 1981. Regular patchy distribution of cytochrome oxidase staining in primary visual cortex of macaque monkey. *Nature* 292:762–764.

Houk, J. C., Adams, J. L., and Barto, A. G. 1995. A model of how the basal ganglia generate and use neural signals that predict reinforcement. In *Models of information processing in the basal ganglia*, eds. J. C. Houk, J. L. Davis, and D. G. Beiser, 249–270. Cambridge, MA: Bradford Books/MIT Press.

Houk, J. C., and Barto, A. G. 1992. Distributed sensorimotor learning. In *Tutorial in motor behavior II*, eds. G. E. Stelmach and J. Requin, 71–100. Amsterdam: Elsevier.

Houk, J. C., Buckingham, J. T., and Barto, A. G. In press. Models of the cerebellum and motor learning. *Behav. Brain Sci.*

Houk, J. C., Gibson, A. R., Harvey, C. F., Kennedy, P. R., and Van Kan, P. L. E. 1988. Activity of primate magnocellular red nucleus related to hand and finger movements. *Behav. Brain Res.* 28:201–206.

Houk, J. C., Keifer, J., and Barto, A. G. 1993. Distributed motor commands in the limb premotor network. *Trends Neurosci.* 16:27–33.

Hounsgaard, J., and Kjaerulff, O. 1992. Ca^{2+}-mediated plateau potentials in a subpopulation of interneurons in the ventral horn of the turtle spinal cord. *Eur. J. Neurosci.* 4:183–188.

House, D. H. 1989. *Depth perception in frogs and toads: A study in neural computing.* Berlin: Springer-Verlag.

Hubel, D. H. 1982. Exploration of the primary visual cortex, 1955–78. *Nature* 299:515–524.

Hubel, D. H., and Wiesel, T. N. 1959. Receptive fields of single neurones in the cat's striate cortex. *J. Physiol.* 148:574–591.

Hubel, D. H., and Wiesel, T. N. 1962. Receptive fields, binocular interaction and functional architecture in the cat's visual cortex. *J. Physiol. (Lond.)* 160:106–154.

Hubel, D. H., and Wiesel, T. N. 1968. Receptive fields and functional architecture of monkey striate cortex. *J. Physiol. (Lond.)* 195:215–243.

Hubel, D. H., and Wiesel, T. N. 1972. Laminar and columnar distribution geniculo-cortical fibers in the macaque monkey. *J. Comp. Neurol.* 146:421–450.

Hubel, D. H., and Wiesel, T. N. 1974. Uniformity of monkey striate cortex: A parallel relationship between field size, scatter and magnification factor. *J. Comp. Neurol.* 158:295–306.

Hubel, D. H., and Wiesel, T. N. 1977. Functional architecture of macaque monkey visual cortex. *Proc. R. Soc. Lond. [B]* 198:1–59.

Hubel, D. H., Wiesel, T. N., and Stryker, M. P. 1978. Anatomical demonstration of orientation columns in macaque monkey. *J. Comp. Neurol.* 166:361–379.

Huberman, B. A., and Lumer, E. 1990. Dynamics of adaptive systems. *I.E.E.E. Trans. Circ. Syst.* 37:547–550.

Hudson, R., and Distel, H. 1987. Regional autonomy in the peripheral processing of odor signals in newborn rabbits. *Brain Res.* 421:85–94.

Hudson, R., Distel, H., and Zippel, H. P. 1990. Perceptual performance in peripherically reduced olfactory systems. In *Chemosensory information processing*, NATO ASI Series, Vol. H 39, ed. D. Schild, 259–269. Berlin: Springer-Verlag.

Hull, C. L. 1943. *Principles of behavior.* New York: Appleton-Century.

Humphrey, N. K. 1970. What the frog's eye tells the monkey's brain. *Brain Behav. Evol.* 3:324–337.

Iberall, A. S. 1978. A field and circuit thermodynamics for integrative physiology: I. Introduction to the general notions. *Am. J. Physiol.* 233:171–180.

Iberall, T., and Arbib, M. A. 1990. Schemas for the control of hand movements: An essay on cortical localization. In *Vision and action: The control of grasping*, ed. M. A. Goodale, 204–242. Norwood, NJ: Ablex Publishing.

Iberall, T., Bingham, G., and Arbib, M. A. 1986. Opposition space as a structuring concept for the analysis of skilled hand movements. In *Generation and modulation of action patterns*, eds. H. Heuer and C. Fromm, 158–173. Berlin: Springer-Verlag.

Ikegami, T., and Kaneko, K. 1992. Evolution of host-parasitoid through homeochaotic dynamics. *Chaos* 2:397–407.

Ilinsky, I. A., Jouandet, M. L., and Goldman-Rakic, P. S. 1985. Organization of the nigrothalamocortical system in the rhesus monkey. *J. Comp. Neurol.* 236:315–330.

Ingber, L. 1982. Statistical mechanics of neocortical interactions: I. Basic formulation. *Physica D* 5:83–107.

Ingle, D. 1968. Visual releasers of prey catching behaviour in frogs and toads. *Brain Behav. Evol.* 1:500–518.

Ingle, D. 1976. Spatial vision in anurans. In *The amphibian visual system*, ed. K. V. Fite, 119–140. New York: Academic Press.

Ingle, D., and Hoff, K.vS. 1990. Visually elicited evasive behavior in frogs: Giving memory research an ethological context. *BioScience* 40(4): 284–291.

Ingle, D. J. 1983. Visual mechanisms of optic tectum and pretectum related to stimulus localization in frogs and toads. In *Advances in vertebrate neuroethology*, eds. J.-P. Ewert, R. R. Capranica, and D. J. Ingle, 177–226. New York: Plenum Press.

Intrator, N., and Cooper, L. N. 1995. BCM theory of visual cortical plasticity. In *The handbook of brain theory and neural networks*, ed. M. A. Arbib, 153–157. Cambridge, MA: Bradford Books/MIT Press.

Ishizuka, N., Weber, J., and Amaral, D. G. 1990. Organization of intrahippocampal projections originating from CA3 pyramidal cells in the rat. *J. Comp. Neurol.* 295:580–623.

Ising, E. 1925. Beitrag zur theorie des ferromagnetizmus. *Z. Physik* 31:253–258.

Israel, M., Lesbats, B., Manaranche, R., Marsal, J., and Mastour-Frachon, P. 1977. Related changes in amounts of ACh and ATP in resting and active torpedo nerve electroplaque synapse. *J. Neurochem.* 28:1259–1267.

Ito, M. 1970. Neurophysiological aspects of the cerebellar motor control system. *Int. J. Neurol.* 7:162–176.

Ito, M. 1972a. Cerebellar control of the vestibular neurons: Physiology and pharmacology. *Prog. Brain Res.* 37:377–390.

Ito, M. 1972b. Neural design of the cerebellar control system. *Brain Res.* 40:80–82.

Ito, M. 1973. The vestibulo-cerebellar relationships: Vestibulo-ocular reflex arc and flocculus. In *Handbook of sensory physiology, vol. 6. Vestibular system*, ed. M. M. Kornhuber, 35. New York: Springer-Verlag.

Ito, M. 1974. The control mechanisms of cerebellar motor systems. In *The neurosciences: Third study program*, eds. F. O. Schmitt and F. Worden, 293–303. Cambridge MA: MIT Press.

Ito, M. 1982. Cerebellar control of the vestibulo-ocular reflex around the flocculus hypothesis. *Annu. Rev. Neurosci.* 5:275–296.

Ito, M. 1984. *The cerebellum and neuronal control.* New York: Raven Press.

Ito, M. 1989. Long-term depression. *Annu. Rev. Neurosci.* 12:85–102.

Ito, M. 1990. A new physiological concept on cerebellum. *Rev. Neurol. (Paris)* 146:564–569.

Ito, M. 1993. Movement and thought: Identical control mechanisms by the cerebellum. *Trends Neurosci.* 16:448–450.

Ito, M., and Kano, M. 1982. Long-lasting depression of parallel fiber Purkinje cell transmission induced by conjunctive stimulation of parallel fibers and climbing fibers in the cerebellar cortex. *Neurosci. Lett.* 33: 253–258.

Ito, M., and Karachot, L. 1990. Receptor subtypes involved in, and time course of, the long-term desensitization of glutamate receptors in cerebellar Purkinje cells. *Neurosci. Res.* 8:303–307.

Ivry, R. B., Keele, S. W., and Diener, H. C. 1988. Dissociation of the lateral and medial cerebellum in movement timing and movement execution. *Exp. Brain Res.* 73:167–180.

Jack, J. J. B., Noble, D., and Tsien, R. W. 1975. *Electrical current flow in excitable cells.* London: Oxford University Press.

Jackson, E. A. 1991. Controls of dynamic flows with attractors. *Physiol. Rev.* 44A:4839–4853.

Jackson, E. A., and Kodogeorgiou, A. 1991. Entrainment and migration controls of two-dimensional maps. *Physica D* 54:253–265.

Jacobson, M. 1970. *Developmental neurobiology.* Chicago: Holt-Rinehart-Winston.

Jacobson, M. 1978. *Developmental neurobiology*, 2d ed. New York: Plenum Press.

Jaffe, D. B., Fisher, S. A., and Brown, T. H. 1994. Confocal laser scanning microscopy reveals voltage-gated calcium signals within hippocampal dendritic spines. *J. Neurobiol.* 25:220–223.

Jahnsen, H., and Llinás, R. 1984. Ionic basis for the electroresponsiveness and oscillatory properties of guinea-pig thalamic neurons in vitro. *J. Physiol. (Lond.)* 349:227–247.

Jakobson, L. S., Archibald, Y. M., Carey, D. P., and Goodale, M. A. 1991. A kinematic analysis of reaching and grasping movements in a patient recovering from optic ataxia. *Neuropsychologia* 29:803–809.

Jansen, J. 1969. On cerebellar evolution and organization from the point of view of a morphologist. In *Neurobiology of cerebellar evolution and development*, ed. R. Llinás, 88–89. Chicago: American Medical Association.

Jansen, J., and Brodal, A. 1940. Experimental studies on the intrinsic fibers of the cerebellum: II. The cortico-nuclear projection. *J. Comp. Neurol.* 73:267–321.

Jansen, J., and Brodal, A. 1942. Experimental studies on the intrinsic fibers of the cerebellum. The cortico-nuclear projection in the rabbit and the monkey (*Macacus rhesus*). *Avh. Norske Vid.-Akad. I. Mat.-Nat. Kl.* 3:1–50.

Jansen, J., and Brodal, A. 1954. *Aspects of cerebellar anatomy.* Oslo: Forlagt Johan Grundt Tanum.

Jasper, H. H. 1949. Diffuse projection systems: The integrative action of the thalamic reticular system. *Electroencephalogr. Clin. Neurophysiol.* 1:405–420.

Jeannerod, M. 1984. The timing of natural prehension movements. *J. Motor Behav.* 16(3):235–254.

Jeannerod, M. 1994. The representing brain: Neural correlates of motor intention and imagery. *Behav. Brain. Sci.* 17:187–245.

Jefferys, J. G. R., and Haas, H. L. 1982. Synchronized bursting of CA1 hippocampal pyramidal cells in the absence of synaptic transmission. *Nature* 300:448–450.

Jeffries, C. 1974. Qualitative stability and digraphs in model ecosystems. *Ecology* 55, 1415–1419.

Jenkins, I. H., Brooks, D. J., Nixon, P. D., Frackowiak, R. S. J., and Passingham, R. E. 1994. Motor sequence learning—a study with positron emission tomography. *J. Neurosci.* 14:3775–3790.

Johnson-Laird, P. N. 1988. *The computer and the mind: An introduction to cognitive science.* London: Fontana Press.

Johnston, D., Magaee, J. C., Colbert, D. M., and Christie, B. R. 1996. Active properties of neuronal dendrites. *Annu. Rev. Neurosci.* 19:165–186.

Johnston, D., Williams, S., Jaffe, D. B., and Gray, R. 1992. NMDA-receptor independent long-term potentiation. *Annu. Rev. Physiol.* 54: 489–505.

Johnston, D., and Wu, S. M-S. 1994. *Foundations of cellular neurophysiology.* Cambridge, MA: MIT Press.

Jones, E. G. 1985. *The thalamus.* New York: Plenum Press.

Jones, E. G., Burton, H., and Porter, R. 1975. Commisural and corticocortical "columns" in the somatic sensory cortex of primates. *Science* 190:572–574.

Jope, R. S. 1979. High affinity choline transport and acetylCoA production in brain and their roles in the regulation of acetylcholine synthesis. *Brain Res. Rev.* 1:313–344.

Juhász, F. 1990. On the characteristic values of non-symmetric block random matrices. *J. Theor. Prob.* 67:199–205.

Juhász, F. 1992. On the asymptotic behavior of the spectra of non-symmetric random (0,1) matrices. *Discr. Math.* 41:161–165.

Kaas, J. H., Krubitzer, L. A., Chio, Y. M., Langston, A. L., Polley, H., and Blair, N. 1990. Reorganization of retinotopic cortical maps in adult mammals after lesions of the retina. *Science* 228:229–231.

Kaczmarek, L. K, and Levitan, I. B. 1987. *Neuromodulation.* Oxford: Oxford University Press.

Kalaska, J. F., and Crammond, D. J. 1992. Cerebral cortical mechanism of reaching movements. *Science* 255:1517–1523.

Kalman, R. E., and Bucy, R. S. 1961. New results in linear prediction and filtering theory. *J. Basic Engr.* (Trans. ASME, Ser. D) 83D:95–100.

Kalman, R. E., Falb, P. L., and Arbib, M. A. 1969. *Topics in mathematical system theory.* New York: McGraw-Hill.

Kandel, E. R. 1976. *Cellular basis of behavior: An introduction to behavioral neurobiology.* San Francisco: Freeman.

Kant, I. 1929. *Critique of pure reason.* Translated by Norman Kemp Smith. London: McMillan.

Kaplan, D., and Glass, L. 1995. *Understanding nonlinear dynamics.* New York: Springer-Verlag.

Kase, C. S., Tronocoso, J. F., Court, J. E., Tapia, J. F., and Mohr, J. P. 1977. Global spatial disorientation: Clinico-pathological correlations. *J. Neurol. Sci.* 34:267–278.

Katchalsky, A. K., Rowland, V., and Blumenthal, R. 1974. *Dynamic patterns of brain cell assemblies. NRP Bull.* 12(1):3–187.

Katsumaru, H., Kosaka, T., Heizmann, C. W., and Hama, K. 1988. Immunocytochemical study of GABAergic neurons containing the calcium-binding protein parvalbumin in the rat hippocampus. *Exp. Brain Res.* 72:347–362.

Kauer, J. S., Neff, S. R., Hamilton, K. A., and Cinelli, A. R. 1991. The salamander olfactory pathway: visualizing and modeling circuit activity. In *Olfaction: A model system for computational neuroscience,* eds. JL. Davis and H. Eichenbaum, 43–68. Cambridge, MA: MIT Press.

Kaufmann, S. A. 1993. *Origins of order: Self-organization and selection in evolution.* Oxford: Oxford University Press.

Kawato, M., and Gomi, H. 1992. The cerebellum and VOR/OKR learning models. *Trends Neurosci.* 15:445–453.

Kawato, M., Isobe, M., and Suzuki, R. 1989. Hierarchical learning of voluntary movement by cerebellum and sensory association cortices. In *Dynamic interactions in neural networks: Models and data. Vol. 1, Research notes in neural computing,* eds. M. A. Arbib and S.-I. Amari, 195–214. New York: Springer-Verlag.

Kawato, M., Miyamoto, H., Setoyama, T., and Suzuki, R. 1988. Feedback-error-learning neural network for trajectory control of a robotic manipulator. *Neural Networks* 1:256–265.

Keating, E. G., and Gooley, S. C. 1988. Saccadic disorders caused by cooling the superior colliculus or the frontal eye fields or from combined lesions of both structures. *Brain Res.* 438:247–255.

Keele, S. W., and Ivry, I. R. 1991. Does the cerebellum provide a common computation for diverse tasks? A timing hypothesis. In *The development and neural bases of higher cognitive functions,* ed. A. Diamond. *Ann. N. Y. Acad. Sci.* 608:179–211.

Keener, J. P. 1981. Infinite period bifurcation and global bifurcation branches. *S.I.A.M. J. Appl. Math.* 41:127–144.

Kelly, D. G. 1990. Stability in contractive nonlinear neural networks. *I.E.E.E. Trans. Biomed. Engineering* 37:231–242.

Kelso, J. A. S. 1995. *Dynamic patterns. The self-organization of brain and behavior.* Cambridge, MA: Bradford Books/MIT Press.

Kepler, T. B., Abbott, L. F., and Marder, E. 1992. Reduction of conductance-based neuron models. *Biol. Cybern.* 66:381–387.

Kermadi, I., and Joseph, J. P. 1995. Activity in the caudate nucleus of monkey during spatial sequencing. *J. Neurophysiol.* 74:911–933.

Kermadi, I., Jurquet, Y., Arzi, M., and Joseph, J. P. 1993. Neural activity in the caudate nucleus of monkeys during spatial sequencing. *Exp. Brain Res.* 94:352–356.

Kerr, F. W. L., and Carey, K. L. 1978. Pain. *Neurosci. Prog. Bull.* 16:1–207.

Kesner, R. P., and Novak, J. M. 1981. Memory for lists of items in rats: Role of the hippocampus. *Soc. Neurosci. Abstr.* 7(80.12):237.

Kievit, J., and Kuypers, H. G. J. M. 1977. Organization of the thalamo-cortical connexions to the frontal lobe in the rhesus monkey. *Exp. Brain Res.* 29:299–322.

Kilmer, W. L., McCulloch, W. S., and Blum, J. 1969. A model of the vertebrate central command system. *Int. J. Man-Mach. Stud.* 1:279–309.

Kimura, M. 1995. Role of basal ganglia in behavioral learning. *Neurosci. Res.* 22:353–358.

Kimura, M., Aosaki, T., and Graybiel, A. 1993. Role of basal ganglia in the acquisition and initiation of learned movement. In *Role of the cerebellum and basal ganglia in voluntary movement,* eds. N. Mano, I. Hamada, and M. R. DeLong, 83–87. Amsterdam: Excerpta Medica.

Kimura, M., Aosaki, T., and Ishida, A. 1993. Neurophysiological aspects of the differential roles of the putamen and caudate nucleus in voluntary movement. *Adv. Neurol.* 60:62–70.

King, C. C. 1991. Fractal and chaotic dynamics in nervous systems. *Prog. Neurobiol.* 36:279–308.

King, R., Barchas, J. D., and Huberman, B. A. 1984. Chaotic behavior in dopamine neurodynamics. *Proc. Natl. Acad. Sci. U.S.A.* 81:1244–1247.

King, R. B. 1983. Chemical applications of topology and group theory 14. Topological aspects of chaotic chemical reactions. *Theor. Chim. Acta (Berl.)* 63:323–338.

Kirkwood, A., Gold, S. M. D. J. T., Aizenman, C., and Bear, M. F. 1993. Common forms of synaptic plasticity in hippocampus and neocortex in vitro. *Science* 260:1518–1521.

Kisvarday, Z. F., Martin, K. A. C., Freund, T. F., Magloczky, Z. S., Whitteridge, D., and Somogyi, P. 1986. Synaptic targets of HRP-filled layer III pyramidal cells in the striate cortex. *Exp. Brain Res.* 44:541–552.

Kling, U. 1971. Simulation neuronaler Impulsrhythmen. Zur Theorie der Netzwerke mit cyclishen Hemmverbindungen. *Kybernetik* 9:123–139.

Kling, U., and Székely, G. 1968. Simulation of rhythmic nervous activities: I. Function of networks with cyclic inhibitions, *Kybernetik* 5:89–103.

Klopf, A. H. 1982. *The hedonistic neuron: A theory of memory, learning, and intelligence.* Washington, DC: Hemisphere.

Klopf, A. H. 1986. A drive-reinforcement model of single neuron function: An alternative to the Hebbian neuronal model. In *Proceedings of the American Institute of Physics: Neural Networks for Computing,* 265–270.

Koch, C., and Ullman, S. 1985. Shifts in selective visual attention: Towards the underlying neural circuitry. *Hum. Neurobiol.* 4:219–227.

Köhler, C., and Steinbusch, H. 1982. Identification of serotonin and non-serotonin-containing neurons of the midbrain raphe projecting to the entorhinal area and the hippocampal formation. A combined immunohistochemical and fluorescent retrograde tracing study in the rat brain. *Neuroscience* 7:951–975.

Kohonen, T. 1972. Correlation matrix memories. *I.E.E.E. Trans. Comput.* C-21:353–359.

Kohonen, T. 1982. Self-organized formation of topologically correct feature maps. *Biol. Cybern.* 43:59–69.

Kohonen, T. 1984. *Self-organization and associative memory.* Berlin: Springer-Verlag.

Kohonen, T. 1988. *Self-organization and associative memory,* 2d ed. Berlin: Springer-Verlag.

Komisaruk, B. R. 1970. Synchrony between limbic system theta activity and rhythmical behavior in rats. *J. Comp. Physiol. Psychol.* 70:182–492.

Konen, W., and von der Malsburg, C. 1994. Learning to generalize from single examples in dynamic link architecture. In *Temporal coding in the brain,* eds. G. Buzsáki, R. Llinás, W. Singer, A. Berthoz, and Y. Christen, 205–219. Berlin: Springer-Verlag.

König, R., and Schillen, T. B. 1991. Stimulus-dependent assembly formation of oscillatory responses: I. Synchronization. *Neural Comput.* 3:155–166.

Konopacki, J., MacIver, M. B., Bland, B. H., and Roth, S. H. 1987. Carbachol-induced EEG "theta" activity in hippocampal brain slice. *Brain Res.* 405:196–198.

Kopell, N. 1988. Toward a theory of modeling central pattern generators. In *Neural control of rhythmic movements in vertebrates,* eds. A. H. Cohen, S. Rossignol, and S. Grillner. New York: Wiley.

Kopell, N., and Ermentrout, G. B. 1990. Phase transition and other phenomena in chains of coupled oscillators. *S.I.A.M. J. Appl. Math.* 50:1014–1052.

Kosaka, T., Katsumaru, H., Hama, K., Wu, J.-Y., and Heizmann, C. W. 1987. GABAergic neurons containing the Ca-binding protein parvalbumin in the rat hippocampus and dentate gyrus. *Brain Res.* 419:119–130.

Kosko, B. 1986. Differential Hebbian learning. In *Proceedings of the American Institute of Physics: Neural Networks for Computing,* 277–282.

Kosko, B. 1990. Unsupervised learning rules. *I.E.E.E. T.N.N.* 1:44–57.

Kotter, R., and Wickens, J. 1995. Interactions of glutamate and dopamine in a computational model of the striatum. *J. Comput. Neurosci.* 2:195–214.

Kreiter, A. K., and Singer, W. 1992. Oscillatory neuronal responses in the visual cortex of the awake macaque monkey. *Eur. J. Neurosci.* 4:369–375.

Kriebel, M. E., Vautrin, J., and Holsapple, J. 1990. Transmitter release: Prepacking and random mechanism or dynamic and deterministic process. *Brain Res. Rev.* 15:167–178.

Kritikos, A., Leahy, C., Bradshaw, J. L., Iansek, R., Phillips, J. G., and Bradshaw, J. A. 1995. Contingent and noncontingent auditory cueing in parkinson's disease. *Neuropsychologia* 33:1193–1203.

Krueger, J. 1983. Simultaneous individual recordings form many cerebral neurons: Techniques and results. *Rev. Physiol. Biochem. Pharmacol.* 98:178–233.

Kubie, L., and Ranck, J. B. 1983. Sensory-behavioral correlates in individual neurons in three situations: Space and content. In *The neurobiology of the hippocampus,* ed. W. Seifert. New York: Academic Press.

Kuramoto, Y. 1984. *Chemical oscillations, waves, and turbulence.* Berlin: Springer-Verlag.

Kuypers, H. G. J. M. 1987. Some aspects of the organization of the output of the motor cortex. In *Motor areas of the cerebral cortex,* eds. G. Bock, M. O'Connor, and J. Marsh. Chichester, UK: Wiley and Sons.

Lábos, E. 1977a. Theoretical considerations of local neuron circuits and their triadic synaptic arrangements (TSA) in subcortical sensory nuclei. *J. Neurosci. Res.* 3:1–10.

Lábos, E. 1977b. Neuronal networks detecting movements of input signals. In *Proceedings of the IFAC Symposium on Control Mechanisms in Bio- and Ecosystems,* Vol. 3, 25–33. Leipzig.

Lábos, E. 1984. Periodic and non-periodic motions in different classes of formal neuronal networks and chaotic like generators. In *Cybernetic and system research,* Vol. 2, ed. R. Trappl, 237–243. Amsterdam: Elsevier North-Holland.

Lábos, E., Hámori, J., and Isomura, G. 1980. On the functional significance of axonal triads in medial cuneate nucleus. *J. Hirnforsch.* 21:569–572.

Lábos, E., Pasik, P., Hámori, J., and Nógrádi, E. 1990. On the dynamics of triadic synaptic arrangements: Computer experiments with formal neural nets of chaotic units. *J. Hirnforsch.* 31:715–722.

Lancet, D. 1992. Olfactory reception: From transduction to human genetics. In *Sensory transduction,* eds. D. P. Corey and S. D. Roper, 73–91. New York: Rockefeller University Press.

Lánský, P., and Lánská, V. 1987. Diffusion approximation of the neuronal model with synaptic reversal potentials. *Biol. Cybern.* 56:19–26.

Lánský, P., and Rospars, J.-P. 1993. Coding of odor intensity. *BioSystems* 31:15–38.

Lara, R., Carmona, M., Daza, F., and Cruz, A. 1984. A global model of the neural mechanisms responsible for visuomotor coordination in toads. *J. Theor. Biol.* 110:587–618.

Larson, J. J., and Lynch, G. 1986. Induction of synaptic potentiation in hippocampus by patterned stimulation involves two events. *Science* 232:985–988.

Larson, J., Xiao, P., and Lynch, G. 1993. Reversal of LTP by theta frequency stimulation. *Brain Res.* 600:97–102.

Lashley, K. S. 1951. The problem of serial order in behavior. In *Cerebral mechanisms in behavior: The Hixon symposium*, ed. L. Jeffress, 112–136. New York: Wiley.

Lawrence, D. G., and Kuypers, H. G. J. M. 1968. The functional organization of the motor system in the monkey: I. The effects of bilateral pyramidal lesions. *Brain* 91:1–14.

Lawrence, P. A. 1992. *The making of a fly: The genetics of animal design.* Oxford: Blackwell Scientific.

LeDoux, J. E. 1992. Brain mechanisms of emotion and emotional learning. *Curr. Opin. Neurobiol.* 2:191–198.

Legendre, P., Tixier-Vidal, A., Brigant, J. L., and Vincent, J. P. 1988. Electrophysiology and ultrastructure of mouse hypothalamic neurons in culture: A correlative analysis during development. *Dev. Brain Res.* 43:273–285.

Leiner, H. C., Leiner, A. L., and Dow, R. S. 1986. Does the cerebellum contribute to mental skills? *Behav. Neurosci.* 100:443–453.

Leiner, H. C., Leiner, A. L., and Dow, R. S. 1987. Cerebro-cerebellar learning loops in apes and humans. *Ital. J. Neurol. Sci.* 425–436.

Leiner, H. C., Leiner, A. L., and Dow, R. S. 1989. Reappraising the cerebellum: What does the hindbrain contribute to the forebrain? *Behav. Neurosci.* 103:998–1008.

Leiner, H. C., Leiner, A. L., and Dow, R. S. 1991. The human cerebro-cerebellar system: Its computing, cognitive, and language skills. *Behav. Brain Res.* 44:113–128.

Lenhossek, M. V. 1891. Zur Kenntnis der Neuroglia des amenschlichen Ruckenmarkes. *Verhandl. Anat. Gesellsch.* 5:93.

Lenhossek, M. V. 1895. *Der feinere Bau des Nervensystems im Lichte neuer Forschungen*, ed. H. Kornfeld. Berlin: Fischers Med. Buchhandlung.

Leon, M., Wilson, D. A., and Guthrie, K. L. 1991. Plasticity in the developing olfactory system. In *Olfaction: A model system for computational neuroscience*, eds. J. L. Davis and H. Eichenbaum, 121–140. Cambridge, MA: MIT Press.

Leresche, N., Lightowler, S., Soltesz, I., Jassik-Gerschenfeld, D., and Crunelli, V. 1991. Low-frequency oscillatory activities intrinsic to rat and cat thalamocortical cells. *J. Physiol. (Lond.)* 441:155–174.

Lettvin, J. Y. 1989. Warren and Walter. In *Collected works of Warren S. McCulloch*, Vol. 3, ed. R. McCulloch, 514–529. Salinas, CA: Intersystems Publications.

Lettvin, J. Y., Maturana, H., McCulloch, W. S., and Pitts, W. H. 1959. What the frog's eye tells the frog brain. *Proc. I.R.E.* 47:1940–1951.

LeVay, S., Hubel, D. H., and Wiesel T. N. 1975. The pattern of ocular dominance columns in macaque revealed by a reduced silver stain. *J. Comp. Neurol.* 159:559–576.

Li, X.-G., Somogyi, P., Ylinen, A., and Buzsáki, G. 1994. The hippocampal CA3 network: An in vivo intracellular labeling study. *J. Comp. Neurol.* 339:181–208.

Li, Z., and Hopfield, J. J. 1989. Modeling the olfactory bulb and its neural oscillatory processings. *Biol. Cybern.* 61:379–392.

Liao, D. Z., Hessler, N. A., and Malinow, R. 1995. Activation of postsynaptically silent synapses during pairing-induced LTP in CA1 region of hippocampal slice. *Nature* 375:400–404.

Liaw, J.-S., and Arbib, M. A. 1993. Neural mechanisms underlying direction-selective avoidance behavior. *Adap. Behav.* 1:227–261.

Liaw, J.-S., Berger, T. W., and Baudry, M. 1995. NMDA receptors: Synaptic, cellular, and network models. In *The handbook of brain theory and neural networks*, ed. M. A. Arbib, 644–647. Cambridge, MA: Bradford Books/MIT Press.

Lichtheim, L. 1885. On aphasia. *Brain* 7:433–484.

Lieblich, I., and Arbib, M. A. 1982. Multiple representations of space underlying behavior. *Behav. Brain Sci.* 5:627–659.

Liljenström, H. 1991. Modeling the dynamics of olfactory coding using simplified network units and realistic architecture. *Int. J. Neural Syst.* 2:1–15.

Liljenström, H., and Hasselmo, M. E. 1993. Acetylcholine and cortical oscillatory dynamics. In *Computation and neural systems*, eds. F. Eeckman and J. M. Bower, 523–530. Dordrecht: Kluwer.

Liljenström, H., and Hasselmo, M. E. 1995. Cholinergic modulation of cortical oscillatory dynamics. *J. Neurophysiol.* 74:288–297.

Linsker, R. 1986. From basis network principles to neural architecture: Emergence of orientation columns. *Proc. Natl. Acad. Sci. U.S.A.* 83:8779–8783.

Linsker, R. 1990. Perceptual neural organization: Some approaches based on network models and information theory. *Annu. Rev. Neurosci.* 13:257–281.

Linster, C., and Gervais, R. 1996. Investigation of the role of interneurons and their modulation by centrifugal fibers in a neural model of the olfactory bulb. *J. Comp. Neurosci.* 3:225–246.

Little, W. A. 1974. The existence of persistent states in the brain. *Math. Biosci.* 19:101–120.

Livingstone, M. S., and Hubel, D. H. 1981. Effects of sleep and arousal on the processing of visual information in the cat. *Nature* 291:554–561.

Livingstone, M. S., and Hubel, D. H. 1988. Segregation of form, color, movement and depth: Anatomy, physiology and perception. *Science* 240:740–749.

Ljungberg, T., Apicella, P., and Schultz, W. 1991. Responses of monkey midbrain dopamine neurons during delayed alternation performance. *Brain Res.* 567:337–341.

Ljungberg, T., Apicella, P., and Schultz, W. 1992. Responses of monkey dopamine neurons during learning of behavioral reactions. *J. Neurophysiol.* 67(1):145–163.

Llinás, R. 1987. "Mindness" as a functional state of the brain. In *Mindwaves*, eds. C. Blakemore and S. Greenfield, 339–358. Oxford: Basel Blackwell.

Llinás, R. 1988. The intrinsic electrophysiological properties of mammalian neurons: Insight into central nervous system function. *Science* 242:1654–1664.

Llinás, R., Ribary, U., Joliot, M., and Wang, X.-J. 1994. Content and context in temporal thalamocortical binding. In *Temporal coding in the brain*, eds. G. Buzsáki, R. Llinás, W. Singer, A. Berthoz, and Y. Christen, 251–272. Berlin: Springer-Verlag.

Llinás, R., and Sugimori, M. 1980a. Electrophysiological properties of *in vitro* Purkinje cell somata in mammalian cerebellar slices. *J. Physiol.* 305:171–195.

Llinás, R., and Sugimori, M. 1980b. Electrophysiological properties of *in vitro* Purkinje cell dendrites in mammalian cerbellar slices. *J. Physiol.* 305:197–213.

Llinás, R., and Yarom, Y. 1981. Properties and distribution of ionic conductances generating electroresponsiveness of mammalian inferior olivary neurons *in vitro*. *J. Physiol.* 315:569–584.

Lopes da Silva, F. H., and Pijn, J. P. 1995. EEG analysis. In *The handbook of brain theory and neural networks*, ed. M. A. Arbib, 348–351. Cambridge, MA: Bradford Books/MIT Press.

Lorente de Nó, R. 1922. La corteza cerebral del ratón (Primera contribución. La corteza acustica). *Trab. Lab. Invest. Biol. University of Madrid* 20:47–78.

Lorente de Nó, R. 1932. The regulation of eye positions and movements induced by the labyrinth. *Laryngoscope* 42:233–330.

Lorente de Nó, R. 1933. Vestibulo-ocular reflex arc. *Arch. Neurol. Psychiatry* 30:245–291.

Lorente de Nó, R. 1934. Studies on the structure of cerebral cortex: II. Continuation of the study of the ammonic system. *J. Physiol. Neurol.* 46:113–177.

Lorente de Nó, R. 1938a. The cerebral cortex: Architecture, intracortical connections and motor projections. In *Physiology of the nervous system*, ed. D. F. Fulton, 291–321. London: Oxford University Press.

Lorente de Nó, R. 1938b. Analysis of the activity of chain of internuncial neurones. *J. Neurophysiol.* 1:207–244.

Loskutov, A. Y. 1993. Dynamics control of chaotic systems by parametric destochastization. *J. Phys. A: Math. Gen.* 26:4581–4594.

Lundberg, A. 1969. Reflex control of stepping. The Nansen Memorial Lecture V, 1–42. Oslo: Universitetsforlaget.

Luria, A. R. 1959. Disorders of "simultaneous perception" in a case of bilateral occipito-parietal brain injury. *Brain* 82:437–447.

Luria, A. R. 1973. *The working brain.* New York: Penguin Books.

Lynch, G., and Baudry, M. 1988. Structure-function relationships in the organization of memory. In *Perspectives in memory research*, ed. M. S. Gazzaniga. Cambridge, MA: MIT Press.

Lynch, G., and Granger, R. 1991. Serial steps in memory processing: Possible clues from studies of plasticity in the olfactory-hippocampal circuit. In *Olfaction: A model system for computational neuroscience*, eds. J. L. Davis and H. Eichenbaum, 141–165. Cambridge, MA: MIT Press.

Lynch, G., and Granger, R. 1992. Variations in synaptic plasticity and types of memory in cortico-hippocampal networks. *J. Cog. Neurosci.* 4:189–199.

Lyons, M. A., and Arbib, M. A. 1989. A formal model of computation for sensory-based robotics. *I.E.E.E. Trans. Robot. Autom.* 5:280–293.

Lytton, W., and Sejnowski, T. J. 1991. Inhibitory interneurons may help synchronize oscillations in cortical pyramidal neurons. *J. Neurophysiol.* 66:1059–1079.

MacIntosh, F. C., and Collier, B. 1976. Neurochemistry of cholinergic terminals. In *Handbook of experimental pharmacology* [new series]. *Vol. 42: Neuromuscular junction*, ed. E. Zaimis, 99–228. Berlin: Springer-Verlag.

MacKay, D. M. 1966. Cerebral organization and the conscious control of action. In *Brain and conscious experience*, ed. J. C. Eccles, 422–440. Berlin: Springer-Verlag.

MacKenzie, C. L., and Iberall, T. 1994. *The grasping hand.* Amsterdam: Elsevier North-Holland.

Macrides, F. 1975. Temporal relations between hippocampal slow waves and exploratory shifting in hamsters. *Behav. Biol.* 14:295–308.

Macrides, F., Eichenbaum, H. B., and Forbes, W. B. 1982. Temporal relationship between sniffing and limbic theta rhythm during odor discrimination reversal learning. *J. Neurosci.* 2:1705–1717.

MacVicar, B. A., and Tse, F. W. 1989. Local neuronal circuitry underlying cholinergic rhythmical slow activity in CA3 area of rat hippocampal slices. *J. Physiol.* 417:197–212.

Maffei, L., and Fiorentini, A. 1977. Spatial frequency rows in the striate visual cortex. *Vis. Res.* 17:257–264.

Makara, G. B., Palkovits, M., and Szentágothai, J. 1980. The endocrine hypothalamus and the hormonal response to stress. In *Selye's guide to stress research*, ed. H. Selye, 280–337. New York: Van Nostrand Reinhold.

Maler, L., and Mugnaini, E. 1993. Organization and function of feedback to the electrosensory lateral line lobe of *Gymnotiform* fish, with emphasis on a searchlight mechanism. *J. Comp. Physiol.* 173:667–670.

Mallot, H. A. 1985. An overall description of retinotopic mapping in the cat's visual cortex areas 17, 18, and 19. *Biol. Cybern.* 52:45–51.

Mandler, G. 1985. *Cognitive psychology: An essay in cognitive science.* Hillsdale, NJ: Lawrence Erlbaum Associates.

Mangold, O. 1931. Das Determinationsproblem: III. Das Wirbel tierauge in der Entwicklung und Regeneration. *Erg. Biol.* 7:193–403.

Marder, E., and Nusbaum, M. P. 1989. Peptidergic modulation of the motor pattern generators in the stomatogastric ganglion. In *Perspectives in neural systems and behavior*, eds. T. J. Carew and D. B. Kelley, 73–91. New York: Alan R. Liss.

Marder, E., and Selverston, A. I. 1992. Modeling the stomatogastric nervous system. In *Dynamic biological networks: The stomatogastric nervous system*, eds. R. M. Harris-Warrick, E. Marder, A. I. Selverston, and M. Moulins, 161–196. Cambridge, MA: MIT Press.

Marr, D. 1969. A theory of cerebellar cortex. *J. Physiol.* 202:437–470.

Marr, D. 1971. Simple memory: A theory for archicortex. *Philos. Trans. R. Soc. [B]* 262:23–81.

Marr, D., and Poggio, T. 1977. Cooperative computation of stereo disparity. *Science* 194:283–287.

Martin, K. A. C. 1988a. From single cells to simple circuits in the cerebral cortex. *Q. J. Exp. Physiol.* 73:637–702.

Martin, K. A. C. 1988b. From enzymes in visual perception: A bridge too far? *Trends Neurosci.* 11:380–387.

Martin, K. A. C., and Whitteridge, D. 1984. Form, function and intracortical projections of spiny neurones in the striate visual cortex of the cat. *J. Physiol.* 353:463–504.

Martin, T., Keating, J. G., Goodkin, H. P., Bastian, A. J., and Thach, W. T. In press. Prism adaptation of human eye-hand coordination: Task specificity and dependency on the olivo-cerebellar system.

Matelli, M., Camarda, R., Glickstein, M., and Rizzolatti, G. 1986. Afferent and efferent projections of the inferior area 6 in the macaque monkey. *J. Comp. Neurol.* 251:281–298.

Matelli, M., Luppino, G., and Rizzolatti, G. 1985. Patterns of cytochrome oxidase activity in the frontal agranular cortex of macaque monkey. *Behav. Brain Res.* 18:125–137.

Matesz, C., and Székely, G. 1977. The dorsomedial group of cranial nerves in the frog. *Acta Biol. Acad. Sci. Hung.* 28:461–474.

Matsumoto, G., Aihara, K., Ichikawa, M., and Tasaki, A. 1984. Periodic and nonperiodic responses of membrane potentials in squid giant axons during sinusoidal current stimulation. *J. Theor. Neurobiol.* 43:1–4.

Matsumura, M., and Kubota, K. 1979. Cortical projection of hand-arm motor area from postarcuate area in macaque monkey: A histological study of retrograde transport of horseradish peroxidase. *Neurosci. Lett.* 11:241–246.

Maturana, H. R., and Varela, F. J. 1980. *Autopoiesis and cognition.* Dordrecht: Reidel.

Maunsell, X. X. 1995. The brain s visual world: Representation of visual targets in cerebral cortex. *Science* 270:764–769.

May, R. M. 1972. Will a large complex system be stable? *Nature* 238:413–414.

May, R. M. 1976. Simple mathematical models with very complicated dynamics. *Nature* 261:459–467.

Mays, L. E., and Sparks, D. L. 1980. Dissociation of visual and saccade related responses in superior colliculus neurons. *J. Neurophysiol.* 43: 207–232.

McBain, C. J. 1994. Hippocampal inhibitory neuron activity in the elevated potassium model of epilepsy. *J. Neurophysiol.* 72:2853–2863.

McBain, C. J., Traynelis, S. F., and Digledine, R. 1993. High potassium induced synchronous bursts and electrographic seizures. In *Epilepsy: Models, mechanisms and concepts,* ed. P. A. Schwartzkoin, 437–461. Cambridge, UK: Cambridge University Press.

McCormick, D. A. 1989. Cholinergic and noradrenergic modulation of thalamocortical processing. *Trends Neurosci.* 12:215.

McCulloch, W. S., and Pitts, W. H. 1943. A logical calculus of the ideas immanent in nervous activity. *Bull. Math. Biophys.* 5:115–133.

McDonald, J., and MacWhinney, B. 1989. Maximum likelihood models for sentence processing. In *A cross-linguistic study of sentence processing,* eds. B. MacWhinney and E. Bates, 397–422. Cambridge, UK: Cambridge University Press.

McNaughton, B. L. 1989. Neural mechanism for spatial computation and information storage. In *Neural connections, mental computation,* eds. L. Nadel, L. A. Cooper, P. Culicover, and R. M. Harish, 285–350. Cambridge, MA: MIT Press.

McNaughton, B. L., Barnes, A., and Andersen, P. 1981. Synaptic efficacy and EPSP summation in granule cells of rat fascia dentate studied in vitro. *J. Neurophysiol.* 46:952–966.

McNaughton, B. L., Barnes, C. A., and O'Keefe, J. 1983. The contribution of position, direction and velocity to single unit activity in the hippocampus of freely moving rats. *Exp. Brain Res.* 52:41–49.

McNaughton, B. L., Knierim, J. J., and Wilson, M. A. 1995. Vector encoding and the vestibular foundations of spatial cognition: A neuro-

physiological and computational hypothesis. In *The cognitive neurosciences,* ed. M. Gazzaniga, 585–595. Cambridge, MA: MIT Press.

McNaughton, B. L., Leonard, B., and Chen, L. 1989. Cortical-hippocampal interactions and cognitive mapping: A hypothesis based on reintegration of the parietal and inferotemporal pathways for visual processing. *Psychobiology* 17:230–235.

McNaughton, B. L., and Nadel, L. 1990. Hebb-Marr networks and the neurobiological representation of action in space. In *Neuroscience and connectionist theory,* eds. M. A. Gluck and D. E. Rumelhart, 1–63. Hillsdale, NJ: Lawrence Erlbaum Associates.

Melzack, R., and Wall, P. D. 1965. Pain mechanism: A new theory. *Science* 50:971–979.

Merzenich, M. M. 1987. Dynamic neocortical processes and the origins of higher brain functions. In *The neural and molecular bases of learning,* eds. J.-P. Changeux and M. Konishi, 337–358. New York: Wiley.

Merzenich, M. M., and Kaas, J. H. 1980. Principles of organization of sensory-perceptual systems in mammals. *Prog. Psychobiol.* 9:1–42.

Merzenich, M. M., Kaas, J. H., Wall, J. T., Nelson, R. J., Sur, M., and Felleman, D. J. 1983. Topographic representation of somatosensory cortical areas 3b and 1 in adult monkeys following restricted deafferentation. *Neuroscience* 8:33–55.

Meynerd, P., Simmers, J., and Moulins, M. 1991. Construction of a pattern-generating circuit with neurons of different networks. *Nature* 351:60–63.

Miall, R. C., Weir, D. J., and Stein, J. F. 1993a. Intermittency in human manual tracking tasks. *J. Motor Behav.* 25(1):53–63.

Miall, R. C., Weir, D. J., Wolpert, D. M., and Stein, J. F. 1993b. Is the cerebellum a Smith predictor? *J. Motor Behav.,* 25. 203–216.

Miall, R. C., and Wolpert, D. M. 1995. The cerebellum as a predictive model of the motor system: A Smith predictor hypothesis. In *Neural control of movement,* eds. W. R. Ferrell and U. Proske, 215–223. New York: Plenum Press.

Miettinen, R., Gulyás, A. I., Baimbridge, K. G., Jacobowitz, D. M., and Freund, T. F. 1992. Calretinin is present in pyramidal cells of the rat hippocampus: II. Coexistence with other calcium binding proteins and GABA. *Neuroscience* 48:29–43.

Miikkulainen, R., and Leow, W. K. 1995. Visual schemas in object recognition and schema analysis. In *The handbook of brain theory and neural networks,* ed. M. A. Arbib, 1029–1031. Cambridge, MA: Bradford Books/MIT Press.

Miller, K. D., Keller, J. B., and Stryker, M. P. 1989. Ocular dominance column development: Analysis and simulation. *Science* 245:605–615.

Miller, R. J. 1991. Metabotropic excitatory amino acid receptors reveal their true colors. *Trends Pharmacol. Sci.* 12:365–367.

Milner, A. D., and Goodale, M. A. 1995. *The visual brain in action.* London: Oxford University Press.

Milner, B. 1962. Les troubles de la memoire accompagnant des lesions hippocampiques bilaterales. In *Physiologie de hippocampe,* ed. P. Passquant, 257–272. Paris: C.N.R.S.

Minsky, M. 1985. *The society of mind.* New York: Simon and Schuster.

Minsky, M. L. 1961. Steps toward artificial intelligence. *Proc. I.R.E.* 49:8–30.

Minsky, M. L. 1965. Matter, mind and models. In *Information processing 1965. Proceedings of IFIP Congress '65*, Vol. 1, 45–59. Washington, DC: Spartan Books.

Minsky, M. L. 1975. A framework for representing knowledge. In *The psychology of computer vision*, ed. P. H. Winston, 211–277. New York: McGraw-Hill.

Mishkin, M. 1982. A memory system in the monkey. *Philos. Trans. R. Soc. Lond. [B]* 298:85–95.

Mishkin, M., Ungerleider, L. G., and Macko, K. A. 1983. Object vision and spatial vision: Two cortical pathways. *Trends Neurosci.* 6:414–417.

Mitchison, G. 1991. Neuronal branching patterns and the economy of cortical wiring. *Proc. R. Soc. Lond. [B]* 245:151–158.

Mitchison, G., and Durbin, R. 1986. Optimal numberings of an N × N array. *S.I.A.M. J. Alg. Disc. Math.* 7:571–581.

Mittelstaedt, M. L., and Mittelsdaedt, H. 1980. Homing by path integration in a mammal. *Naturwissenschaften* 67S:566.

Mitz, A. R., Godshalk, M., and Wise, S. P. 1991. Learning-dependent neuronal activity in the premotor cortex. Activity during the acquisition of conditional motor associations. *J. Neurosci.* 11(6):1855–1872.

Mizunori, S. J. Y., McNaughton, B. L., Barnes, C. A., and Fox, K. B. 1989. Preserved spatial coding in hippocampal CA1 pyramidal cells during reversible suppression of CA3 output: Evidence for pattern completion in hippocampus. *J. Neurosci.* 9:3915–3928.

Monaghan, D. T., and Cotman, C. W. 1985. Distribution of N-methyl-D-aspartate-sensitive L-[3H]glutamate-binding sites in rat brain. *J. Neurosci.* 5(11):2909–2919.

Montgomery, J. C., and Bodznick, D. 1994. An adaptive filter that cancels self-induced noise in the electrosensory and lateral line mechanosensory systems of fish. *Neurosci. Lett.* 174:145–148.

Moore, J. W., and Blazis, D. E. J. 1989. Stimulation of classically conditioned response: A cerebellar neural network implementation of the Sutton-Barto-Desmond model. In *Neural models of plasticity: Experimental and theoretical approaches*, eds. J. H. Byrne and W. O. Berry, 187–207. San Diego: Academic Press.

Moore, J. W., Desmond, J. E., and Berthier, N. E. 1989. Adaptively timed conditioned responses and the cerebellum: A neural network approach. *Biol. Cybern.* 62:17–28.

Moran, J., and Desimone, R. 1985. Selective attention gates visual processing in the extrastriate cortex. *Science* 229:782–784.

Morest, D. K. 1965. The laminar structure of the medial geniculate body of the cat. *J. Anat.* 99:143–160.

Morris, R. G., and Willshaw, O. J. 1989. Must what goes up come down? *Nature* 339:175–176.

Morris, R. G., Downes, J. J., Sahakian, B. J., Evenden, J. L. Heald, A., and Robbins, T. W. 1988. Planning and spatial working memory in Parkinson's disease. *J. Neurol. Neurosurg. Psychiatry* 51:757–766.

Morris, R. G. M. 1984. Developments of a water-maze procedure for studying spatial learning in the rat. *J. Neurosci. Methods* 11:47–60.

Morrison, R. S., and Bassett, D. L. 1945. Electrical activity of the thalamus and basal ganglia in decorticate cats. *J. Neurophysiol.* 8:309–314.

Moruzzi, G., and Magoun, H. W. 1949. Brainstem reticular formation and activation of the EEG. *Electroencephalogr. Clin. Neurophysiol.* 1:455–473.

Moss, F. 1994. Chaos under control. *Nature* 370:596–597.

Mountcastle, V. B. 1957. Modalities and typographic properties of single neurones of the cat's sensory cortex. *J. Neurophysiol.* 20:408–434.

Mountcastle, V. B., Lynch, J. C. G. A., Sakata, H., and Acuna, C. 1975. Posterior parietal association cortex of the monkey: Command functions for operations within extrapersonal space. *J. Neurophysiol.* 38:871–908.

Mpitsos, G. J., Burton, R. M., Creech, H. C., and Soinila, S. O. 1988. Evidence for chaos in spike trains of neurons that generate rhythmic motor patterns. *Brain Res. Bull.* 21:529–538.

Muakkassa, K. F., and Strick, P. L. 1979. Frontal lobe inputs to primate motor cortex: Evidence for four somatotopically organized "premotor" areas. *Brain Res.* 177:176–182.

Mugnaini, E. 1983. The length of cerebellar parallel fibers in chicken and rhesus monkey. *J. Comp. Neurol.* 220:7–15.

Muller, R. U., and Kubie, J. L. 1987. The effects of changes in the environment on the spatial firing of hippocampal complex spike cells. *J. Neurosci.* 7:1951–1968.

Muller, R. U., Kubie, J. L., Bostock, E. M., Taube, J. S., and Quirk, G. J. 1991. Spatial firing correlates of neurons in the hippocampal formation of freely moving rats. In *Brain and space*, ed. J. Paillard, 296–333. London: Oxford University Press.

Mumford, D. 1991. On the computational architecture of the neocortex: I. The role of the thalamo-cortical loop. *Biol. Cybern.* 65:135–145.

Mumford, D. 1992. On the computational architecture of the neocortex: II. The role of the cortico-cortical loops. *Biol. Cybern.* 6:241–251.

Mumford, D. 1995. Thalamus. In *The handbook of brain theory and neural networks*, ed. M. A. Arbib, 981–984. Cambridge, MA: Bradford Books/MIT Press.

Munoz, D. P., Pelisson, D., and Duhamel, G. 1991. Movement of neural activity on the superior colliculus motor map during gaze shifts. *Science* 251:1358–1360.

Murphy, J. T., MacKay, W. A., and Johnson, F. 1973a. Differences between cerebellar mossy and climbing fibre responses to natural stimulation of forelimb muscle proprioceptors. *Brain Res.* 55:263–289.

Murphy, J. T., MacKay, W. A., and Johnson, F. 1973b. Responses of cerebellar cortical neurons to dynamic proprioceptive input from forelimb muscles. *J. Neurophysiol.* 36:711–723.

Murphy, J. T., and Sabah, N. H. 1970. The inhibitory effect of climbing fiber activation on cerebellar Purkinje cells. *Brain Res.* 19:486–490.

Murphy, M. G., and O'Leary, M. 1971. Neurological deficits in cats with lesions of olivocerebellar system. *Arch. Neurol.* 24:145.

Murray, J. D. 1989. *Mathematical biology*. Heidelberg: Springer-Verlag.

Murthy, V. N., and Fetz, E. E. 1992. Coherent 25–35 Hz oscillations in the sensorimotor cortex of the awake behaving monkey. *Proc. Natl. Acad. Sci. U.S.A.* 89:5670–5674.

Mushiake, H., and Strick, P. L. 1995. Pallidal neuron activity during sequential arm movements. *J. Neurophysiol.* 74:2754–2758.

Nagao, S., and Ito, M. 1991. Subdural application of hemoglobin to the cerebellum blocks vestibuloocular reflex adaptation. *Neuroreport* 2:193–196.

Nagumo, J., Arimoto, S., and Yoshizawa, S. 1962. An active pulse transmission line simulating nerve axons. *Proc. I.R.E.* 50:2061–2070.

Narendra, K. S. 1995. Identification and control. In *The handbook of brain theory and neural networks*, ed. M. A. Arbib, 477–480. Cambridge, MA: Bradford Books/MIT Press.

Neisser, U. 1976. *Cognition and reality: Principles and implications of cognitive psychology.* San Francisco: W. H. Freeman.

Nelson, J. I. 1975. Globality and stereoscopic fusion in binocular vision. *J. Theor. Biol.* 49:1–88.

Newberry, N. R., and Nicoll, R. A. 1985. Comparison of the action of baclofen with aminobutyric acid on rat hippocampal pyramidal cells in vitro. *J. Physiol. (Lond.)* 360:161–185.

Newell, A. 1990. *Unified theories of cognition.* Cambridge, MA: Harvard University Press.

Nicolis, J. S. 1986. Chaotic dynamics applied to information processing. *Rep. Prog. Phys.* 49:1109–1196.

Nicoll, R., and Jahr, C. E. 1982. Self-excitation of olfactory bulb neurones. *Nature* 196:441–444.

Nicoll, R. A. 1994. Cajal's rational psychology. *Nature* 368:808–809.

Noda, H., Sugita, S., and Ikeda, Y. 1990. Afferent and efferent connections of the oculomotor region of the fastigial nucleus in the macaque monkey. *J. Comp. Neurol.* 302:330–348.

Nowycky, M. C., Mori, K., and Shepherd, G. M. 1981. GABAergic mechanisms of dendrodendritc synapses in isolated turtle olfactory bulb. *J. Neurophysiol.* 46:639–648.

Nunzi, M. G., Gorio, A., Milan, F., Freund, T. F., Somogyi, P., and Smith, A. D. 1985. Cholecystokinin immunoreactive cells form symmetrical synaptic contacts with pyramidal and non-pyramidal neurons in the hippocampus. *J. Comp. Neurol.* 237:485–505.

Obermayer, K., Blasdel, G. G., and Schulten, K. 1991. A neural network model for the formation and for the spatial structure of retinotopic maps, orientation and ocular dominance columns. In *Artifical neural networks. Vol. 1*, eds. T. Kohonas, K. Mäkisara, O. Simsla, and J. A. Kangar, 505–511. Amsterdam: Elsevier North-Holland.

Obermayer, K., Ritter, H., and Schulten, K. 1990. A principle for the formation of the spatial structure of cortical feature maps. *Proc. Natl. Acad. Sci. U.S.A.* 87:8345–8349.

Obermayer, K., Ritter, H., and Schulten, K. 1991. Development and spatial structue of cortical feature maps: A model study. In *Advances inneural information processing systems*, Vol. 3, eds. R. P. Lippmann, J. Moody, and D. S. Touretzky, 11–17. San Mateo, CA: Morgan Kaufmann.

Obermayer, K., Sejnowski, T., and Blasdel, G. G. 1995. Neural pattern formation via a competitive Hebbian mechanism. *Behav. Brain Res.* 66:151–160.

O'Dell, T. J., and Kandel, E. R. 1994. Low-frequency stimulation erases LTP through an NMDA receptor mediated activation of protein phosphatases. *Learning and Memory* 1:129–139.

Ogden, J. A. 1985. Autotopagnosia: Occurrence in a patient without nominal aphasia and an intact ability to point to parts of animals and objects. *Brain* 108:1009–1022.

O'Keefe, J. 1991. The hippocampal cognitive map and navigational strategies. In *Brain and space*, ed. J. Paillard, 273–295. New York: Oxford University Press.

O'Keefe, J., and Burgess, N. 1995. Geometric determinants of hippocampal place fields. *Soc. Neurosci. Abstr.* 21:944, Abstract 376.6.

O'Keefe, J., and Conway, D. H. 1978. Hippocampal place units in the freely moving rat: Why they fire when they fire. *Exp. Brain Res.* 31:573–590.

O'Keefe, J., and Conway, D. H. 1980. On the trail of the hippocampal engram. *Physiol. Psychol.* 8:229–238.

O'Keefe, J., Conway, D. H., and Schenk, F. 1983, manuscript submitted. Learning and memory in a cue controlled environment: The effects of spatial configuration of the cues, delay interval, and damage to the hippocampal system.

O'Keefe, J., and Dostrovsky, J. 1971. The hippocampus as a spatial map. Preliminary evidence from unit activity in the freely-moving rat. *Brain Res.* 34:171–175.

O'Keefe, J., and Nadel, L. 1978. *The hippocampus as a cognitive map.* Oxford: Clarendon Press.

O'Keefe, J., and Recce, M. 1993. Phase relationship between hippocampal place units and the EEG theta rhythm. *Hippocampus* 3:317–330.

Oldfield, R. C., and Zangwill, O. L. 1942–1943. Head's concept of the body schema and its application in contemporary British psychology. *Br. J. Psychol.* 32:267–286; 33:58–64ff.

Olton, D. S. 1979. Mazes, maps and memory. *Am. Psychol.* 34:588–596.

Olton, D. S., Becker, J. T., and Handelmann, G. E. 1979. Hippocampus, space and memory. *Behav. Brain Sci.* 2:313–365.

Olton, D. S., and Samuelson, R. J. 1976. Remembrance of places passed: Spatial memory in rats. *J. Exp. Psychol. Anim. Behav. Proc.* 2:97–116.

Ono, T., Nakamura, K., Fukuda, M., and Tamura, R. 1991. Place recognition responses of neurons in monkey hippocampus. *Neurosci. Lett.* 121:194–198.

Onsager, L. 1944. Crystal statistics I. A two-dimensional model with an order-disorder transition. *Phys. Rev.* 65:117–149.

Optican, L. 1982. Saccadic dysmetria. In *Functional basis of ocular mobility disorders*, eds. G. Lennerstrand, D. Zee, and E. Keller, 441–451. Oxford: Pergamon Press.

Orlovskii, G. N. 1970. Influence of the cerebellum on the reticulo-spinal neurons during locomotion. *Biophysics* 15:928–936.

Orlovskii, G. N. 1972a. Activity of vestibulospinal neurons during locomotion. *Brain Res.* 46:85–98.

Orlovskii, G. N. 1972b. The effect of different descending systems on flexor and extensor activity during locomotion. *Brain Res.* 40:359–371.

Oscarsson, O. 1969. The sagittal organization of the cerebellar anterior lobe as revealed by projection patterns of the climbing fiber system. In *Neurobiology of cerebellar evolution and development*, ed. R. Llinás, 525–537. Chicago: American Medical Association.

Oscarsson, O. 1973. Functional organization of spinocerebellar paths. In *Handbook of sensory physiology: Vol. 2, Somatosensory system*, ed. A. Iggo, 339–380. Berlin: Springer-Verlag.

Ott, E., Greborgi, C., and Yorke, J. A. 1990. Controlling chaos. *Physiol. Rev. Lett.* 64:1196–1199.

Otto, T., Eichenbaum, H., Wiener, S. I., and Wible, C. G. 1991. Learning-related patterns of CA1 spike trains parallel stimulation parameters optimal for inducing hippocampal long-term potentiation. *Hippocampus* 1:181–192.

Ottoson, D. 1959. Studies of slow potentials in the rabbit's olfactory bulb and nasal mucosa. *Acta. Physiol. Scand.* 47:136–148.

Overton, K. J., and Arbib, M. A. 1982a. System matching and topographic maps: The branch-arrow model (BAM). In *Competition and cooperation in neural nets. Vol. 45, Lecture notes in biomathematics*, eds. S. Amari and M. A. Arbib, 202–225. Berlin: Springer-Verlag.

Overton, K. J., and Arbib, M. A. 1982b. The extended branch-arrow model of the formation of retino-tectal connections. *Biol. Cybern.* 45: 157–175.

Paillard, J. 1991. Knowing where and knowing how to get there. In *Brain and space*, ed. J. Paillard, 461–481. London: Oxford University Press.

Palkovits, M., Magyar, P., and Szentágothai, J. 1971a. Quantitative histological analysis of the cerebellar cortex in the cat: I. Number and arrangement in space of the Purkinje cells. *Brain Res.* 32:1–13.

Palkovits, M., Magyar, P., and Szentágothai, J. 1971b. Quantitative histological analysis of the cerebellar cortex in the cat: II. Cell numbers and densities in the granular layer. *Brain Res.* 32:15–30.

Palkovits, M., Magyar, P., and Szentágothai, J. 1971c. Quantitative histological analysis of the cerebellar cortex in the cat: III. Structural organization of the molecular layer. *Brain Res.* 34:1–18.

Palkovits, M., Mezey, É., Hámori, J., and Szentágothai, J. 1977. Quantitative histological analysis of the cerebellar cortex in the cat: I. Numerical data on cells and on synapses. *Exp. Brain Res.* 28:189–209.

Palm, G. 1982. Rules for synaptic changes and their relevance for the storage of information in the brain. In *Cybernetics and system research*, ed. R. Trappl, 277–280. Amsterdam: Elsevier North-Holland.

Palm, G., and Braitenberg, V. 1979. Tentative contributions of neuroanatomy to nerve net theories. In *Progress in cybernetics and system research*, eds. R. Trappl, G. J. Klir, and L. Ricciardi, 211–228. New York: Wiley.

Pascualleone, A., Wassermann, E. M., Grafman, J., and Hallet, M., 1996. The role of the dorsolateral prefrontal cortex in implicit procedural learning. *Exp. Brain Res.* 107:479–485.

Pasik, P., Pasik, T., and Hámori, J. 1976. Synapses between interneurons in the lateral geniculate nuclei of the monkey. *Exp. Brain Res.* 25:1–13.

Pasik, P., Pasik, T., Hámori, J., and Szentágothai, J. 1973a. Dendrites with synaptic vesicles of Golgi type II neurons in the lateral geniculate nuclei of the monkey. *Trans. Am. Neurol. Assoc.* 97:331–334.

Pasik, P., Pasik, T., Hámori, J., and Szentágothai, J. 1973b. Golgi II type interneurons in the neuronal circuit of the monkey lateral geniculate nucleus. *Exp. Brain Res.* 17:18–34.

Paulignan, Y., Jeannerod, M., MacKenzie, C., and Marteniuk, R. 1991a. Selective perturbation of visual input during prehension movements: 2. The effects of changing object size. *Exp. Brain Res.* 87:407–420.

Paulignan, Y., MacKenzie, C., Marteniuk, R., and Jeannerod, M. 1991b. Selective perturbation of visual input during prehension movements: 1. The effects of changing object position. *Exp. Brain Res.* 83:502–512.

Paulin, M. G. 1989. A Kalman filter theory of the cerebellum. In *Dynamic interactions in neural networks: Models and data*, eds. M. A. Arbib and S. I. Amari, 239–259. New York: Springer-Verlag.

Paulin, M. G. 1993. The role of the cerebellum in motor control and perception. *Brain Behav. Evol.* 41:39–50.

Pavlides, C., Greenstein, Y. J., Grudman, M., and Winston, J. 1988. Long-term potentiation in the dentate gyrus is induced preferentially on the positive phase of the theta rhythm. *Brain Res.* 439:383–387.

Pavlides, C., and Winson, J. 1989. Influences of hippocampal place cell firing in the awake state on the activity of these cells during subsequent sleep episodes. *J. Neurosci.* 9:2907–2918.

Pearce, R. A. 1993. Physiological evidence for two distinct GABA responses in rat hippocampus. *Neuron* 10:189–200.

Penfield, W., and Roberts, L. 1959. *Speech and brain mechanisms.* Princeton: Princeton University Press.

Perenin, M. T., and Vighetto, A. 1988. Optic ataxia: A specific disruption in visuomotor mechanisms: I. Different aspects of the deficit in reaching for objects. *Brain* 111:643–674.

Peretto, P. 1984. Collective properties of neural networks: A statistical physics approach. *Biol. Cybern.* 50:51–62.

Peretto, P. 1992. *An introduction to the modeling of neural networks.* London: Cambridge University Press.

Perrett, D. I., Mistlin, A. J., and Chitty, A. J. 1987. Visual neurones responsive to faces. *Trends Neurosci.* 10:358–364.

Peters, A., and Sethares, C. 1991. Layer IVA of Rhesus monkey primary visual cortex. *Cereb. Cortex* 1:445–462.

Petsche, H., Stumpf, C., and Gogolak, G. 1962. Significance of the rabbit's septum as a relay station between the midbrain and the hippocampus: I. The control of hippocampus arousal activity by septum cells. *Electroencephalogr. Clin. Neurophysiol.* 14:202–211.

Piaget, J. 1971. *Biology and knowledge.* Ediburgh: Edinburgh University Press.

Pinker, S., and Bloom, P. 1990. Natural language and natural selection. *Behav. Brain Sci.* 13:707–784.

Pinsky, P. F., and Rinzel, J. 1994. Intrinsic and network rhythmogenesis in a reduced Traub model for CA3 neurons. *J. Comput. Neurosci.* 1:39–60.

Pitler, T. A., and Alger, B. E. 1992. Cholinergic excitation of GABAergic interneurons in the rat hippocampal slice. *J. Physiol.* 450:127–142.

Pitler, T. A., and Alger, B. E. 1994. Differences between presynaptic and postsynaptic GABA mechanisms in rat hippocampal pyramidal cells. *J. Comp. Neurol.* 72:2317–2327.

Pitts, W. H., and McCulloch, W. S. 1947. How we know universals: The perception of auditory and visual forms. *Bull. Math. Biophy.* 9: 127–147.

Plaitakis, A., ed. 1992. *Cerebellar degeneration: Clinical neurobiology.* Norwell, MA: Kluwer.

Plaut, D. C., and Shallice, T. 1993. Deep dyslexia: A case study of connectionist neuropsychology. *Cogn. Neuropsychol.* 10:377–500.

Pongrácz, F., Poolos, N. P., Kocsis, J. D., and Shepherd, G. M. 1992. A model of NMDA receptor mediated activity in dendrites of hippocampal CA1 pyramidal neurons. *J. Neurophysiol.* 68:2248–2259.

Popper, K. R., and Eccles, J. C. 1977. *The self and its brain.* Berlin: Springer-Verlag.

Pouget, A., and Sejnowski, T. J. 1995. Dynamic remapping. In *The handbook of brain theory and neural networks,* ed. M. A. Arbib, 335–338. Cambridge, MA: Bradford Books/MIT Press.

Preissl, M. Aertsen, A., and Palm, G. 1990. Are fractal dimensions a good measure for neural activity? In *Parallel processing in neural systems and computers,* eds. R. Eckmiller, G. Harman, and G. Hauske, 83–86. Amsterdam: Elsevier North-Holland.

Price, J. L., Carmichael, S. T., Carnes, K. M., Clugnet, M.-C., Kuroda, M., and Ray, J. P. 1991. Olfactory input to the prefrontal cortex. In *Olfaction: A model system for computational neuroscience,* eds. J. L. Davis and H. Eichenbaum, 101–120. Cambridge, MA: MIT Press.

Pryer, W. 1885. *Die spezielle Physiologie des Embryos.* Leipzig: Griebens Verlag.

Purpura, D. P. 1970. Operations and processes in thalamic and synaptically related neural subsystems. In *The neurosciences: Second study program,* ed. F. O. Schmitt, 458–470. New York: Rockefeller University Press.

Purves, D., Riddle, D. R., and La Mantia, A. S. 1992. Iterated patterns of brain circuitry (or how the cortex gets its spots). *Trends Neurosci.* 15:362–368.

Pyragas, K. 1992. Continuous control of chaos by self-controlling feedback. *Phys. Lett.* 170A:421–428.

Pyragas, K., and Tamasevicius, A. 1993. Experimental control of chaos by delayed self-controlling feedback. *Phys. Lett.* 180A:99–102.

Quillian, M. R. 1968. Semantic memory. In *Semantic information processing,* ed. M. L. Minsky, 216–270. Cambridge, MA: MIT Press.

Rager, G. 1983. Structural analysis of fiber organization during development. *Prog. Brain Res.* 85:313–319.

Rajesekar, S., and Lakshmanan, M. 1994. Bifurcation, chaos and suppression of chaos in FitzHugh-Nagumo nerve conduction model equation. *J. Theor. Biol.* 166:275–288.

Rakic, P. 1971. Neuron-glial relationship during granule cell migration in developing cerebellar cortex. A Golgi and electron microscopic study in macacus rhesus. *J. Comp. Neurol.* 14:283–312.

Rakic, P. 1975. Local circuit neurons. *Neurosci. Res. Prog. Bull.* 13:245–446.

Rakic, P. 1981. Neuron-glial interaction during brain development. *Trends Neurosci.* 4:184–187.

Rakic, P. 1982. Development and modifiability of the cerebral cortex. *Neurosci. Res. Prog. Bull.* 20:439–454.

Rakic, P. 1988. Specification of cerebral cortical areas. *Science* 241:170–176.

Rall, W. 1962. Electrophysiology of a dendritic neuron model. *Biophys. J.* 2:145–167.

Rall, W. 1967. Distinguishing theoretical synaptic potentials computed for different soma-dendritic distribution of synaptic inputs. *J. Neurophysiol.* 30:1138–1168.

Rall, W. 1977. Core conductor theory and cable properties of neurons. In *Handbook of physiology: The nervous system,* eds. E. R. Kandel, J. M. Brookhardt, and V. B. Mountcastle, 39–98. Baltimore: William & Wilkins.

Rall, W. 1989. Cable theory for dendritic neurons. In *Methods in neuronal modeling,* 9–62. Cambridge, MA: MIT Press.

Rall, W. 1995. Perspective on neuron model complexity. In *The handbook of brain theory and neural networks,* ed. M. A. Arbib, 728–732. Cambridge, MA: Bradford Books/MIT Press.

Rall, W., and Shepherd, G. 1968. Theoretical representation of field potentials and dendro-dendritic synaptic interaction in olfactory bulb. *J. Neurophysiol.* 31:884–915.

Ramón y Cajal, S. 1888. Estructura de los centros nerviosos de las aves. *Rev. Trimest. Histol. Norm. Pat.*

Ramón y Cajal, S. 1893. Estructura del asta de Ammon y fascia dentata. *Ann. Soc. Esp. Hist. Nat.* 22.

Ramón y Cajal, S. 1894. Les nouvelles idees sur la structure du Systeme nerveux chez l'homme et les vertebres. Paris: C. Reinwald et Cie.

Ramón y Cajal, S. 1899. Estudio sobra la corteza cerebral humana. *Rev. Trimest. Microscopia* 4:1–63.

Ramón y Cajal, S. 1909. *Histologie du systeme nerveux de l'homme et des vertebres,* Vol. 1. Paris: A. Maloine.

Ramón y Cajal, S. 1911. *Histologie du systeme nerveux.* Paris: A. Maloine.

Ramón-Moliner, E., and Nauta, W. J. H. 1966. The isodendritic core of the brainstem. *J. Comp. Neurol.* 126:311–335.

Ranck, J. B., Jr. 1973. Studies on single neurons in dorsal hippocampal formation and septum in unrestrained rats: I. Behavioral correlates and firing repertoires. *Exp. Neurol.* 41:461–535.

Rapp, P. E. 1994. A guide to dynamical analysis. *Integr. Physiol. Behav. Sci.* 29:311–327.

Rapp, P. E., Zimmerman, I. D., Albano, A. M., deGuzman, G. C., and Greenbaum, N. N. 1985. Dynamics of spontaneous neural activity in the simian motor cortex: The dimension of chaotic neurons. *Phys. Lett.* 110A:335–338.

Ratcliff, G., and Davies-Jones, G. A. B. 1972. Defective visual localization in focal brain wounds. 95:49–60.

Ratcliff, G., and Newcombe, F. 1973. Spatial orientation in man: Effects of left, right, and bilateral posterior cerebral lesions. *J. Neurol. Neurosurg. Psychiatry* 36:448–454.

Rensing, L., an der Heiden, U., and Mackey, M. C. 1987. *Temporal disorder in human oscillatory systems.* Berlin: Springer-Verlag.

Rescorla, R. A., and Wagner, A. R. 1972. A theory of Pavlovian conditioning: Variations in the effectiveness of reinforcement and non-reinforcement. In *Classical conditioning II*, eds. A. Black and W. Prokasy, 64–99. New York: Appleton-Century-Crofts.

Réthelyi, M. 1976. Central core in the spinal gray matter. *Acta Morph. Acad. Sci. Hung.* 24:64–70.

Réthelyi, M. 1977. Preterminal and terminal axon arborizations in the substantia gelatinosa of cat's spinal cord. *J. Comp. Neurol.* 172:511–528.

Réthelyi, M., and Szentágothai, J. 1969. The large synaptic complexes of the substantia gelatinosa. *Exp. Brain Res.* 258–274.

Retzius, G. 1891. Zur Kenntnis des Ependymiellen der Zentral organe. *Verhandl. Biol. Vereins.*

Rexed, B. 1954. A citoarchitectonic atlas of the spinal cord in the cat. *J. Comp. Neurol.* 100:297–379.

Reyher, C. K. H., Luebke, J., Larsen, W. J., Hendrix, G. M., Shipley, M. T., and Baumgarten, H. G. 1991. Olfactory bulb granule cell aggregates: Morphological evidence for interperikaryal electrotonic coupling via gap junctions. *J. Neurosci.* 11:1485–1495.

Ribak, C. E., Nitsch, R., and Seress, L. 1990. Proportion of parvalbumin-positive basket cells in the GABAergic innervation of pyramidal and granule cells of the rat hippocampal formation. *J. Comp. Neurol.* 271:67–78.

Ribak, C. E., Seress, L., and Amaral, D. G. 1985. The development, ultrastructure and synaptic connections of the mossy cells of the dentate gyrus. *J. Neurocytol.* 14:835–857.

Ricciardi, L. M. 1994. Diffusion models of single neurones' activity. In *Neural modeling and neural networks*, ed. F. Ventriglia, 129–162. Oxford: Pergamon Press.

Riedel, H., and Schild, D. 1992. The dynamics of Hebbian synapses can be stabilized by a nonlinear decay term. *Neural Networks* 5:454–463.

Rinzel, J. 1987. A formal classification of bursting mechanisms in excitable systems. In *Mathematical topics in population biology, morphogenesis and neurosciences: Vol. 71, Lecture notes in biomathematics*, eds. E. Teramoto and M. Yamaguti, 267–281. Berlin: Springer-Verlag.

Riseman, E. M., and Hanson, A. R. 1987. A methodology for the development of general knowledge-based vision systems. In *Vision, brain and cooperative computation*, eds. M. A. Arbib and A. R. Hanson, 285–328. Cambridge, MA: Bradford Books/MIT Press.

Risold, P. Y., and Swanson, L. S. 1996. Structural evidence for functional domains in the rat hippocampus. *Science* 272:1484–1486.

Risser, J. M., and Slotnick, B. M. 1987. Nipple attachment and survival in neonatal olfactory bulbectomized rats. *Physiol. Behav.* 40:545–550.

Ritchie, L. 1976. Effects of cerebellar lesions on saccadic eye movements. *J. Neurophysiol.* 39:1246–1256.

Ritter, H., and Schulten, K. 1986. On the stationary state of Kohonen's self-organizing sensory mapping. *Biol. Cybern.* 54:99–106.

Ritz, R., Gerstner, W., Fuentes, U, and van Hemmen, J. L. 1994. A biologically motivated and analytically soluble model of collective oscillation in the cortex. II. Application to binding and pattern segmentation. *Biol. Cybern.* 71:349–358.

Rizzolatti, G., Camarda, R., Fogassi, L., Gentilucci, M., Luppino, G., and Matelli, M. 1988. Functional organization of inferior area 6 in the macaque monkey: II. Area F5 and the control of distal movements. *Exp. Brain Res.* 71:491–507.

Rizzolatti, G., Fadiga, L., Gallese, V., and Fogassi, L. 1996. Premotor cortex and the recognition of motor actions. *Cog. Brain Res.* 3:131–141.

Rizzolatti, G., and Gentilucci, M. 1988. Motor and visual-motor functions of the premotor cortex. In *Neurobiology of neocortex*, eds. P. Rakic and W. Singer, 269–284. Chichester, UK: Wiley.

Rizzolatti, G., Gentilucci, M., and Matelli, M. 1985. Selective spatial attention: One center, one circuit, or many circuits? In *Attention and performance XI*, eds. M. I. Posner and O. S. M. Marin, 251–265. Hillsdale, NJ: Lawrence Erlbaum Associates.

Robins, T. W., Giardini, V., Jones, G. H., Reading, P. J., and Sahakian, B. J. 1990. Effects of dopamine depletion from the caudate-putamen and nucleus accumbens septi on the acquisition and performance of a conditional discrimination task. *Behav. Brain Res.* 38:243–261.

Robinson, D. A. 1964. The mechanics of human saccadic eye movement. *J. Physiol.* 174:245–264.

Robinson, D. A. 1972. Eye movement evoked by collicular stimulation in the alert monkey. *Vis. Res.* 12:1795–1808.

Robinson, D. A. 1975. Oculomotor control signals. In *Basic mechanisms of ocular motility and their clinical implications*, eds. G. Lennerstrand and P. Bach-y-Rita, 337–374. Oxford: Pergamon Press.

Robinson, D. A. 1981. The use of control systems analysis in the neurophysiology of eye movements. *Annu. Rev. Neurosci.* 4:463–503.

Rockland, K. S., and Lund, J. S. 1983. Intrinsic laminar lattice connections in primate visual cortex. *J. Comp. Neurol.* 216:303–318.

Roland, P. E. 1993. *Brain activation*. New York: Wiley-Liss.

Rolls, E. T. 1987. Information representation, processing, and storage in the brain: Analysis at the single neuron level. In *The neural and molecular bases of learning*, eds. J.-P. Changeux and M. Konishi, 503–540. New York: Wiley.

Rolls, E. T. 1994. Neurophysiology and cognitive functions of the striatum. *Rev. Neurol.* 150:648–660.

Roman, F. Staubli, U., and Lynch. G. 1987. Evidence for synaptic potentiation in a cortical network during learning. *Brain Res.* 418:221–226.

Romanes, G. J., ed. 1991. *Cunningham's textbook of anatomy*, 12th ed. London: Oxford University Press.

Rose, R. M., and Hindmarsh, J. L. 1985. A model of a thalamic neuron. *Prog. R. Soc. Lond. [B]* 225:161–193.

Rosen, R. 1981. Pattern generation in networks. *Prog. Theor. Biol.* 6:161–209.

Rosenblatt, F. 1962. *Principle of neurodynamics*. Washington, DC: Spartan Books.

Rössler, O. E. 1983. The chaotic hierarchy. *Z. Naturfursch.* 38a:788–801.

Rozin, P. 1976. The evolution of intelligence and access to the cognitive unconscious. *Prog. Psychobiol. Physiol. Psych.* 6:245–280.

Rumelhart, D. E., and McClelland, J. L., eds. 1986. *Parallel distributed processing: Explorations in the microstructure of cognition*. Cambridge, MA: Bradford Books/MIT Press.

Rumelhart, D. E., Smolensky, P., McClelland, J. L., and Hinton, G. E. 1986. Schemata and sequential thought processes in PDP models. In *Parallel distributed processing: Explorations in the microstructure of cogni-*

tion, Vol. 2, eds. J. L. McClelland and D. E. Rumelhart. Cambridge, MA: Bradford Books/MIT Press.

Rumelhart, D. E., and Zipser, D. 1986. Feature discovery by competitive learning. In *Parallel distributed processing: Explorations in the microstructure of cognition*, Vol. 1, eds. J. L. McClelland and D. E. Rumelhart. Cambridge, MA: Bradford Books/MIT Press.

Sakaguchi, H. 1988. Oscillatory and excitable behaviors in a population of model neurons. *Prog. Theor. Phys.* 79:1061–1068.

Sakata, H., Shibutani, H., Ito, Y., Tsurugai, K., Mine, S., and Kusunoki, M. 1994. Functional-properties of rotation sensitive neurons in the posterior parietal association cortex of the monkey. *Exp. Brain Res.* 101:183–202.

Sakata, H., Taira, M., Mine, S., and Murata, A. 1992. Hand-movement related neurons of the posterior parietal cortex of the monkey: Their role in visual guidance of hand movements. *Exp. Brain Res.* 22(suppl.): 185–198.

Sakmann, B., and Neher, E., eds. 1983. *Single-channel recording*. New York: Plenum Press.

Schank, R., and Abelson, R. 1977. *Scripts, plans, goals and understanding: An inquiry into human knowledge structures*. Hillsdale, NJ: Lawrence Erlbaum Associates.

Schechter, B. 1996. How the brain gets rhythm. *Science* 274:339–340.

Scheibel, M. E., and Scheibel, A. B. 1958. Structural substrates for integrative patterns in the brain stem reticular core. In *Reticular formation of the brain*, eds. H. H. Jasper, L. P. Proctor, R. S. Knighton, W. C. Noskay, and R. T. Costello, 31–68. Boston, MA: Little, Brown.

Scheibel, M. E., and Scheibel, A. B. 1970. Elementary processes in selected thalamic and cortical subsystem—the structural substrates. In *The neurosciences: Second study program*, ed. F. O. Schmitt, 443–457. New York: Rockefeller University Press.

Schiff, S. J., Jerger, K., Duong, D. H., Chang, T., Spano, J. L., and Ditto, W. L. 1994. Controlling chaos in the brain. *Nature* 370:615–620.

Schillen, T. B., and König, P. 1991. Stimulus-dependent assembly formation of oscillatory responses: II. Desynchronization. *Neural Comput.* 3:167–178.

Schmidt, R. A. 1975. A schema theory of discrete motor skill learning. *Psychol. Rev.* 82:225–260.

Schmidt, R. A. 1976. The schema as a solution to some persistent problems in motor learning theory. In *Motor control: Issues and trends*, ed. G. E. Stelmach, 41–65. New York: Academic Press.

Schmidt, R. A., Zelaznik, H. N., and Frank, J. S. 1977. Motor output variability: An alternative interpretation of Fitts' law. In *Big 10 Symposium on Information Processing in Motor Learning and Control*, University of Wisconsin at Madison.

Schmitt, F. O., Dev, P., and Smith, B. 1976. Electronic processing of information by brain cells. *Science* 193:114–120.

Schöner, G., Jiang, W., and Kelso, J. A. S. 1990. A synergetic theory of quadrupedal gaits and gait transitions. *J. Theor. Biol.* 142:359–393.

Schultz, W., Apicella, P., and Ljungberg, T. 1993. Responses of monkey dopamine neurons to reward and conditioned stimuli during successive steps of learning a delayed response task. *J. Neurosci.* 13(3):900–913.

Schultz, W., Ljungberg, T., Apicella, P., Romo, R., Mirenowicz, J., and Hollerman, J. R. 1993. Primate dopamine neurons: From movement to motivation and back. In *Role of the cerebellum and basal ganglia in voluntary movement*, eds. N. Mano et al., 89–97. Amsterdam: Elsevier Science.

Schultz, W., and Romo, R. 1992. Role of primate basal ganglia and frontal cortex in the internal generation of movements: 1. Preparatory activity in the anterior striatum. *Exp. Brain Res.* 91(3):363–384.

Schuster, H. G. 1984. *Deterministic chaos*. Weinheim: Physik Verlag.

Schuster, H. G., and Wagner, P. 1990a. A model for neuronal oscillations in the visual cortex: I. Mean-field theory and derivation of the phase equations. *Biol. Cybern.* 64:77–82.

Schuster, H. G., and Wagner, P. 1990b. A model for neuronal oscillations in the visual cortex; II. Phase description of the feature dependent synchronization. *Biol. Cybern.* 64:83–85.

Schuster, P., and Sigmund, K. 1983. Replicator dynamics. *J. Theor. Biol.* 100:333–338.

Schwartz, A. B. 1987. Responses of interposed and dentate neurons to perturbations of the locomotor cycle. *Exp. Brain Res.* 67:323–338.

Schwartz, E. L. 1977. Afferent geometry in the primate visual cortex and the generation of neuronal trigger features. *Biol. Cybern.* 25:181–194.

Schwartz, E. L. 1980. Computational anatomy and functional architecture of striate cortex: A spatial mapping approach to perceptual coding. *Vis. Res.* 20:645–669.

Schweighofer, N., Arbib, M. A., and Dominey, P. F. 1996a. A model of adaptive control of saccades: I. The model and its biological stustrate. *Biol. Cybern.* 75:19–28.

Schweighofer, N., Arbib, M. A., and Dominey, P. F. 1996b. A model of adaptive control of saccades: II. Simulation results. *Biol. Cybern.* 75:29–36.

Schweighofer, N., Arbib, M. A., and Thach, W. T. 1994. Modeling the role of cerebellum in prism adaptation. In *From animals to animats 3*, eds. S. Wilson, J.-A. Meyer, and D. Cliff. Cambridge, MA: Bradford Books/MIT Press.

Schweighofer, N., Spoelstra, J., Arbib, M. A., and Kawato, M. 1997. Role of the cerebellum in reaching quickly and accurately: II. A detailed model of the intermediate cerebellum, *European J. Neurosci.*, in press.

Scott, J. W., and Harrison, T. A. 1987. The olfactory bulb: Anatomy and physiology. In *Neurobiology of taste and smell*, eds. T. E. Finger and W. L. Silver, 151–178. New York: Wiley.

Scoville, W. B., and Milner, B. 1957. Loss of recent memory after bilateral hippocampal lesions. *J. Neurol. Neurosurg. Psychiatry* 20:11–21.

Scudder, C. A. 1988. A new local feedback model of the saccadic burst generator. *J. Neurophysiol.* 59:1455–1475.

Sechenov. 1965. *Reflexes of the brain*. English translation by S. Belsky. Cambridge, MA: MIT Press.

Segraves, M., and Goldberg, M. E. 1987. Functional properties of corticotectal neurons in the monkey's frontal eye field. *J. Neurophysiol.* 58:1387–1419.

Seitz, R. J., and Roland, P. E. 1992. Learning of sequential finger movements in man: A combined kinematic and positron emission tomography study. *Eur. J. Neurosci.* 4:154–165.

Sejnowski, T. J. 1977. Storing covariance with nonlinearly interacting neurons. *J. Math. Biol.* 4:303–321.

Sejnowski, T. J., and Tesauro, G. 1990. Building network learning algorithms for Hebbian synapses. In *Brain organization and memory cells, systems, and circuit*, eds. N. M. McGaugh, N. M. Weinberger, and G. Lynch, 338–355. New York: Oxford University Press.

Selemon, L. D., and Goldman-Rakic, P. S. 1985. Longitudinal topography and interdigitation of corticostriatal projections in the rhesus monkey. *J. Neurosci.* 5:776–794.

Self, D. W., and Nestler, E. J. 1995. Molecular mechanisms of drug reinforcement and addiction. *Annu. Rev. Neurosci.* 18:463–495.

Selverston, A. I., and Moulins, M. 1987. *The crustacean stomatogastric system.* Berlin: Springer-Verlag.

Sepulchre, J. A., and Babloyantz, A. 1993. Controlling chaos in a network of oscillators. *Physiol. Rev.* 48:945–950.

Serafin, M., Khateb, A., Dewale, C., Vidal, P. P., and Mahletha, M. 1992. Medial vestibular nucleus in guinea-pig NMDA-induced oscillations. *Exp. Brain Res.* 88:187–192.

Serra, R., and Zanarini, G. 1990. *Complex systems and cognitive processes.* Berlin: Springer-Verlag.

Shallice, T. 1988. *From neuropsychology to mental structure.* London: Cambridge University Press.

Shannon, C. E., and McCarthy, J., eds. 1956. *Automata studies.* Princeton: Princeton University Press.

Sharp, P. E. 1991. Computer simulation of hippocampal place cells. *Psychobiology* 19:103–115.

Shatz, C. J. 1990. Impulse activity and the patterning of connections during CNS development. *Neuron* 5:745–756.

Shatz, C. J., Lindstrom, S., and Wiesel, T. N. 1977. The distribution of afferents representing the right and left eyes in the cat's visual cortex. *Brain Res.* 131:103–116.

Shepherd, G. M. 1991. Computational structure of the olfactory system. In *Olfaction: A model system for computational neuroscience*, eds. J. L. Davis and H. Eichenbaum, 3–41. Cambridge, MA: MIT Press.

Sherman, M., and Koch, C. 1986. The control of retinogeniculate transmission in the mammalian LGN. *Exp. Brain Res.* 63:1–20.

Sherrington, C. S. 1906. *The integrative action of the nervous system.* New Haven: Yale University Press.

Sherrington, C. S. 1910. Flexion-reflex of the limb, crossed extension-reflex, and reflex stepping and standing. *J. Physiol. (Lond.)* 40:28–121.

Shik, M. L., Severin, F. V., and Orlovskii, G. N. 1966. Control of walking and running by means of electrical stimulation of the mid-brain. *Biophysics* 11:756–765.

Shik, M. L., Severin, F. V., and Orlovsky, G. N. 1967. Structures of the brain stem responsible for evoked locomotion. *Fiziol. Zh. SSSR.* 12:660–668.

Shinbrot, T., Greborgi, C., Ott, E., and Yorke, J. A. 1993. Using small perturbations to control chaos. *Nature* 363:411–417.

Shofer, R. J., Pappas, G. D., and Purpura, D. P. 1964. Radiation induced changes in morphological and physiological properties of immature cerebellar cortex. In *Response of the nervous systems to ionizing radiation*, eds. J. J. Hayley and R. Ader, 201–223. Boston: Little, Brown.

Sidman, R. L. 1970. Cell proliferation, migration, and interaction in the developing mammalian central nervous system. In *The neurosciences: Second study program*, ed. F. O. Schmitt, 100–107. New York: Rockefeller University Press.

Sik, A., Penttonen, M., Ylinen, A., and Buzsaki, G. 1995. Hippocampal CA1 interneurons: An in vivo intracellular labeling study. *J. Neurosci.* 15:6651–6665.

Sík, A., Tamamaki, N., and Freund, T. F. 1993. Complete axon arborization of a single CA3 pyramidal cell in the rat hippocampus, and its relationship with postsynaptic parvalbumin-containing interneurons. *Eur. J. Neurosci.* 5:1719–1728.

Singer, W. 1990. Search for coherence: A basic principle of cortical self-organization. *Concepts Neurosci.* 1:1–26.

Skarda, C. A., and Freeman, W. J. 1987. How brains make chaos in order to make sense of the world. *Behav. Brain. Sci.* 10:161–195.

Skinner, B. F. 1971. *Beyond freedom and dignity.* New York: Knopf.

Slotnick, B. M., and Katz, H. M. 1974. Olfactory learning-set formation in rats. *Science* 185:796–798.

Smart, J. C. 1981. Physicalism and emergence. *Neuroscience* 6:109–113.

Smith, O. J. M. 1959. A controller to overcome dead time. *I.S.A. J.* 6:28–33.

Smythe, J. W., Colom, L. V., and Bland, B. H. 1992. The extrinsic modulation of hippocampal data depends on the coactivation of cholinergic and GABAergic medial septal inputs. *Neurosci. Biobehav. Rev.* 16:289–308.

Snider, R. S., and Eldred, E. 1952. Cerebro-cerebellar relationships in the monkey. *J. Neurophysiol.* 15:27–40.

Snider, R. S., and Stowell, A. 1944. Receiving areas of the tactile, auditory, and visual systems in the cerebellum. *J. Neurophysiol.* 7:331–357.

Sodickson, D. L., and Bean, B. P. 1996. GABA-B receptor activated inwardly rectifying potassium current in dissociated hippocampal CA3 neurons. *J. Neurosci.* 16:637–646.

Soemmering, S. T. 1788. *Vom Hirn und Rückenmark.* Mainz.

Solomon, P. R., Vander Schaaf, E. R., Thompson, R. F., and Weisz, D. J. 1986. Hippocampus and trace conditioning of the rabbit's classically conditioned nictitating membrane response. *Behav. Neurosci.* 100:729–744.

Soltesz, I., Lightowler, S., Leresche, N., Jassik-Gerschenfeld, O., Pollard, C. E., and Crunelli, V. 1991. Two inward currents and the transformation of low frequency oscillations of rat and cat thalamocortical cells. *J. Physiol. (Lond.)* 441:175–197.

Somogyi, G., Hajdú, F., and Tömböl, T. 1978. Ultrastructure of the anterior ventral and anterior medial nuclei of the cat thalamus. *Exp. Brain Res.* 31:417–431.

Somogyi, P. 1977. A specific axonal interneuron in the visual cortex of the rat. *Brain Res.* 136:345–350.

Somogyi, P. 1978. The study of Golgi stained cells and of experimental degeneration under the electron microscope. *Neuroscience* 3:167–180.

Somogyi, P. 1991. Molecular neuroanatomy of synapses, cells and systems in the brain. In *Neurocytochemical methods*, NATO ASI Series, Vol. H58, eds. A. Lalas and D. Eugene, 117–135. Heidelberg: Springer-Verlag.

Somogyi, P., and Cowey, A. 1981. Combined Golgi and electron microscopic study on the synapses formed by double bouquet cells in the visual cortex of cat and monkey. *J. Comp. Neurol.* 195:547–566.

Somogyi, P., Cowey, A., Kisvarday, Z., Freund, T. F., and Szentágothai, J. 1982. Retrograde transport of gamma-amino [³H] butyric acid reveals specific interlaminar connections in the striate cortex of monkey. *Proc. Natl. Acad. Sci. U.S.A.* 80:2385–2398.

Somogyi, P., Hodgson, A. J., and Smith, A. D. 1979. An approach to tracing neuron networks in the cerebral cortex and basal ganglia. Combination of Golgi staining, retrograde transport horseradish peroxidase and anterograde degeneration of synaptic boutons in the same material. *Neuroscience* 4:1805–1852.

Somogyi, P., Kisvarday, Z. F., Matin, K. A. C., and Whitteridge, D. 1983a. Synaptic connections of morphologically identified and physiologically characterised large basket cells in the striate cortex of the cat. *Neuroscience* 10:261–294.

Somogyi, P., Nunzi, M. G., Gorio, A., and Smith, A. D. 1983b. A new type of specific interneuron in the monkey hippocampus forming synapses exclusively with the axonal initial segment of pyramidal neurons. *J. Neurosci.* 3:1450–1468.

Sompolinsky, H., Crisanti, A., and Sommers, H. J. 1988. Chaos in random neural networks. *Physiol. Rev. Lett.* 63:259–262.

Soong, A. C. K., and Stuart, C. I. J. M. 1989. Evidence of chaotic dynamics underlying the human alpha-rhythm electro-encephalogram. *Biol. Cybern.* 62:55–62.

Sparks, D. L., and Jay, M. F. 1985. The functional organization of the primate superior colliculus: A motor perspective. *Prog. Brain Res.* 64:235–242.

Sparks, D. L., and Mays, L. E. 1980. Movement fields of saccade-related burst neurons in the monkey superior colliculus. *Brain Res.* 190:39–50.

Speakman, and O'Keefe. 1990.

Sperry, R. W. 1943a. Visuomotor coordination in the newt *(Triturus viridescens)* after regeneration of the optic nerve. *J. Comp. Neurol.* 79:33–55.

Sperry, R. W. 1943b. Effect of 180 degree rotation of the retinal field of visuomotor coordination. *J. Exp. Zool.* 92:263–279.

Spillman, L., and Werner, J. S., eds. 1990. *Visual perception: The neurophysiological foundations.* San Diego: Academic Press.

Sporns, O., Gally, J. A., Reeke, G. N., and Edelman, G. M. 1989. Reentrant signaling among simulated neuronal groups leads to coherency in their oscillatory activity. *Proc. Natl. Acad. Sci. U.S.A.* 86:7265–7269.

Sporns, O., Tononi, G., and Edelman, G. M. 1991. Modeling perceptual grouping and figure-ground segregation of means of active reentrant connections. *Proc. Natl. Acad. Sci. U.S.A.* 88:129–133.

Squire, L. R. 1986. Mechanisms of memory. *Science* 232:1612–1619.

Squire, L. R., Cohen, N. J., and Zouzounis, J. A. 1984. Preserved memory in retrograde amnesia. *Neuropsychologia* 22:145–152.

Squire, L. R., Slater, P. C., and Chace, P. M. 1975. Retrograde amnesia: Temporal gradient in very long-term memory following electroconculsive therapy. *Science* 187:77–79.

Stanton, G. B., Goldberg, M. E., and Bruce, C. J. 1988a. Frontal eye field efferents in the macaque monkey: I. Subcortical pathways and topography of striatal and thalamic terminal fields. *J. Comp. Neurol.* 271:473–492.

Stanton, P. K., and Sejnowski, T. J. 1989. Associative long-term depression in the hippocampus induced by Hebbian covariance. *Nature* 339:215–218.

Staubli, U., Fraser, D., Faraday, R., and Lynch, G. 1987. Olfaction and the "data" memory systems in rats. *Behav. Neurosci.* 101:757–765.

Staubli, U., and Lynch, G. 1987. Stable hippocampal long-term potentiation elicited by theta pattern stimulation. *Brain Res.* 45:227–234.

Staubli, U., and Lynch. G. 1990. Stable depression of potentiated synaptic responses in the hippocampus with 1–5 Hz stimulation. *Brain Res.* 53:113–118.

Stein, B. E., and Meredith, M. A. 1993. *The merging of the senses.* Cambridge, MA: MIT Press.

Steinbuch, K. 1961. Die Lernmatrix. *Kybernetik* 1:36–45.

Stent, G. S. 1981. Strength and weakness of genetic approach to the development of the nervous system. *Annu. Rev. Neurosci.* 4:163–194.

Steriade, M., Contreras, D., Curr'Dossi, R., and Nunez, A. 1993. The slow (<1 Hz) oscillation in reticular thalamic and thalamocortical neurons: Scenario of sleep rhythm generation in interacting thalamic and neocortical networks. *J. Neurosci.* 13:3284–3299.

Steriade, M., and Deschenes, M. 1984. The thalamus as a neuronal oscillator. *Brain Res. Rev.* 8:1–63.

Steriade, M., Jones, E. G., and Llinás, R. R. 1990. *Thalamic oscillations and signalling.* New York: Wiley.

Steriade, M., and Llinás, R. R. 1988. The functional states of the thalamus and the associated neuronal interplay. *Physiol. Rev.* 68:649–742.

Steriade, M., McCormick, D. A., and Sejnowski, T. J. 1993. Thalamocortical oscillations in the sleeping and aroused brain. *Science* 262:679–685.

Steriade, M., Nunez, A., and Amzica, F. 1993a. A novel slow (<1 Hz) oscillation of neocortical neurons in vivo: Depolarizing and hyperpolarizing components. *J. Neurosci.* 13:3252–3265.

Steriade, M., Nunez, A., and Amzica, F. 1993b. Intracellular analysis of relations between the slow (<1 Hz) neocortical oscillations and other sleep rhythms of the electroencephalogram. *J. Neurosci.* 13:3266–3283.

Stevens, C. F. 1990. Neurobiology—a depression long awaited. *Nature* 347:16.

Steward, O. 1976. Topographical organization of the projection from entorhinal area to the hippocampal formation of the rat. *J. Comp. Neurol.* 167:285–314.

Stewart, M., and Fox, S. E. 1989. Two populations of rhythmically bursting neurons in rat medial septum are revealed by atropine. *J. Neurophysiol.* 61:982–993.

Strata, P. 1987. Inferior olive and motor control. In *Cerebellum and neuronal plasticity*, ed. M. Glickstein, 209–224. New York: Plenum Press.

Stryker, M. P., and Harris, W. A. 1986. Binocular impulse blockade prevents the formation of ocular dominance columns in cat visual cortex. *J. Neurosci.* 6:2117–2133.

Suga, N., and Kanwal, J. S. 1995. Echolocation: creating computational maps via parallel-hierarchical processing. In *The handbook of brain theory and neural networks*, ed. M. A. Arbib, 344–348. Cambridge, MA: Bradford Books/MIT Press.

Sutton, R. S., and Barto, A. G. 1981. Toward a modern theory of adaptive networks: Expectation and prediction. *Psychol. Rev.* 88:135–170.

Suzuki, S. S., and Smith, G. K. 1988. Spontaneous EEG spikes in the normal hippocampus: II. Relations to synchronous burst discharges. *Electroencephalogr. Clin. Neurophysiol.* 69:532–540.

Swanson, L. W., and Cowan, W. M. 1975. Hippocampo-hypothalamic connections: Origin in subicular cortex not Ammon's horn. *Science* 189: 303–304.

Swanson, L. W., and Cowan, W. M. 1977. An autoradiographic study of the organization of the efferent connections of the hippocampal formation in the rat. *J. Comp. Neurol.* 172:49–84.

Swanson, L. W., and Köhler, C. 1986. Anatomical evidence for direct projections from the entorhinal area to the entire cortical mantle in the rat. *J. Neurosci.* 6(10):3010–3023.

Swanson, L. W., Köhler, C., and Björklund, A. 1987. The limbic region: I. The septohippocampal system. In *Handbook of chemical neuroanatomy: Vol. 5, Integrated systems of the CNS, part I*, eds. A. Björklund, T. Hokfelt, and L. W. Swanson. New York: Elsevier.

Swanson, L. W., Sawchenko, P. E., and Cowan, W. M. 1981. Evidence for collateral projections by neurons in Ammon's horn, the dentate gyrus, and the subiculum: A multiple retrograde labeling study in the rat. *J. Neurosci.* 1:548–559.

Swindale, N. V. 1982. A model for the formation of orientation columns. *Proc. R. Soc. Lond. [B]* 215:211–230.

Swindale, N. V. 1990. Is the cerebral cortex modular? *Trends Neurosci.* 13:487–492.

Székely, G. 1965. Logical networks for controlling limb movements in Urodela. *Acta Physiol. Acad. Sci. Hung.* 27:285–289.

Székely, G. 1968. Development of limb movements: Embryological, physiological and model studies. In *Growth of the nervous system*, CIBA Foundation Symposium, eds. G. E. W. Wolstenholme and M. O'Connor.

Székely, G. 1989. Ontogeny and morphology of neural structures controlling tetrapod locomotion. In *Complex organismal functions: Integration and evolution in vertebrates*, eds. P. B. Wake and G. Roth, 117–131. New York: Wiley.

Székely, G. 1990. Problems of the neuronal specificity concept in the development of neural organization. *Concepts Neurosci.* 1:165–197.

Székely, G., and Czeh, G. 1971. Activity of spinal cord fragments and limbs deplanted in the dorsal fin of Urodele larvae. *Acta Physiol. Acad. Sci. Hung.* 40:303–312.

Székely, G., Czeh, G., and Vörös, G. 1969. The activity pattern of limb muscles in freely moving normal and deafferented newts. *Exp. Brain Res.* 9:53–62.

Székely, G., and Matesz, C. 1989. Comparative anatomy of the neural control of mastication. In *Complex organismal functions: Integration and evolution in vertebrates*, eds. P. B. Wake and G. Roth, 41–52. New York: Wiley.

Székely, G., and Szentágothai, J. 1962. Experiments with "model nervous system." *Acta Biol. Acad. Sci. Hung.* 12:253–269.

Szentágothai, J. 1952. An attempt at a "natural" systematization of nervous elements. *Magy. Tud. Akad. Biol. Orv. Tud. Osztl. Közl.* 3:365–412.

Szentágothai, J. 1962. On the synaptology of the cerebral cortex [in Russian]. In *Structure and function of the nervous system*, ed. S. A. Sarkissov, 6–14. Moscow: Medgiz.

Szentágothai, J. 1963. New data on the functional anatomy of synapses. *Magy. Tud. Akad. Biol. Orv. Tud. Osztl. Közl.* 6:212–227.

Szentágothai, J. 1964. Propriospinal pathways and their synapses. *Prog. Brain Res.* 11:155–177.

Szentágothai, J. 1965. The use of degeneration methods in the investigation of short neuronal connections. *Prog. Brain Res.* 14:1–32.

Szentágothai, J. 1967. The anatomy of complex integration units in the nervous system. In *Recent development of neurobiology in Hungary: I. Results in neuroanatomy, neuropharmacology and neurophysiology*, ed. K. Lissak, 9–45. Budapest: Akadémiai Kiadó.

Szentágothai, J. 1969. Architecture of the cerebral cortex. In Basic mechanisms of the epilepsies, eds. H. H. I. Jasper, A. A. Ward, Jr., and A. Pope, 13–28. Boston: Little, Brown.

Szentágothai, J. 1975. The module concept in cerebral cortex architecture. *Brain Res.* 95:475–496.

Szentágothai, J. 1978a. Specificity versus (quasi-) randomness in cortical connectivity. In *Architectonics of the cerebral cortex connectivity*, eds. M. A. B. Brazier and H. Petsche, 77–97. New York: Raven Press.

Szentágothai, J. 1978b. The neuron network of the cerebral cortex: A functional interpretation. *Proc. R. Soc. Lond. [B]* 201:219–248.

Szentágothai, J. 1981. Principles of neural organization. In *Advances in physiological science: I. Regulatory functions of the CNS—principles of motion and organization*, eds. J. Szentágothai, M. Palkovits, and J. Hamori, 1–56. Oxford: Pergamon Press.

Szentágothai, J. 1982. Too "much" and too "soon". A lifetime of inquiry into the functional organization of the nervous system. *Acta Biol. Hung.* 33:107–126.

Szentágothai, J. 1983. The modular architectonic principle of neural centers. *Rev. Physiol. Biochem. Pharmacol.* 98:11–61.

Szentágothai, J. 1984. Downward causation? *Annu. Rev. Neurosci.* 7:1–11.

Szentágothai, J. 1985. Functional anatomy of the visual centers as cues for pattern recognition concepts. *Pontificiae Acad. Sci. Scripta Varia.* 54:39–52.

Szentágothai, J. 1987a. The architecture of neural centers and understanding neural organization. In *Advances in Physiological Research*, eds. M. McLennan, S. R. Ledisome, C. S. M McIntosh, and P. R. Jones, 111–129. New York: Plenum Press.

Szentágothai, J. 1987b. The "brain-mind" relation: A pseudoproblem. In *Mindwaves*, eds. C. Blakemore and S. Greenfield, 323–336. Oxford: Basil Blackwell.

Szentágothai, J. 1989. Organizzazione neuronale cerebrale e cerebellare. In *Enciclopedia del novecento*, Vol. 8, 764–790.

Szentágothai, J. 1990. "Specificity versus (quasi-) randomness" revisited. *Acta Morphol. Hung.* 38:159–167.

Szentágothai, J. 1993. Self-organization: The basic principle of neural functions. *Theor. Med.* 14:101–116.

Szentágothai, J., and Arbib, M. 1974. Conceptual models of neural organization. *Neurosci. Res. Progr. Bull.* 121:307–479.

Szentágothai, J., and Arbib, M. A. 1975. *Conceptual models of neural organization*. Reprint. Cambridge, MA: MIT Press.

Szentágothai, J., and Érdi, P. 1989. Self-organization in the nervous system. *J. Soc. Biol. Struct.* 12:367–384.

Szentágothai, J., Hámori, J., and Tömböl, T. 1966. Degeneration and electron microscope analysis of the synaptic glomeruli in the lateral geniculate body. *Exp. Brain Res.* 2:283–301.

Szentágothai, J., and Kiss, T. 1949. Projection of dermatomes in the substantia gelatinosa. *Arch. Neurol. Psychiatry* 62:734–744.

Szentágothai, J., and Réthelyi, M. 1973. Cyto- and neuropil architecture of the spinal cord. In *New developments in electromyography and clinical neurophysiology*, Vol. 3, ed. J. E. Desmedt, 20–37. Basel: Karger.

Szentágothai, J., and Székely, G. 1956a. Elementary nervous mechanisms underlying optokinetic responses, analyzed by contralateral eye grafts in urodele larvae. *Acta Physiol. Acad. Sci. Hung.* 10:43–55.

Szentágothai, J., and Székely, G. 1956b. Zum Problem der Kreuzung der Nervenbahnen. *Acta Biol. Acad. Sci. Hung.* 6:215–229.

Taira, M., Mine, S., Georgopoulos, A. P., Murata, A., and Sakata, H. 1990. Parietal cortex neurons of the monkey related to the visual guidance of hand movement. *Exp. Brain Res.* 83:29–36.

Tanaka, S. 1990. Theory of self-organization of cortical maps: Mathematical framework. *Neural Networks* 3:62–640.

Tanaka, S. 1991. Theory of ocular dominance column formation. Mathematical basis and computer simulation. *Biol. Cybern.* 64:263–272.

Tanji, J., and Kurata, K. 1985. Contrasting neuronal activity in supplementary and premotor cortex of monkeys. I. Responses to instructions determining motor responses to forthcoming signals of different modalities. *J. Neurophysiol.* 53:129–141.

Tanji, J., and Shima, K. 1994. Role for supplementary motor areas in planning several movements ahead. *Nature* 371:412–416.

Tank, D. W., and Hopfield, J. J. 1987. Neural computation by concentrating information in time. *Proc. Natl. Acad. Sci. U.S.A.* 84:1896–1900.

Taube, J. S., Muller, R. U., and Ranck, J. B., Jr. 1987. A quantitative analysis of head-direction cells in the postsubiculum. *Soc. Neurosci. Abstr.* 13:1332.

Taube, J. S., Muller, R. U., and Ranck, J. B., Jr. 1990. Head-direction cells recorded from the postsubiculum in freely moving rats; I. Description and quantitative analysis. *J. Neurosci.* 10:420–435.

Taylor, C. P., and Dudek, F. E. 1982. Synchronous neural afterdischarges in rat hippocampal slices without active chemical synapses. *Science* 218:810–812.

Thach, W. T. 1968. Discharge of Purkinje and cerebellar nuclear neurons during rapidly alternating arm movements in the monkey. *J. Neurophysiol.* 31:785–797.

Thach, W. T. 1996. On the specific role of the cerebellum in motor learning and cognition: Clues from PET activation and lesion studies in man. *Behav. Brain Sci.*

Thach, W. T., Goodkin, H. G., and Keating, J. G. 1992. The cerebellum and the adaptive coordination of movement. *Annu. Rev. Neurosci.* 15:403–442.

Thelen, E., and Smith, L. B. 1994. *A dynamic system approach to the development of cognition and action.* Cambridge, MA: MIT Press.

Thompson, R. F. 1986. The neurobiology of learning and memory. *Science* 233:941–947.

Thompson, R. F. 1990. Neural mechanisms of classical conditioning in mammals. *Philos. Trans. R. Soc. Lond. [B]* 329:161–170.

Thompson D'Arcy, W. 1961. *On growth and form.* Abridged from the 1917 original by J. T. Bonner. London: Cambridge University Press.

Thomson, J. R., Zhang, Z., Cowan, W., Grant, M., Hertz, J. A., and Zuckermann, M. J. 1990. A simple model for pattern formation in primate visual cortex for the case of monocular deprivation. *Physica Scripta* T33:102–109.

Tolman, E. C. 1932. *Purposive behavior in animals and man.* New York: Century. Tolman, E. C. 1948. Cognitive maps in rats and men. *Psychol. Rev.* 55:189–208.

Tömböl, T. 1978. Comparative data on the Golgi architecture of interneurons of different cortical areas in cat and rabbit. In *Architectonics of the cerebral cortex*, International Brain Research Organization Monograph Series, Vol. 3, eds. M. A. B. Brazier and H. P. Petsche, 59–76. New York: Raven Press.

Tononi, G. 1994. Reentry and the problem of cortical integration. *Int. Rev. Neurobiol.* 37:127–152.

Tootell, R. B., Silverman, M. S., and DeValois, R. L. 1981. Spatial frequency columns in primary visual cortex. *Science* 214:813–815.

Tóth, J. 1985. A mass action kinetic model of neurochemical transmission. In *Dynamic phenomena in neurochemistry and neurophysics: Theoretical aspects*, ed. P. Érdi, 52–55. Budapest: KFKI.

Tóth, K., Borhegyi, Z., and Freund, T. 1993. Postsynaptic targets of GABAergic hippocampal neurons in the medial septum diagonal band of Broca complex. *J. Neurosci.* 13:3712–3724.

Tóth, K., and Freund, T. F. 1992. D-containing nonpyramidal cells in the rat hippocampus: Their immunoreactivity for GABA and projection to the medial septum. *Neuroscience* 49:807–817.

Tóth, T., and Crunelli, V. 1992a. Computer simulations of the pacemaker oscillations of thalamocortical cells. *Neuroreport* 3:65–68.

Tóth, T., and Crunelli, V. 1992b. Modelling of pacemaker oscillations in thalamocortical neurones. In *Cybernetics and systems '92*, ed. R. Trappl, 749–756. Singapore: World Scientific.

Touretzky, D. S., and Redish, A. D. 1996. A theory of rodent navigation based on interacting representations of space. Tech. rep. Pittsburgh: Carnegie-Mellon University.

Tovee, M. J., and Rolls, E. T. 1992. Oscillatory activity is not evident in the primate temporal visual cortex with static stimuli. *Neuroreport* 3:369–372.

Traub, R. D., and Jefferys, J. G. R. 1994. Mechanisms responsible for epilepsy in hippocampal slices predispose the brain to collective oscillations. In *Neural modeling and neural networks*, ed. F. Ventriglia, 111–127. Oxford: Pergamon Press.

Traub, R. D., Jefferys, J. G. R., and Miles, R. 1994. Common principles in three experimental epilepsies. In *Temporal coding in the brain*, eds. G. Buzsáki, R. Llinás, W. Singer, A. Berthoz, and Y. Chrisen, 173–183. Berlin: Springer-Verlag.

Traub, R. D., Jefferys, J. G. R., Miles, R., Whittington, M. A., and Tóth, K. 1994. A branching dendritic model of a rodent CA3 pyramidal neurons. *J. Physiol.* 481:79–95.

Traub, R. D., and Miles, R. 1991. *Neuronal networks of the hippocampus.* London: Cambridge University Press.

Traub, R. D., and Miles, R. 1992. Modeling hippocampal circuitry using data from whole cell patch clamp and dual intracellular recordings in vitro. *Semin. Neurosci.* 4:27–36.

Traub, R. D., Miles, R., and Jefferys, J. G. R. 1993. Synaptic and intrinsic conductances shape picrotoxin-induced synchronized afterdischarges in the guinea-pig hippocampal slice. *J. Neurophysiol.* 461:525–547.

Traub, R. D., Miles, R., Muller, R. U., and Gulyás, A. I. 1992. Functional organization of the hippocampal CA3 region: Implications for epilepsy, brain waves and spatial behavior. *Network* 3:465–488.

Traub, R. D., Miles, R., and Wong, R. K. S. 1989. Model of the origin of rhythmic population oscillations in the hippocampal slice. *Science* 243:1319–1325.

Traub, R. D., and Wong, R. K. S. 1982. Cellular mechanism of neuronal synchronization in epilepsy. *Science* 216:745–747.

Traub, R. D., Whittington, M. A., Stanford, I. M., and Jefferys, J. G. R. 1996. A mechanism for generation of long-range synchronous fast oscillation in the cortex. *Nature* 303:621–624.

Traub, R. D., Wong, K. S., and Miles, R. 1987. In vitro models of epilepsy. In *Neurotransmitters and epilepsy*, eds. P. C. Jobe and H. E. Laird II, 161–190. Clifton, NJ: Humana Press.

Traub, R. D., Wong, R. K. S., Miles, R., and Michelson, H. 1991. A model of a CA3 hippocampal neuron incorporating voltage-clamp data on intrinsic conductances. *J. Neurophysiol.* 66:635–650.

Träven, H., Brodin, L., Lansner, A., Ekeberg, O., Wallén, P., and Grillner, S. 1993. Computer simulations of NMDA and non-NMDA receptor-mediated synaptic drive: Sensory and supraspinal modulation of neurons and small network. *J. Neurophysiol.* 70:695–709.

Traynelis, S. F., and Dingledine, R. 1988. Potassium-induced spontaneous electrographic seizures in the rat hippocampus slice. *J. Neurophysiol.* 59:259–276.

Trisler, D. 1982. Are molecular markers of cell position involved in the formation of neural circuits? *Trends Neurosci.* 5:306–310.

Trombley, P. O., and Shepherd, G. M. 1991. Norepinephrine inhibits mitral cells evoked EPSPs in mammalian olfactory bulb granule cells in culture. *Soc. Neurosci. Abstr.* 17:103.12.

Troy, W. C. 1976. Oscillation phenomena in the Hodgkin-Huxley equations. *Proc. R. Soc. Edinb.* 74A:299–310.

Ts'o, D., Gilbert, C. D., and Wiesel, T. N. 1986. Relationship between horizontal and functional architecture in cat striate cortex as revealed by cross-correlation analysis. *J. Neurosci.* 6:1160–1170.

Tsuda, I. 1991. Chaotic itinerancy as a dynamical hermeneutics in brain and mind. *World Futures* 32:167–184.

Tsuda, I. 1992. Dynamic link of memory—chaotic memory map in monequilibrium neural networks. *Neural Networks* 5:313–326.

Tsuda, I., Iwanaga, H., and Takara, T. 1992. Chaotic pulsation in human capillary vessels and its dependence on mental and physical conditions. *Int. J. Bifurc. Chaos* 21:313–326.

Tsukahara, N. 1972. The properties of the cerebello-pontine reverberating circuit. *Brain Res.* 40:67.

Tucek, S. 1983. Acetylcoenzyme-A and the synthesis of acetylcholine in neurons. Review of recent progress. *Gen. Physiol.* B2:313–324.

Tucek, S. 1993. Short-term control of the synthesis of acetylcholine. *Prog. Biophys. Molec. Biol.* 60:59–69.

Tuckwell, H. C. 1988. *Introduction to theoretical neurobiology: Vol. 2, Nonlinear and stochastic theories.* London: Cambridge University Press.

Tulving, E. 1983. *Elements of episodic mewmory.* New York: Oxford University Press.

Turányi, T. 1990. Sensitivity analysis of complex kinetic systems. Tools and applications. *J. Math. Chem.* 5:203–248.

Turner, D. A., Li, X.-G., Pyapali, G. K., Ylinen, A., and Buzsáki, G. 1995. Morphometric and electrical properties of reconstructed hippocampal CA3 neurons recorded in vivo. *J. Comp. Neurol.* 356:580–594.

Tyson, J. J. 1975. Classification of instabilities in chemical reaction systems. *J. Chem. Phys.* 62:1010–1015.

Ungerleider, L. G., and Mishkin, M. 1982. Two cortical visual systems. In *Analysis of visual behavior*, eds. D. J. Ingle, M. A. Goodale, and R. J. W. Mansfield. Cambridge, MA: MIT Press.

Uttley, A. M. 1975. The informon in classical conditioning. *J. Theor. Biol.* 49:355–376.

van der Kooy Fishell, G., Krushel, L. A., and Johnston, J. G. 1987. The development of striatal compartments: From proliferation to patches. In *The basal ganglia: II. Structure and function—current concepts*, eds. M. B. Carpenter and A. Jayaraman, 81–98. New York: Plenum Press.

Vanderwolf, C. H. 1969. Hippocampal electrical activity and voluntary movement in the rat. *Electroencephalogr. Clin. Neurophysiol.* 26:407–418.

Vanderwolf, C. H., and Leung, L. W. S. 1983. Hippocampal rhythmical slow activity: A brief history and the effects of entorhinal lesions and phencyclidine. In *Neurobiology of the hippocampus*, ed. W. Seifert, 225–302. London: Academic Press.

van Gisbergen, J. A. M., Robinson, D. A., and Gielen, S. 1981. A quantitative analysis of generation of saccadic eye movements by burst neurons. *J. Neurophysiol.* 45:417–442.

Van Hoesen, G. W., Pandya, D. N., and Butters, N. 1972. Cortical efferents to the entorhinal cortex of the rhesus monkey. *Science* 175:1471–1473.

Vanier, M., and Caplan, D. 1990. CT scan correlates of agrammatism. In *Agrammatic aphasia*, eds. L. Menn and L. Obler, 97–114. Amsterdam: Benjamins.

van Riemsdijk, H., and Williams, E. 1986. *Introduction to the theory of grammar*. Cambridge, MA: MIT Press.

Van Vreeswijk, C., Abbot, L. E., and Ermentrout, G. B. 1994. When inhibition, not excitation, synchronizes neural firing. *J. Comp. Neurosci.* 1:313–321.

Ventriglia, F. 1974. Kinetic approach to neural systems. *Bull. Math. Biol.* 36:534–544.

Ventriglia, F. 1988. Computational simulation of cortical-like neural systems. *Bull. Math. Biol.* 50:143–185.

Ventriglia, F. 1990. Activity in cortical-like neural systems: Short-range effects and attention phenomena. *Bull. Math. Biol.* 52:397–429.

Ventriglia, F. 1994. Toward a kinetic theory of cortical-like neural fields. In *Neural modeling and neural networks*, ed. F. Ventriglia, 217–249. Oxford: Pergamon Press.

Vicq d'Azyr, F. 1786. *Traité d'anatomie et de physiologie*. Paris.

Vogt, O., and Vogt, C. 1919. Allgemeine Ergebnisse unserer Hirnforschung. *J. Psychol. Neurol.* 251:279–461.

von Bonin, G. 1944. Architecture of the precentral motor cortex and some adjacent areas. In *The precentral motor cortex*, ed. P. Bucy, 7–82. Urbana: University of Illinois Press.

von der Malsburg, C. 1973. Self-organization of orientation sensitive cells in the striate cortex. *Kybernetik* 14:85–100.

von der Malsburg, C. 1979. Development of ocularity domains and growth behavior of axon terminals. *Biol. Cybern.* 32:49–62.

von der Malsburg, C. 1981. *The correlation theory of brain functions*. Internal rep. no. 81–2. Göttingen: Department of Neurobiology, Max Planck Institute of Biophysics and Chemistry.

von der Malsburg, C. 1985. Nervous structures with dynamical links. *Ber. Bunsen Ges. Phys. Chem.* 89:700–709.

von der Malsburg, C., and Buhmann, J. 1992. Sensory segmentation with coupled neural oscillators. *Biol. Cybern.* 67:233–242.

von der Malsburg, C., and Singer. 1988. Principles of cortical network organization. In *Neurobiology of the neocortex*, eds. P. Rakic and W. Singer, 69–99. New York: John Wiley and Sons.

von Economo, C. 1929. *The cytoarchitectonics of the human cerebral cortex*. London: Oxford University Press.

von Neumann, J. 1958. *The computer and the brain*. New Haven: Yale University Press.

von Seelen, W., Mallot, H. A., and Giannakopoulos, F. 1987. Characteristics of neuronal systems in visual cortex. *Biol. Cybern.* 56:37–49.

Voogd, J. 1969. The importance of fiber connections in the comparative anatomy of the mammalian cerebellum. In *Neurobiology of cerebellar evolution and development*, ed. R. Llinás. Chicago: American Medical Association.

Waddington, C. H. 1957. *The strategy of the genes*. London: Allen & Unwin.

Wallenstein, G. V. 1994. Simulation of GABA$_B$-receptor mediated K$^+$ current in thalamocortical relay neurons: Tonic firing, bursting, and oscillations. *Biol. Cybern.* 71:271–280.

Walsh, J. P., Cepeda, C., Hull, C. D., Fisher, R. S., Levine, X. X., and Buchwald, A. N. 1989. Dye-coupling in the neostriatum of the rat: II. Decreased coupling between neurons during development. *Synapse* 4:238–247.

Walsh, J. P., and Dunia, R. In press. Synaptic activation of NMDA receptors induces short-term potentiation at the corticostriatal synapse of the rat.

Walter, W. G. 1953. *The living brain*. London: Duckworth.

Weilhmuller, F. B., Ulas, J., Nguyen, L., Cotman, C. W., and Marshall, J. F. 1992. Elevated NMDA receptors in Parkinsonian striatum. *Neuroreport* 3:997–980.

Weiner, M. J., Hallet, M., and Funkenstein, H. H. 1983. Adaptation to lateral displacement of vision in patients with lesions of the central nervous system. *Neurology* 33.

Weiskrantz, L. 1974a. The interaction between occipital and temporal cortex in vision: An overview. In *The neurosciences: Third study program*, eds. F. O. Schmitt and F. G. Worden, 189–204. Cambridge, MA: MIT Press.

Weiskrantz, L. 1974b. Brain research and parallel processing. *Physiol. Psychol.* 2:53–54.

Weiss, P. 1934. In vitro experiments on the factors determining the course of the outgrowing nerve fiber. *J. Exp. Zool.* 113:397–461.

Weiss, P. 1939. *Principles of development*. New York: Holt.

Weiss, P. 1950. The deplantation of fragments of neuron system in amphibians. *J. Exp. Zool.* 113:397–461.

Weitzenfeld, A. 1991. NSL: Neural simulation language, Vers. 2.1. *Technical report 91-05*. Los Angeles: Center for Neural Engineering, University of Southern California.

Weitzenfeld, A., and Arbib, M. 1991. A concurrent object-oriented framework for the simulation of neural networks. Proceedings of the ECOOP/OOPSLA '90 Workshop on Object-Based Concurrent Programming. *SIGPLAN, OOPS Messenger (Apr)* 2(2):120–124.

Wellis, D. P., and Scott, J. W. 1990. Intracellular responses of identified rat olfactory bulb interneurons to electrical and odor stimulation. *J. Neurophysiol.* 64:932–947.

Wernicke, C. 1874. *Die aphasische Symptomencomplex*. Breslau.

West, B. 1985. *An essay on the importance of being nonlinear*. Berlin: Springer-Verlag.

White, J., Hamilton, K. A., Neff, S. R., and Kauer, J. 1992. Emergent properties of odor information coding in a representational model of the salamander olfactory bulb. *J. Neurosci.* 12:1772–1780.

Whitelaw, V. A., and Cowan, J. D. 1981. Specificity and plasticity of retinotectal connections: A computational model. *J. Neurosci.* 1:1369–1387.

Whittington, M. A., Traub, R. B. and Jefferys, J. 1995. Synchronized oscillations in interneuron networks driven by metabotropic glutamate receptor activation. *Nature* 370:612–615.

Wickens, J. R. 1993. Corticostriatal interactions in neuromotor programming. *Hum. Move. Sci.* 12:17–35.

Wickens, J. R., Hyland, B., and Anson, G. 1994. Cortical cell assemblies: A possible mechanism for motor programs. *J. Motor Behav.* 26:66–82.

Widrow, B., and Hoff, T. 1960. Adaptive switching circuits. *Inst. Radio Eng. WESCON Conv. Rec.* 4:96–104.

Widrow, B., and Lehr, M. A. 1995. Perceptrons, adalines and backpropagation. In *The handbook of brain theory and neural networks*, ed. M. A. Arbib, 719–724. Cambridge, MA: Bradford Books/MIT Press.

Wiener, N. 1948. *Cybernetics: Or control and communication in the animal and the machine.* New York: Technology Press/Wiley.

Wiener, N. 1949. *Extrapolation, interpolation, and smoothing of stationary time* [series]. New York: Technology Press/Wiley.

Wiener, S. I., Paul, C. A., and Eichenbaum, H. 1989. Spatial and behavioral correlates of hippocampal neuronal activity. *J. Neurosci.* 9:2737–2763.

Wiesel, T. N. 1982. Postnatal development of the visual cortex and the influence of environment. *Nature* 299:583–591.

Wigner, E. P. 1959. Statistical properties of real symmetric matrices with many dimensions. In *Proceedings of the Fourth Canadian Mathematics Congress*, ed. M. S MacPhail, 174–184. Toronto: University Toronto Press.

Wilkins, K., and Wakefield, J. 1995. Brain evolution and neurolinguistic preconditions. *Behav. Brain Sci.*

Williams, T. L., and Sigvardt, K. A. 1995. Generation of locomotor patterns by the lamprey spinal cord. In *The handbook of brain theory and neural networks*, ed. M. A. Arbib. Cambridge, MA: Bradford Books/MIT Press.

Willshaw, D. J., and Dayan, P. 1990. Optimal plasticity from matrix memories: What goes up must come down. *Neural Comput.* 2:85–93.

Willshaw, D. J., and Buckingham, J. T. 1990. An assessment of Marr's theory of the hippocampus as a temporary memory store. *Philos. Trans. R. Soc. Lond. [B]* 329:205–215.

Willshaw, D. J., Buneman, O. P., and Longuet-Higgins, H. C. 1969. Nonholographic associative memory. *Nature* 222:960–962.

Willshaw, D. J., and von der Malsburg, C. 1976. How patterned neural connections can be set up by self-organization. *Proc. R. Soc. Lond. [B]* 194:431–445.

Willshaw, D. J., and von der Malsburg, C. 1979. A marker induction mechanism for the establishment of ordered neural mappings: Its application to the retinotectal problem. *Philos. Trans. R. Soc. Lond. [B]* 287:203–243.

Wilson, C. J. 1995. The contribution of cortical neurons to the firing pattern of striatal spiny neurons. In *Models of information processing in the basal ganglia*, eds. J. C. Houk, J. L. Davis, and D. G. Beiser, 29–50. Cambridge, MA: Bradford Books/MIT Press.

Wilson, H. R., and Cowan, J. 1972. Excitatory and inhibitory interactions in localized populations of model neurons. *Biophys. J.* 12:1–24.

Wilson, H. R., and Cowan, J. 1973. A mathematical theory of the functional dynamics of cortical and thalamic neurons tissue. *Kybernetik* 13:55–80.

Wilson, M., Bhalla, U. S., Uhley, J. D., Bower, J. M. 1989. GENESIS: A system for simulating neural networks. In *Advances in neural information processing systems*, ed. D. S. Touretzky, 485–492. San Mateo, CA: Morgan Kaufmann.

Wilson, M., and Bower, J. M. 1988. A computer simulation of olfactory cortex with functional implications for storage and recognition of olfactory information. In *Neural information processing systems*, ed. D. Z. Anderson, 114–126. New York: American Institute of Physics.

Wilson, M., and Bower, J. M. 1989. The simulation of large-scale neural networks. In *Methods in neural modeling: From synapses to networks*, eds. C. Koch and I. Segev, 291–334. Cambridge, MA: MIT Press.

Wilson, M., and Bower, J. M. 1992. Cortical oscillations and temporal interactions in a computer simulation of pirifom cortex. *J. Neurophysiol.* 67:981–995.

Wilson, M. A., and McNaughton, B. L. 1993. Dynamics of the hippocampal ensemble code for space. *Science* 261:1055–1058.

Wilson, M. A., and McNaughton, B. L. 1994. Reactivation of hippocampal ensemble memories during sleep. *Science* 265:676–679.

Wing, A., and Kristofferson, A. 1973. Response delays and the timing of discrete motor responses. *Percept. Psychophys.* 14:5–12.

Wirtschafter, D., Asin, K. E., and Kent, E. W. 1979. Median raphe lesions impair the acquisition and performance of an 8-arm maze task. *Soc. Neurosci. Abstr.* 5:282.

Witter, M. P., Griffoen, A. W., Joritsma-Byhan, B. R., and Krinjen, J. L. M. 1988. Entorhinal projections to the hippocampal CA1 region in the rat: An underestimated pathway. *Neurosci. Lett.* 85:193–198.

Wolpert, L. 1969. Positional information and the spatial pattern of cellular differentiation. *J. Theor. Biol.* 25:1–47.

Wolpert, L. 1971. Positional information and pattern formation. *Top. Dev. Biol.* 6:183–224.

Wolpert, L. 1981. Positional information and pattern formation. *Philos. Trans. R. Soc. Lond. [B]* 295:441–450.

Wong-Riley, M. 1979. Columnar cortico-cortical interactions within the visual system of the squirrel and macaque monkeys. *Brain Res.* 162:201–217.

Wong-Riley, M. T. 1989. Cytochrome oxidase: An endogenous metabolic marker for neuronal activity. *Trends Neurosci.* 12:94–101.

Wright, J. J., and Liley, D. T. J. 1996. Dynamics of the brain at global and microscopic scales: Neural networks and the EEG. *Behav. Brain Sci.* 19:285–295, 310–320.

Wu, X., and Liljenström, H. 1994. Regulating the nonlinear dynamics of olfactory cortex. *Network* 5:47–60.

Wurtman, R. J., Hefti, F., and Melamed, E. 1981. Precursor control of neurotransmitter synthesis. *Pharmacol. Rev.* 32:315–335.

Yamada, J., and Noda, H. 1987. Afferent and efferent connections of the oculomotor cerebellar vermis in the macaque monkey. *J. Comp. Neurol.* 265:224–241.

Yamada, W. M., Koch, C., and Adams, P. R. 1989. Multiple channels and calcium dynamics. In *Methods of neuronal modeling*, eds. C. Koch and I. Segev, 97–134. Cambridge, MA: MIT Press.

Yates, F. E. 1980. Physical causality and brain theories. *Am. J. Physiol.* 238:R277–R290.

Yeckel, M. F., and Berger, T. W. 1990. Feedforward excitation of the hippocampus by afferents from the entorhinal cortex: Redefinition of the role of the trisynaptic pathway. *Proc. Natl. Acad. Sci. U.S.A.* 87:5832–5836.

Ylinen, A., Bragin, A., Nadasdy, Z., Jando, G., Szabo, I., Sik, A., and Buzsáki, G. 1995a. Sharp wave associated high-frequency oscillation (200 Hz) in the intact hippocampus: Network and intracellular mechanisms. *J. Neurosci.* 15:30–46.

Ylinen, A., Soltesz, I., Bragin, A., Penttonen, M., Sik, A., and Buzsáki, G. 1995b. Intracellular correlates of hippocampal theta rhythm in identified pyramidal cells, granule cells, and basket cells. *Hippocampus* 5:78–90.

Yuille, A. L., and Geiger, D. 1995. Winner-take-all mechanisms. In *The handbook of brain theory and neural networks*, ed. M. A. Arbib, 1056–1060. Cambridge, MA: Bradford Books/MIT Press.

Záborsky, L., Palkovits, M., Flerkó, B. 1992. A life-time adventure with the brain. An appreciation of his eightieth birthday. *J. Comp. Neurol.* 326:1–6.

Zador, A., Koch, C., and Brown, T. H. 1990. Biophysical model of a Hebbian synapse. *Proc. Natl. Acad. Sci. U.S.A.* 87:6718–6722.

Zak, M. 1988. Terminal attractors for associative memory in neural networks. *Phys. Lett.* 133A:18–22.

Zak, M. 1990. Creative dynamics approach to neural intelligence. *Biol. Cybern.* 64:15–21.

Zeki, S., and Shipp, S. 1988. The functional logic of cortical connections. *Nature* 335:311–317.

Zipser, D. 1986. A model of hippocampal learning during classical conditioning. *Behav. Neurosci.* 100:764–776

Zucker, R. S. 1989. Short-term synaptic plasticity. *Annu. Rev. Neurosci.* 12:13–31.

Zurif, E. 1984. Psycholinguistic interpretations of the aphasias. In *Biological perspectives on language*, eds. D. Caplan, A. R. Lecours, and A. Smith, 158–171. Cambridge, MA: MIT Press.

Index

Six-layered neocortex, 206
Skeleton model of olfactory bulb, 120, 126
Skill, 179, 183
Sleep cycle, 91
Sleeping brain, 229
Sleep state, 229
Slow inhibition, 151
Slow oscillation, 134, 231
  imposed on olfactory bulb, 119
  in olfactory system, 119
Small sharp spikes (SSS), 149
Smith predictor approach to long delays, 293
Sniff cycle, 119, 121, 133, 154
Somatosensory cortex, 203
Somatosensory system, 194
Somatotopic architecture, principle of, 25
Somatotopy, 223
Spatial attention, 245
Spatial behavior, 183
Spatial memory, 164, 248, 314
Spatial orientation
  of dendrites, 22
  neurophysiology of, 164
  of neuropil, 22
  in rats, 160
Spatial representation, 164
Spatiotemporal activity pattern, 230
Spatiotemporal coherence, 74
Spatiotemporal pattern formation, 113, 115
Specificity, 96
Specific nuclei of thalamus, 187
Speed-accuracy relationship, 65
Spike-and-wave discharge, 231
Spike generation, somatic and dendritic, 272
Spinal cord, 12, 13, 20, 186, 195
Spinal locomotor network, 157
Spinal motor pattern generator during locomotion, 281
Spindle oscillation, 83, 126, 229, 230, 231
Spinothalamic pathway, 197
Spiny stellate cell, 212
Spontaneous activity, 225
Spreading-activation hypothesis, 342
Stable, qualitatively, 81
State space, 69
Static structures, 71
Stellate cell, 261
Stepping rhythm, 73
Stereopsis, Dev model, 49, 50
Stimulus-induced activity, 119
Stimulus-matching, 50
Stiosome, 307
Stochastic model
  development of ordered neural structures, 95
  for generation of electrocortical activity, 91
Stochastic neurodynamics, 79
Storage of temporal sequences, 107
Strange attractor, 72, 87, 105, 114, 122, 348
Striatopallidal system, 202
Striatum, 160, 303, 304
  organization of, 305

patch-matrix organization of, 307
Structural organization of cerebellar cortex and nuclei, 268
Structural overview of cerebral cortex, 205
Structure, 330
Structure-function problem, 80
Styles of modeling, 155
Subcortical connections, 146
Subicular cell, 177
Subicular complex, 146
Subiculum, 145, 172, 184
Sublayers (strata) in hippocampus, 142
Subschema, 49
  neural localization, 46
Substantia nigra, 303, 304
  pars compacta (SNc), 303
  pars reticulata (SNr), 303
Subthalamic nucleus (STN), 303
Subthalamus, 186
Sulci, 211
Superficial short-axon cells (SSA), 116
Superior colliculus (SC), 57, 58, 184, 203, 237, 259, 294
Superior parietal lobule, 203
Supplementary motor area, 203
Symmetry detection, 102
Synaptic connectivity of cortical neurons, 214
Synaptic currents, 75
Synaptic glomeruli, 26, 190
Synaptic level, 78
Synaptic matrix, 101, 103, 172
  heteroassociative, 170
Synaptic matrix model, 101, 179
  of hippocampus, 172
Synaptic modification induced transitions, 132
Synaptic organization of olfactory bulb, 116
Synaptic plasticity, 108, 109, 134, 135, 280, 292, 297
  BCM rule of, 157
  and physiological patterns, 154
Synaptic transmission, cholinergic suppression of, 131
Synaptic triad, 190
Synchronization, 82, 149, 334
  in CA3 network, 152
  mediated by excitatory connections, 148
  neural mechanisms, 154
Synchronized burst, 149, 157, 181
Synchronized low-frequency activity, 229
Synchronized multiple burst, 149
Synchronized oscillation, 83
  by inhibitory coupling, 126
Synchronized rhythmic activity, 134, 154, 232
  in hippocampus, 153
Synchronized spindle oscillation, 231
Synergetics, 39, 74
Synergic linkage, 283
Synergy, 281
Synthetic PET imaging, 246, 247, 248

2-1/2 D sketch, 223
Target location, 248
Taxon system, 163
Tectum, 45, 96